NURSING AND THE AGED

NURSING AND THE AGED

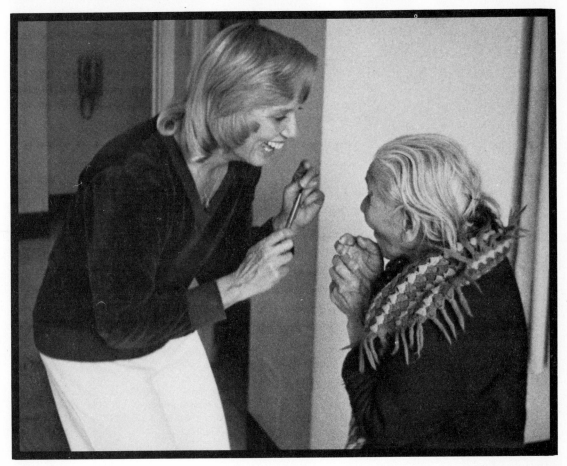

SECOND EDITION

EDITED BY
Irene Mortenson Burnside, R.N., M.S.

Research Associate
Gerontological Nurse Specialist Program
San Jose State University
San Jose, California

McGRAW-HILL BOOK COMPANY

New York St. Louis San Francisco Auckland Bogotá Hamburg Johannesburg London Madrid
Mexico Montreal New Delhi Panama Paris São Paulo Singapore Sydney Tokyo Toronto

234567890 DODO 8987654321

**This book was set in Serifa by Bi-Comp, Incorporated.
The editors were David P. Carroll and Moira Lerner;
the production supervisor was Robert A. Pirrung;
the designer was Robin Hessel.
The drawings were done by J & R Services, Inc.
R. R. Donnelley & Sons Company was printer and binder.**

Library of Congress Cataloging in Publication

Main entry under title:

Nursing and the aged.

    Bibliography: p.
    Includes indexes.
    1. Geriatric nursing. I. Burnside, Irene
Mortenson, date   [DNLM: 1. Geriatric nursing.
2. Nurse-Patient relations. WY152 N976]
RC954.N87 1981   610.73'65   80-11056
ISBN 0-07-009211-7

NOTICE

Medicine is an ever-changing science. As new research and clinical experience broaden our
knowledge, changes in treatment and drug therapy are required. The editors and the publisher of
this work have made every effort to ensure that the drug dosage schedules herein are accurate
and in accord with the standards accepted at the time of publication. Readers are advised,
however, to check the product information sheet included in the package of each drug they plan to
administer to be certain that changes have not been made in the recommended dose or in the
contraindications for administration. This recommendation is of particular importance in regard to
new or infrequently used drugs.

ACKNOWLEDGMENTS

American Nurses' Association: Two resolutions approved by the ANA House of Delegates, copyright 1978 by American Nurses' Association. Reprinted with permission of American Nurses' Association.

Rosemary Brant: "Across the Broken Pavement," reprinted courtesy of the Mental Health Association, 1800 N. Kent St., Arlington, VA 22209.

Lorraine Bridge: "Crumbs for My Heart," reprinted from *The Lutheran Standard,* copyright 1977, by permission of Augsburg Publishing House.

Irene M. Burnside: Selected lines from "Baroque Pearls," in "Touching is Talking," by Irene M. Burnside, copyright December 1973, The American Journal of Nursing Company. Reprinted with permission.

Thomas Cole: "Portrait of a Lady," from *The Various Light,* edited by Dr. C. Muses, copyright Lausanne 1958. Reprinted with permission.

Alice J. Davis: "How It Is with Me Now," in *Helping Each Other in Widowhood,* edited by Phyllis Silverman et al., published by Health Sciences Publishing Corp., 1974. Reprinted with permission.

Mardelle Dressler Dobbins: "Notes from an Old Church Member," copyright May 1974. Reprinted by permission.

T. S. Eliot: From *The Family Reunion,* copyright 1939 by T. S. Eliot, renewed 1967, by Esme Valerie Eliot. Reprinted by permission of Harcourt Brace Jovanovich, Inc.

T. S. Eliot: Selected lines from the play *Murder in the Cathedral.* Reprinted by permission of Harcourt Brace Jovanovich, Inc.

Harold G. Henderson: "Parting," from *An Introduction to Haiku,* copyright 1958 by Harold G. Henderson. Reprinted by permission of Doubleday & Company, Inc.

Harold G. Henderson: "Haze," from *An Introduction to Haiku,* copyright 1958 by Harold G. Henderson. Reprinted by permission of Doubleday & Company, Inc.

A. E. Housman: Selected lines from *The Collected Poems of A. E. Housman,* copyright 1936 by Barclays Bank Ltd., copyright 1964 by Robert E. Symons. Reprinted by permission of Holt, Rinehart and Winston, and the Society of Authors as the literary representative of the Estate of A. E. Housman and Jonathan Cape Ltd., publishers of A. E. Housman's *Collected Poems.*

Ross Allen McClelland: Selected lines from "Fantasy," from *The Errant Dawn,* copyright 1969. Published by Olivant Press, Homestead, Florida. Reprinted with permission.

Audrey McGaffin: "Inertia," from *New Poems,* edited by R. Humphries, Ballantine Books, 1953. Reprinted with permission.

Elise Maclay: Selected lines from the poem "I Don't Hear as Well as I Used To," from *Green Winter, Celebrations of Old Age,* copyright 1977. Published by Reader's Digest Press, New York. Reprinted with permission.

Arthur Miller: Selected lines from the play *Death of a Salesman,* Viking Press, New York. Reprinted with permission.

Rainer Maria Rilke: Selected lines from *The Duino Elegies,* copyright 1957. Published by Peter Pauper Press, Mount Vernon, New York. Reprinted with permission.

Rainer Maria Rilke: Selected lines from *Selected Poems,* copyright 1940. Reprinted with permission of the University of California Press.

Florida Scott-Maxwell: Lines from *Measure of My Days,* copyright 1968. Published by Alfred A. Knopf, Inc., New York. Reprinted with permission.

Muriel Spark: Selected lines from "Elementary," from *Collected Poems: I.* Published by Alfred A. Knopf, Inc., 1968. Reprinted with permission of Harold Ober Associates, Inc., New York.

Carol Staudacher: "Old Man," from *Creative Writing in the Classroom,* copyright 1968 by Fearon-Pitman Publishers, Inc., Belmont, California. Reprinted with permission.

For my children, Mark and Mary, Tonya, and Clark

CONTENTS

PART FOUR
ORGANIC BRAIN SYNDROME: THEORY AND THERAPY

PART FIVE
SPECIAL CONCERNS OF THE AGED: THEORY AND THERAPY

PART SIX
ASSESSMENT OF THE ELDERLY CLIENT

PART SEVEN
IMPORTANT CONSIDERATIONS OF THE ELDERLY ADULT

LIST OF CONTRIBUTORS

June C. Abbey, R.N., Ph.D., F.A.A.N.
Professor and Director of the Physiological
  Nursing Programs
College of Nursing
University of Utah
Salt Lake City, Utah

Robert C. Atchley, Ph.D.
Director, Scripps Foundation Gerontology
  Center
Miami University
Oxford, Ohio

Vern L. Bengtson, Ph.D.
Professor of Sociology
University of Stockholm
Stockholm, Sweden

David I. Berland, M.D.
Child Psychiatrist
Children's Division of the Menninger Foundation
Topeka, Kansas

Dorothy Rinehart Blake, R.N., M.Ed., F.N.P.
Department of Nursing
Sonoma State University
Rohnert Park, California

Ruth Bright, Mus. Bac., C.M.T.
Music Therapist
Lidcombe Hospital
Health Commission of New South Wales,
  Australia

Carol A. Brink, R.N., M.P.H.
Nurse Clinician, Home Healthcare Team
Visiting Nurse Service of Rochester and
  Monroe County
Adjunct Assistant Professor of Nursing
  (Gerontology)
School of Nursing
University of Michigan
Ann Arbor, Michigan

Irene Mortenson Burnside, R.N., M.S.
Research Associate
Gerontological Nurse Specialist Program
San Jose State University
San Jose, California

Michael A. Caggiano, M. Arch.
Vice President, DMT International USA, Inc.
Burbank, California

Caleb E. Finch, Ph.D.
Professor, Biological Sciences and Gerontology
Chief, Neurobiology Laboratory
Ethel Percy Andrus Gerontology Center
University of Southern California
Los Angeles, California

Kathy Gribbin, Ph.D.
Chief Psychologist, Geriatric Unit
Department of Psychiatry
Maricopa County General Hospital
Phoenix, Arizona

David A. Haber, Ph.D.
Program Specialist
Institute of Gerontology
University of the District of Columbia
Washington, D.C.

John J. Herr, Ph.D.
Research Clinical Associate
Family Interaction Center
Mental Research Institute
Palo Alto, California

Ronald C. Kayne, Pharm. D.
Director of Professional Services
Beverly Enterprises
Pasadena, California

Patricia Ann King, R.N., M.A., M.S.N.
Instructor, College of Nursing
University of Arizona
Tucson, Arizona

Gerald A. Larue, Th.D.
Professor of Religion, School of Religion
University of Southern California
Los Angeles, California

Barbara A. Moehrlin, R.N., M.S.
Coordinator, Senior Health Promotion Project
Blossom Hill Public Health
San Jose, California

Sharon Y. Moriwaki, Ph.D.
Assistant Director, Hawaii Gerontology Center
University of Hawaii
Honolulu, Hawaii

Robert J. Newcomer, Ph.D.
Associate Director, Aging Health Policy Center
School of Nursing
University of California
San Francisco, California

Virgil Parsons, R.N., D.N.Sc.
Assistant Professor and Curriculum Coordinator
Department of Nursing
San Jose State University
San Jose, California

Raymond G. Poggi, M.D.
Staff Psychiatrist, C. F. Menninger Memorial
    Hospital
Topeka, Kansas

Janet E. Porter, M.O.T., O.T.R.
Director, Institute for Independent Living —
    Geriatrics Unit
Western State Hospital
Fort Steilacoom, Washington

Theodore J. Rasmussen, L.P.N., A.T.A.
R.N. Student, Tacoma Community College
Tacoma, Washington

Valerie L. Remnet, R.N., M.S.W.
Mental Health Project Director
Division of Educational Development

Ethel Percy Andrus Gerontology Center
University of Southern California
Los Angeles, California;
Lecturer, Department of Nursing
California State University
Long Beach, California

Sharon L. Roberts, R.N., M.S.
Associate Professor, School of Nursing
California State University
Long Beach, California

Linda Dold Robinson, R.N., M.S., D.N.S. candidate
Associate Chief, Nursing Service for Geriatrics
Geriatric Research, Education, and Clinical
    Center
Veterans Administration Medical Center
Little Rock, Arkansas

Billie J. Robison, B.S.N., M.H.S., F.N.P.
ANA Certified Family Nurse Practitioner in
    Joint Practice with Family Practice Physician
Fremont, California

Isadore Rossman, Ph.D., M.D.
Medical Director, Department of Home Care
    and Extended Services
Montefiore Hospital and Medical Center;
Associate Professor, Medicine and Community
    Medicine
Albert Einstein Medical School
New York, New York

Dorothy R. Scarbrough, R.N., M.S.
Chief, Reality Orientation Training Program
Veterans Administration Medical Center
Tuscaloosa, Alabama

James A. Severson, Ph.D.
Postdoctoral Fellow, Laboratory of Neurobiology
Ethel Percy Andrus Gerontology Center
University of Southern California
Los Angeles, California

Ann Herbert Shanck, R.N., M.S., M.A.
Associate Professor, School of Nursing
California State University
Hayward, California

Bernita M. Steffl, R.N., M.P.H.
Professor, College of Nursing
Arizona State University
Tempe, Arizona

John H. Weakland, Ch.E.
Research Associate and Associate Director
Brief Therapy Center
Mental Research Institute
Palo Alto, California;
Clinical Instructor, Department of Psychiatry
    and Behavioral Sciences
Stanford University School of Medicine
Stanford, California

Ruth B. Weg, Ph.D.
Associate Professor of Biology and Gerontology
Leonard B. Davis School of Gerontology
Ethel Percy Andrus Gerontology Center
University of Southern California
Los Angeles, California

Thelma J. Wells, R.N., Ph.D.
Associate Professor
School of Nursing
University of Michigan
Ann Arbor, Michigan

Mary Opal Wolanin, R.N., B.A., M.P.A.
Consultant and Educator, Geratric
    Nursing
Associate Professor Emeritus
University of Arizona
Tucson, Arizona

PREFACE

Elderly patients on the nursing scene are not a recent happening, but there are so many more of them and they are so much older that they sometimes seem to be a recent phenomenon. Old people have long resided in the back wards of state hospitals; they have wandered away from home and hospital; they have been climbing over bed rails all the years I have been nursing. Many of the problems of the elderly patient or client that I saw as a neophyte nurse in the 1940s are still with us—lack of decision-making by the elderly, lack of privacy, broken hips and bedsores, nasty falls, confusional states, wandering, subjection to restraints, and a dearth of dignity in both their lonely living and lonely dying. If this second edition does not make any changes toward increasing preventive care, improving the sad conditions mentioned above, or increasing the holistic nursing care of aged people, it will have failed its goals.

Recently there has been a proliferation of gerontological nursing textbooks written or edited by nurses. Frustrated teachers are often driven to compiling a textbook after having searched for materials which are scattered in a variety of likely (and unlikely) places. That selfish motive was behind my first edition of this text. At the time the first edition was assembled, there was only one gerontological program at the master's level in the United States, two nurse practitioner programs in gerontology, and a smattering of summer classes; this edition should reflect the changes that have been made in gerontological nursing since then. There are now gerontological nurse practitioners carrying caseloads. There are classes in continuing education about care of the older adult. The growth and development model for teaching includes the aged person on the continuum. And student nurses placed in long-term settings are changing and improving the care. There are new programs beginning and new grants being funded all across the United States.

My purpose is to present a comprehensive multidisciplinary textbook, written for nurses and nursing students, which includes a variety of ways to view and care for the aged person.

The fact that the first edition was used as a text by disciplines other than nursing came as a surprise and a delight to me. I was delighted because it meant that the multidisciplinary approach of the book was successful and accepted. I took that approach because I believe that, just as no individual can be separated into his physical, psychological, and sociological components, so no problem in aging belongs solely to one discipline. I have continued that multidisciplinary approach in this second edition.

Nursing still tends to overemphasize the decremental model in the study of the aged and often focuses on physical care. This book offers many facets of the aging process for nurses to consider in the holistic care of the elderly—retirement, ethnicity, religion, and the environment.

I have tried to emphasize psychosocial care and the mental health of the aged because these components in nursing care of the elderly still receive short shrift. Aspects of care not covered here in depth can be found in *Psychosocial Nursing Care of the Aged* (McGraw-Hill, 1980), a small companion book to this one; the books were revised concurrently so that they might complement each other.

Although the book is divided into sections on psychology, geropsychiatry, physiology, and sociology for editorial purposes, I hope it is clear throughout the book that the entire range of an individual's problems, the interplay of one problem upon the other, should be considered in the care of the elderly person. This textbook handles as many of the complicated, interrelated problems which concern nursing the aged client as space permits.

If this second edition is not a great improvement over the first, it is not because the reviewers did not carefully and critically review the original book. I thank each of them for their most helpful critiques; their suggestions have resulted in an extensive overhaul.

Some of the changes which have, I hope, improved this edition are as follows:

- Twenty-one new chapters have been added (33 chapters are written by nurses).
- Sections were extensively reorganized, and new ones have been added on such topics as organic brain syndromes, assessment of the elderly person, special problems, and older women.
- Learning objectives for the student have been included at the beginning of each chapter.
- A list of additional resources has been added at the end of some chapters, if any could be found.
- The range of coverage on the following subjects has been greatly expanded: (1) assessment, (2) confusional states, (3) depression, (4) dying and death, (5) organic brain syndromes, (6) paranoia, and (7) suicide.
- In four disciplines I have added contributions by professionals: (1) a music therapist, (2) family therapists, (3) psychiatrists, (4) an occupational therapist, plus chapters by nurse practitioners.

The editor of a book finds the list of people to be thanked incredibly long; so it is for me.

My four years at the Andrus Gerontology Center, University of Southern California, left their mark on me. This book began in that environment, and I was greatly influenced by working in a multidisciplinary team there. I am most grateful to Dr. James E. Birren and the late Dr. Albert B. Feldman for showing me the necessity of the multidiscipline approach to gerontology

and sharing with me their insights. Many of the contributors were originally USC faculty who gave lectures in my nursing classes there; those lectures subsequently became important chapters in this book.

I feel special, warm gratitude to Professor Marion Kalkman and Dean Helen Nahm, of the University of California in San Francisco, for their steady encouragement and support during my graduate study. They have been, and continue to be, tremendous role models.

Students are seldom aware of how much they teach instructors—partly, I suppose, because we are reluctant to tell them so. I would like to acknowledge how much my students taught me as they struggled with the problems of the elderly. I am also grateful to the many nurses and administrators who welcomed me into their facilities through the years, either as a volunteer or an instructor.

I would also like to thank a very special team who helped me with this revision:

- Marsella Smith helped out with the exacting task of objective writing.
- Ed Biglin helped me improve my syntax time and again and never questioned me about how I got through Freshman English.
- Pearl Bladek willingly typed and typed and typed.
- Evelyn Butorac and Audrey McGaffin were tenacious in getting permissions for all the various items needing permission. They both offered me much support.
- Dave Carroll was my friend from McGraw-Hill throughout the trying times.
- Diane Miller started with me on the first edition of *Nursing and the Aged*. Three books later, she is still doing the detailed, careful work manuscripts require. Her steadiness during my occasional confusional states certainly helped the progress of the book and improved my own mental health.
- Milt Northway came through with cartoons under pressure and contended with my finicky instructions.
- Anthony Skirlick, Jr., found his way into a variety of institutions and also many old persons' hearts as he took photographs in all parts of the United States.

The book belongs to the above team, as well

as to the contributors. To say that I am grateful to each of them and needed them all is surely an understatement.

Throughout the many years that I have been a nurse and the many positions I have held, I have learned from the elderly; it is inevitable that what they so patiently taught me has found its way into this book. I am haunted by Mr. Shirley, the 103-year-old man in a county nursing home who plaintively said, "I do not know how to grow old gracefully, but I do know how to grow old quietly." I am deeply grateful to Mr. Shirley and many other old people because the aged themselves have been some of my best teachers about the aging process. Basho said that to learn about the pine, one must study pine trees!

Irene Mortenson Burnside

NURSING AND THE AGED

ONE

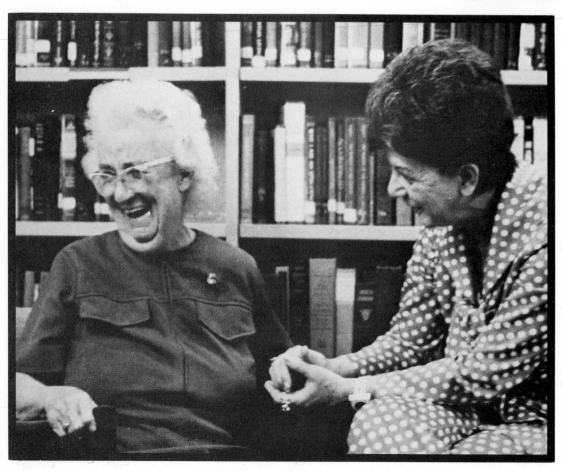

Diane E. Miller

AGING AND NURSING

A great deal of talent is lost in the world from want
of little courage. Every day sends to their graves
obscure men whom timidity prevented from making
a first effort; who if they could have been induced to
begin, would have in all probability gone great
lengths in the career of same. The fact is that to do
anything in the world worth doing we must not
stand back shivering and thinking of the cold and
danger but jump in and scramble through as well as
we can.

Richard Cardinal Cushing

GERONTOLOGICAL NURSING

Irene Mortenson Burnside

We are made wise not by the recollections of our past, but by the responsibilities of our future.
George Bernard Shaw

LEARNING OBJECTIVES

- Compare and discuss the terms *geriatric* and *gerontology.*
- List at least three factors contributing to the negative view generally held of the aged.
- Discuss three levels of gerontological nursing.
- Identify and compare the crucial components in the care of the elderly.
- Discuss two important areas that influence student attitudes toward nursing care of the elderly.
- Identify eight goals of gerontological nursing education to better prepare students for elder care.

Gerontology is a new field and is still in the pioneering phase in many ways. Gerontology is the science concerned with the process of aging. Studies appeared sporadically in the scientific literature, but not until 1939 did a presentation appear; it was Cowdry's book, *Problems in Aging,* and was a summary of the literature on all the various aspects of aging. The American Geriatric Society was formed in 1942, and the Gerontological Society began in 1945. The first meeting of the International Association of Gerontology was held in Liège, Belgium, in 1950. Ninety-five participants from 14 countries attended that meeting. Only 22 years later the International Congress of Gerontology, held in Kiev, U.S.S.R., was attended by over 2000 professionals, representing 45 countries!

Shock (1973) notes a change in gerontological research and writes that there is a "shift from descriptive studies to investigation and mechanisms which produce age changes or age differences." He describes research in cell biology as a recent advance and then states, "Although I do not regard extension of life span as a worthy goal for gerontological research, many do."

Science that deals with aging is gerontology; it focuses on old age. About 1903 the term *gerontology* was originated by Ilya Mechnikov (Gruman, 1978).

Gunter and Miller (1977) define nursing gerontology as ". . . the scientific study of the nursing care of the elderly. It is characterized as an applied science, since its aim is to use knowledge of the aging process to design nursing care and services which provide for health, longevity, and independence—or highest level of functioning possible—in the aging, and aged." *Geriatrics* is the term applied to the medical treatment of old age and the diseases common in later life.

Physicians and nurses differ in choice of terms, and physicians will continue to use the term *geriatrics,* but nurses who are in the field of aging lean toward the definition provided by Gunter and Miller. The pioneer in the field, Doreen Norton (1965) of the United Kingdom, defined geriatric nursing as a positive approach to preserve and to restore abilities in later life. For teaching purposes, she further differentiated the care into two divisions: physical management of the patient, and knowledge of social aspects and the problems of the aged who reside in the community. She went so far as to describe two different categories in practice—(1) rehabilitation, when possible, and (2) care of the irremediable persons who will need nursing care as long as they live.

Nurses apparently find the term *geriatric* too constrictive, too pejorative, and so have begun to use *gerontological nursing* in titles of programs (e.g., gerontological nurse specialist), to establish master's degrees in gerontological nursing, and to christen one professional journal, *Journal of Gerontological Nursing;* the division title of the American Nurses' Association (ANA) is known as Division on Gerontological Nursing Practice, and the certification of two levels are the Gerontological Nurse Certification and the Gerontological Nurse Practitioner (ANA, 1979).

Geriatric nursing may be a term still heard. Medical doctors still practice geriatric medicine, and chairs of geriatric medicine are still endowed in universities. Nurses have chosen the word *gerontology* to better describe their role and functions as they care for elderly clients. Professionally, we seem to have opted for different terminology for what we do. Gunter and Miller (1977) have added it as a third applied field based on Havighurst (1971), who stated that gerontology was an applied science and divided it into medical and social gerontology. Physicians, however, still call themselves *geriatricians,* not *medical gerontologists,* and nurses now identify themselves as *gerontological nurses,* not *geriatric nurses.* Perhaps this is but one more attempt to move out of the physicians' shadows, which hid many nurses for so long.

HEALTH NEEDS OF ADULTS WILL INCREASE

If one studies population projections, one can see that planning for the health needs of many older people will be required in the very near future. There were only 3.1 million people aged 65 and older in the United States in 1900. By 1940 the number had tripled to 9.0 million, and in the next 30 years it more than doubled to 20.2 million in 1970. The number increases by about 300,000 to 400,000 per year. By the year

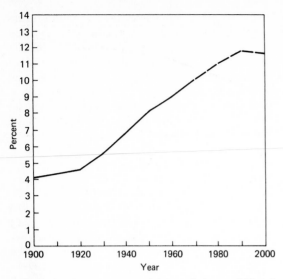

FIGURE 1-1 The percentage of the population aged 65 and older has increased. (*National Center for Health Statistics.*)

2000, it is expected that there will be about 29 million persons 65 or older (see Figure 1-1).

The size of the population can be predicted with a fair degree of accuracy because the people who will be age 65 or older in the year 2000 are for the most part already living in the United States. Those people who will have their 65th birthday in the year 2000 were born in 1935 and will have their 40th birthday this year—1975. Unless there is a great increase in immigration of persons age 40 and older, there will be few additions to this population. Unless there are radical changes in the death rates, 77 percent of those having their 40th birthday this year will survive to age 65. (US Department of Health, Education, and Welfare,[1] 1976, p. 542)

About one-third of the older population is very old, 75 years or above. This proportion will stay about the same for the foreseeable future if mortality rates remain constant.

---

[1] When a separate Department of Education was formed in 1979, this department was renamed the Department of Health and Human Services.

. . . If mortality rates decline, however, the number of the very old may grow as high as 16 or 18 million. A 65-year-old man can now expect, on the average, to live to 78; a woman of 65, to 82. By the year 2000, life expectancies for 65-year-olds may increase by another two to five years. (Neugarten and Maddox, 1978, p. 1) (See Figure 1-2)

GAINS IN LONGEVITY CONTINUE

During 1977, the average length of life for the resident population of the United States reached an all-time high of 73 years, and both sexes shared in the gains. The expectation of life at birth increased to 69.2 years for newborn males and to 76.9 years for females. The longevity of the total population has improved by 2.3 years since 1969–1971, and by 13.8 years since 1929–1931, when the average was 59.2 years (*Metropolitan Life Statistical Bulletin,* 1978).

The gains in longevity in recent years are due to a general reduction in mortality throughout the life-span. The greatest improvement has

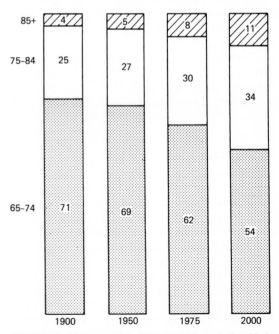

FIGURE 1-2 The proportion of the very old among the elderly is increasing. (*National Center for Health Statistics.*)

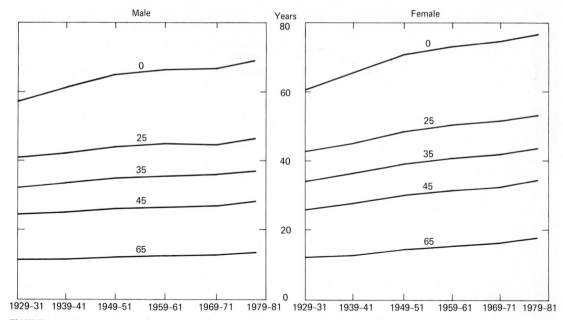

FIGURE 1-3   Expectation of life (in years) at selected ages: United States, 1929–1977. Figures for 1929–1931 estimated from data for whites and blacks. (*Figures for 1929–1931 to 1976 from the National Center for Health Statistics; 1977 computed by the Statistical Bureau of the Metropolitan Life Insurance Company.*)

taken place in the first few years of life. The infant death rate dropped from 20.0 per 1000 live births in 1969–1971 to 15.1 in 1976 and fell by an additional 7 percent to a new low of 14.0 in 1977. Declining mortality from ischemic heart disease, the cerebrovascular diseases, pneumonia, and influenza also contributed to the improvement in longevity (*Metropolitan Life Statistical Bulletin,* 1978). See Figure 1-3 for expectation of life (in years) at various ages.

PATTERNS OF IMMIGRATION

Another historical factor which influenced the nursing care and treatment of the elderly in the United States was the pattern of immigration. In the 1800s, large numbers of immigrants came to the United States from many countries; most could not speak English. Even today there are areas in the United States where a language barrier still exists, e.g., in Southwestern states, where Spanish is the language of many people, or in San Francisco's Chinatown, where elderly Chinese still speak their own language. It is, therefore, not uncommon to find elderly people

in hospitals and nursing homes who cannot speak English. Recently a director of nurses discussed her concern about a Japanese patient who attempted suicide while in the extended care facility. She spoke no English so that the problem of communicating with her had to be solved. In Maine a director of nursing of a long-term care facility talked about language problems; all her residents spoke French because of the proximity of the facility to the Canadian border.

The rapidity of the industrial and technological changes has also influenced care of the aged population. The new medical advances and new drugs and treatments have vastly affected the medical, nursing, and related professions. Furthermore, it is increasingly difficult for the practitioner to keep abreast of the many recent trends and treatments and publications.

HOME HEALTH CARE PROGRAMS

Shanas et al. (1968) estimate that, in the over-65 population, 14 percent are limited in mobility, bedfast, or homebound for some reason.

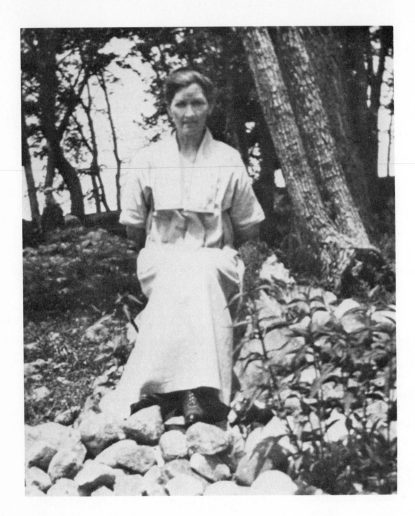

FIGURE 1-4 This woman was an immigrant from Sweden in the 1800s. She left her homeland at the age of 19 to marry and to spend the rest of her life in the United States. For financial reasons she was never able to revisit her homeland, where all her relatives remained. (*Courtesy of May Belle Nelson.*)

Rossman (1973) has described home care programs in New York City which offer effective services for such persons and are cheaper than hospitalization. Such services also use the time of the health professional to better advantage, which increases the economy of such programs. One of the recommendations of the White House Conference of 1971 was to maintain elderly people in their own homes as long as possible; the recommendation still holds, but it is difficult to know if much progress has been made toward that end (Post–White House Conference on Aging Reports, 1973). Nurses can be influential in disposition decisions, but often they are not included in the decision making or do not wish to accept such responsibility.

In past years old people were often sent to what was then known as "the poor farm" or sometimes "the old people's home." Many who died there were buried in cemeteries known as "potter's fields." State hospital patients with no relatives and/or no one to pay for a funeral were also buried in such cemeteries. The stigma of the poor farm is still with us, and many old people feel that institutionalization is the end of the road for them. The elderly in the United States, who were accustomed to a Judeo-Christian work ethic, dislike being dependent on others, and many detest welfare help. It is not uncommon for old people in nursing homes to wander about the home asking who is paying for their care. One concerned administrator writes a

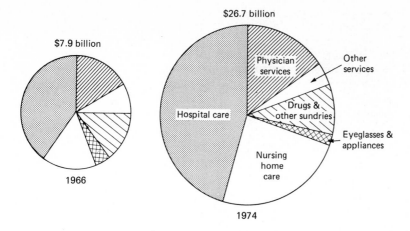

$26.7 billion

$7.9 billion

Physician services

Other services

Hospital care

Drugs & other sundries

Eyeglasses & appliances

Nursing home care

1966

1974

FIGURE 1-5 Expenditures for medical care for the elderly have more than tripled since 1966. (*National Center for Health Statistics.*)

"paid in full" receipt for such patients to carry in their pocket at all times to keep them from feeling indebted (Patton, 1974).

EVOLUTION OF GERONTOLOGICAL NURSING

The evolution of gerontological nursing in the United States has been slow and gradual. As stated in the preface of the book, nurses have always taken care of old people, but they are doing so more today because of the increased number of people over age 65 and because many of them are now reaching advanced ages of 90 and 100 and over.

In 1935 the Social Security Act was passed, and money became available to the aged poor, provided they did not live in an institution. There was an increase in the number of boarding homes to accommodate these oldsters; and since retired and widowed nurses often converted their homes into such living quarters, these women became the first geriatric nurses and their homes the first nursing homes in the United States. There are now over 1 million nursing home beds in this country.

Nurses of the past did not think of themselves as geriatric nurses even though they cared for elderly people. Barbara Allen Davis gave an address on this subject at the American Geriatric Society; she was the first nurse ever to speak before this group (Davis, 1968).

In 1961 a committee of the American

Nurses' Association (ANA) recommended a geriatric nursing group. "In the spring of 1962, 70 pioneering nurses attended the first national ANA meeting of a Conference Group on Geriatric Nursing Practice, in Detroit, Michigan. They were still so uncertain of their identity that the main item on their agenda was their name" (Davis, 1968).

ANA developed Divisions on Nursing Practice; June 1966 was the first time that a geriatric nurse was considered to be as important as the other nursing specialists. The pamphlet *Standards of Geriatric Nursing Practice* was first published in 1970 and was recently revised; all nurses working with aged clientele need to familiarize themselves with the standards because they are written so that the knowledge base in aging can be applied to nursing to enhance and improve the care of the aged person.

For an outstanding chapter on the historical background of gerontological nursing, the reader is referred to "Nursing Committed to the Elderly" by Thelma Wells (1979).

INCOMPLETE DATA

The changing funding of programs for gerontological nurses makes it difficult to keep a current list of programs in the United States. A list is available from the U.S. Department of Health, Education, and Welfare (1979), but it is not complete. I tried during the preparation of this book to compile such a list, but the list was changed and already outdated by the time the book was ready to go to press. We do need an improved data base about the location of gerontology programs, the degrees offered, the number of nurses graduating, and the number of nurses working in various settings with the elderly.

In spite of what many nurses still believe, there is a body of knowledge regarding the care of the older adult. The knowledge base is slowly growing, as can be seen by the increasing publications by nurses. Gerontological nurses, of course, still borrow from other disciplines. They also must interact with a variety of disciplines to provide holistic health care for elderly clients.

GERONTOLOGICAL NURSE PRACTITIONER

Currently two types of gerontological nurses are being educated in the United States. One is the gerontological nurse practitioner (GNP), and the other is the gerontological nurse clinical specialist.

Entry requirements for programs for the gerontological nurse practitioner may vary from registered nurse to master's degree level. The ANA describes a nurse practitioner as one who has advanced skills in the assessment of the physical and psychosocial health-illness status of individuals, families, or groups in a variety of settings through health and development history taking to physical examination. They are prepared either by formal continuing education which adheres to ANA-approved guidelines or by a baccalaureate nursing program.

GERONTOLOGICAL CLINICAL NURSE SPECIALIST

The gerontological nurse specialist is educated at the master's degree level. ANA describes a clinical nurse specialist as primarily a clinician with a high degree of knowledge, skill, and competence in a specialized area of nursing. Clinical nurse specialists hold a master's degree in nursing, preferably with an emphasis in clinical nursing. (These nurses may have more re-

search education and experience in their programs than the GNPs who have not been through a master's program. The GNP will have physical assessment skills par excellence concerning the older adult.) The reader is referred to a study by Brody et al. about nurse practitioners in the extended care facility (Brody et al., 1976).

NURSE CLINICIANS

Nurse clinicians have well-developed competencies in utilizing a broad range of cues. They demonstrate expertise in nursing practice and ensure ongoing development of expertise through clinical experience and continuing education. Minimal preparation for this role is the baccalaureate degree.

ROLES IN PRACTICE

Practitioners of professional nursing are registered nurses who provide direct care to clients, utilizing the nursing process in arriving at decisions. They work in a collegial and collaborative relationship with other health professionals to determine health care needs and assume responsibility for nursing care (ANA, 1975).

The lack of physicians to care for elderly clients is one reason that gerontological nurse practitioners should have an important role in health delivery for the aged clients. Estes (1977) states,

> The elderly patient faces many problems in seeking assistance for health and illness problems. First, a physician may not be available. Second, the patient usually has several medical problems (e.g., hypertension, prostatic hypertrophy, and glaucoma, and each of these problems may require the services of a different specialist). Third, he has difficulty in obtaining guidance in matters of general hygiene and the application of techniques to prevent illness (e.g., dietary measures, exercise), as well as in obtaining advice for minor day-to-day illnesses, due to the lack of primary care physicians, or the

crowding of the physician's schedule or both.

CERTIFICATION

The best information available about numbers of gerontological nurses at this writing concerns the certification of nurses who have clinical skills in gerontological nursing. The first nurses were certified in 1972. The test has been revised and updated twice since then. Certification is handled by the ANA. Most nurses who have been certified work in long-term care. Candidates must demonstrate that their current practice is beyond requirements for licensure. Certification is granted for 5 years; the individual may submit evidence of practice and credentials for renewal.

CONTINUING EDUCATION

A major educational program was undertaken in 1972 when the Department of Health, Education, and Welfare funded a continuing education curriculum. The curriculum was taught in 44 sites in the country under the aegis of the ANA (Shields, 1978).

At this writing, 19 states have mandatory continuing education for relicensure. That is one of the bright spots in improving the care of the elderly. Another hopeful change is the requirement in some states, for example, in California, that nurse's aides be taught basic information about aging and that they be certified also.

GERONTOLOGICAL NURSING LEADERS

Doris Schwartz was one of the early leaders in the development of the gerontological nurse practitioner program, and her background with the Primex Nursing Program at Cornell University was helpful at that time. Virginia Stone of Duke University headed the first master's program for clinical nurse specialists in gerontol-ogy; her students were the first specialists to graduate. Delores Alford and Jacqueline Heppler also headed programs for practitioners in the early seventies.

Laurie Gunter was one of the first nurses in the United States to present papers at the meetings of the International Congress of Gerontology, both here and abroad. On the national scene, there are now enough nursing papers presented to warrant a special section of gerontological nurse practitioners in one recent annual society meeting.

Two nurses have been honored as the Gerontological Nurse of the Year by the *Journal of Gerontological Nursing*. The first was Janet Specht and the second was Dorothy Moses.

The renowned pioneer in the United Kingdom is Doreen Norton whose work *An Investigation of Geriatric Nursing Problems in Hospital* (Norton et al., 1962) is now a classic in the field of nursing the aged.

EMERGENCE OF GEROPSYCHIATRIC NURSING

We still have a dearth of nurses who are skilled in geropsychiatric nursing. There are to date no programs that focus on teaching these skills to nurses. The physical assessment has taken off well, but there also needs to be an emphasis on the psychological or psychosocial assessment.

> The one deficiency in gerontological nursing training has been inadequate preparation in the psychological sphere. Once this is added, a gerontological or geropsychiatric nursing practitioner might serve as a linchpin of geriatric services. (Birren and Sloan, 1977)

It is possible that geropsychiatric nurses will emerge within the next decade. If not, then others in psychology, theology, and psychiatric social work may well carry the load of mental health care of the aged. Or perhaps a new discipline may be formed to train professionals in mental health and aging (Butler, 1975).

NURSE SHORTAGE

The shortage of nurses prepared at the graduate level is still critical. The need is great because this is the cadre of nurses from which teachers, consultants, administrators, and clinical specialists are drawn. The need for doctorally prepared nurses for higher echelons of administrative jobs, teaching positions, and for research is also acute.

There are more nursing home beds (1,235,404) in the United States than there are general and surgical hospital beds (1,006,951) ("Nursing Home Care in the United States," Senate Special Subcommittee on Aging, November 1974). The shortage of nurses to work in nursing homes can be seen in Table 1-1, in which the level of skill of the person in charge is noted. The lack of registered nurses in charge for all three shifts is quite apparent in that table (USDHEW, 1974).

TABLE 1-1
NURSING HOMES WITH CHARGE PERSONS ON DUTY FOR THREE SHIFTS, BY LEVEL OF SKILL

Level of Skill of Charge Persons*	Homes with Charge Persons for Three Shifts†	
	No.	%
All levels of skill	12,600	100.0
RNs in charge for three shifts	3,600	28.7
Combination of RNs and LPNs in charge for three shifts	4,300	34.2
LPNs in charge for three shifts		
Nurse's aides in charge for three shifts		
Other combinations of skills in charge for three shifts	3,500	28.2

* A person in charge of a shift is on duty, awake, dressed, and routinely serving the residents.

† Excludes 3600 homes having a charge person on duty less than three shifts a day.

SOURCE: *Monthly Vital Statistics Report,* DHEW, Sept. 5, 1974.

NEGATIVE VIEWS OF THE AGED

Instructors must constantly battle the pervasive negative attitude in our society about the aged. Nurses are not immune to this attitude. Mass media bombard our youth with images of the beautiful young people.

Sometimes nurses have to defend their interest in the aged. Freud's statement about people over 50 not being amenable to therapy has not helped the pessimistic view of psychotherapy with the aged. Freud (1949) wrote that at about the age of 50, people lack the elasticity of the mental process needed for psychotherapy. He felt that not only were old people uneducable, but that there was so much material to be handled that the treatment would last indefinitely.

The pessimistic view has permeated psychiatric nursing just as it has psychiatry. I once had to defend my choice of a 55-year-old man for a one-to-one relationship. He had been diagnosed as schizophrenic and had spent 30 years of his life in a state hospital; my preceptor wondered why I had selected him. My peers, of course, had all selected young patients.

Butler's (1978) term *ageism* refers to the devaluation of older people simply because they are old. Nurses continue to have problems with their own personal feelings. Butler (1978, p. 6) also makes the powerful point ". . . that ageism is the only form of prejudice in which you *become* that which you despise."

Nursing as a profession certainly has not been immune to society's negative views of the aged. This becomes even more apparent if one looks at the nursing curricula in our schools of nursing. Moses and Lake (1968) had written about the lack of interest in the aged by the profession and document the paucity of gerontology courses in undergraduate nursing curricula throughout the United States. In another study about specialty preferences, it was shown that few baccalaureate students expressed a preference for geriatric nursing (De Lora and Moses, 1969). Gillis (1973) studied attitudes of nursing personnel toward the aged. She found that "the age variable was not related to nursing personnel's attitudes toward the aged, but educational level did seem to have some effect, i.e., licensed practical nurses were more positive in their attitudes toward the aged than baccalaureate nurses" (p. 530).

Another aspect of the present problem in nursing is that there are still not enough prepared and qualified instructors to teach gerontological nursing courses at all the various levels of nursing which exist. We still lack role models.

The negativistic attitude in the profession is also manifested in the subtle and not-so-subtle treatment of nurses who choose to work with the aged. For some time now, nurses who work in nursing homes, long-term care facilities, or geriatric units have stated they are tired of being regarded as second-class nurses. The low salaries received by some would also indicate that they are not as qualified as the nurses who are employed in other settings. One nurse who had worked in an intensive care unit (ICU) became a director of nursing in an extended care facility; a friend asked her what had caused her to slide so far backward!

The lack of interest in the aged by nurses and the shortage of nurses may in some instances create the problem of poorly qualified and inexperienced nurses caring for the aged. Hard-pressed nursing home administrators, who are forced to abide by laws which become increasingly stringent, justifiably grumble about having to pay someone simply for being a registered nurse while often being poorly qualified.

Some instructors feel that it is easier to teach gerontology to students who have had a positive relationship with an aged person. But with the increase of nuclear families, with the mobility of both parents and grandparents, and with an increasing number of the aged population living in areas specifically designated for older persons, some nursing students have little contact with aged people. (See Table 1-2 for special interest groups in state associations.)

While we must continue to educate "new" nurses, there must also be a concerted effort to help diploma nurses with their continuing education because many of them are employed in long-term care facilities. Furthermore, registered nurses still complain about how difficult it is for them to obtain a baccalaureate degree.

Student nurses sometimes say that they got their negative attitudes about the care of the aged from initial unpleasant, traumatic assignments. Nurse educators are hard-pressed to find enough "good" learning experiences, and it seems to be generally agreed that exposure to an alert elderly person who does not overwhelm the student with complex nursing problems is preferred for a neophyte nursing student in gerontology.

PROFESSIONAL RESPONSIBILITIES

There are some responsibilities regarding gerontological nursing under the aegis of the nursing profession. As nurses, we can ill afford to downgrade the importance of gerontological nurses. Gerontological nurses, and especially those employed in nursing homes, carry much responsibility. The myth that it does not take much skill or expertise to take care of old people unfortunately still prevails, and old people are still viewed as needing custodial care more than anything else.

The profession will have to accept more responsibility in getting gerontology content into nursing curricula at all levels of education and in sharing their knowledge with those in other disciplines. How do we increase the articulateness of nurses? How do we encourage nurses to write about their skills and experiences with older clients? Some very skilled nurses remain incredibly inarticulate. If we decry the quality of materials in the literature, what then shall we do to improve the body of literature on nursing care of the aged? Pressure on the editors of nursing journals is one method. Letters also need to be sent to the editor when excellent studies or articles do appear in the literature. Instructors must encourage and positively reinforce student writing and publication. Students *do* expend great effort and energy to improve nursing care as they acquire their education, but get little credit or reward for doing so. Projects required for classes should not be "busy work." (See Figure 1-6 for a cartoonist's view regarding publishing and the professionals!)

The need for nurses to begin to publish their findings and expertise in care of the aged is becoming more apparent as nursing lags behind other disciplines. In *Gerontology: A Core List of Significant Works* (Edwards and Flynn, 1978), only three works are by nurses. See Chapter 45

TABLE 1-2
CONFERENCE AND SPECIAL INTEREST GROUPS IN STATE AND TERRITORIAL NURSES' ASSOCIATIONS, 1975

State or Territory	Advanced Practice Areas Combined	Community Health	Gerontological	Maternal/Child Health	Medical/Surgical	Psychiatric/Mental Health	Educational Administrators, Consultants, and Teachers	Nursing Service Administration	Occupational Health	Operating Room Nursing Practice	Private Duty	School Nurse	Other
Total	5	18	22	21	18	20	7	12	7	6	6	10	17
Alabama													
Alaska	(1)	(1)	(1)	(1)	(1)	(1)	(1)	(1)	(1)	(1)	(1)	(1)	(1)
Arizona		[2]X					X	X			X	X	[3]X
Arkansas		[4]X	[4]X	[4]X	[4]X	[4]X							[5]X
California													
...													
Colorado						X							
Connecticut													
Delaware		X	X	X	X	X					X		
District of Columbia													
Florida													
Georgia		X	X	X	X		X		X				[5]X
Guam	(1)	(1)	(1)	(1)	(1)	(1)	(1)	(1)	(1)	(1)	(1)	(1)	(1)
Hawaii													[6]X
Idaho													
Illinois			X	[7]X	X								
Indiana	[8,9]X	X	X	X	[10]X	X		X	X	X	X	X	[11,12]X
Iowa		X	X	X	X	X		X					
Kansas		X	X	X	X	X		X					
Kentucky			[4]X	[4]X		[4]X							[11]X
Louisiana													
Maine		X		X		X							
Maryland	[13]X			[14]X	[14]X				X		X		[15]X
Massachusetts	(1)	(1)	(1)	(1)	(1)	(1)	(1)	(1)	(1)	(1)	(1)	(1)	(1)
Michigan	[16]X		X	X	X	[17]X				X			[18]X
Minnesota			X	X	X	[19]X				X		X	[20,21,22,23]X
Mississippi		X	[4]X	[4]X	[4]X	[4]X	X					X	
Missouri		X	X	X	X	X					X	X	
Montana		[24]X	[4]X	[4]X				X				X	
Nebraska													
Nevada	(1)	(1)	(1)	(1)	(1)	(1)	(1)	(1)	(1)	(1)	(1)	(1)	(1)
New Hampshire		[25]X	X	X									
New Jersey		(1)	(1)	(1)	(1)	(1)	(1)	(1)	(1)	(1)	(1)	(1)	(1)
New Mexico	(1)	(1)	(1)	(1)	(1)	(1)	(1)	(1)	(1)	(1)	(1)	(1)	(1)
New York	(1)	(1)	(1)	(1)	(1)	(1)	(1)	(1)	(1)	(1)	(1)	(1)	(1)

State												
North Carolina	...	...	...	...	X						X
North Dakota	X	X	...	...	X	X	X	X	X	X	...
Ohio	...	...	...	[26]X	[26]X	[26]X	[26]X	[26]X	[26]X	...	[26,27,28]X
Oklahoma	[24]X	...	...	X	X	X	X	X	X	X	...
Oregon	[4]X	[4]X	[4]X	X	X	X	X	X	X	X	[29]X
Pennsylvania	...	...	...	...	...	...	...	...	[30]X	...	[31]X
Rhode Island	X	X	X	X	X	...	...	...	...	...	...
South Carolina	...	...	...	...	...	...	...	...	...	...	...
Tennessee	[4]X	[4]X	X	X	X	X	X	X	X	X	[32]X
Texas	[4]X	[4]X	[4]X	X	X	X	X	X	X	X	[5]X
Utah	[24]X	[24]X	...	...	...	...	...	...	...	...	[33]X
Vermont	(34)	(34)	(34)	(34)	(34)	(34)	(34)	(34)	(34)	(34)	(34)
Virginia	X	X	[35]X	X	X	X	X	X	X	X	[13,26]X
Virgin Islands	(1)	(1)	(1)	(1)	(1)	(1)	(1)	(1)	(1)	(1)	(1)
Washington	X	X	...	...	X	...	...	...	...	...	...
West Virginia	[8]X	...	...	...	...	...	...	...	...	...	...
Wisconsin	...	X	X	X	X	...	X	X	X	X	[37]X
Wyoming	...	...	...	...	...	...	...	...	...	...	...

SOURCE: American Nurses' Association, Statistics Department, "State Nurses' Association Report to American Nurses' Association as of June 1975." Reprinted from *Facts about Nursing*, pp. 74–75, American Nurses' Association, Kansas City, Mo., 1974.

[1] No report.
[2] Ambulatory care nurses in extended roles occupational interest group.
[3] Inservice and continuing education educators occupational interest group.
[4] Includes both a clinical practice and an advanced practice conference group.
[5] Nursing education.
[6] Manpower.
[7] Includes both a maternal/child health conference group and a pediatric nurse associate special interest group.
[8] Clinical nurse specialists.
[9] Primary care.
[10] Includes both a nursing care of the adult and an intensive and coronary care conference group.
[11] Emergency health preparedness.
[12] Nurses as change agents.
[13] Nurse practitioners.
[14] Ostomy.
[15] Research and studies.
[16] Nurses in expanded practice.
[17] Child psychology.
[18] Quality assurance.
[19] Includes both psychiatric/mental health and a developmentally disabled conference group.
[20] Head nurse.
[21] Manager's branch.
[22] Inservice educators.
[23] Chemical dependency.
[24] Advanced practice conference group.
[25] Includes both a public health nurse and a community health conference group.
[26] Occupational forum.
[27] General duty nurse occupational forum.
[28] Public health occupational forum.
[29] Public health nurse.
[30] College nurse.
[31] Continuing education forum.
[32] General duty nurse.
[33] Bicentennial.
[34] Information not available.
[35] Includes both a medical/surgical and a critical care conference group.
[36] Continuing education.
[37] Patient care review coordinators.

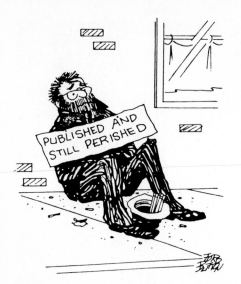

FIGURE 1-6 *NRTA Journal, 1978. Copyright by the National Retired Teachers Association. Reprinted with permission.*

for an update on gerontological nursing research.

EMPATHY AND SENSITIVITY: CRUCIAL COMPONENTS IN CARE OF ELDERLY

The importance of empathy when caring for the aged needs to be underscored. As one elderly lady said to a young student desperately trying to understand the woman's plight, "The trouble is I've been young, but you have never been old." A study by Mansfield (1973) on empathy has relevance for geriatric nurses. Mansfield studied behavior between a psychiatric nurse and schizophrenic patients. There is still a long way to go to increase empathy in the care of the aged. Nurses have not taken the role of advocacy very seriously.

It is a real challenge then for teachers in gerontological nursing to increase the sensitivity in the student nurse about the feelings, needs, and rights of the aged individual. Recently a director of nursing took me on a tour of her locked facility. We walked into a large dormlike seven-bed ward. Elderly women lay curled up in their beds; all the bed rails were

raised. The room was very quiet, and I was struck with the whiteness and sterility of it all. The nurse in her loud, gruff voice said, "And this is our terminal ward; we bring all of our dying patients here." At that moment I could only hope that all seven of the old ladies were very hard-of-hearing. Later I learned that plans were in the offing to transfer a problem (but not dying) patient to this room to see if it would "straighten her out." This is an extreme example of insensitivity, to be sure, but it brings home the responsibilities of upgrading the quality of nurses in leadership positions, and the need for developing and nurturing empathy and sensitivity in nurses who care for the aged.

If we have difficulty teaching sensitivity and empathy, then instructors really do carry a tremendous responsibility to be excellent role models for the students and for the employees of the various agencies where the instructor supervises. And, of course, instructors, too, will have to prove themselves competent in the care of the aged. The effort expended in keeping one's clinical practice current pays dividends in teaching student nurses; instructors can be more effective if they have an awareness of the current multiple and difficult problems that face the students.

A slower pace and a different attitude are necessary for the nurse who works with the elderly; all nurses are not prepared for this type of nursing any more than all nurses make excellent maternal-child nurses. Sometimes nurses view geriatric wards and units as the least desirable place to work. To be assigned to a geriatric unit is viewed as a punitive measure by some employees.

Gerontological nursing instructors should consider the following in planning courses:

1. A positive first learning experience for the student (placement of students in long-term care facilities, especially nursing homes, for the learning of basic skills is generally considered to be a disservice to both the aged client and the student).
2. Normal aging changes should be taught early in the course or curriculum.
3. Faculty should be prepared in gerontology (and should have worked with aged clients).
4. The needs of well and ambulatory aged need

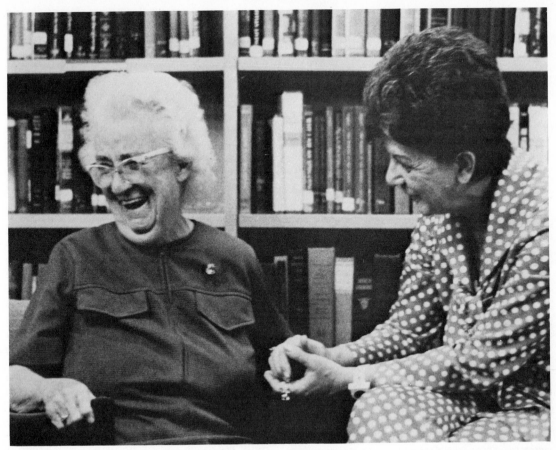

FIGURE 1-7 Instructors carry the responsibility of role modeling for students. Here an instructor is teaching interview techniques to a group of nurses in the library of a retirement home. (*Courtesy of Diane E. Miller.*)

to be considered as well as those of the ill and the frail elderly.

5. A multidisciplinary and interdisciplinary approach to the care is required.
6. Aged clients should assist in teaching whenever possible.
7. Library materials should contain the classics in gerontological nursing, e.g., the work of Doreen Norton in the United Kingdom.
8. Students may need help with their own ageism.
9. Role models are needed both in the classroom and in the agencies selected for clinical experience.

The following resolutions were approved by the ANA House of Delegates at the 1978 bien-

nial convention and are important to include in this chapter because they serve as a succinct and accurate summary.

EDUCATIONAL PREPARATION IN GERONTOLOGICAL NURSING[2]

WHEREAS, the American Nurses' Association promotes knowledgeable nursing care for all segments of the population, and

[2] Resolutions approved by the ANA House of Delegates, 1978. Reprinted with the permission of American Nurses' Association. Copyright by American Nurses' Association.

WHEREAS, the numbers and percentage of the elderly segment of the population are increasing, and

WHEREAS, the elderly clients present themselves in all settings where registered nurses practice, and

WHEREAS, comprehensive nursing care of elderly clients requires a definitive knowledge based in gerontological nursing, and

WHEREAS, this knowledge base can best be assured through universally identifiable gerontological nursing content in schools of nursing curricula, and

WHEREAS, this universality can be assured only with an adequate cadre of faculty prepared in gerontological nursing, and

WHEREAS, registered nurses providing nursing care for elderly clients are not generally prepared in basic gerontological nursing; therefore be it

RESOLVED, that the American Nurses' Association encourage universal inclusion of gerontological nursing content in the curricula of basic nursing educational programs, and be it

RESOLVED, that the American Nurses' Association encourage graduate programs in gerontological nursing to assure adequate numbers of faculty to teach gerontological nursing and of gerontological nurse researchers to expand the scientific base for gerontological nursing practice, and be it

RESOLVED, that the American Nurses' Association encourage continuing education programming in gerontological nursing to supplement the preparation of practicing registered nurses who have not had gerontological nursing in basic preparation.

I like what Hamner (1977, p. 18) has given as a charge to the gerontological nurse instructors. "If we as nursing instructors will be more diligent in providing experiences which enable the young health professional to begin the process of developing a positive philosophy of aging, we will make a valuable contribution toward upgrading the health care of the aged client."

REFERENCES

American Nurses' Association: Biennial convention, Honolulu, 1978.

————: *Nursing and Long-Term Care: Toward Quality Care for the Aging,* Publication G-E-4 3m, Kansas City, Mo., April 1975.

————: *Outline of Certification Offerings,* Kansas City, Mo., May 1979.

Birren, James E., and R. Bruce Sloan: *Manpower and Training Needs in Mental Health and Illness of the Aging,* Andrus Gerontology Center, University of Southern California, Los Angeles, 1977.

Brody, Stanley J., Linda Cole, Patrick Storey, and Nancy J. Wink: The geriatric nurse practitioner: A new medical resource in the skilled nursing home, *Journal of Chronic Disease,* **29:**537–543, 1976.

Butler, Robert N.: The future psychiatric care of older people, *Journal of the National Association of Private Psychiatric Hospitals,* **10**(1):4–9, fall 1978.

————: *Why Survive? Being Old in America,* Harper & Row, New York, 1975.

Cowdry, M. R.: *Problems in Aging,* Williams & Wilkins, Baltimore, 1939.

Davis, Barbara Allen: Coming of age: A challenge for geriatric nursing, *Journal of the American Geriatrics Society,* **16**(10):1100–1106, October 1968.

De Lora, Jack R., and Dorothy V. Moses: Specialty preferences and characteristics of nursing students in baccalaureate programs, *Nursing Research,* **18:**137–144, March–April 1969.

Edwards, Willie M., and Frances Flynn: *Gerontology: A Core List of Significant Works,* Institute of Gerontology, University of Michigan, Wayne State University, 1978.

Estes, E. Harvey: Health experience in the elderly, in Ewald W. Busse and Eric Pfeiffer (eds.), *Behavior and Adaptation in Late Life,* 2d ed., Little, Brown, Boston, 1977, p. 107.

Freud, Sigmund: *Collected Papers,* vol. IV, Ernest Jones (ed.), Joan Riviere (translator), Hogarth, London, 1949.

Gillis, Marion, Sister: Attitudes of nursing personnel toward the aged, *Nursing Research,* **22:**517–520, November–December 1973.

Gruman, Gerald J.: Cultural origin of present day age-ism, in *Aging and the Elderly: Humanistic Perspectives in Gerontology,* Humanities Press, Atlantic Highlands, N.J., 1978.

Gunter, Laurie M., and Jeanne C. Miller: Toward a nursing gerontology, *Nursing Research,* **26**(3):208–221, May–June 1977.

Hamner, Mildred Louise: Symbols of aging as perceived by the young, *Journal of Gerontological Nursing,* **3**(4):18, July–August 1977.

Havighurst, Robert J.: A world view of gerontology, in C. C. Vedder (ed.), *Gerontology, A Book of Readings,* Charles C Thomas, Publisher, Springfield, Ill., 1971, pp. 20–28.

Mansfield, Elaine: Empathy: Concept and identified psychiatric nursing behavior, *Nursing Research,* **22:**525–529, November–December 1973.

Metropolitan Life Statistical Bulletin: Gains in longevity continue, **59**(3):7–8, July–September 1978.

Moses, Dorothy V., and Carolyn S. Lake: Geriatrics in the baccalaureate nursing curriculum, *Nursing Outlook,* **16**:41–43, July 1968.

Neugarten, Bernice L., and George L. Maddox: *Our Future Selves,* Department of Health, Education, and Welfare, publication no. NIH 78-1444, GPO, Washington, 1978, p. 1.

Norton, Doreen: Nursing in geriatrics, *Gerontologia Clinica,* **7**:51–60, 1965.

——, Rhoda McLaren, and N. Exton-Smith: *An Investigation of Geriatric Nursing Problems in Hospital,* National Corporation for the Care of Old People, 1962. Reprinted by Churchill Livingstone, Edinburgh, 1962; 1975.

Nursing Home Care in the United States, Senate Special Subcommittee on Aging, Washington, November 1974.

Patton, Florence: Personal communication, 1974.

Post-White House Conferences on Aging Reports, Washington, 1973, p. 65.

Rossman, Isadore: Alternatives to institutional care, *Bulletin of the New York Academy of Medicine,* 2d series, **49**:1084–1092, December 1973.

Shanas, Ethel, et al.: *Old People in Three Industrial Societies,* Atherton, New York, 1968.

Shields, Eldonna: Statement on the education of nurses in gerontological nursing, House Select Committee on Aging, May 17, 1978.

Shock, Nathan: Congressional Debates of the 93rd Congress, Record Proceedings and First Session Addresses at the Dedication of the Ethel Percy Andrus Gerontology Center, Los Angeles, Feb. 12, 1973, p. 56.

U.S. Department of Health, Education, and Welfare: *A Directory of Expanded Programs for Registered Nurses,* DHEW publication no. HRA 79-10, Division of Nursing, Hyattsville, Md., Government Printing Office, Washington, 1979.

——: *Health: United States, 1975,* Public Health Service, DHEW publication no. HRA 76-1232, Rockville, Md., 1976, p. 542.

——: *Monthly Vital Statistics Report,* Sept. 5, 1974.

Wells, Thelma: Nursing committed to the elderly, in Adina M. Reinhardt and Mildred D. Quinn (eds.), *Current Practice in Gerontological Nursing,* Mosby, St. Louis, 1979.

TWO

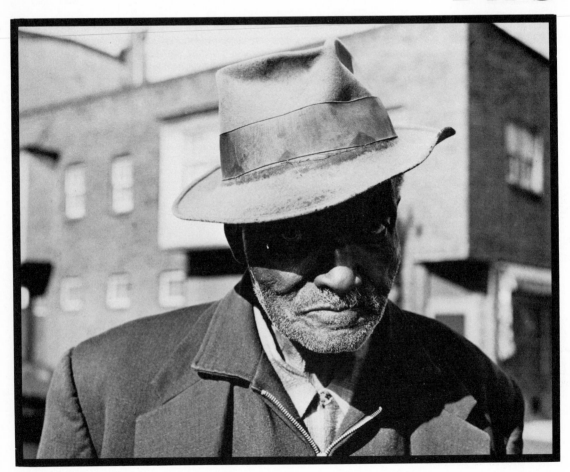

Harvey Finkle

AGING CHANGES

If to see more is to really become more, then we
should look closely at man in order to increase our
capacity to live.

Père Teilhard de Chardin

TWO

BIOLOGICAL THEORIES OF AGING

Caleb E. Finch
James A. Severson

If old age weakens most of our facilities, it is far from paralyzing them all; and rigorous observation shows us that in certain ways the organs of the aged acquit themselves of their tasks with quite as much energy as those of the adult.
Jean M. Charcot, 1881

LEARNING OBJECTIVES

- Recognize sources of endocrine changes during aging.
- Describe three phenomena generally observed in humans during the aging process.
- Define lipofuscin.

It is very difficult to establish the true facts about aging. There is probably greater confusion even in the minds of professionals and experts about the nature of the aging process than any other single aspect of human development. For example, it has been a part of folklore that during aging men inevitably become impotent; yet the sober studies of Masters and Johnson (1966) as well as their predecessors in the Kinsey report (1948) have shown quite clearly that the capacity for a full sexual response is not lost during aging, in either men or women.

Why is it so difficult to find out the facts about aging? Certainly most of us have ample opportunity for first-hand observation on aging, for example, from our parents and grandparents. It is not as though aging changes were hidden and unobservable. One of the major reasons for this confusion in our opinion is the difficulty in distinguishing between changes caused by aging and those which are secondary to disease. Consider, for example, the question of memory loss and intelligence during aging. It has long been axiomatic that older people slowly lose intellectual functions and the ability to remember recent events, whereas their ability to remember times long past may be much less impaired (Craik, 1977). However, those individuals most prone to deficits of mental function are subjects with high blood pressure or other deteriorative vascular diseases. In a study at Duke University, Wilkie and Eisdorfer (1971) followed a number of men aged 50. These researchers found that there was minimal evidence of impairment in the memory and intelligence performance in men with normal blood pressure, whereas those with high blood pressure manifested marked declines. As expected, mortality was higher in the group with the high blood pressure. Because high blood pressure is a major cause associated with strokes or cerebral accidents which impair the blood circulation of the brain, it seems likely that much of the physiolog-

ical loss of memory during aging occurs in a subpopulation of those individuals who are at particular risk for strokes and other similar changes.

How would strokes affect recent memory and not long-term memory? It is known that a part of the brain called the *hippocampus* is crucial for the incorporation of new information. The hippocampus is more sensitive to oxygen deficits than other tissues of the brain. Thus, it is no surprise to find that individuals with strong evidence of memory impairment showed abnormal electrical activities in the hippocampus (Drachman and Hughes, 1970). It is possible that a series of minor strokes might not even be perceived as a single event; such strokes could cause cumulative damage to this system of the brain, which might not be manifested in other parts of the brain. Also, there is an age-related loss of the neurotransmitter synthetic enzyme choline acetyltransferase in the human hippocampus (Davies, 1978) which implies that there is a loss of cholinergic nerve cells in this region. The cholinergic system in the hippocampus has been shown to be important in memory incorporation. Possibly, the loss of cholinergic cells, compounded with damage from minor strokes, would worsen memory deficits in the aged. Although at the present time the precise localization of memory in the brain is unclear, the major storage of old memories or previous memory appears to occur outside the hippocampus and would, therefore, be at least somewhat protected in individuals with high blood pressure who are prone to stroke. This example also emphasizes that there are some parts of the body that are more sensitive to damage during aging than are others. Another part of the body with high sensitivity to oxygen debt is the myocardium, or heart muscle, which, like the brain, cannot regenerate after early development. As is well known, myocardial infarctions, or occlusions of the coronary arteries, produce irreversible damage to the heart muscles. With these examples in mind, it is clear that many of the phenomena of aging may not occur universally or to the same extent in all human beings. This is not to say that such pathological changes lack importance in the aging process, but it is necessary to keep in perspective the individualistic nature of their occurrence and impact.

The authors wish to acknowledge the patience of Diane Miller in preparing this chapter and the generous support of the National Institutes of Health (HD-07359, Training Grant #157 to the Andrus Gerontology Center) and the National Science Foundation (GB-35236). Contribution XIX from the Laboratory of Neurobiology.

EXAMPLES OF SELECTIVE AGE CHANGES

With this information as background, some current theories of aging now may be considered. Let us start with some considerations of phenomena generally observed in humans and other mammals during aging. It is well established, for example, that the ability of the body to resist stress of many different origins is reduced. For instance, older people have a much higher mortality rate during heat waves (Shattuck and Hilferty, 1932). Similar decreased resistance to exposure to cold in humans (Krag and Kountz, 1950) and in laboratory animals (Finch, Foster, and Mirsky, 1969) has been well documented. The ability to react rapidly to sounds and other external stimuli is lessened during aging (Corso, 1977). The ability to withstand fluctuations in the pH (acidity and alkalinity) of the blood is reduced (Shock and Yiengst, 1950). All these changes may be summarized as a declining homeostatic capacity during aging.

Why does the body lose its ability to react to stimuli and to buffer or absorb fluctuations? The answer probably may not be found in any single cause. There are many systems in the body which must function perfectly for homeostasis to be achieved. For example, the loss of ability to regulate temperature during extremes of heat or cold involves the "thermometers" in the central nervous system, which alter the flow of the blood, the action of the heart, and the capacity to produce heat or to shut off metabolic machinery making heat. The thyroid hormones are major stimulants of body metabolism and heat production. Circulating thyroid hormones decline in aged humans and rodents. Recent evidence indicates that the capacity of the rodent pituitary to respond to direct stimulation by thyrotropin-releasing hormone (TRH) is unaltered during aging (Chen and Walfish, 1978; Klug and Adelman, 1979). These data suggest that the inability of aged rodents to adapt to cold exposure is a failure of higher brain centers to stimulate hypothalamic TRH release. Another fascinating aspect of this research is the possibility that the aged pituitary secretes "false hormones." The pituitary of aged rats secretes a molecule that in some hormone assay systems registers a false-positive reading for thyroid-stimulating hormone (TSH). However, direct assays for biologic activity reveal that this molecule inhibits thyroid gland activity (Klug and Adelman, 1977). In old rats, TSH may thus have an *opposite* effect to its normal function. If other pituitary hormones have corresponding false hormones that act as inhibitors of function in aged humans and rodents, we may be required to alter our thoughts on hormonal control of body processes during aging.

Another example of selective changes in the homeostatic system is the adrenal cortex. This gland forms the steroids, such as cortisol and corticosterone, which are normally produced during responses to stress. The basal hormone output of the adrenal cortex is indeed less in older people; e.g., cortisol production is decreased by about 25 percent (Romanoff et al., 1958), whereas pregnanediol output is decreased by 75 percent (Romanoff, Thomas, and Baxter, 1970). However, these decreases do not determine the ability of the adrenal cortex to respond to the hormones which stimulate it. A number of studies have shown very clearly that injections of adrenocorticotropic hormone (ACTH), the pituitary hormone which acts upon the adrenal cortex, can stimulate a high production of adrenal steroids in both old and young (Romanoff et al., 1969). This implies that the cause of lower adrenal steroid production is lower pituitary ACTH output.

The same argument may be applied to many other functions in the body which show a decline; however, many systems appear to show normal competence with direct stimulation. Let us consider another example. Changes in heart function are for many people the major basis of their loss of activity during aging. Most of the changes of heart function during aging reflect arteriosclerosis. However, a number of major functions of the heart do not show impairment. In fact, ironically, one of those functions which is revealed during coronary artery disease is the ability of the heart to increase in size, or to hypertrophy, to compensate for damage to other regions of the heart. Experimental studies with mice (Florini, Saito, and Manowitz, 1973) have shown no limitations on the ability of the hearts of aging mice to hypertrophy. Because the heart consists of cells which do not divide during adult life-span, this hypertrophy results from an enlargement of the individual cells of the heart. Large amounts of new muscle protein must be laid down and assembled properly for a successful hypertrophy to occur. Here then is an interesting case of an organ which shows deficits in function during aging, especially when associated with disease, but which on the other hand does not show at some levels of cellular functions a serious impairment. Thus, it is of great importance in considering the aging process to realize that there are indeed many cells in the body whose functions do not change even under stressful conditions. It is important to account for these selective changes of aging in constructing any theories of aging.

There are, however, certain general changes of aging in cells and tissues. One of the best-documented general changes concerns the accumulation of aging pigments, lipofuscins. These are found in cells and increase more or less in proportion to the age of the individual (Strehler, 1977). The rate of accumulation of course varies from cell to cell. Lipofuscins may be found in the heart, in the liver, and in the ovary; their function and the meaning of this accumulation are completely unknown. Curiously, they are even found in the heart of the newborn human (Goldfischer and Bernstein, 1969). One of the long-standing theories of aging is the autointoxication (self-poisoning) theory; i.e., cells cannot rid themselves of their waste products which accumulate and thereby ultimately poison or autointoxicate their function. The gradual accumulation of aging pigments seems an apt illustration of this theory. Regardless of their age, neurons in the locus ceruleus of monkey brain contain less norepinephrine when lipofuscin is present in the cell (Sladek and Sladek, 1978). Although this study implies an impairment caused by lipofuscin, no measurements of actual cellular norepinephrine in lipofuscin-containing cells were taken. It is possible that this loss of norepinephrine in lipofuscin-containing cells represented a cellular component that is seldom used; therefore, normal function remained unaltered. Despite over 80 years of theorizing, no cellular dysfunction has been clearly demonstrated for the accumulation of the aging pigment in any cell type.

One very interesting point about aging pigments is that the rate of accumulation is adjusted in proportion to the life-span of the species. Dogs accumulate aging pigments about five times faster per year than do humans (Few and Getty, 1967), a rate which is increased in rough proportion to the shorter life-span of the dog. This suggests that there is some yet unknown control mechanism which adjusts the rate of aging to the life-span. At present, aging pigments represent the best example of a time-dependent change during aging. We emphasize that the functional consequences of accumulation of aging pigment are still unknown.

REPRODUCTIVE SENESCENCE

Most other phenomena that can be observed appear to be more or less dependent on endocrine or other physiological changes. The best and clearest example of endocrine-related changes is the change that takes place in the reproductive system of women during aging. Menopause is an inevitable event and occurs irreversibly by the age of 60 (Talbert, 1977). This age of cutoff of the reproductive functions stands in marked contrast to that of men who apparently do not have an upper age limit of fertility; paternity is possible for men even in their nineties (Seymour, Duffy, and Koerner, 1935). One of the most characteristic changes of aging in women after menopause is the tendency for the mucosa and epithelium of the vagina and uterus to atrophy (Lin et al., 1973; Talbert, 1977). This is undoubtedly the result of a major loss of estrogen and progestins which occurs after the ovary ceases its monthly cycle of hormonal production (Finch and Flurkey, 1977). However, the uterus of postmenopausal women and of aged rodents is still capable of responding to treatment with exogenous estrogens (Finch and Flurkey, 1977). This is consistent with observations, at least in rodents, that the estrogen receptor, the initial mediator of estrogen response in the cell, is unaltered with age in the uterus and vagina.

There are many consequences of the loss of estrogen, probably involving nearly every cell in the body which is sensitive. One may ask why the ovary loses its functions during aging. It is well known that during aging the ovary irreversibly loses its oocytes, or egg cells, which are necessary for fertility (Block, 1953; Talbert, 1977). Oocytes are necessary for the stimulation of hormone production in the follicles around them. However, oocytes are not completely depleted at the cessation of regular estrous cycles in rodents (Talbert, 1977). Also, postmenopausal women possess residual oocytes and primordial follicles (Costoff and Mahesh, 1975). This does not discount the possibility, however, that there exists a critical number of oocytes below which reproductive cycles cease.

Other factors also may be involved in cycling losses, such as the loss of cycles of hormones which stimulate the ovary. Ovariectomy in young rodents results in a dramatic increase in the plasma levels of pituitary gonadotropins. This rise results from the removal of the inhibitory influence of the ovary on gonadotropin secretion. Aged rodents do not respond to ovariectomy with nearly as great a rise in plasma gonadotropins (Meites et al., 1978). This suggests that a deficit may exist in the ability of the hypothalamus and pituitary to respond to feedback information from either the periphery or higher centers. In human females, the rise in plasma follicle-stimulating hormone (FSH) following menopause is less than that of premenopausal women who were ovariectomized to treat ovarian and uterine disorders (Chakravarti et al., 1977). Experiments in rats have shown that old ovaries may sometimes be transplanted to young rats and that the ovary of an old rat in a young host may be stimulated to new cycles (Ascheim, 1964; Peng and Huang, 1972). This also suggests that there are changes in the hormone system regulating the ovary (i.e., the pituitary and hypothalamus) as well as the changes within the ovary. Ultimately, the hormones which control the ovary are produced in the hormone-controlling centers of the brain, e.g., in the hypothalamus and preoptic region, which regulate a cyclic production of pituitary gonadotropins that, in turn, cyclicly stimulate the ovary. If we pursue the loss of functions in the ovary, we find that destruction of cells in these brain regions can mimic aging changes in female rats (Clemens and Bennett, 1977) and that certain drugs can reactivate the ovary in old rats (Quadri, Kledzik, and Meites, 1973). It is possible that changes in certain discrete regions of the brain may influence cellular activities throughout the entire body, thereby serving as pacemakers of aging (Finch, 1976).

There are other changes of hormones with age which ultimately may be traced to the brain. Among those are the regulation of ACTH, the regulation of the thyroid by TSH, the regulation of growth hormone (which influences carbohydrate metabolism and fat metabolism) (Andres and Tobin, 1977), and, finally, the regulation of the autonomic nervous system (Frolkis, 1977), since both the parasympathetic and sympathetic branches are controlled by centers in the brain. It is unknown now how many phenomena of aging may ultimately be traced to the brain, but there are numerous examples which indicate this possibility. The best is the example of reproductive aging in female mammals, providing an excellent illustration of changes in the brain which may influence other parts of the body. In turn, the loss of cells in the ovary that produce hormones (estrogens and progestins) shows that peripheral tissues can also influence functions in the central regulating machinery.

THEORIES OF AGING

What theories of aging can account for changes in the regulation of hormones? We have just mentioned the importance of their loss as being one contribution. But what about changes in the functions of nerve cells, ultimately the seats of hormone control? One change which may play a role is accumulation of aging pigment, although nothing is known about how aging pigment affects the functions of cells. Another often-mentioned change is the loss of nerve cells. This phenomenon may be one of those associated more with diseases of aging than with aging per se. There are reports claiming losses of brain cells during aging. However, many of the older observations do not include careful selection of material to eliminate specific diseases of aging (e.g., Parkinson's disease, Huntington's disease, and Alzheimer's type senile dementia) which can seriously distort the overall picture. Individuals suffering from these diseases show large losses of nerve cells from brain regions that are characteristic of each disease. Nonetheless, some brain regions show neuronal losses which cannot be ascribed to disease consequences (Brody, 1976). The age-related onset of neurological diseases also suggests that an aging component is involved in their etiology. For example, Alzheimer's type senile dementia, which is characterized clinically by cognitive alteration, shows a distinctive alteration in brain morphology. Microscopic examination of brains from individuals with Alzheimer's disease reveals a complex degeneration pattern of neuritic plaques, neurofibrillary tangles, and granulovacular degeneration. Each separate lesion ultimately results in a loss of cellular function; however, neuritic plaques and neurofibrillary tangles involve presynaptic elements, and granulovascular degeneration results from degeneration of postsynaptic cells. The frequency of these type lesions in nondemented individuals increases with age.

Although the data at the present are far from complete, it is very clear that not all regions of the brain show a major loss of neurons. For example, the inferior olivary nucleus, which processes auditory stimuli, does not show any loss of neurons at all in human beings (Monagle and Brody, 1974). On the other hand the precentral gyrus in the cerebral cortex, which is involved in the control of movement, does show substantial nerve cell loss in apparently healthy adults (Brody, 1973). Cell losses have also been reported in the putamen, another region linked to motor control (Bugiani et al., 1978). It still is unknown whether there is a loss of neurons in the parts of the brain which regulate hormones, but this is a question of great interest. If there are losses of neurons in these brain regions, then a simple explanation of losses of endocrine regulation could be derived. But if these regions of the brain do not show losses of neurons, then a far more complicated view of aging may be needed. In the latter case, it may require an analysis of how all the components of the body interact. It is possible that a type of "cascade" occurs during aging in which changes in one part of the body influence another distant part of the body, which in turn further alters the "clockwork" (Finch, 1976). The analogy with a clock may be very appropriate, because the whole system behaves as an interrelated set of wheels and gears without any one wheel or gear being the ultimate pacemaker for aging. In this sense, aging may be compared very reasonably to some of the earlier stages of development, in which at one time or another a given hormone or given cell type sets the stage for regulating the pace of development. However, all parts of the system may be essential, because if one were to remove the pituitary, puberty would not occur. On the other hand, puberty seems to be an interactive phenomenon which occurs at a particular height and body weight. Thus, the most fruitful point of view may be to consider aging as an extension of development in which one may trace chains of influences from one cell type to another.

CONCLUSION

The points of view articulated in the above analysis stand at loggerheads to a widespread point of view that aging is a degenerative and deteriorating process intrinsic to every cell. The latter theory is represented by the autointoxication theory or the belief that there are accumulations of errors or mutations in the chromosomes or DNA (Szilard, 1959; von Hahn and Fritz, 1966). The data for such changes are at the present time very limited. This is not to say that intrinsic cellular changes do not have a role, but their roles are incompletely shown. Ultimately it may prove possible to formulate a general theory of aging, but at this time, absence of data prohibits this. Our own best guesses are that there may be at certain stages of aging a dominance of the physiological mechanisms involving hormones and neuroendocrine-control mechanisms, whereas at much later ages the time-dependent changes represented by aging-pigment accumulation or mutation accumulation may dominate. It is simply not known how much either process contributes to functional changes at any age. On the practical side, it must be recognized that a large number of functions of cells remain proficiently intact so that under normal circumstances no deficit is obvious. This point is of great consequence to the design of treatment and therapy for older people, because it is clear that many of the prejudices which exist in the medical community about the uselessness of careful treatment of the elderly are poorly founded. A great deal of rehabilitation may be accomplished if it is recognized that many, if not most, components of the body have the capacity for normal function.

How many of our convalescent homes are crowded with people who are mistreated or inadequately treated because of the professional attitude that little can actually be done to improve their condition? For example, the opinion that brain cell loss universally occurs on a large scale is so firmly entrenched that it is extremely difficult to separate organic damage from the severe depression that often strikes older people as they become physically infirm and as they become separated from their friends in the world which they lived in before their "senescence." The effect of environmental deprivation on the functions of the mind and the emotional state is so well established that it is entirely possible to achieve much greater convalescence, rehabilitation, and reengagement of the individuals with society than is accomplished at present. The contributions that researchers can make to the area of aging thus may start at a very practical level, even though we cannot explain very fully what the aging process is at the present time.

REFERENCES

Andres, R., and J. Tobin: Endocrine systems, in C. E. Finch and L. Hayflick (eds.), *Handbook of the Biology of Aging,* Van Nostrand, New York, 1977, pp. 357– 378.

Ascheim, P.: Rèsultats fournis par la greffe hètèrochrone des ovarie dans l'ètude de la règulation hypothalamo-hypophyso-ovarienne de la ratte sènile, *Gerontologia,* 10:65– 75, 1964.

Block, E.: A quantitative morphological investigation of the follicular system in newborn female infants, *Acta Anatomica,* 17:201– 206, 1953.

Brody, H.: Aging of the vertebrate brain, in M. Rockstein (ed.), *Development and Aging in the Central Nervous System,* Academic, New York, 1973.

_____: An examination of cerebral cortex and brainstem aging, in R. D. Terry and S. Gershon (eds.), *Aging,* 3:177– 182, *Neurobiology of Aging,* Raven Press, New York, 1976.

Bugiani, O., et al.: Nerve cell loss in aging in the putamen, *European Neurology,* 17:286– 291, 1978.

Chakravarti, S., et al.: Endocrine changes and symptomatology after oophorectomy in premenopausal women, *British Journal of Obstetrics and Gynecology,* 84:769– 775, 1977.

Chen, H. J., and P. G. Walfish: Effects of age and ovarian function on the pituitary-thyroid systems in female rats, *Journal of Endocrinology,* 78:225– 232, 1978.

Clemens, J. A., and D. P. Bennett: Do aging changes in the preoptic area contribute to loss of cyclic endocrine function? *Journal of Gerontology,* 32:19– 24, 1977.

Corso, J. F.: Auditory perception and communication, in J. E. Birren and K. W. Schaie (eds.), *Handbook of the Psychology of Aging,* Van Nostrand Reinhold Co., New York, 1977, pp. 535– 553.

Costoff, A., and V. B. Mahesh: Primordial follicles with normal oocytes in the ovaries of postmenopausal women, *Journal of the American Geriatrics Society,* 23:193– 196, 1975.

Craik, F. I. M.: Age differences in human memory, in J. E. Birren and K. W. Schaie (eds.), *Handbook of the Psychology of Aging,* Van Nostrand Reinhold, New York, 1977, pp. 384– 420.

Davies, P.: Loss of choline acetyltransferase activity in normal aging and in senile dementia, in C. E. Finch, D. E. Potter, and A. D. Kenny (eds.), *Advances in Experimental Medicine and Biology,* vol. 113, *Parkinson's Disease—II, Aging and Neuroendocrine Relationships,* Plenum Press, New York, 1978, pp. 251– 256.

Drachman, D. A., and J. R. Hughes: Memory and the hippocampal complexes: III. Aging and temporal EEG abnormalities, *Neurology,* 21:1– 14, 1970.

Few, A., and R. Getty: Occurrence of lipofuscin as related to aging in the canine and porcine nervous system, *Journal of Gerontology,* 22:357– 367, 1967.

Finch, C. E.: The regulation of physiological changes during mammalian aging, *Quarterly Review of Biology,* 51:49– 83, 1976.

_____, J. R. Foster, and A. E. Mirsky: Aging and the regulation of cell activities during exposure to cold, *Journal of General Physiology,* 54:690– 712, 1969.

_____, and K. Flurkey: The molecular biology of estrogen replacement therapy, *Contemporary Obstetrics and Gynecology,* 9:97– 107, 1977.

Florini, J. R., Y. Saito, and E. J. Manowitz: Effect of age on thyroxin-induced cardiac hypertrophy in mice, *Journal of Gerontology,* 28:293– 297, 1973.

Frolkis, V. V.: Aging of the autonomic nervous system, in J. E. Birren and K. W. Schaie (eds.), *Handbook of the Psychology of Aging,* Van Nostrand Reinhold, New York, 1977, pp. 177– 189.

Goldfischer, S., and J. Bernstein: Lipofuscin (aging) pigment granules of the newborn human liver, *Journal of Cell Biology,* 42:253– 261, 1969.

Kinsey, A. C., W. B. Pomeroy, and C. E. Martin: *Sexual Behavior in the Human Male,* Saunders, Philadelphia, 1948.

Klug, T. L., and R. C. Adelman: Altered hypothalamic-pituitary regulation of thyrotropin in male rats during aging, *Endocrinology,* **104:**1136–1142, 1979.

———, and ———: Evidence for a large thyrotropin and its accumulation during aging in rats, *Biochemical and Biophysical Research Communications,* **77:**1431–1437, 1977.

Krag, C. L., and W. B. Kountz: Stability of body function in the aged: I. Effect of exposure of the body to cold, *Journal of Gerontology,* **5:**227–235, 1950.

Lin, T. J., et al.: Clinical and cytologic responses of postmenopausal women to estrogen, *Obstetrics and Gynecology,* **41:**97–107, 1973.

Masters, W. H., and V. Johnson: *Human Sexual Response,* Little, Brown, Boston, 1966.

Meites, J., H. H. Huang, and J. W. Simpkins: Recent studies on neuroendocrine control of reproductive senescence in rats, in E. L. Schneider (ed.), *The Aging Reproductive System,* vol. 4, Raven, New York, 1978, pp. 213–235.

Monagle, R. D., and H. Brody: The effects of age upon the main nucleus of the inferior olive in the human, *Journal of Comparative Neurology,* **155:**61–66, 1974.

Peng, M. T., and H. H. Huang: Aging of hypothalamic-pituitary-ovarian function in the rat, *Fertility and Sterility,* **23:**535–542, 1972.

Quadri, S. K., G. S. Kledzik, and J. Meites: Reinitiation of estrous cycles in old constant estrous rats by central acting drugs, *Neuroendocrinology,* **11:**248, 1973.

Romanoff, L. P., et al.: Effect of ACTH of the metabolism of pregnenolone 7-αH^3 and cortisol-r-C^{14} in young and elderly men, *Journal of Clinical Endocrinology and Metabolism,* **28:**819–830, 1969.

——— et al.: The urinary secretion of tetrahydrocortisol, 3α-allotetrahydrocortisol, and tetrahydrocortisone in young and elderly men and women, *Journal of Clinical Endocrinology and Metabolism,* **18:**1285–1293, 1958.

———, A. W. Thomas, and M. N. Baxter: Effect of age on pregnanediol excretion by men, *Journal of Gerontology,* **25:**98–101, 1970.

Seymour, F. I., C. Duffy, and A. Koerner: A case of authenticated fertility in a man of 94, *Journal of the American Medical Association,* **105:**1423–1424, 1935.

Shattuck, G. C., and M. M. Hilferty: Sunstroke and allied conditions in the United States, *American Journal of Tropical Medicine and Hygiene,* **12:**223, 1932.

Shock, N. W., and M. J. Yiengst: Age changes in the acid-base equilibrium of the blood of males, *Journal of Gerontology,* **5:**1–4, 1950.

Sladek, J. R., Jr., and C. D. Sladek: Relative quantitation of monoamine histofluorescence in young and old non-human primates, in C. E. Finch, D. E. Potter, and A. D. Kenny (eds.), *Advances in Experimental Medicine and Biology,* vol. 113, *Parkinson's Disease—II. Aging and Neuroendocrine Relationships,* Plenum, New York, 1978, pp. 231–239.

Strehler, B. L.: *Time, Cells, and Aging,* Academic Press, New York, 1977.

Szilard, L.: On the nature of the aging process, *Proceedings of the National Academy of Science (USA),* **45:**30–45, 1959.

Talbert, G.: Aging of the female reproductive system, in C. E. Finch and L. Hayflick (eds.), *Handbook of the Biology of Aging,* Van Nostrand, New York, 1977, pp. 318–358.

Von Hahn, H. P., and E. Fritz: Age-dependent alterations in the structure of DNA: III. Thermal stability of rat liver DNA, related to age, histone content and ionic strength, *Gerontologia,* **12:**237–250, 1966.

Wilkie, F., and C. Eisdorfer: Intelligence and blood pressure in the aged, *Science,* **172:**959–962, 1971.

HUMAN AGING CHANGES

Isadore Rossman

The sixth age shifts
Into the lean and slipper'd pantaloon
With spectacles on nose and pouch on side,
His youthful hose well sav'd a world too wide
For his shrunk shank . . .
William Shakespeare
As You Like It

LEARNING OBJECTIVES

- Describe the exterior physical changes attributable to the aging process.
- Describe the interior physical changes attributable to the aging process.
- Contrast Rossman's view of loss of neurons during aging with Finch's in the previous chapter.
- List at least five pathological events.
- Define at least five pathological events.

The human body is the most complex creation we have knowledge of. Its structure is a source of admiration because of its adaptability and infinite complexity, but it is also a source of despair because of its obvious defects, pathology, and retrogressive changes. The latter regularly occur with aging, and it is clear that when one talks about the human body, one must specify whose body and at what age. From infancy on to old age, all manner of aging changes take place. It is not only that the body ages obviously, but that a variety of cyclic aging changes on a lesser level are constantly occurring within. Thus blood cells go through approximate 120-day cycles, ending up with their dissolution and followed by scavenging, particularly of iron—an admirable example of recycling. The epithelial cells lining the intestine and the skin go through a similar cycle, eventually to die and be cast off. These irreversible cellular cycles of birth, maturation, and death go on within a major organism that is recognizably the same year in and year out, but which, too, is going through a slow aging evolvement which is as surely irreversible. Aging changes of the body as a whole are a matter of everyday observation, and have been for many thousands of years. Thus the classic riddle of the Sphinx was based on the fact that man creeps on all fours in infancy, and walks with the aid of a cane in old age. This altered mobility reflects an altered anatomy, and all who are seriously concerned with the human body, therapeutically or otherwise, must necessarily concern themselves with its aging changes.

But what are true aging changes? We tend to judge the age of our patients at a glance by such grossly visible ectodermal changes as wrinkling or graying of hair. But there are some who show little wrinkling or little graying, yet are surely aging by a number of other more discerning criteria. Indeed, it has been established that much wrinkling of the skin is pathological, especially when it reflects solar exposure to which we subject ourselves variably. Thus, to understand a common aging change such as wrinkling, one would have to discriminate between two variables: (1) an intrinsic and perhaps unmodifiable one, and (2) exposure to elements specific to that individual's life history. The concept that internally generated events can interact with factors from outside is crucial

to a clear understanding of aging. An example would be sclerotic phenomena in arteries. Once regarded as inevitable aging changes, these changes are now recognized as predominantly due to a number of such external factors as diets and even such seemingly remote factors as cigarette smoking. Even if a very large majority of us develop atherosclerosis, it is by no means clear that this is an inevitable or true aging change. It may be more accurate to regard it as a process which occurs with the passage of time in many human beings in a particular society, but is distinct from aging.

Another example, still more subtle, is the demineralization of bone that occurs with aging. This leads to a rarefaction, generally referred to as osteoporosis. Some degree of osteoporosis seems to be inevitable with aging, but it is clinically more severe in women than in men and in whites as compared with blacks. An "idiopathic" form, which may be marked, is sometimes seen in the middle years. Everything else being equal, its advent is hastened by a low calcium diet, by inactivity, and by early menopause, surgical or otherwise. Here again one must discriminate an interaction between the external and the internal. Furthermore, excessive secretions from such varied glands as the thyroid, the parathyroid, and the adrenal alone may produce or aggravate osteoporosis. Similarly, hypofunction of the thyroid may intensify atherosclerosis.

As these examples indicate, aging changes are often due to a complex of interacting forces, and in some sites, it may be difficult to be sure what are intrinsic and inevitable changes and what are changes imposed on the tissue by common or uncommon external forces. When common, these external forces might be designated as time-related pathological events, which are variable from person to person and perhaps basically controllable in their manifestations. To the extent that this is the case, some aging changes offer more hope for control or reversibility than had been thought to be the case until recent years. It is quite possible, therefore, that some aliquot of such changes as wrinkling, hardening of arteries, loss of bone substance, perhaps even cataract formation, may turn out to be far less certain aging changes than we have been led to suppose; however, in this present chapter, we will consider all these varied aging changes without further consideration of a theoretical basis for controllability.

LOSS IN HEIGHT

A majority of older people are short, and many aged women are well under 5 feet. We are often surprised, after taking care of bedridden patients who later become ambulatory, to observe how short they are when they get up and about. This short stature is due not only to a shrinkage associated with aging but also to the fact that many older patients were short to start with. It seems reasonably established that the stature of many Americans has increased by about 2 inches during the course of the twentieth century. Anthropologists refer to this as a secular increase in height, which might be looked upon as a fuller achievement of one's genetic potential, primarily attributable to better nutrition.

A number of studies indicate that distinct losses in height occur during later life. By ages 50 to 55, a decrease perhaps on the order of $\frac{1}{2}$ to $\frac{3}{4}$ inch occurs which is ascribable to a shrinkage in the fibroelastic disks between the vertebrae. Subsequently, major losses in height occur because of osteoporosis. In osteoporosis, there is a loss of matrix, both of protein and deposited calcium, from bones and especially vertebrae. This produces a reduction of height caused by shortening of the spine. Loss of height is further accentuated by a bowing in the vertebral column, most marked in the thoracic region. The degree of thoracic curvature varies, but in older women marked kyphosis is unfortunately quite common. Some decalcification can be demonstrated in the skull and the bones of the extremities also, but this does not contribute to loss in height. As a result of this differential, elderly people seem to have unduly long extremities. In fact, the fingertip-to-fingertip span does not change appreciably as a result of osteoporosis. Since height roughly equals span at full growth, the span of elderly individuals continues to give evidence of their height at maturity, even when they are bowed and short. Heights 2 to 4 inches less than spans are not unusual in many elderly women. More complicated methods, used by physical anthropologists, are based upon such measurements as tibial height, which also bears a fixed relationship to height at maturity. A few series of longitudinal measurements, span determinations, estimations of degrees of bowing due to osteoporosis, and measurements on collections of human skeletons going back more than a century all confirm the fact that the major loss in height with aging is due to a progressive decrement in length of the vertebral column, particularly in the thoracic portion.

CHANGES IN SKIN AND SUBCUTANEOUS TISSUE

Among the major changes in the skin with aging are thinning of the epithelial and subcutaneous fatty layers. There are multiple factors that determine the amount of fat in the subcutaneous tissue, including a genetic potential inherited as type of body build, and states of nutrition—specifically, obesity and undernutrition. However these individual variations tend to mask the process, one can observe a trend which consists of a loss of fatty tissue, particularly from the periphery. In older individuals, this progresses to a point where little subcutaneous fat is seen over the legs or the forearms. This may be the case even in the presence of abundant abdominal and hip fat. Skin-fold measurements indicate that diminution of subcutaneous fat in the region of the upper tibia regularly occurs by age 45 and thereafter. This loss in the lower extremities is sometimes masked by other processes, such as edema, and by the fact that, in some persons in the middle years, fat may be deposited around the ankle joints. In the upper extremities, fatty tissue loss contributes to the characteristic hands of old age, with their prominent tendons, veins, and knuckles. As with other atrophic processes associated with aging, probably the more one starts with, the less frank is the loss, despite the impact of aging. But even with initially obese individuals, aging produces a quite general loss of fat from the subcutaneous tissue. This makes for prominence of bony markings, such as the thoracic cage, scapulas, trochanters, and knees, and loss of this valuable padding predisposes to bedsores. One also observes a deepening of hollows, such as those in the supraclavicular and axillary regions, and increased boniness of the face. With disappearance of covering fat, muscle markings may become more prominent so that origins and insertions of muscle, such as the deltoid, are plain to see.

Other constituents of the skin also undergo regression, including the collagen and elastic fibers, and the epithelial layer also shrinks in thickness. Sweat gland counts indicate that these, too, diminish in number. The net effect is to leave the skin of the elderly in a thin, dry, and inelastic state. Picked up between the fingers, it tends to remain there and only slowly flattens down, in contrast to the springiness found in youthful skin. Loss of sweat glands makes for an important change in regulation of body temperature. Since elderly people cannot sweat freely, they are more subject to heat exhaustion. They are also more likely to complain of dryness and itchiness of the skin, especially in wintertime. But perhaps more than anything else, they complain bitterly of cold. Sensitivity to cold is due to loss of insulating fat and to the diminished peripheral circulation which accompanies regressive changes in any organ. Among the cellular losses are the melanocytes which contribute pigmentation. Thus, the skin of the typical Caucasian tends to become whiter with age, and sometimes the pallor incorrectly makes one think of anemia. This is further accentuated by the loss of ruddiness, that component of skin hue due to the smaller blood vessels. Graying of the hair, also a failure of pigment cells, is doubtless the best known of aging changes.

In general, old people tend to become hairless. Not only is there a more or less marked thinning out of scalp hair, but also a loss in such hairy areas as the pubis and axilla. Older women find they no longer need to shave their armpits. Particularly over the extremities, hair loss may be quite complete. Oddly, along with this undesired loss from such areas as the scalp, there may be a growth of hairs on the face. This is more noteworthy in elderly women and is thought to be due to changes in the androgen/estrogen ratio. Facial hairs are often bristly and may be sufficiently numerous and disturbing as to require shaving or depilation.

Wrinkles are permanent infoldings of the epithelium and the subepithelial tissue, more or less linear or curvilinear in shape. They are most marked on the face and are due in part to repeated stresses on the skin produced by the activity of the muscles of expression. As we frown, laugh, wrinkle our foreheads, or grimace, the skin is pulled in characteristic and repetitive ways which lead to permanent changes. Other processes are superimposed on the effect of muscle action, especially loss of elasticity plus the pulls of gravity. Thus with aging, the skin undergoes sagging. One specific place to observe this is the earlobe, which is not correctible by plastic surgery, the "face lift." By the fifties, the lobes of the ears have become fuller and more dependent, resulting in an elongation of the ear. This may be associated with an oblique wrinkle of the lobe or a number of crumpled-looking wrinkles. The elongation of the lobe is subject to variable progression; but in some older persons, the earlobes dangle like pendants.

In addition to wrinkles produced by use, they also result from atrophic changes in the subcutaneous tissue. On the face this may lead to a myriad of fine wrinkles, sometimes paralleling each other or sometimes intersecting in a crisscross fashion. Exposure to the sun is the single most important factor in producing wrinkles or hastening their advent. Thus, wrinkling is more severe in those exposed to the elements and has become more common in women since the parasol was discarded in favor of sun bathing. Protection of the skin from sun is conferred by pigmentation, and its value is to be seen in the black and yellow races in whom wrinkling appears to be less marked and occurs later in life.

The neck is perhaps an even more reliable area in which to observe aging changes. Most of the wrinkling here is produced by the platysma muscle and tends to become quite obvious by the fifties. It sometimes presents as two curvilinear parallel lines ("railroad tracks"), extending from the clavicles up toward the chin, also as finer transverse wrinklings, a crumpled paperlike appearance, or various combinations thereof. Other common sites for wrinkling due to age are the curvilinear parallel wrinkles above each eyebrow, produced by the action of the occipitofrontalis (epicranius) muscle, and the multiple wrinkles radiating outwards from the lips, reminiscent of the wrinkling produced when a purse string is pulled closed. These are due to the action of the orbicularis oris muscle which contracts the opening of the mouth.

OCULAR CHANGES

A number of changes in the eyes are regularly encountered, but are variable in onset. Thus some individuals develop cataracts in their fifties, others not until several decades later. An early cataract is detectable only by an ophthalmoscope or other special instrument. The more advanced cataracts of clinical interest, however, are readily seen by shining a light into the pupil of the eye, whereupon one observes a grayish or whitish opacity of variable density. Another quite common change is the deposition of a whitish material on the periphery of the cornea. The deposit may first appear as a dotlike or slightly curved infiltrate and has been observed as early as the twenties and thirties. As the infiltrate progresses, it tends to completely encircle the cornea, becomes thickened, and even slightly elevated. This whitish arc or circle consists of a fatty material and is called the *arcus senilis*. Since it may sometimes be found in individuals in their twenties and thirties, this is a bit of a misnomer. It also may be seen relatively early in life in individuals with elevated blood cholesterol, but bears no constant relation to the level of the blood fats. Despite some assertions to the contrary, there is no clearcut relationship of arcus senilis to coronary artery disease or to the extent of atherosclerosis.

A further common change associated with aging is in the pupil of the eye, which becomes smaller, sometimes strikingly so, and occasionally irregular. It is ascribed to long-standing effects of parasympathetic tone, and as such is to be contrasted to the large pupils seen in youthful eyes. A drooping of the lids, a change comparable to the elongation of the earlobes and the formation of jowls, is often seen. Occasionally the drooping upper lid comes down so far over the cornea as to interfere with vision. The lid may evert (ectropion) or less commonly become inverted (entropion), changes that are associated with chronic infections of the lids and with scarring. The lacrimal glands, like the salivary glands to which they are related, exhibit involution or loss of function with aging, contributing to dryness and a loss of luster of the eyes.

DENTAL CHANGES

One occasionally sees individuals in their seventies with the 32 teeth nature gave them. Most often one sees the teeth the dentist gave them. Unlike the tooth loss of earlier years which is due to caries, tooth loss in the middle and later years results from inflammatory bone resorption around the teeth and what is known as the "bone factor," essentially a degree of osteoporosis. The teeth that remain are likely to exhibit some flattening of their surfaces because of use. Resorption of gum tissue around the base of the tooth exposes more of it, hence the expression "long in the tooth." Removal of the teeth tends to aggravate the process of osteoporosis, hence the desirability of dental procedures which are conservative and maintain the teeth in the jaw as long as possible. When the edentulous state has been of long standing, resorption of bone of the mandible and maxilla leads to a shortening of the distance between chin and nose and a pulling inward of the lips. In the tongue, a major change with aging is a progressive decrease in taste buds. This may be the basis for the frequent complaint that food has lost its taste.

Taking the pulse of old individuals gives us some insight as to what happens to the arterial system generally in aging. The artery is felt more readily, not alone because of loss of supporting tissue, but because of increased stiffness of its wall. One may also note increased tortuosity of the radial artery, and in some patients, hardness to a degree which bespeaks calcification, the so-called pipestem radial. In thin individuals, one may observe the same changes in the brachial artery further up the arm. These represent the aging changes referred to as *arteriosclerosis*. This is more accurately divided into a combination of atherosclerosis, deposit of fatty materials in the intima of the artery, and a calcification of the middle coat of the vessel, known also as *Mönckeberg sclerosis*. Medial calcification does not interfere with the blood flow through arteries in the obstructive sense that atherosclerotic deposition does. Elongation and increased tortuosity of arteries with stiffening of their walls tend to go on throughout the body with aging. Since arteries tend to be fixed at their points of origin, elongation generally leads to tortuosity or kinking. This is often observed on plain x-ray films of the chest where widening of the aortic shadow and deposits of calcium are frequently seen by middle age. The whole process is abetted by hypertension. A further change occurs in osteoporotic elderly women whose thoracic spines have partially collapsed; the aorta and its arch will be brought up closer into the neck. In fact, one can often palpate the innominate artery under these circumstances by inserting one's finger behind the supraclavicular notch.

CHANGES BENEATH THE SKIN

It is clear from a glance at elderly persons that what one sees going on in the integument are regressive and atrophic changes. The question one may then raise is whether similar changes may not be going on in other parts of the body, in deeper structures such as muscles, viscera, brain, and the like. Both brain and skin are formed from the same germ layer and in fact regression, manifested by shrinkage and loss of cells, occurs also in the brain with aging. It has long been known that the brains of older people are generally lighter than the brains of younger people, a process which may be associated with flattening of the gyri and sulci and an increase in the size of the ventricles. Cellular loss in the brain is thought to occur by the thirties and to continue in a steady fashion thereafter. It has been estimated that 50,000 to 100,000 brain cells are lost every day, starting in the mid-twenties. Despite this relatively large cellular loss, there is a huge number of functioning cells in the human brain. Many cells seem to have no identifiable function and perhaps are to be regarded as a contingency reserve. Significant loss of neurons

seems to go on for decades without gross interference with functioning.

It is also a matter of everyday observation that the muscles of older people, even those who work hard, become smaller and stringier with age. Gross weighing of muscles indicates that this phenomenon is quite marked by the sixth decade and progresses thereafter. Under the microscope there is shrinkage of individual cells, infiltration with connective tissue and fatty cells, and other evidences of regression. As has been noted above, the bones become lighter through a loss of calcified matrix and the trabeculae shrink in size so that the bones become porous in gross appearance. Thus, if one weighs such organs as the liver, the pancreas, and the kidneys, these, too, are found to weigh less in old age than in youth or the middle years. Figure 3-1 illustrates this for a number of organs.

A new way of quantifying these aging changes, and detecting them earlier than would otherwise be the case, has been made possible by the use of isotope counting. The technique is based upon the fact that potassium is almost exclusively an intracellular element within the body. The largest such potassium-containing tissue is muscle. Potassium is also the chief ion found within all the other differentiated cells, whether they be neurons, heart cells, or cells of the thyroid or any other organ. All these tissues contain a naturally occurring radioisotope of potassium (^{40}K) which is a gamma emitter. Thus the body is weakly radioactive. It is possible to quantitate the radioactivity by placing people inside large cylinders and arranging counting devices in such a manner as to record the radiations (counts) emanating from within the enclosure. This technique is known as *total body counting*. Since fat cells contain very little cytoplasm, the fat cell in essence being a large globule of fat, marked changes in body weight representing ups and downs in fat content do not significantly change the radioactive counts. Hence, the counts can be used as an index to what has been termed the *lean body mass* (LBM) which can be defined as the functioning mass of the body, including organs, heart, muscles and tendons, brain and nervous system, etc. The LBM as demonstrated by counting techniques steadily diminishes with age, starting in the thirties,

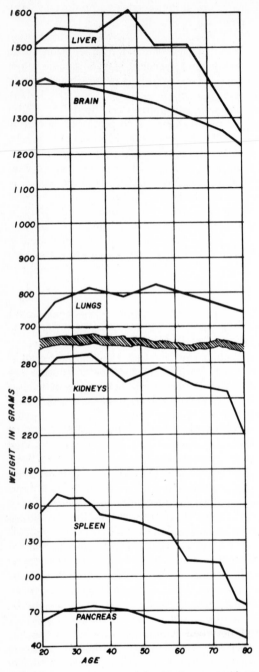

WEIGHT IN GRAMS

FIGURE 3-1 Decrease in weight of body organs with aging. With few exceptions—the prostate and occasionally the heart in hypertension—all organs shrink with age. [Based on data of R. Rössle and F. Roulet, 1932, in I. Rossman (ed.), Clinical Geriatrics, J. B. Lippincott, Philadelphia, 1979.]

and this becomes increasingly more marked past the age of 50. In short, whether one uses naked-eye observation, gross anatomic methods, such as weighing muscles and organs, or sophisticated techniques, such as the whole body counter, it is clear that with aging there is a loss of functioning tissue from all vital organs and that this is a uniform and predictable event. See Figure 3-2.

To be sure, there are a few exceptions which perhaps prove the rule. Some of these are well known and are clearly pathological rather than normal. The prostate, for example, is notorious for enlargement in the later years, and this often produces urinary obstruction. It is generally agreed that prostatic hypertrophy is to be regarded as a form of benign tumor to which not all men are subject.

Similarly the heart sometimes enlarges with aging, generally in association with hypertension of some degree or with other processes associated with heart failure. In old age not complicated with cardiovascular disease, the heart is often strikingly smaller than normal, and its cells are filled with a brownish "old age" pigment, the lipofuscin granules. In these older individuals free of hypertension, the myocardium has clearly undergone atrophy, also. Similarly the lungs may or may not undergo shrinkage with aging, depending upon whether variable degrees of emphysema are present.

There is as yet no explanation for the loss of cells and resultant shrinkage of tissues that mark the aging process. Among the explanatory theories that have been entertained are the chance occurrence of damaging events within cells with the passage of time, the using up of some nonreproducible material, errors in the DNA-RNA synthesis system. There have even been speculations that the whole process is programmed in view of its universality in the biological kingdom. It has been shown that cells explanted into tissue culture have a predictable number of cell divisions before they die, with the number of multiplications characteristic of each species and roughly correlated with the life of the species (e.g., mouse 18, human 55). Exceptions to this have occurred only when the cultured cells spontaneously undergo a neoplastic transformation, in which they develop an unlimited proliferative capacity.

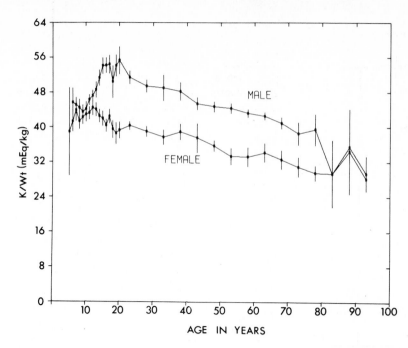

FIGURE 3-2 Decline in body potassium with aging as determined by whole body counting. [*Courtesy of R. N. Pierson, Jr., D. H. Y. Lind, and R. A. Phillips, American Journal of Physiology, 226(1):206–212, 1974.*]

OSTEOPOROSIS

An interesting aspect of bony tissue is the balance in bone resorption and bone formation due to the constant activity of osteoclasts and osteoblasts. The immediacy of the potential for change is illustrated by the prompt loss of bone that occurs in the patient put to bed or in a limb immobilized in a cast. In the latter decades there is a shift in the balance toward resorption in apparently healthy ambulatory persons. When sufficiently marked, this produces brittleness of bone, with increased tendency to fracture, referred to as *senile osteoporosis.* In women the disturbed balance seems to come on promptly after the menopause and has been related to estrogen deprivation. It is, therefore, often called *postmenopausal osteoporosis.* Its earlier onset in females accounts for "dowager's hump," which can progress to a frank, often severe, curvature of the spine. Osteoporosis of the femur is the background to the common and serious group of fractures in women. To some extent osteoporosis may be regarded as a tissue loss comparable with declines in the cellular content of other tissues in the body. However,

osteoporosis can be favorably affected, with slowing of its rate of progression, by high calcium intake plus vitamin D administration, and perhaps also with fluoride and hormonal administration.

What with loss of calcium and bone, shrinkage of muscle and organ tissue, frequently with declines in total weight, the gross composition of the body in old age is markedly different from that in youth. This is illustrated by Figure 3-3. Among other changes one notes the decline in specific gravity of the human body with aging. Since the only body tissue lighter than water is fat, one may infer that the amount of fat relative to lean body tissue has risen. At first this seems to be in contradiction to the seeming loss of fat that one observes in the extremities and elsewhere in aged individuals. The explanation for the paradox is that fat has increasingly accumulated between muscle fibers and within and around the viscera, while the lean body mass has shrunk. This results in a rising percentage of fat into old age. Fat is a primitive tissue as compared with specialized tissues such as muscles or organs, and in this sense the process may be regarded as a substitution of primitive cells for sophisticated cells.

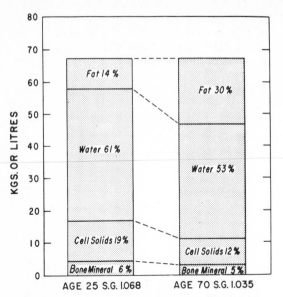

FIGURE 3-3 Changes in body composition with aging. A 25-year-old male with a body specific gravity of 1.068 is compared with a 70-year-old male whose specific gravity has decreased to 1.035. Both men have the same body weight. [*Reprinted with permission from J. H. Fryer in N. W. Shock (ed.), Biological Aspects of Aging, Columbia University, New York, 1962.*]

DECREMENT IN FUNCTION WITH AGING

Since aging leads to a decrease in the size and weight of most organs and other body constituents, it is not unexpected that a decrease in functional capacity also occurs. Thus, a decrease in grip strength past age 50 is an invariable aging change. It progresses steadily in successive decades and thus parallels the shrinking muscle mass. In some organs the loss of function greatly exceeds what one would anticipate on purely anatomic grounds. In the kidneys, the filtration through the glomeruli decreases 46 percent and the renal blood flow 53 percent from age 20 to age 90. The cardiac output decreases 30 to 40 percent from the third to the seventh decade. This decreased output, in association with changes in the lungs themselves, leads to a reduction in oxygen consumption under stress by about 50 percent. The cardiorespiratory changes that have occurred by the time old age is reached may not be obvious with the subject at rest or under little stress, but are quickly ap-

parent when dyspnea and other symptoms are produced by light work or stress testing on the treadmill. Similarly, although the excretory capacity of the kidneys is adequate to meet ordinary needs, it, too, may be unable to handle an increased workload such as may be presented by sudden water or salt loading. The digestive system, in contrast, tolerates aging changes better than do other organ systems. Hydrochloric acid production by the stomach diminishes in many older people; past age 60, more than one-quarter of all subjects tested with histamine fail to secrete free hydrochloric acid. However, because of protein-digesting backup systems furnished by the pancreas and the intestine itself, there is no significant impairment. The effects of aging on the various organ systems are discussed in detail in Chapters 18 to 22.

TIME-RELATED PATHOLOGICAL EVENTS

As we have seen, aging involves an atrophy or regression in many specialized tissues of the body. On the other hand, hardening of arteries, once considered to be a concomitant of aging, is now more accurately regarded as a pathological phenomenon in which fatty materials are deposited within the arterial wall. This varies considerably from person to person and is known to be affected by such factors as diet, hypertension, inborn metabolic errors such as familial hypercholesterolemia, and sex (male is "bad," female "good"). One should, therefore, regard arterial hardening as a common pathological event which shows a variable increase with the passage of the decades, but is not a true aging change since it lacks universality. Changes of this kind have been termed *time-related pathological events.* A number of others seem to fall into the same category.

Osteoarthritis Osteoarthritis is a variable but seldom-escaped phenomenon in which the bone around a joint undergoes changes, generally of a proliferative type. In the spine the bony growths are called *osteophytes,* as an example, and produce lipping at the intervertebral surface. In advanced stages, there is bridging between the vertebrae, which limits motion considerably. The phenomenon is sufficiently regularly encountered after age 40 so that one can make an estimate of the age of an individual simply by looking at x-rays of the spine. The most positive correlations are to be found in the cervical spine, particularly in its lowermost portion. A common, easily visible form of osteoarthritis occurs in the distal finger joints where the thickening is termed *Heberden's nodes.* It is more common in women, has a hereditary aspect, and generally appears in the forties. In more advanced cases involving the proximal joints, *Bouchard's nodes* are seen. Osteoarthritis of the hips is clinically perhaps the most significant form of osteoarthritis, as it may produce pain and a limitation of motion requiring surgical intervention. Similar events may occur in the knee joint, and in both regions, the burden of obesity is considered an aggravating factor.

Dupuytren's Contracture A nodular thickening of the palmar fascia is seen in 10 percent or more of the aging population. The nodules appear as firm, discrete thickenings in the palm and are composed of fibrous tissue in association with which the lateral fingers may be pulled toward the palm. Full extension of the involved fingers becomes increasingly difficult or impossible. The contraction is more common in diabetic than nondiabetic persons and, like Heberden's nodes, has no relationship to use or trauma.

Hearing Loss Degenerative changes in the cochlea regularly lead to diminution in hearing in aging individuals. It has been said that these changes do not occur in parts of the world where there is relatively little noise. Conversely, hearing loss is well known to be aggravated by acoustic trauma, whether over a short- or long-term period.

Elasticity of the Lens Loss of elasticity of the lens accounts for the fact that most people need the help of reading glasses by about age 40. In contrast, children are able to focus on a line of print whether it is only a few inches away or at a more conventional distance. This loss of elasticity of the lens has been shown to occur early in life, probably in the teens, and its slow progression is the major reason that most of us need increasingly stronger lenses for reading with the passage of the decades.

Other Skin Changes Although the essential aging change in the skin is shrinkage or atrophy, there may be a concomitant superimposition of a number of growths and other changes. So-called senile telangiectasias are tiny, scarlet growths scattered over the skin, which seem to increase slowly in number over the middle years. Deposits of pigmentation (melanotic freckles, lentigines) are also to be seen, although the skin overall may be getting paler. In addition, seborrheic hyperkeratoses, brown to blackish plaquelike growths about the size of a dime, appear increasingly past age 50. They may be multiple and considered disfiguring, but they are generally harmless. Not to go unmentioned are a number of cancers of the skin, most commonly seen on exposed surfaces, of which basal-cell carcinoma is perhaps the most common. For these growths an almost linear relationship to solar exposure can be demonstrated. Very often on histological section, it can be demonstrated that the neoplasm has developed in an area of obviously atrophic epithelium.

The relationship between aging and disease has given aging a worse name than it deserves. Also, in a society in which our older citizens generally come to a bad end, speaking psychiatrically, socially, and fiscally, it would be predictable that aging would be associated with highly negative attitudes. These attitudes have increased our fears about aging by increasing our anxiety over the appearance of the first wrinkle or gray hairs. It also is disruptive to interpersonal relationships by tending to cloud our feelings even toward our own parents and grandparents. It is true that aging is essentially a regression affecting the structure, size, and functioning of most of our organs, but many of them are usually compensated for by the use of devices as elementary as eyeglasses or power steering. Although no one can be happy over the alleged daily loss of neurons, judgment, wisdom, and capacity to add to one's accumulated facts and information can go right on. Behind the trappings of the gray hair and the wrinkling, there is such an entity as healthy old age, and with reasonable luck most of us will attain it. All of us must make our peace with aging processes, and the first step is to know what they are and to accept them. Spinoza put it succinctly: "Freedom is the recognition of necessity."

REFERENCES

Annals of the New York Academy of Sciences (entire volume devoted to body composition and aging changes), vol. 110, 1963.

Bourliere, F.: *The Assessment of Biological Age in Man,* Public Health Papers No. 37, World Health Organization, Geneva, 1970, p. 67.

Moore, F. D.: *The Body Cell Mass and its Supporting Environment,* Saunders, Philadelphia, 1963, p. 535.

Rossman, Isadore: Anatomic and body composition changes with aging, in *Handbook of Biology of Aging,* Van Nostrand Reinhold, New York, 1977, pp. 189–216.

————: The anatomy of aging, in Isadore Rossman (ed.), *Clinical Geriatrics,* (2d ed.) Lippincott, Philadelphia, 1979.

OTHER RESOURCES

The Osteoporosis of Aging, Richard W. Smith, M.D., and Harold M. Frost, M.D., Henry Ford Hospital, Detroit, Michigan, 16 mm, color (animation), and sound; running time 20 minutes. This animated film employs current teaching techniques to identify the osteoporotic process. Its nature is defined, its course determined, and the latest treatment presented. A review of normal bone development is presented in order to explain the nature of skeletal wasting. The remodeling process of bone and its regulators are discussed with regard to their role in the development of osteoporosis.

FOUR

COGNITIVE PROCESSES IN AGING

Kathy Gribbin

Thou shalt neither abuse nor neglect old age, rather shalt thou pray to attain it, for age is a blessing wherein the gates of wisdom open.
Morton Leeds
"Decalogue of the Elder," in *The Gerontologist's Notebook*, **1971**

LEARNING OBJECTIVES

- List five processes involved in dealing with information on the cognitive level.
- Discuss at least six factors relevant to learning and memory and elaborate on their importance.
- Describe the difference between fluid and crystal intelligence.
- Describe the research methodologies used to study developmental change.

Today there are over 20 million persons over the age of 65 in the United States. Although most older people have at least one chronic condition, this does not severely hamper their functioning in everyday life. In fact, less than 5 percent of all people over 65 live in institutions. An even better indicator of health impairment is short-term hospitalization. In the year from July 1965 to June 1966, 87 percent of the aged in the United States had no hospital episodes, which differs very little from the 90 percent figure of the total population.

Nurses tend to see only the sick older people, making an easy generalization to "all old people are sick." As can be seen above, this is not necessarily the case. In order to judge more accurately the implications of illness on behavior, one should have a general idea of how the individual functions in good health. That is the intent of this chapter—to present the cognitive functioning of the normal older person. The plan of the chapter is to begin with a discussion of methodology. Some methodological problems are unique to the study of aging; therefore, a basic understanding of the procedures used to develop knowledge in this area is extremely important. Next will be a discussion of intelligence. A great deal of effort has been devoted to research in this area and the findings have been fruitful. Long-held beliefs, which have been shown to be inaccurate, will be discussed as will the usefulness of studying intelligence to predict longevity. This will be followed by a discussion of rigidity and cautiousness, which are often felt to increase with age, and then by learning and memory. In conclusion, some implications for nursing will be put forth.

METHODOLOGY

The most common approach for studying age differences is the *cross-sectional method*. This procedure compares the performance of people who are of different ages at the time the research is conducted. For the researcher who is interested in what happens to the same individual over time, however, this method is unsuitable because there is no assurance that the young people being tested are similar to the older people who were tested when they were young. Consequently, the cross-sectional method measures only age differences in performance.

In order to observe the changes that occur with age, one must employ the *longitudinal method*. This approach studies the same persons over a period of time, and, thus, the changes individuals undergo as they age can be observed. Even this method has its drawbacks, however, because it presumes that young people today will experience the same sociocultural environment as did the older people and, therefore, will age in much the same manner. We know our environment has rapidly changed over the past years; e.g., the advent of television has drastically changed the environment of today's children as opposed to that of their grandparents when they were children. Since such environmental differences may affect the development of the individual, we must also tease out the influence of the environment which may contribute to differences among the various generations. In combination with the other two methods, the approach which does this is the *time-lag method* (Schaie and Gribbin, 1975).

In summary, we want to know not only how individuals change as they age, but also how generations differ in these changes. When we have an idea of what factors are important in influencing these changes, we will be in a better position to suggest intervention techniques for the maintenance of behavior in old age.

COGNITIVE PROCESSES

When we discuss cognitive processes, we are concerned with how one deals with information. Intelligence is a very important factor, but many other processes are involved. Some of these processes include (1) how information is interpreted, (2) how it is stored and retrieved from memory, (3) how it is evaluated, (4) how hypotheses are generated, and (5) how one reasons. *Although popular opinion generally presumes that cognitive processes decline with age, research evidence indicates that this is not necessarily the case.*

INTELLIGENCE

Tests of intelligence have recently been attacked because what they measure is not always relevant to the purpose for which the test is being used. Minority groups question the use of traditional IQ tests because they are designed to measure the skills of the white middle class and not necessarily to measure intrinsic ability. An analogous argument may be made for older people in that IQ tests involve items more relevant to children or young adults. When intelligence tests comprise items more related to the needs of adults, scores tend to rise through the middle and later years, even though the scores of the same people may decline on conventional tests (Demming and Pressey, 1957). However, such findings may also be the result of only one type of intelligence being measured—that which makes use of previous knowledge and experiences.

TYPES OF INTELLIGENCE

There are actually several types of intelligence. With advancing age, these "intelligences" vary in different ways and to different extents. One way of looking at the dimensions of intelligence is to distinguish between *fluid* and *crystallized* intelligence. Fluid intelligence depends upon species-specific, and probably biologically mediated, functions. Crystallized intelligence, on the other hand, is assumed to be a function of experience and is, therefore, reflective of individual differences in experiential processes which occur as a result of acculturation.

As one ages, fluid and crystallized abilities change in different ways. Fluid intelligence shows a steady decline from the teens on, while crystallized intelligence seems to increase through adulthood and shows a slight decline only in old age. Looking at intelligence as composed of fluid and crystallized abilities is a relatively recent approach. Although the evidence for these differential age trends is not conclusive, support for this approach is growing (Schaie and Gribbin, 1975).

More traditional approaches to studying intelligence and aging are not quite so complex. A number of abilities, such as vocabulary, word fluency, space, number, reasoning, and memory, may be examined and the differences which occur with age may be measured. In general, cross-sectional studies show that subtests which primarily emphasize verbal skills show little, if any, decline, while those which require psychomotor performance decline a great deal (Botwinick, 1973, 1977).

CROSS-SECTIONAL VERSUS LONGITUDINAL FINDINGS

Cross-sectional findings have been seriously challenged, however, by longitudinal studies. Whereas cross-sectional studies suggest an early performance decrement, longitudinal studies show stability even into late adulthood. Inconsistent findings such as these are somewhat difficult to resolve; however, recall the section on methodology and the discussion of sociocultural change.

Cross-sectional studies may actually be measuring differences between generations, while longitudinal studies are measuring changes in a single generation. Recent research utilizing the time-lag method seems to be quite successful in resolving these differences (Schaie and Labouvie-Vief, 1974; Schaie, Labouvie, and Buech, 1973). Much of the conflicting literature can be explained by differential abilities among the generations. Probably as a result of a more enriched environment (e.g., the younger generations have a greater opportunity to receive much more education), younger generations seem to be getting smarter! Consequently, if we compare younger and older generations, the older generations will be at a disadvantage on our measure of intellectual performance, and we can in no way infer changes. For instance, even if the older person's ability on some measure is increasing over time, a younger person may score as high or higher as a result of his environmental advantage. Our interpretation would be no age difference, or even a differential age decline, whereas actually the older person may still be improving. Such confounding factors demonstrate some of the difficulties in interpreting what happens to intellectual abilities with increasing age.

Existing studies suggest that measurable declines for many abilities occur at much later ages than results from earlier cross-sectional studies had shown. In general, such declines, although statistically significant, may be relatively small in magnitude.

It should be noted that the results presented above refer to group data. Patterns may differ for specific individuals; however, it is felt that people who do well when young will tend also to do well when old.

ENVIRONMENTAL CHARACTERISTICS INFLUENCING INTELLIGENCE

One very important area of current research involves identifying which components of the environment contribute to the observed differences in intelligence. Factors, such as personality characteristics, physical vigor, socioeconomic status, years of education, activities, etc., have been found to influence intellectual ability. One hopes that more detailed investigations in this area, including specific information on the individual's life-style, will give us some idea of the critical variables or combination of variables which contribute to the increase, maintenance, or decline of the aging individual's complex cognitive functioning.

PREDICTING LONGEVITY FROM INTELLECTUAL PERFORMANCE

One problem in drawing conclusions about intellectual change with age which was not discussed above concerns subject attrition, i.e., the selective dropout of individuals over time. Dropouts occur because of death, lack of further interest, moving away, etc., and create a tremendous problem to longitudinal research. It has been found that the initially more able are usually those who are still around for retesting (Riegel, Riegel, and Meyer, 1968; Schaie, Labouvie, and Barrett, 1973). This factor confounds our interpretation of changes over time because these results really may be referring primarily to those individuals who had more ability to begin with. Nevertheless, some very useful information can be gleaned from such findings. *Several studies have now found that there is a drop or deterioration in performance which occurs shortly before death* (Jarvik and Blum, 1971; Riegel and Riegel, 1972). Performance on tests which require a speed component are normally seen to decline continuously over later adulthood and do not show a relationship to a death-related drop. Performance on tests of verbal abilities and information storage, however, do display this "terminal-drop." Since this decline in function is most likely indicative of some form of pathological condition, with further research we someday may be able to use psychological tests to diagnose pathology before a medical diagnosis is possible. Such an advance may then enable medical professionals to intervene and to effect a cure or at least to retard the progress of various debilitating diseases.

Already some progress has been made in achieving such a goal. For example, Wilkie and Eisdorfer (1971) found that an elevated diastolic blood pressure was related to a decline in intellectual ability over a 10-year period among those subjects who were first tested at the ages of 60 to 69. Those of the same age with normal or slightly elevated blood pressure showed no loss and some even showed a gain. Of those first tested at ages 70 to 79, none who had high blood pressure was around to be retested 10 years later, and those with normal or slightly elevated pressures showed some loss of intellectual function. Such results suggest a relationship between disease and intellectual functioning, but do not suggest an early way of intervening (other than avoiding hypertension, which we know is desirable). A recent study, however, by Abrahams and Birren (1973) has shown that subjects with a personality predisposing them to coronary heart disease performed more poorly on a test which measured their speed of response than did subjects of a different personality type. The critical feature of this study, for our purposes, is that the medical diagnosis of these individuals did not indicate any evidence of coronary heart disease, but the psychological tests were able to differentiate performance. Studies such as these may someday be of a tremendous aid to the medical profession.

RIGIDITY

A commonly held belief is that older people are more rigid than younger ones. There is an old saying, "You can't teach an old dog new tricks." This saying does not necessarily suggest that older people cannot learn, but that it is more difficult for them to "unlearn" their already well-established ways of doing things. This may be so even when the old way is no longer effective. For example, older nurses returning to school may find that they have much to unlearn. The procedures and techniques they learned as young nurses are now outmoded or have changed considerably.

Rigidity involves resistance to change. However, just because people are rigid in one respect does not necessarily mean that they are rigid in another. Research on aging and rigidity has shown it to be a very complex and ambiguous problem. Most research supports the contention that rigidity is more a function of intelligence than of age. Naturally then, if old and young people are compared, the older people will seem more rigid. This rigidity, however, similar to what we found with intelligence, is determined by cultural and experiential factors—not by age! Consequently, in the future, older people are less likely to seem rigid than are older people of today. In fact, they may not seem any more rigid than people younger than they (Botwinick, 1973).

CAUTIOUSNESS

Cautiousness seems to increase with age. This is apparently the result of discomfort with uncertainty and the expectation and fear of failure. Viewed in this way, cautiousness is a defense mechanism.

Older people want certainty in a situation before they are willing to make a response. Since there is a decline in many abilities with age, and since older people normally need a stimulus of greater intensity before perceiving it than do younger people, such caution may be a precautionary measure. That is, older people proceed more cautiously because they are not receiving as much information about the environment as are younger people, and impulsive behavior may result in some degree of risk. (See Chapter 34 for a discussion of elderly persons misperceiving their environment.)

Experimental studies of cautiousness have shown that if some risk is unavoidable, old and young people do not differ in their cautiousness. However, if given the opportunity to totally avoid risk, older people are reluctant to take any action. Thus, older people seem to differ from young ones in their desire to avoid risky situations in the first place, even when there is very little risk involved (Botwinick, 1973).

Such behavior on the part of old people has been shown to have practical consequences in the health profession. During the traditional audiological examination, people are presented with a very low level sound. They are expected to report whether or not they have heard the sound. Since older people are reluctant to report that they have heard the sound unless they are certain that they have heard it, they may score lower than is necessary in the hearing test. In an experiment designed to test this assumption, it was concluded that the magnitude of sensory deficits in older people may be overestimated by traditional hearing tests (Rees and Botwinick, 1971). The possibility remains that such behavior may have implications for countless other situations that have not yet been identified.

LEARNING AND MEMORY

LEARNING

In previous sections we have discussed the importance of sociocultural change as a factor influencing the performance of older people. This effect has not been investigated with relation to learning and memory, so that the particular contribution of this effect is presently unknown. Consequently, our discussion is limited to describing the age differences which are found in present generations.

Learning refers to the acquisition of skills or information. Birren (1964) has stated that there is little decrease with advancing age in the primary capacity to learn. Those differences which do appear are attributed to perception, set, attention, motivation, and the physiological state (including disease) of the person. This really comes down to a difference between learning *ability* as an abstract process and learning *performance* as an observable phenomenon. All we can measure is performance and thereby infer what has been learned. As can be seen by Birren's discussion, however, we may actually be looking at the effect of these other factors.

Such a distinction is very important, because once we are able to identify these factors, we may be able to suggest techniques which will minimize the typically observed learning deficit in old age.

PACING

One factor found to be a very important contributor to observed age deficits in learning is the speed at which the material to be learned is presented. *In general, older people learn better when working at their own pace. When the pace is determined by someone else, the performance of older people is seen to decline.* This can happen even if the required pace is exactly the same as when older people are working at their own pace. Consequently, for older people to perform well, they should not be rushed, but should be permitted to proceed at a speed which is comfortable for them. This has real importance in the teaching and learning of older patients, e.g., in learning to give themselves insulin shots, take care of their own colostomy dressings, and the like.

MOTIVATION

Another extremely important factor affecting performance is motivation. To perform well, one must be motivated to do so. It is commonly felt that older people are less motivated to learn than are younger people, particularly in a laboratory situation, and this results in their poorer performance. Actually, this may not be correct. There is some evidence that older people may be highly involved in the task and that this involvement is detrimental to their performance. Although this explanation seems somewhat paradoxical, consider a situation where you are

very anxious to do a certain task well. The harder you try, the worse you do. You may be experiencing a situation where instead of your increased motivation helping you perform better, you are performing worse! In short, you are "overaroused." There seems to be an optimum level of arousal for good performance. To exceed the optimal level leads to poorer performance, just as does not achieving it. The issue of the motivation levels of older people is by no means clear. Some studies seem to suggest that older people are underaroused, while others suggest that they are overaroused (Botwinick, 1973). It may well be that older people have more difficulty in maintaining "optimum levels of motivation." However, our knowledge in this area is too limited to draw firm conclusions at this point. It might be interesting for nurses to study the lack of motivation, since they often become so exasperated with the unmotivated oldster.

Task Meaningfulness Meaningfulness of the task is a factor related to age differences in performance. Since many psychological testing laboratory procedures are not relevant to the personal needs of the elderly, these people may tend not to get involved in the task and, consequently, might perform poorly. In general, this is what is found. Older people perform better on meaningful tasks than they do on tasks which are less meaningful. For example, Arenberg (1968) studied the performance of young and old people on tasks which required the identification of concepts by logical analysis. He presented subjects with nine stimuli—three different forms (e.g., square, circle, triangle), three colors (e.g., red, blue, and yellow), and three numbers (e.g., 1, 2, 3). One element from each category was presented at a single time. This constituted one trial. The subject was to go through several trials, after each of which Arenberg provided the information "yes" or "no." The task of the subject was to discover which element the experimenter had in mind. Based on this information and using the process of elimination, the concept could be attained. This task was so difficult for older people that only a few could do it. However, when he used food items instead of the abstract categories of form, color, and number, and gave the information "lived" or "died" instead of "yes" or "no," older people were able to identify the "poisoned food" and solved many of the problems, although their overall performance still did not equal that of younger subjects.

One problem in interpreting this study is that not only did Arenberg make the task more meaningful, he also made it easier. Older people perform disproportionately more poorly as tasks increase in difficulty than do younger people. Consequently, the improved performance of older people may also have been the result of an easier task. Nevertheless, for our purposes here, *it should be remembered that if one can simplify the demands of the task and make it meaningful, older people will do relatively well.* This information should be kept in mind when designing nursing-care plans for the elderly, or teaching them self-care or rehabilitation techniques.

Irrelevant Information   Another factor which taxes the ability of older people concerns irrelevant information. It has been shown that as the amount of irrelevant information being presented is increased, the performance of older as opposed to younger people disproportionately declines (Rabbitt, 1965). A practical, although extreme, example of how this can affect older people has been related by Burnside (1974). An elderly gentleman who required several different types of medication was given a list to help him remember how many pills to take and on what schedule. See medication schedule below:

Medication Schedule

1. Take 2 blue pills before breakfast.
2. Take 1 white pill at bedtime.
3. Take 1 yellow pill at breakfast, dinner, and supper time.
4. Take 1 pink and gray pill as needed for your pain.

Following the instructions as he read them, the old man took 1 blue pill, 2 white pills, 3 yellow pills, and 4 pink and gray pills. Fortunately, the error was discovered before any great harm resulted; nevertheless, it does illustrate the influence of irrelevant information. The numerical order of the list had no relevance to the number of pills required and only served to confuse the man. Needless to say, the addition of irrelevant information normally will not lead to such severe consequences, but it is important to note that it can impede good performance in older people.

Other Relevant Factors   A factor that appears to put some older people at a disadvantage is the organization of information. A task becomes easier when the information can be organized into larger units; however, many older people are not able to take advantage of this. When instructions are given describing how best to organize material, many elderly, particularly those with low verbal facility, are seen to improve. This suggests that information on how to organize material for learning and recall is more important for older than for younger people.

Mediational techniques (e.g., word associations, forming mental pictures) and note taking are other useful types of aids to improve learning and memory; however, the aged do not tend to make use of them. When they are instructed to use mediators, older people's performance is seen to improve. Note taking, on the other hand, does not seem to help the elderly. What little research there is on the topic suggests that the aged do not make use of their notes, if instructed to take them, and see no reason for writing them.

LEARNING AND MEMORY DISTINGUISHED

Thus far we have discussed some of the factors which influence learning performance in the aged, but have not mentioned memory. Although conceptually different, learning and memory are inextricably linked. For example, how does one remember something that has not been learned? Along this line, *the more one has learned, the greater the possibility of remembering more of the information.* Since the learning performance of older people is normally less than that of younger people, one would expect that older people would not remember as much as would the young. Consequently, to establish that older people do not remember as well as younger ones, either we must establish that they have indeed learned the task as well as the young, or else we must compare the relative loss between age groups of that material which was originally learned.

There is much confusion regarding when "learning" ends and "memory" begins. Also when does short-term memory end and long-term memory begin? Most of the distinctions are arbitrary and are distinguished by various time bases. Learning refers to a change from one trial to another, while memory normally refers to the temporal interval between the trials.

MEMORY

Recent work in memory and aging has focused on information-processing models. These models usually involve three stages: (1) sensory memory, which is modality-specific; (2) primary memory, a short-term storage system where the material to be retained is still at the focus of attention; and (3) secondary memory, a long-term storage system. Present thought is that the quantitative aspects of secondary memory are the same whether the time period elapsed is a minute, months, or years. It is felt that minimal age differences are observed in primary memory; however, age differences are observed in secondary memory (Craik, 1977).

It is often felt that old people are well able to recall important events which occurred in the past. Our knowledge of age differences in these "old" memories is slight because it is very difficult to establish the needed experimental controls. Nevertheless, the evidence which is available seems to indicate that aging leads to little, if any, impairment of old memory.

Such memories would be involved in reminiscence. Although the assumption is commonly held that older people typically engage in reminiscence, *empirical studies find no evidence that older people engage in thinking about the past more than the present. It seems to be a characteristic of only some older people.* When reminiscence does occur, however, it is thought to be adaptive. In fact, Butler (1963) defines the life review as a "naturally occurring, universal mental process . . . prompted by the realization of approaching dissolution and death, and the inability to maintain one's sense of personal invulnerability." As such, the life review is an important step, as one ages, to prepare for eventual death. (See Chapter 8 for an elaboration of reminiscing.)

It should be remembered that all types of memory involve several stages: (1) registration, which refers to the stimulus entering the memory system; (2) retention, which is the ability to maintain registration over time; and (3) recall, which is the retrieval of that material registered and retained.

Factors Influencing Age Differences in Memory It is important to ascertain where differences in primary and secondary memory exist and to identify factors that may account for the observed decrements. Just as is found with learning, age deficits in memory are normally found on tasks which are paced and tasks which are not meaningful. *Deficits are also seen to occur when the task demands a constant switching of attention or requires a change of set. It has also been found that older people are disproportionately impaired on visual as opposed to auditory memory tasks* (Schaie and Gribbin, 1975).

An area of research which has results that nurses can put into practice concerns age differences in free recall versus recognition. Free recall can be likened to a fill-in-the-blank or completion test when the right answer must be supplied by the individual; recognition is like a multiple choice test where one must choose the right answer from those supplied. Age differences in memory are found with tasks that require free recall, but are greatly reduced or even disappear on recognition tasks. Essentially what this demonstrates is that older people have "stored" the memory, but have difficulty in retrieving it. Such a finding suggests that the use of "cues" may be extremely helpful as an aid for improving memory performance in the aged. It is interesting to note that the age differences in recognition of material presented verbally appears to be less than that of material presented pictorially (Schonfield and Robertson, 1966; Harwood and Naylor, 1969). Such findings suggest that nurses should use large charts and many visual aids in teaching and counseling the elderly in conjunction with verbal explanations.

Among the concepts used by psychologists to explain age differences in learning and memory, perhaps the most frequently used is *interference*. This refers to the idea that people do not learn well or do not retain what they have learned because of the competition of other previously learned information. Much laboratory evidence suggests that a great deal of the age-related deficits in performance may be attributed to interference effects. It has been found that in order to minimize interference effects for older people, the initial task should be well learned and at a slow pace.

INTERVENTION TECHNIQUES

In general, it has been found that older people do not perform as well as younger people in learning and memory tasks, and several factors have been identified which seem to contribute to the observed decrements. The possibility of intervention techniques, however, still remains a question. Practice or repeated testing may lead to improvement in the memory of older people, but there is no evidence that the elderly benefit any more than the young.

Attempts to improve learning RNA memory functions by the administration of yeast have not been successful; however, in one study pentylenetetrazol administration was found to lead to improvement (Leckman et al., 1971). In addition, experiments with older people in hyperbaric chambers suggest that hyperoxygenation may lead to improvement (Jacobs, Winter, and Alvis, 1969), although impairment of function has also been found (Goldfarb et al., 1972). Needless to say, much more work is needed before any conclusions may be drawn about the effectiveness of any particular intervention technique. Nevertheless, the results are encouraging.

IMPLICATIONS FOR NURSING

This chapter described the cognitive processes of the "normal" older person. Any such broad generalization is necessarily lacking when applied to a specific individual, and this is definitely so in the case of the elderly. Older people have had a lifetime to accumulate many different and varied experiences. They have exercised their abilities and capabilities in a multitude of ways. In addition, older people are physiologically very different from one another. It is very possible that older people are the most hetero-geneous age group as concerns variations in functioning. Some older people may be extremely intelligent and perform far better on a variety of tasks than most young people, but the reverse may also be true.

Perhaps *one of the most important ideas to be brought out in this chapter is that old age is not necessarily a process of decline.* This is particularly true with regard to intellectual changes over the life-span. Maintenance or stability of intellectual functioning seems to be the rule, at least until shortly before death. This has relevance for the nurse caring for the terminally ill person, because when one finds that an older person's intellectual performance is declining, one should look for other causes to account for it than "old age." It may be a precursor to a death-related decline; however, it may also be the result of a depression. Identification of the specific cause may be an extremely important factor in caring for the patient.

Rigidity is also not necessarily concomitant with aging. If one encounters rigidity when trying to get a patient to change some behavior, the blame for it should not be the age of the patient, for even young people can be rigid. It should be realized that rigidity is probably more a function of lack of education or lesser intellectual ability. Possibly providing information in a very organized manner may aid in eliciting the desired behavior.

Increased cautiousness may be very adaptive to aging because the environment is necessarily more of a threat to older people. Since older people are slower to respond, they are unable to compensate quickly if their action results in some risk. Consequently, proceeding cautiously may be an important factor for older people in order to avoid physical danger. Nurses should be aware of this tendency toward caution in order to deal more effectively with the elderly patient.

Probably one of the most useful sections for nurses to put into practice is that of learning and memory. Understanding the factors which are most conducive to an effective learning situation for the aged may be most beneficial for good nursing practice. Allowing people to proceed at their own pace, making the task meaningful, avoiding irrelevant information, keeping the task as simple as possible, providing cues—all are very important factors to consider if one wishes to improve the learning and memory performance of the elderly.

The usefulness of collaborative efforts between psychologists and health professionals is only beginning to be explored. Several such endeavors were described in this chapter. Hopefully, continued effort in this direction will lead to beneficial results for nursing practice in the near future.

REFERENCES

Abrahams, Joel P., and James E. Birren: Reaction time as a function of age and behavioral predisposition to coronary heart disease, *Journal of Gerontology,* **28:**471–478, 1973.

Arenberg, David.: Concept problem solving in young and old adults, *Journal of Gerontology,* **23:**279–282, 1968.

Birren, James E.: *The Psychology of Aging,* Prentice-Hall, Englewood Cliffs, N.J., 1964.

Botwinick, Jack: *Aging and Behavior,* Springer, New York, 1973.

———: Intellectual abilities, in James E. Birren and K. W. Schaie (eds.), *The Handbook of the Psychology of Aging,* Van Nostrand Reinhold, New York, 1977, pp. 580–605.

Burnside, Irene M.: Personal communication, 1974.

Butler, Robert N.: The life review: An interpretation of reminiscence in the aged, *Psychiatry,* **26**(1):65–76, 1963.

Craik, F. I. M.: Age differences in human memory, in James E. Birren and K. W. Schaie (eds.), *The Handbook of the Psychology of Aging,* Van Nostrand Reinhold, New York, 1977, pp. 384–414.

Demming, J. A., and S. L. Pressey: Tests "indigenous" to the adult and older years, *Journal of Counseling Psychology,* **2:**144–148, 1957.

Goldfarb, Alvin I., Neil J. Hochstadt, Julius H. Jacobson, and Edwin A. Weinstein: Hyperbaric oxygen treatment of organic mental syndrome in aged persons, *Journal of Gerontology,* **27**(2):212–217, 1972.

Harwood, E., and G. F. K. Naylor: Recall and recognition in elderly, and young subjects, *Australian Journal of Psychology,* **21:**251–257, 1969.

Jacobs, E. A., P. M. Winter, and H. J. Alvis: Hyperoxygenation effect on cognitive functioning in the aged, *New England Journal of Medicine,* **28:**753–757, 1969.

Jarvik, Lissy F., and June E. Blum: Cognitive declines as predictors of mortality in twin pairs: A twenty-year longitudinal study of aging, in E. Palmore and F. C. Jeffers (eds.) *Prediction of Life-Span,* Heath, Boston, 1971.

Leckman, J., J. V. Ananth, T. A. Ban, and H. E. Lehman: Pentylenetetrazol in the treatment of geriatric patients with disturbed memory function, *Journal of Clinical Pharmacology and New Drugs,* **11:**301–303, 1971.

Rabbitt, P. M. A.: An age decrement in the ability to ignore irrelevant information, *Journal of Gerontology,* **20:**233–238, 1965.

Rees, J. N., and Jack Botwinick: Detection and decision factors in auditory behavior of the elderly, *Journal of Gerontology,* **26:**133–136, 1971.

Riegel, Klaus F., and Ruth M. Riegel: Development, drop, and death, *Developmental Psychology,* **6:**306–319, 1972.

———, ———, and G. Meyer: The prediction of retest resisters in research on aging, *Journal of Gerontology,* **23:**370–374, 1968.

Schaie, K. Warner, and Kathy Gribbin: Adult development and aging, in *The Annual Review of Psychology,* Annual Reviews Incorporated, Palo Alto, Calif. 1975.

———, and Gisela Labouvie-Vief: Generational versus ontogenetic components of change in adult cognitive behavior: A fourteen-year cross-sequential study, *Developmental Psychology,* **10:**305–320, 1974.

———, Gisela V. Labouvie, and T. J. Barrett: Selective attrition effects in a fourteen-year study of adult intelligence, *Journal of Gerontology,* **28:**328–334, 1973.

———, ———, and Barbara U. Buech: Generational and cohort-specific differences in adult cognitive functioning: A fourteen-year study of independent samples, *Developmental Psychology,* **9:**151–166, 1973.

Schonfield, David, and Elizabeth A. Robertson: Memory storage and aging. *Canadian Journal of Psychology,* **20:**228–236, 1966.

Wilkie, Frances L., and Carl Eisdorfer: Intelligence and blood pressure in the aged, *Science,* **172:**959–962, 1971.

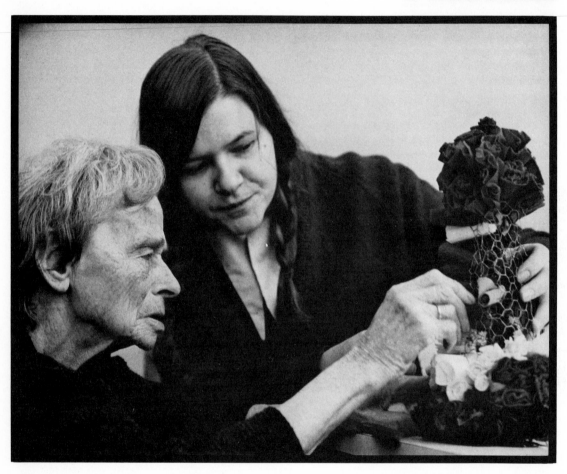

E. Schwab, reprinted with permission
of the World Health Organization

MENTAL HEALTH: THEORY AND THERAPY

One might speak to great length of the three corners
of reality—what was seen, what was thought to be
seen, and what was thought ought to be seen.

Marvin Bell
"Things We Dreamt We Died For"

FIVE

MENTAL HEALTH AND THE AGED

Irene Mortenson Burnside

The advancing edge of knowledge that will eventually cut through the thick wall of pathology accounting for the many psychiatric problems of the aged is moving ahead slowly, but surely.
E. W. Busse

LEARNING OBJECTIVES

- State four causes for the problems of conceptualization of mental health.
- State three factors which are associated with life satisfaction and/or morale in the elderly.
- List seven positive characteristics of mental health.
- Discuss the magnitude of mental health problems in nursing homes.
- Define iatrogenic mental illness.
- Define anxiety.
- Define a freeze action.
- List four cues to anxiety in bedridden patients.
- Define overload as it relates to communication.
- List two nursing interventions when anxiety cues are observed in an older patient.
- List four possible reasons for loneliness in the elderly.

MENTAL HEALTH: DIFFICULT TO DEFINE

Researchers have expended great effort to define various mental illnesses carefully and precisely, but what is mental health? *Mental health* as a concept does not have a precise definition with a wide consensus. Williams (1972, p. 3) defines it "as a particular field of human endeavor, in which people are doing things in describable and relatively organized ways." Ramshorn (1978) states that practitioners and teachers alike have problems in the conceptualization of mental health. She offers these possible reasons: (1) boundaries of mental health are diffuse and fluid, and imprecise adjectives are used; (2) the major focus in the health care systems has been directed toward diagnosis, treatment, and restoration of health and function; (3) there are cultural variations in the definition of mental health and labeling mental illness; and (4) professionals hold one view of normality and friends and families may have another.

In writing about mental health and the aged, one is caught between the euphemistic view of mental health as being "a repository for virtues and the good life" (Williams, 1972, p. 3) and the harsh vision of mental illness—the grossly disabling disorders that can occur in behavior. Not only does disabling behavior affect old people (and middle-aged clients, if we consider the tragic effects of presenile dementia), but the suffering, expense, and sorrow that are created for family members often jeopardize their own mental health. The mental health of the family must always be considered in the care of the mentally impaired elderly.

WHAT CONSTITUTES MENTAL HEALTH?

Studies to determine the factors associated with life satisfaction and morale among the aged have usually isolated three variables: health, income, and activity (Gubrium, 1971). These findings generally emerged out of the statistical cross-tabulation of theoretically significant factors. Respondents usually were not asked directly about the conditions which affected their mental health. The factors found to be strongly related, statistically, to life satisfaction and morale have been said to be the conditions which influenced mental health (Gubrium, 1971).

Gubrium (1971) states that, although studies have been highly consistent in the factors identified as influencing the mental health of old people, one must not infer from this that the aged themselves are aware of these relationships.

Mental health at any age surely implies more than the mere absence of mental disturbances. Positive characteristics of mental health must be sought, e.g., qualities such as zest; confidence; the ability to learn, to communicate, to share with others; various skills and competencies; and a receptivity to experience (Kastenbaum, 1974). Often we fail to find, or we neglect, the positive characteristics in the aged client.

MENTAL HEALTH PROBLEMS OF THE AGED

This chapter focuses on two important mental health problems of the aged—anxiety and loneliness. The chapter begins with an introduction to the magnitude of the mental health problems of the aged and then discusses anxiety and loneliness. These two particular aspects of mental health were selected because the qualities are pervasive, they may occur in any setting, and nurses frequently will need to intervene in the anxiety or lonely states of aged clients. There are many old people who are well-adjusted and are neither anxious nor lonely, but they very rarely need a nurse.

WHO ARE THE MENTALLY ILL AGED?

People over age 65 are the most susceptible to mental illness (Butler, 1974; Jaro, 1960). Goldfarb (1975) states that individuals can carry into old age any of the psychiatric problems of youth. It is a well-known fact that the proportion of successful suicides increases with age

(Payne, 1975) and that men over 65 have suicide rates five times as high as young adult men [Group for Advancement of Psychiatry (GAP), 1971]. (See Chapter 12 for a discussion of suicide in the elderly.) Table 5-1 presents some statistics on the chronically ill elderly.

TABLE 5-1
SOME STATISTICS ON CHRONICALLY ILL ELDERLY

- In 1974, there were 3.3 million "mentally ill aged" over 65—greater than the total population of the aged (3 million) in 1900.
- In 1972, 25.9 million persons were limited to some degree because of chronic disease impairment.
- Of these, 6.5 million were limited in mobility.
- In 1970, 7.3 million of these were confined to the house except in an emergency.
- Of the millions of elderly chronically ill, at least 2.5 million are out of the mainstream of life and are in mental institutions (111,000), nursing homes (900,000), and related facilities.
- 1.5 million are estimated as requiring home care; .5 million, constant care.

While the increase of the older population and the complexity of their needs are becoming highly publicized, significant figures also emerge for those under 65 requiring long-term care—and these figures are conservative.

- There are 113,218 in nursing homes, of whom approximately one-half have lived in a nursing home over $1\frac{1}{2}$ years and receive only routine nursing or personal care. Approximately 40% have a mental disorder or impairment.
- There are 300,000 under 65 in psychiatric hospitals, retardation facilities, and children's facilities.

The NCHS Health Interview Survey gives us some idea of the potential need for long-term care resulting from chronic disabilities. In 1973, 13.5% of the noninstitutionalized, civilian population reported some degree of activity limitation due to "chronic conditions"; this ranged from 3.4% for those under 17 years, 8.5% for the 17- to 44-year age group, 23.3% for the 45- to 64-year age group, and 44.1% for those 65 and over.

SOURCE: Department of Health, Education, and Welfare, "Excerpts from Health, United States, 1975," PHS, Health Resources Administration, National Center for Health Services Research of National Center for Health Statistics, January 1976.

We can only guess at the extent of mental health problems in the elderly since so many of them live outside the range of medical, psychiatric, and social care systems (Butler, 1974). But there are more than a million persons over age 65 in institutions, most of them in nursing homes, and well over 50 percent of these aged persons have some type of psychiatric symptomatology or mental impairment (Butler, 1974).

Teeter et al. (1976) found psychiatric disorders in 85 percent of 74 patients in two skilled nursing homes studied. Schmidt et al. reported in 1977 that one-third of nursing home patients had a psychiatric diagnosis—more than one-half were psychotic! Eisdorfer (1977) states that psychiatric problems probably could be found in 60 percent of nursing home residents.

IATROGENIC MENTAL ILLNESS

Some authors discuss the mental changes caused by institutionalization and have named them *iatrogenic mental illnesses*. The deinstitutionalization of mental health services is the subject of a comprehensive and excellent paper by Bassuk and Gerson (1978) in *Scientific American*. These authors describe the difficulties following deinstitutionalization and the complex interactions of financial, professional, political, and administrative factors. Most nursing homes have more than 100 beds and yet offer only custodial care. In a 1974 national survey of the patients 65 years and over, a third had chronic brain disease and a tenth were diagnosed as being neurotic or psychotic. Placing patients in nursing home beds means that those persons with chronic physical illness stay longer in general hospitals.

Leonard Schmidt et al. (1977) describe the nursing homes in the community as the new back wards. (*Back wards* formerly referred to the wards of state hospitals where patients received little treatment.) The dramatic drop in state hospital populations has caused many psychiatric patients ultimately to end up in nursing homes. The reason for the mass move has been a financial one. The states could shift the burden of care to the federal government. Butler (1978, p. 7) states, "The real story behind the transfer

TABLE 5-2

PERCENT CHANGE IN THE NUMBER AND RATE PER 100,000 POPULATION OF ADMISSIONS WITH NO PRIOR INPATIENT CARE WHO WERE ADMITTED TO STATE AND COUNTY MENTAL HOSPITALS, UNITED STATES: 1962, 1965, 1969, 1972, AND 1975

Sex and Age at Admission	Percent Change							
	Number of First Admissions				Rate per 100,000 Population			
	1962–1965	1965–1969	1969–1972	1972–1975	1962–1965	1965–1969	1969–1972	1972–1975
Both sexes, all ages:	+ 11.1	+ 13.8	− 14.1	− 14.3	+ 6.4	+ 9.3	− 16.9	− 16.3
Under 15	+ 30.3	+ 45.3	+ 16.9	+ 8.4	+ 25.0	+ 46.7	+ 22.7	+ 14.8
15–24	+ 32.9	+ 44.9	− 6.4	+ 2.1	+ 15.2	+ 29.1	− 16.9	− 3.5
25–34	+ 12.6	+ 3.9	+ 4.3	+ 0.6	+ 12.7	− 6.0	− 6.8	− 11.2
35–44	+ 10.9	+ 19.9	− 21.8	− 30.2	+ 11.0	+ 26.0	− 20.2	− 30.4
45–54	+ 10.2	+ 16.4	− 20.5	− 33.2	+ 5.9	+ 10.6	− 22.0	− 33.6
55–64	+ 9.9	+ 25.1	− 33.8	− 13.7	+ 4.5	+ 16.5	− 36.9	− 16.6
65+	− 6.1	− 26.4	− 26.0	− 43.3	− 10.5	− 31.3	− 31.2	− 47.0
Males, all ages:	+ 13.6	+ 19.8	− 3.2	− 16.2	+ 8.7	+ 16.0	− 6.5	− 18.1
Under 15	+ 27.0	+ 35.8	+ 66.3	− 22.0	+ 22.8	+ 38.1	+ 73.1	− 17.7
15–24	+ 35.5	+ 46.9	+ 7.9	− 0.9	+ 15.8	+ 33.1	− 7.2	− 6.9
25–34	+ 16.7	+ 14.1	+ 9.0	+ 13.5	+ 16.5	+ 2.9	− 3.4	− 0.3
35–44	+ 14.2	+ 17.0	+ 2.0	− 34.5	+ 14.1	+ 23.0	+ 4.0	− 34.7
45–54	+ 11.1	+ 32.2	− 26.9	− 33.3	+ 7.5	+ 26.7	− 28.1	− 34.2
55–64	+ 13.2	+ 16.9	− 13.5	− 31.7	+ 8.2	+ 10.1	− 16.9	− 34.3
65+	− 6.6	− 15.0	− 30.3	− 39.9	− 9.1	− 18.7	− 33.3	− 43.2
Females, all ages:	+ 7.9	+ 5.8	− 30.8	− 10.3	+ 3.3	− 1.0	− 33.0	− 12.3
Under 15	+ 37.3	+ 63.5	− 62.3	+ 223.7	+ 33.3	+ 67.3	− 60.9	+ 244.1
15–24	+ 29.3	+ 42.1	− 28.0	+ 8.9	+ 13.4	+ 24.6	− 34.0	+ 3.5
25–34	+ 7.7	− 9.2	− 3.1	− 22.7	+ 8.3	− 17.6	− 12.7	− 31.6
35–44	+ 6.7	+ 23.8	− 52.3	− 18.2	+ 7.2	+ 29.9	− 51.3	− 18.4
45–54	+ 8.9	− 7.3	− 6.8	− 32.9	+ 4.2	− 12.6	− 8.8	− 33.1
55–64	+ 5.4	+ 37.4	− 59.6	+ 35.5	− 0.5	+ 26.6	− 61.7	+ 31.2
65+	− 5.6	− 38.3	− 19.9	− 47.5	− 11.5	− 43.5	− 27.2	− 51.3

SOURCE: *Mental Health Statistical Note* no. 146, Department of Health, Education, and Welfare, NIMH, DHEW Publication no. (ADM) 78–158, March 1978.

TABLE 5-3

RESIDENT PATIENT POPULATION IN 1975 AS A PERCENT OF THE 1965 RESIDENT POPULATION, STATE AND COUNTY MENTAL HOSPITALS, UNITED STATES

Age	Both Sexes	Males	Females
All ages	40.3	44.2	36.5
Under 15	69.9	68.3	74.2
15–24	75.1	82.6	61.8
25–34	61.0	70.3	47.3
35–44	35.1	41.2	28.8
45–54	31.6	32.4	30.8
55–64	33.6	32.8	34.5
Over 65	38.6	39.9	37.7

NOTE: The resident population of state and county mental hospitals experienced a dramatic reduction over the interval 1965–1975. The total number of resident patients decreased from 475,202 in 1965 to 191,391 in 1975—a decrease of 60 percent. As can be seen above, the resident population for all ages in 1975 represents only 40 percent of what it was in 1965. Upon closer examination, each age-sex group is observed as having experienced a decrease in number over the 1965–1975 interval, the greatest decrease occurring in the 45- to 64-year age groups for males and in the 35- to 44-year age group for females.

SOURCE: *Mental Health Statistical Note* no. 146, Department of Health, Education, and Welfare, NIMH, DHEW Publication no. (ADM) 78-158, March 1978, p. 1.

of patients to the community is that it has been extraordinarily convenient to the states. State governors and legislators recognized home care or foster care under the Supplemental Security Income of Medicaid programs, rather than paying state funds for state hospitals directly caring for older people." See Tables 5-2 and 5-3.

SEEKING HELP HAS PROBLEMS

Several problems frequently arise in the seeking of help for old people with mental problems; among them are:

1. Psychiatrically trained professionals still hold the nihilistic therapeutic view of aged; that view originated long ago with Freud, who felt that people over 50 were not treatable and not amenable to psychotherapeutic interventions (Freud, 1949).
2. Mental health workers still lack adequate training in the therapeutic techniques necessary to work with older persons.
3. Medicare pays for only a small portion of a psychiatrist's fees, and few old people are able to afford the cost of psychotherapy at $50 (or more) per hour.
4. Many individuals caring for the aged, especially the caretakers who spend the most time with the elderly (e.g., home health aides and nurse's aides) lack knowledge of psychosocial care, psychodynamics, and gerontology.

Reidun Ingebretsen (1978) has observed, "It is a well-known problem that some of the elderly most in need of help keep away from health and welfare centers and different social agencies." Although this therapist was discussing her home country, Norway, her observation applies to the United States as well.

Older people do not go to the psychiatrist or to mental health workers. They do not often admit to having mental problems (or physical ones, for that matter), and they are, in fact, sometimes unaware of the problems. The clever ones can occasionally convince the nurse trying to help that the nurse is the one with a problem, not them!

Davidson (1976, p. 35) reminds us that there is a tendency to make an easy assumption that an old person "is mentally ill rather than ill in some other way [and this] is usually a sign of emotional rejection by those taking care of him."

For an outstanding review of behavioral and dynamic psychotherapy, the reader is referred to a chapter by Gunnar Götestam (1980).

COMMUNITY HEALTH CENTERS AND LONG-TERM CARE FACILITIES

There is a great need for community mental health centers and long-term care facilities to begin developing programs in which they share their expertise with one another. For some time now, the pressure has been on community mental health centers (CMHC) because of poor track records in care of the elderly since the inception of CMHCs in the 1960s. It has been well documented that CMHCs have treated only about three percent of people over age 65. CMHCs and long-term care facilities need one another because each can share the expertise of the other. That is, the mental health concepts need to be better taught and better understood in long-term care facilities; mental health workers could expedite such learning. Mental health workers who are employed in community mental health centers could be "gerontologized" by nursing home staffs and could learn more about normal aging and pathology from those trained in long-term care. Jonathan L. York (1977) has written an excellent handbook about beginning such a joint program.

GEROPSYCHIATRY PROGRAMS

In the area of mental health and aging in the United States a handful of psychiatrists have been the pacesetters when it comes to studying,

describing, researching, and writing about mental health problems of the elderly. They have consistently testified at White House hearings and have long been active in regional, national, and international gerontology societies. They have produced numerous excellent textbooks (Verwoerdt, 1976; GAP, 1971; Wells, 1977; Busse and Pfeiffer, 1973, 1969). At this writing there are now five medical geropsychiatric programs in the United States; there are no geropsychiatric nursing programs. Another development is the program in the National Institute of Mental Health (NIMH) called the Distinguished Senior Scholar Program. A person 65 years or older serves as a consultant in mental health; this program was initiated by Dr. Jack Weinberg, a well-known geropsychiatrist.

Psychiatric nursing in general has not accepted the challenge of care for the elderly, yet the need for geropsychiatric nursing becomes increasingly apparent as nurses grapple with the behavioral problems of their clients. See Tables 5-4 and 5-5. Miller (1976) wonders if adequate preparation is given in geropsychiatric nursing to handle the ever-increasing numbers of old people with dementia. At this writing one would have to say that little preparation is offered, as we have few geropsychiatric nurses. Dorothy Moses has been the pioneer in geropsychiatric nursing.

Anxiety and loneliness are mental states of the elderly in which nurses can effectively intervene once they have made the nursing diagnosis. Each is discussed below.

ANXIETY

Rollo May (1975) pointed out that the word *anxiety* is almost impossible to find in the Greek literature of the fifth century B.C., a time when the symbols and the myths of Greek society were unified. He argues that anxiety and alienation developed during the second and first centuries B.C., when their symbols and myths were no longer orienting the Greeks to their world or to each other (Parker, 1978).

Søren Kierkegaard (1944) wrote that learning about anxiety is an adventure and that everyone has to deal with it. He felt that the

TABLE 5-4
NUMBER OF REGISTERED NURSES EMPLOYED IN MENTAL HEALTH FACILITIES, JANUARY 1974

Type of Facility	Number of Facilities		Number of Registered Nurses Employed			
	Total	Re-porting	Total	Full-time	Part-time	Trainee
Total	*3,596*	*3,180*	*39,228*	*30,104*	*5,551*	*3,573*
State and county mental hospitals	324	304	15,422	13,221	1,045	1,156
Private mental hospitals	182	176	3,469	2,290	888	291
VA psychiatric services	190	179	4,958	4,178	460	320
General hospital psychiatric inpatient and outpatient services	991	783	9,419	6,347	1,973	1,099
Outpatient psychiatric clinics	1,092	996	976	509	252	215
Community mental health centers	400	360	4,148	2,983	776	389
Residential treatment centers for emotionally disturbed children	340	312	337	170	125	42
Other	77	70	499	406	32	61

SOURCE: U.S. Department of Health, Education, and Welfare, Public Health Service, Alcohol, Drug Abuse, and Mental Health Administration, National Institute of Mental Health, Biometry Branch, Survey and Reports Section, 1975.

TABLE 5-5

PROJECTED MANPOWER POOL FOR EACH
PROFESSIONAL DISCIPLINE

Discipline	1975		1980	
	Required	Expected*	Required	Expected
Psychiatry†	86,235	30,300	91,004	38,700
Psychology‡	86,235	30,000	91,004	44,800
Social work§	86,235	25,400	91,004	36,600
Nursing¶	86,235	35,900	91,004	51,300

* The source for these data was the Division of Manpower and Training Programs, National Institute of Mental Health.
† One or more years of psychiatric training.
‡ M.A. or Ph.D. with training in mental health field.
§ M.A. with training in mental health field.
¶ Some training in psychiatric nursing.
SOURCE: Morton Kramer, Carl A. Taube, and Richard Redick, "Patterns of use of psychiatric facilities by the aged: Past, present, and future," in Carl Eisdorfer and M. Powell Lawton (eds.), *The Psychology of Adult Development and Aging,* American Psychological Association, Washington, 1973, p. 486.

person who has learned to be "rightly" anxious has learned a very important thing. Smith (1965) wrote, "The human heart is star-crossed, its tension will never completely go." Nurses who aspire to be skilled and sensitive practitioners must know how to handle their own anxiety. Nathan Rickles and Betty Finkle (1973) spell out some of the issues that could increase a nurse's anxiety. Anxiety-producing situations include: (1) caring for a patient who develops a serious medical problem, (2) being directly involved with a combative patient, and (3) a return of previous anxiety-laden experiences during the care of a client. Nurses may need to ask themselves what specifically tends to heighten their own anxiety about care of the aged. Students may need help in identifying their anxiety when in clinical settings with elderly persons.

One nurse who studied anxiety in two elderly men during a one-to-one therapeutic relationship with them wrote,

The clinical experience was the writer's first "in depth" exposure to the aged and their anxieties. Never has this writer shared the present and past through an aged person's eyes. Never has she heard the future expressed so bleakly. This writer realizes that the aged have so much to share: their memories, knowledge, advice, love, fears, and anxieties. She is also aware that she has something to offer the aged—not only by being a nurse who is interested in reducing their anxieties but by being [one] who cares and can give of self. (Nuzzillio, 1972a)

THIRD EMERGENCY REACTION

Lissy Jarvik and Dan Russell (1979) point out that severe anxiety is not common among the aged. That is, in contrast to depressive states. These authors propose that people who live long develop strategies to handle stress, and one strategy is "a passive stance, termed 'freeze,' and that 'freeze' is a third emergency reaction." The usual paradigm of emergency reactions is based on fight-flight responses.

OTHER MANIFESTATIONS OF ANXIETY

Fromm-Reichmann (1960) wrote that anxiety may be subjectively experienced as a most unpleasant interference with thinking processes and concentration. In a mild form, anxiety may be seen objectively by shift in tone of voice and/or tempo of speech; by change of posture, gesture, and motion; and also by intellectual or emotional preoccupation or blocking of communication. However, one must remember that there is a change in the larynx in normal aging, and changes in the aged person's voice might not be so easy to detect as a manifestation of anxiety as are voice changes in a younger person.

Anxiety is common in old age and may be present intermittently or chronically. Manifestations of anxiety change with advancing age and may be manifested by somatic complaints, insomnia, denial, complaining, restlessness, fatigue, incompetence, fantasizing, hostile or dependent behavior, and isolation (Busse and Pfeiffer, 1969). Peplau (1966) has written extensively about anxiety and rates anxiety 1+ to 4+ (the latter, a state of panic). She points out the positive quality of a 1+ anxiety.

An example of the way a hospitalized aged person copes with anxiety by isolation comes from a student's process recording: "The first two years I was here I acted as if I was dead—it was a terrible thing—I felt I dropped out of the world—and was living but really dead—I practically lived in bed" (Nuzzillio, 1972b). Another nurse, observing anxiety in group members, noted in initial group meetings a voluminous number of physical complaints (Burnside, 1969). Psychosomatic complaints can be used to cover up anxiety or some prevailing concern, or both. McWhorter (1980) also describes this coping device in her group psychotherapy. Abbey (1974) discusses the great need for the aged to conserve energy. Because of their efforts to conserve energy, their manifestations of anxiety are subtler. Cues may not be so obvious as those seen in younger individuals, which can make assessment difficult. The aged who pace and are agitated are readily noticed, it is true, and are usually quickly tranquilized if they are in institutions, but in the pretranquilizer era, the state

hospital back wards were full of agitated, pacing, elderly people. (I recall one elderly lady in a back ward, who had been a bareback rider in a circus. She jumped on the radiator used for heating the ward and pretended she was still galloping on a horse in the circus.)

Loss of mental acuity is often a bitter one to accept, and this loss causes much embarrassment and anxiety (Burnside, 1970). One old man told the nurse-therapist,

My memory and my mind aren't so good as they used to be. I have moments when I forget what I was going to say [speech slower and lower]. I am afraid that my mind is going to be affected—I am always thinking about this possibility—at times I am afraid to talk to other people—they may notice how poor my memory is getting. (Nuzzillio, 1972b)

Anxiety-producing situations may produce insomnia. The sleep patterns of the elderly differ from those of younger people, and they often experience insomnia. New patients in facilities may have difficult times at night until they "settle in." Dying patients have told me how they dread the quiet isolation of nights. Night staff should be taught how to effectively intervene in the special nursing problems of that particular shift (Burnside, 1973b).

Nowlin (1974) studied 279 subjects aged 45 to 71 for anxiety during medical examination and gives three primary sources of discomfort: "Concern—concern over what the physician might find. Manipulation—discomfort at having someone push and press over your body. Exposure—embarrassment at having to undress."

Some of the more obvious signs of anxiety include (1) chain smoking; (2) pacing; (3) restlessness; (4) inability to sit still; (5) fidgeting and nervous mannerisms; and (6) physiological signs such as increased pulse rate, elevated blood pressure, and frequency and urgency of urination. I have noticed that increased respiration is a sign of great anxiety; as anxiety decreases, respiration becomes slower. I have found my physical closeness helps, and I hold the person's hand. The squeeze of the hand, the tremor, the unwillingness to release the hand from mine are all valuable clues in anxiety assessment. In observing people closely, one discovers that the cues to their anxieties will often be shown in the extremities, e.g., wringing hands, trembling hands, pulling on a finger, opening and clenching of fists, moving a foot, crossing and uncrossing legs, picking at clothing or bedclothes. Greenberg (1972) demonstrated the effectiveness of touch as a nursing intervention to diminish psychotic behavior in elderly institutionalized aged. Her study has implications for ameliorating anxiety states in the mentally disturbed elderly. How then do elderly persons confined to bed or wheelchair manifest their anxiety?

CUES TO THE ANXIETY OF BED PATIENTS

Aged patients confined to their beds will often cope with their anxiety by the following behavior: turn their heads away, close their eyes, look out the window or door, or watch television (often quite intently). Such behavior is a means of avoiding eye contact, and lack of eye contact is one simple way to reduce anxiety. Sometimes they fidget with their bedclothes, their fingers and hands, jewelry (which few of them seem to have), so that watching hand movements is important. If the bedclothes are tucked in tightly (which they often are), there is little chance for the aged to move their extremities. Bed patients are often debilitated, frail, with little extra energy to expend.

On a few occasions, I found that the semantics or content changes drastically when the aged person is being interviewed and anxiety is mounting rapidly. One 105-year-old woman talked sanely and sensibly for the first 10 minutes of each of our interviews, but then would lapse into hopeless "word salad" (psychiatric term for unrelated words strung together) about "mud and sticks and stones and the ceiling up there," etc. Since her voice normally crackled, it did not serve as a gauge for anxiety, and since she was so old, she usually lay very still. The cue in this instance was the sudden change in verbal content, which no longer made sense.

Overloading is a common way for the aged to handle anxiety. In this context, to overload means to *verbalize too much, too fast,* so that the person listening cannot absorb all of it. This is commonly seen in anxious elderly persons; however, another reason for overloading by the aged person could be a dread of the time when the listener will leave. "Conversation deprivation" (my term) may be very acute in lonely elderly persons and could well be a nursing diagnosis to use in nursing-care plans. Occasionally overloading is a lifetime habit; some oldsters have always said too much too fast!

CUES TO ANXIETY OF AMBULATORY PATIENTS

Manifestations of anxiety in the ambulatory aged individual are, of course, the easiest to recognize. Pacing is commonly seen in agitated elderly, and is especially observed in "wanderers" who are determined to go home and forever seem to be seeking ways to escape. Incidentally, the police or fire department, or both, should be regarded as the nurse's best friend. Police are helpful in locating wanderers, and fire departments also have rescue squads. These persons are responsive, available, and provide services without charge. It behooves nurses working with elderly clients to have the phone numbers of both the police and fire departments readily accessible. Nurses should also make sure the phone numbers are given to elderly clients who live alone in their own homes.

Ambulatory aged usually are freer to smoke than bedridden or wheelchair patients and are sometimes chain smokers. If one carefully observes smokers in institutions, the days seem to be spent searching for cigarette butts and matches or lights from someone else's cigarette or asking staff members for cigarettes. In one locked facility, several patients would often interrupt group meetings to obtain a light from the men in the group who were smoking. This could, of course, have been a sign of boredom as well as anxiety. Fire hazards are rampant with elderly smokers; Steffl speaks to this in Chapter 32.

Each person has some way of decreasing anxiety, and an intervention that is effective for one person may not work for another. It is difficult to detect anxiety in older people for any number of reasons. For one thing, they have lived for a long time and their defenses have served them well through the years. Many of them also lived in an era in which one was supposed to be stoic and not show one's true feelings. Many aged persons are simply not accustomed to expressing their feelings and are unable to say, "I am depressed" or "I am excited." Another reason that cues to anxiety can be missed is that overt cues are expected. The subtler ones, as previously explained, are due to the patients' limited energy and thus are frequently missed. Terminal patients with great anxiety may conserve energy and attend to the dying process and "letting go."

One of the best things that can be done to alleviate the extreme tensions and feelings of anxiety in the aged is to sit with them and to listen attentively to them. Attentive listening is always important in a nurse-client relationship, but it is crucial in working with the aged. Attentive listening is described in detail by Wilson (1970). Unfortunately, old people in our society are often not taken very seriously, and I recall the surprise of an aged man when I reflected on what he said. "You're the only one who ever really listens to me," he told me.

Kissel (1965) has shown that the mere presence of other persons, especially friendly others, helps to reduce anxiety. And, of course, Lowenthal and Haven (1968) have written of the beneficial effects of a confidante for the elderly.

An aged person who may have to go to surgery or to the hospital for a special examination or into some other new situation that may be frightening needs an attentive listener or someone present. For example, during a summer institute class at the Andrus Gerontology Center, a prominent geropsychiatrist planned to interview elderly persons for a class. Miss H., a 95-year-old, agreed to go to the class to be interviewed. She was extremely anxious when I went to the "L" facility (light-mental, long-term facility) to get her. The unknown had created many qualms for her. The real clue to her anxiety was her heavy breathing, which was most unusual for her. I immediately slowed my pace, even though I knew we were going to be late for the class. We sat down and had a cup of coffee together; I again carefully explained what would ensue and reassured her that I knew

with certainty that she would do well. (Every time I interview elderly persons for a class I am impressed with their fears of not performing well. One is constantly aware of the frequency of negative views of society, which have been internalized by the aged.) I reassured her that I would not leave her there, because she had the fear of being abandoned. When Miss H.'s breathing slowed, we slowly went out to the car and drove to the center. As we were driving to the center, she told me she had been in the facility for 9 years and had never been out of it, so that she had not ridden in a car for that length of time either. How well she had coped under the stress! The elderly are too often underestimated in their superior ability to cope under duress (Burnside, 1978).

Sullivan (1953, p. 310) said, "The greater the degree of maturity, the less will be the interference of anxiety with living, and therefore the less nuisance value one has for oneself and for others." This is also true of the aged and for personnel and caretakers. As stated earlier, nurses must understand their own anxiety to effectively intervene in other people's.

LONELINESS

Loneliness has long been a subject for novelists, poets, and songwriters, but it is now a concern of health care providers also. There are only a few articles about loneliness in the elderly (see Table 5-6). Smith (1975) feels that the greatest problem faced by aged people in and out of nursing homes is the feeling of isolation, of loneliness and hopelessness (see Figure 5-1). And a publication from the Department of Health, Education, and Welfare, *Partnership for Older Americans,* states that, "Isolation and loneliness are related to nutrition." Nutrition is discussed in Chapter 23.

Postmen in Germany (following Sweden's example) are now being used as social workers for elderly and lonely people along their route. See *Security in Old Age* in "Other Resources" at the end of the chapter.

An intensive course was given to the mailmen in a geriatric center to equip them for this work. Their chief function in this role is to assess

TABLE 5-6
JOURNAL ARTICLES ON LONELINESS AND THE ELDERLY

Burnside, Irene Mortenson	Loneliness in old age, *Mental Hygiene*, **55**(3):391–396, July 1971.
Conti, Mary	The loneliness of old age, *Nursing Outlook*, (8):28–30, August 1970.
Curtin, Sharon R.	In praise of old people: In outrage at their loneliness, *Bulletin of the N.Y. Academy of Medicine*, **49**(12):1164–1167, December 1973.
Da Silva, Guy	The loneliness and death of an old man, *Journal of Geriatric Psychiatry*, **1**(1):5–27, Fall 1967.
Faunce, Frances Avery	Loneliness in a nursing home, in Gordon Moss and Walter Moss (eds.), *Growing Old*, Pocket Books, New York, 1975.
Fidler, Joan	Loneliness—The problems of the elderly and retired, *Royal Society of Health Journal*, **96**(1):39–41+, February 1976.
Frances, G., et al.	Long-term residence and loneliness: Myth or reality?, *Journal of Gerontological Nursing*, **5**(1):9–11, January/February 1979.
Jacobs, B. P.	Loneliness. When age brings a crisis, the nurse can restore hope, *Nursing Mirror*, p. 1, **147**:25–27, Oct. 12, 1978.
Kivett, Vira R.	Discriminators of loneliness among the rural elderly: Implications for intervention, *The Gerontologist*, **19**(1):108–115, February 1979.
Lopata, Helen Zaniecki	Loneliness: Forms and components, *Social Problems*, **17**(2):248–262, Fall 1969.
Tannenbaum, David E.	Loneliness in the aged, *Mental Hygiene*, **51**(1):91–99, January 1967.
Thompson, M. K.	Adaptations to loneliness in old age, *Proceedings of the Royal Society of Medicine*, **66**(9):887, September 1973.
Tunstall, Jeremy	*Old and Alone: A Sociological Study of Old People*, Routledge, London, 1966.
Wilson, G. S.	. . . But where is my mince?, *Journal of Long Term Care Administration*, **6**:51–55, Winter 1978.

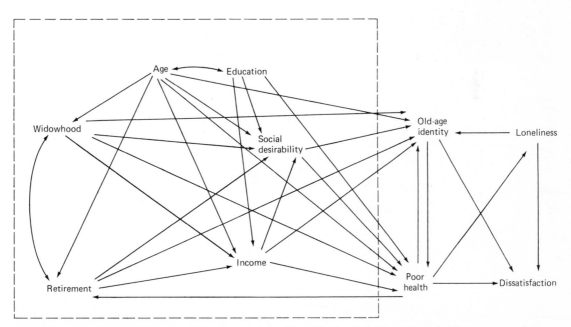

FIGURE 5-1 Path model showing assumed causal network for old age identity. Variables within dashed line are assumed also to influence loneliness and dissatisfaction. [*Elizabeth Mutran and Peter J. Burke, Personalism as a component of old age identity, Research on Aging, 11(1):37–64, March 1979, p. 45. Reprinted by permission of Sage Publications, Inc.*]

and transmit the needs and wishes of older people along their route to the proper authorities. They will also report anything unusual—such as unemptied mail boxes, broken windows, etc. They will provide their clients with coupons permitting them to request a geriatric nurse, emergency food rations, or counseling. The program is operating on an experimental basis in two areas and, if successful, will be expanded across the country.

Two nurses, Gloria Francis and Shirley Odell (1979), measured loneliness in a sample of 42 persons residing in a home for the aged in Virginia. They defined loneliness, from the works of Clark Moustakas (1961) and Harry Stack Sullivan (1953), as the reactive response to separation from persons and things in which one has invested oneself and one's energy. Francis and Odell found that their sample were not lonely, both by objective measures and by the subjective assessment by the elderly.

INTERVENTION IS DIFFICULT

Intervention in the loneliness of the aged is difficult. And just as with anxiety and grief, before we can do anything about the loneliness in old people, we have to be able to handle our own loneliness. One can be lonely even when there are others around or when in the midst of a large crowd. It must be like that for many old people in nursing homes or large institutions. And even though they are surrounded by many people, if one observes them closely they do not interact with the others. If people do not feel some warmth and friendship or input from those about them, they must experience a deep sense of loneliness and isolation. Some have been removed from familiar surroundings and may have left their home permanently. They may have also lost the people in their lives who were important to them and gave their lives meaning. The meaninglessness of their lives is a common complaint of the elderly (Burnside, 1973a).

In the words of Moustakas (1961),

Elder citizens in our society are particularly affected by the social and cultural changes and by the separation, urbanization, alienation, and automation in modern living.

There is no longer a place for old age, no feeling of organic belonging, no reverence or respect or regard for the wisdom and talent of the ancient. Our elder citizens so often have feelings of uselessness, so often experience life as utterly futile. Old age is fertile soil for loneliness and the fear of a lonely old age far outweighs the fear of death in the thinking of many people. Loss of friends and death of contemporaries are realities. The mourning and deep sense of loss are inevitable, but the resounding and lasting depression which results and the emptiness and hopelessness are all a measure of the basic loneliness and anxiety of our time.

CAUSES OF LONELINESS IN THE ELDERLY

1. The death of a spouse certainly increases the loneliness and the bereftness of an aged person. Loss of a sibling, a close neighbor, or a roommate can leave an aged person feeling lonely and without anyone who cares. When a person's last sibling dies, he or she often will talk out the feelings of having outlived all the others. This excerpt is from the letter of an 82-year-old man written to a lifelong friend:

It has been a sad holiday season for us. Tom passed away the fifteenth, although I had been expecting it, it was rough to take when it happened, at least his suffering is over and he has had a lot of it in the past two years. That leaves me the last of the seven Clauson brothers, the closest Clauson relative I now have is one first cousin, living in Wisconsin. Tom was three years younger than I am, he has had a long life considering the heart condition he has had ever since the first World War, he beat it for a long time. I didn't go for his funeral, they were Christian Science; they had a memorial service, he was cremated; I guess that is their religious belief. Tom suggested to me the last time he was here that we not attend the funeral of which ever one went first and also at this time of the year with travel the way it is, and my ability to get around, I was afraid it was too much of an ordeal for me.

2. Pets are very important to some old persons. Loss of a pet an aged person has had for a long time can make life lonelier. One elderly woman could not bury her mynah bird after it died; she wrapped it in foil and put it in her deep freeze for a long while. (See the chapter on pets entitled, "Caring and Care Giving in the Later Years," in Burnside, 1979.)

3. Persons who cannot understand the English language often feel isolated and lonely and brighten up so much if someone can speak the same language they do, and they will enjoy it. Abarca (1980) has written about the results of a one-to-one relationship with a non-English-speaking aged client.

4. Pain can make people very lonely (Burnside, 1971). Old people sometimes think that back pain and aches from rheumatism and arthritis are just a normal part of growing old; sometimes they do not even ask for anything for their pain. Every effort should be made to make them as comfortable as possible, and often an over-the-counter medication can help make them more comfortable. Nurses should always check location of the pain, its severity, and whether a physician has been seen about it.

5. For some people there are certain times of the day that are harder to bear than others, and many say that nighttime or sundown is very difficult for them and they feel lonely. This is commonly handled poorly by the staff. On the 4:00 P.M. to midnight shift, it was not uncommon for me to have to run after some elderly resident who wandered off because of deciding at sundown to go home. Perhaps if we knew the times of day persons experience lonely feelings, we could assist the lonely persons and their peers to know each other. This is not easy to do if the person is withdrawn and quiet; perseverance and patience and not expecting too rapid results are necessary in the care taker.

Nursing care of the lonely aged is not simple to put into practice, for it takes time (which is sometimes precious) and patience (which can run out quickly), and it takes effort (which sometimes one does not have because energies are drained by other tasks). But if one has the time, the patience, and the energy, try the following suggestions.

1. Nurses need to be attentive listeners so that they hear what aged people are trying to tell. The degree of loneliness, the grief, like the level of anxiety, can best be assessed by "attentive listening" and astute observation of behavior.

2. Experiment. If one thing does not work, try something else. Do not give up if a patient refuses a cup of coffee one time, for the next time he or she may accept. Perseverance is important because the negativism that sometimes is encountered might just be a chance to say no to something that the aged person knows will not get him into trouble. Old people do not often get a chance to say no, especially if they are in a situation where they are expected to be compliant most of the time. The "good" patient or client is still often the favored one.

3. Share with peers and ancillary workers what a particular client enjoys. If the client likes to play cribbage, then share the information with the other members who work with the person, so that they can try it also. The needs and wants of older persons are often surprisingly simple and many times bear no resemblance to what we think they need or want or, worst of all, what is "good for them." And so often, staff members know very little about the talents and/or interests of their patients.

4. Nurses should learn to handle their own anxiety, grief, and loneliness.

5. Be creative in approaches to old people. Think of some new ways to approach subjects which may have been previously ignored or handled routinely. What would happen if you brought a lonely, grieving old man a sexy magazine or took an elderly woman, who had given up, to lunch and to get her hair done? Old people do respond to interest, creativity, and spontaneity, and they can be creative, too, if they are given the chance.

The problems in mental health of the aged are very broad; this chapter has offered some statistics to emphasize the problem and then focused on only two states of mental health—anxiety and loneliness. Both are areas in which nurses may have to intervene. Other mental health problems are covered in subsequent chapters. But nurses can also promote better mental health through consultation with non-professionals, especially in nursing homes, and by educating the elderly so they do not have to think of themselves as "crazy" before they will

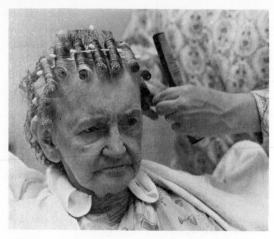

FIGURE 5-2 The important relationship of self-esteem and grooming needs to be underscored. The shabby, disheveled old person who appears that way because of lack of care by nursing personnel continues to reflect a lack of holistic approach to care. (*Courtesy of Harvey Finkle.*)

seek and/or accept help. Nurses can also intervene by stabilizing the milieu (or changing it if necessary) and by continually seeking to find more creative and more therapeutic approaches to the multiple problems in the mental health of the elderly population.

REFERENCES

Abarca, Maria C.: One-to-one relationship therapy: a case study, in Irene M. Burnside (ed.), *Psychosocial Nursing Care of the Aged,* 2d ed., McGraw-Hill, New York, 1980.

Abbey, June C.: Physiology of aging: Implications for nursing, paper presented to class, Andrus Gerontology Center, University of Southern California, March 28, 1974.

Bassuk, Ellen L., and Samuel Gerson: Deinstitutionalization and mental health services, *Scientific American,* **238**(2):46–53, February 1978.

Burnside, Irene M.: Caring and care giving in the later years, in I. Burnside, P. Ebersole, and H. Monea (eds.), *Psychosocial Caring throughout the Life Span,* McGraw-Hill, New York, 1979.

———: Eulogy for Ms. Hogue, *American Journal of Nursing,* **78**(4):624–626, April 1978.

———: Group work among the aged, *Nursing Outlook,* **17**:68–72, June 1969.

———: Loneliness in old age, *Mental Hygiene,* **55**:391–397, July 1971.

———: Loss: A constant theme in group work with the aged, *Hospital and Community Psychiatry,* **21**:173–177, June 1970.

———: Mental health and the aged, in Richard H. Davis (ed.), *Aging: Prospects and Issues,* Andrus Gerontology Center, University of Southern California, 1973a.

———: Multiple losses in the aged: Implications for nursing care, *The Gerontologist,* **13**:157–162, summer 1973b.

Busse, Ewald W., and Eric Pfeiffer: *Mental Illness in Later Life,* American Psychiatric Association, Washington, 1973.

——— and ——— (eds.): *Behavior and Adaptation in Late Life,* Little, Brown, Boston, 1969, pp. 188 and 196–199.

Butler, Robert N.: The future psychiatric care of older people, *Journal of the National Association of Private Psychiatric Hospitals,* **10**(1):4–9, Fall 1978.

———: Mental health and aging: Life cycle perspectives, *Geriatrics,* **29**(11):59–60, November 1974.

Davidson, Robert: Who is to judge what makes behavior "odd"?, *Medical Opinion,* **5**(2):34–39, February 1976.

Eisdorfer, Carl: *Behavioral Problems in Aged,* Sandoz Pharmaceuticals, East Hanover, New Jersey, 1977.

Francis, Gloria, and Shirley Odell: Long-term residence and loneliness: Myth or reality?, *Journal of Gerontological Nursing,* **5**(1):9–11, January–February 1979.

Freud, Sigmund: *Collected Papers,* vol. IV, Ernest Jones (ed.), Joan Riviere (translator), Hogarth, London, 1949.

Fromm-Reichmann, Frieda: Psychiatric aspects of anxiety, in Maurice Stein et al. (eds.), *Identity and Anxiety,* Free Press, New York, 1960, p. 129.

Goldfarb, Alvin I.: Integrated services, in John C. Howells (ed.), *Modern Perspectives in the Psychology of Old Age,* Brunner/Mazel, New York, 1975, pp. 540–569.

Götestam, K. Gunnar: Behavioral and dynamic psychotherapy with the elderly, in James E. Birren and Bruce Sloan (eds.), *Handbook on Mental Health and Aging,* Prentice-Hall, New York, 1980.

Greenberg, Barbara M.: "Therapeutic Effects of Touch on Alteration of Psychotic Behavior in Institutionalized Elderly Patients," unpublished master's thesis, Duke University, Durham, N.C., 1972.

Group for Advancement of Psychiatry: *The Aged and Community Mental Health: A Guide to Program Development,* **8**(81): November 1971.

Gubrium, Jaber F.: Self-conceptions of mental health among the aged, *Mental Hygiene,* **55**(3):398–403 July 1971.

Ingebretsen, Reidun: Psychological services for the elderly, paper presented at the 11th International Congress of Gerontology, Tokyo, Aug. 22, 1978.

Jaro, Gartley: *The Social Epidemiology of Mental Disorders,* Russell Sage Foundation, New York, 1960.

Jarvik, Lissy F., and Dan Russell: Anxiety, aging and the third emergency reaction, *Journal of Gerontology,* **34**(2):197–200, January/February 1979.

Kastenbaum, Robert: . . . Gone tomorrow, *Geriatrics,* **29**(11):127–134, November 1974.

Kierkegaard, Søren: *The Concept of Dread,* Walter Lowrie (translator), Princeton University, Princeton, N.J., 1944.

Kissel, S.: Stress-reducing properties of social stimuli, *Journal of Personality and Social Psychology,* **2**:378–384, 1965.

Lowenthal, Marjorie Fiske, and C. Haven: Interaction and adaptation: Intimacy as a crucial variable, *American Sociological Review,* **31**(1):20–30, February 1968.

McWhorter, Julie M.: Group therapy for high utilizers of clinic facilities, in Irene M. Burnside (ed.), *Psychosocial Nursing Care of the Aged,* 2d ed., McGraw-Hill, New York, 1980.

May, Rollo: Values, myths, and symbols, *American Journal of Psychiatry,* **132**(6):703–706, July 1975.

Miller, A. E.: Geriatrics in psychiatry, *Nursing Mirror,* **142**(23):52–55, June 3, 1976.

Moustakas, Clark E.: *Loneliness,* Prentice-Hall, Inc., Englewood Cliffs, N.J., 1961, p. 26.

Nowlin, John B.: Anxiety during a medical examination, in Erdman Palmore (ed.), *Normal Aging II,* Duke University, Durham, N.C., 1974.

Nuzzillio, Annuzito: Anxiety in the aged, unpublished manuscript, 1972a.

———: Process recordings from class, University of California, San Francisco, 1972b.

Parker, Gordon: *The Bonds of Depression,* Angus & Robertson, Sydney, Australia, 1978.

"Partnership for Older Americans," Department of Health, Education, and Welfare, no. SRS 73-20051, Government Printing Office, Washington, 20402, n.d.

Payne, Edmund C.: Depression and suicide, in John C. Howells (ed.), *Modern Perspectives in the Psychology of Old Age,* Brunner/Mazel, New York, 1975, pp. 290–312.

Peplau, Hildegarde: A working definition of anxiety, in Shirley Burd and Margaret Marshall (eds.), *Some Clinical Approaches to Psychiatric Nursing,* Macmillan, New York, 1966.

Ramshorn, Mary T.: Mental health services, in Judith Haber, Anita M. Leach, Sylvia M. Schudy, Barbara Flynn Sideleau (eds.), *Comprehensive Psychiatric Nursing,* McGraw-Hill, New York, 1978, pp. 10–17.

Rickles, Nathan S., and Betty C. Finkle: Anxiety: Yours . . . and your patient's, *Nursing '73,* **3**:23–26, March 1973.

Schmidt, Leonard J., Adina M. Reinhardt, Robert L. Kane, and Donna M. Olsen: The mentally ill in nursing homes, *Archives of General Psychiatry,* **34**(6):687–691, June 1977.

Smith, Bert Kruger: *Mental Health in Nursing Homes,* The Hogg Foundation for Mental Health, University of Texas, Austin, 1975.

Smith, Huston: *Condemned to Meaning,* Harper & Row, New York, 1965.

Sullivan, Harry S.: *The Interpersonal Theory of Psychiatry,* Norton, New York, 1953, p. 310.

Teeter, Ruth B., Floyd K. Garetz, Winston Teeter, R. Miller, and William Herlaid: Psychiatric disturbances of aged patients in skilled nursing homes, *American Journal of Psychiatry,* **133**(12):1430–1432, December 1976.

Verwoerdt, Adrian: *Clinical Geropsychiatry,* Williams & Wilkins, Baltimore, 1976.

Wells, Charles E. (ed.): *Dementia,* 2d ed., Davis, Philadelphia, 1977.

Williams, Richard Hay: *Perspectives in the Field of Mental Health,* National Institute of Mental Health, Rockville, Md., 1972.

Wilson, Lucille M.: Listening, in Carolyn E. Carlson (ed.), *Behavioral Concepts and Nursing Intervention,* Lippincott, Philadelphia, 1970.

York, Jonathan L.: *Community Mental Health Centers and Nursing Homes: Guidelines for Cooperative Programs,* St. Lawrence Hospital, Lansing, Michigan, 1977.

OTHER RESOURCES

The Psychology of Aging, Stanley Cabanski, Ph.D., and Robert L. Kahn, Ph.D. The strategies of old age are outlined: changes in recall, disengagement, dependence, crises of old age. *Video Nursing,* Black and white, sound, 30 minutes, 16-mm film, videocassette, videotape, audiocassette, 1970.

Security in Old Age, 16 mm/color/24 minutes. Produced by the Swedish National Board of Health and Welfare and the Postal Administration; shows how the community tries in different ways to provide increased security for the elderly, one example being to enlist the aid of rural postmen. Film may be borrowed free of charge from Post film, S-105 00, Stockholm, Sweden.

SIX

ONE-TO-ONE RELATIONSHIP THERAPY WITH THE AGED

Irene Mortenson Burnside

We are all much more simply human than otherwise, be we happy and successful, contented and detached, miserable and mentally disordered, or whatever.

Harry Stack Sullivan

LEARNING OBJECTIVES

- Define relationship therapy.
- Define contract.
- List three criteria in relationship therapy.
- List three behaviors expected of the nurse in the relationship.
- List three guidelines to assist in use of nonverbal content of an interview.
- Describe four modifications necessary in an interview with the aged client.
- Describe three strategies for lowering anxiety in the client.
- Describe the findings of one research study about the health of the aged and pets.
- Define force-field analysis.
- List 10 characteristics of older learners.
- List interventions in learning situations with older adults which may facilitate the learning process.

- Define behavior which may appear during termination.
- Define terminal behavior of a client in a relationship.
- List four purposes of an interview.
- List 10 questions to ask oneself regarding one's own interviewing skills.

This chapter is about one-to-one relationship therapy with the aged and includes guidelines for interviews, modifications of this therapeutic relationship necessary to adapt it to help aged clients, and special aspects of the care of the aged which should be considered, such as the importance of pets and the use of telephone therapy. I will also discuss the implications for instructional methods of certain characteristics of senior adults, since the student nurse must often teach the elderly client during the one-to-one relationship.

GEROPSYCHIATRIC NURSING LITERATURE

Because we still do not have much literature in geropsychiatric nursing, this chapter draws heavily from geropsychiatric literature. The terms *geropsychiatric nursing* did not appear in *The Cumulative Index to Nursing and Allied Health Literature* until 1977. In that year there were a total of 32 articles on the subject. Through October 1978, there were 29 articles published in the English-speaking countries of Australia, Great Britain, and the United States. Consequently, it is not surprising to find that the literature reveals only very scanty information on the use of relationship therapy by nurses with aged clients. There is some discussion of it, however, and it is worth noting that relationship therapy has been an accepted method of psychotherapy, used by psychiatrists, social workers, and psychologists, for many years (Kalkman and Davis, 1974).

One article (Gollicker, 1973) is a case study describing a relationship with a paranoid patient, written when its author was a student nurse. Tyler (1969) reported a study of a nurse influencing the orientation status of a 70-year-old institutionalized man. Another case study by Burnside (1971) described relationship therapy with a 79-year-old man on a back ward of a state hospital. Two other articles deserve mention. Bancroft (1971) wrote a descriptive paper about visits as a volunteer with an 87-year-old woman. Marram (1969), using Tudor's theoretical framework of mutual withdrawal, described the plight of a 72-year-old woman hospitalized in an acute psychiatric ward. Other journal articles (Dominick, 1968; Brown and Ritter, 1972; Rynerson, 1972), which do not deal specifically with one-to-one therapy, are useful as supplemental reading.

The Helping Relationship, by Lawrence M. Brammer, is recommended reading for all who want to better understand the process of helping and to become aware of the skills needed for that process. In his chapter on the characteristics of helpers, Brammer explains that helpers should develop these personal characteristics: (1) awareness of self and values, (2) ability to analyze the helper's own feelings, (3) ability to be a role model and influence, (4) altruism, and (5) a strong sense of responsibility to others. All these characteristics are invaluable to nurses who use relationship therapy with the aged.

DEFINITION

Travelbee (1969) offers a definition of relationship therapy: "The one-to-one relationship is a goal to be achieved. It is the end result of a series of planned purposeful interactions between two human beings, a nurse and a patient. It is also a series of learning experiences for both participants during which they develop increased interpersonal competence." In this chapter *nurse-patient relationship, one-to-one relationship,* and *relationship* are all used synonymously. Details of a one-to-one relationship are described by Travelbee (1969) and Kalkman and Davis (1974).

A student's relationship with an aged person may not be a prolonged period of contact. One reason is that the designated quarter and semester systems in the schools prevent long relationships. Occasionally a student might be able to continue the relationship if instructors cooperate, facilities remain flexible, and the student is desirous of the educational opportunity to improve interpersonal skills and to continue to learn about the aging process.

Gedan et al. (1973) describe staff nurses working as nurse therapists. One of the thrusts of Gedan's paper is that the greatest problem for nurse therapists was unrealistic expectations. This is especially true of student nurses working with aged patients. Goals existing in the student's mind which cannot be fulfilled by the aged patient result in disappointment for both. Sometimes students experience a sense of failure, and at such times need a supportive listener. *Mutually designed goals are a must in relationship therapy with the aged client.*

However, the paper of Gedan et al., like most of the literature on this subject, does not include any case studies of aged clients. They discussed patients who were 22, 23, 25, and 43 years old.

CONTRACT

Students should make contracts for both individual relationships and group work with the elderly. The contract should include the following: (1) the time of day, (2) day of the week, (3) meeting place, (4) expectations of both persons, (5) length of the relationship (this is particularly true if a student has only a 10- or 16-week period for the relationship), and (6) fee, which is also a part of the contract in some instances if the nurse is not a student. Writing the contract information on white paper, using a black felt-tipped pen, helps prevent mixed-up communication. (Because so many elderly persons have failing eyesight, a nurse should get in the habit of using a black felt-tipped pen for written communications with them.) Also, the contract may have to be repeated at each interview until the client grasps the details.

Two important criteria to be met in relationship therapy are goal direction (and the goals should be agreed on by both the nurse and the aged client) and therapist control. The word *control* is often offensive to students, but in this case it is meant to suggest responsibility, concern, and structure more than absolute control. Structure helps to decrease anxiety for both the student and the client and needs to be presented early in the relationship with the aged. The same is true for the student; the preceptor should offer enough structure to decrease the student's anxiety so that the student functions better. Control is also important with confused elderly and manipulative elderly persons. The student needs to learn the setting of limits in the early interviews; for example, elderly persons who experience conversation deprivation are often reluctant to let student therapists leave.

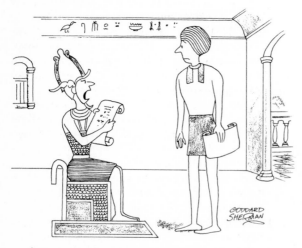

"YOU CALL THIS A CONTRACT? WHY, IT'S NOT WORTH THE PAPYRUS IT'S WRITTEN ON!"

FIGURE 6-1

CLIENT-NURSE RELATIONSHIPS

To establish a therapeutic relationship with an aged client, the nurse must gain rapport early in the interview, be supportive, and be an active listener. One must remember that "even the most garrulous and rambling patient communicates more than any specific answer can provide and the mute patient may declare in his silence, his fear, anger, uncertainty or mistrust of the interviewer. The interviewer should be particularly aware exactly when nonverbal cues, i.e., a tremor, tears, choking voice, etc., are apparent. Timing is very important" (McLeod, 1978).

Listen to the form of thought—is it logical, circumstantial, talking around the point, blocking, perseveration? Listen also to the content—are there ruminations, obsessions, delusions, or hallucinations?

It is also important to pay attention to the behavior, appearance, talk, and affect—is it appropriate or otherwise? What is the range of affect? It is the sign of a sophisticated interviewer to be able to bring together the verbal and nonverbal information offered by the client (McLeod, 1978).

If one is interviewing an elderly client, particular attention must be paid to these three areas: (1) orientation with respect to time, place, and person; (2) memory for recent and distant past events; and (3) insight and judgment.

The following general guidelines[1] to use in the therapeutic setting may be helpful to nurses who have little interviewing experience.

Guidelines for the Interview

1. Edicts are not therapeutic—pontifications tell more about the therapist than the client.
2. Encourage the use of the first person singular; use *I* and not *we* or *one.*
3. Many people confuse *feel* with *think,* and so they ask how someone feels when they want to know what someone thinks about something. Use *feel* when you are asking about feelings. Feelings have to do with

sadness, joy, anger, anxiety, etc., and are always accompanied by physical manifestations. Clients, when asked how they feel, may respond that they feel "rotten," "fine," "good," "strong," etc., which are reports on the state of their physical/psychological health.

4. Encourage "I" messages and avoid telling clients where they are with "you" messages, e.g., "You are now . . . ." Encourage the client to begin sentences with *I.*
5. Change the vague to the definite and the abstract to the concrete; e.g., change *they* to someone specific, *somewhere* to a specific place.
6. Change the negative to the positive and the outdated to the current, e.g., the "there and then" to the "here and now." "I didn't feel sad," leads to "But what do you feel now?"
7. Watch changes in posture, emphasis, gesture, modulation of voice or emotion, or topics under discussion.
8. Avoid doing for the client what the client can do better alone. If the client asks a question, ask the client to change the question to a statement. The answer to the question will often then be self-evident. (For example, "Should I move in with my children?" might be restated, "I do not want to move in with my children.") Respect clients. Request that they do as much as possible for themselves. The solutions provided that way are likely to be more effective than those of the interviewer because expectations of the interviewer regarding background, financial position, ethical codes, etc., are rarely those of the client.
9. Statements of guilt are often also statements of resentment; sometimes it is appropriate to invite the client to explore the feelings behind these statements. (This is particularly true in grief reactions after loss of a spouse.)
10. "Why" questions are often unanswerable for they are usually countered by another "why." The answers either become metaphysical or lead to defensive posturing.
11. Do not be afraid to confess ignorance.
12. Do not gossip, i.e., discuss persons who are absent.
13. Note unsolicited affirmation or denials.

---

[1] Adapted from W. R. McLeod, 1978.

14. Whenever using the word *it,* consider that *I* might well be more appropriate; e.g., "It is difficult" then becomes "I am difficult."

15. We may be easily beguiled by a client's assertions of helplessness, timidity, etc. Such statements are often made from well-defended positions of strength. Patients who declare, "I am just hanging on" have often been just doing so for years.

MODIFICATIONS NECESSARY FOR THE AGED CLIENT

All the above are the basic principles of one-to-one relationships, but they need to be adapted in several ways to fit the needs of the aged or very old client. The sensory losses of the aged, and particularly of the very old, are an important factor which must be considered. Nurses must learn to communicate effectively in spite of clients' difficulties such as loss of hearing, diminished sight or total blindness, diminished tactile sensations, and edentulousness impairing speech. Aphasia can pose another communication problem with poststroke patients, who also may be very depressed. A distinct gentleness seems to be necessary for working with centenarians, and nurses working with clients suffering from chronic brain syndrome must take into account their shortened attention span.

Astute attention to physical problems and symptoms should increase the nurse's therapeutic effectiveness with the elderly. Changes in physical health, for example, may necessitate changes in the scheduling of interviews. And physical problems may have to be taken care of before an interview can get off the ground. A patient with severe emphysema may need medication for that condition to be able to carry on an interview, for instance, or a patient who has pain may need pain medication prior to the interview. Such a holistic approach places much responsibility on the skill and sensitivity of the nurse in assessing an elderly client. The danger of this approach is that the client will see the nurse as interested solely in physical problems; the nurse should remember to reinforce the psychological aspects of the interview as well. Nurses themselves may lose sight of the psychological impact when they dwell on physical complaints.

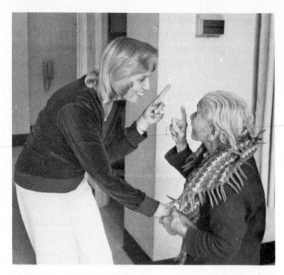

FIGURE 6-2 Old people do respond well to psychotherapeutic intervention, but modifications in the therapeutic technique are needed. The activity and spontaneity of the nurse is important, especially with frail elderly, as seen in this photo. (*Courtesy of Anthony J. Skirlick, Jr.*)

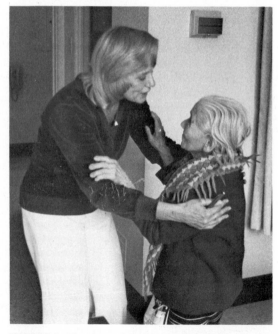

FIGURE 6-3 The generous use of touch during interactions is important. Even though this elderly woman is Japanese and her culture does not use as much touch as some, it is obvious she is comfortable with the nurse. (*Courtesy of Anthony J. Skirlick, Jr.*)

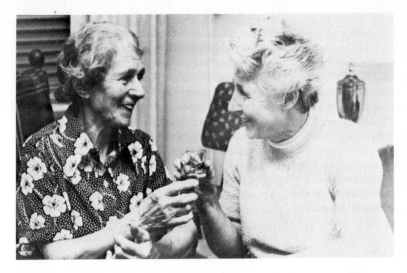

FIGURE 6-4 The nurse may sometimes be in the pseudofamily role or be a confidante. "Twenty-five percent of older people have no relatives or significant others. . . . [That] means that out of the present 23 million persons over 65, about 6 million are without significant others" (Robert Butler, on "Over Easy" TV program, October 30, 1978). (*Courtesy of Lea Meyer.*)

Pfeiffer (1973) offers some basic concepts which he has written for physicians, but an eclectic nurse will quickly take some of those basic ideas and tailor them to fit the needs of aged clients. The nurse must realize that old people do respond very well to medical and psychotherapeutic intervention. A second principle is that they respond well only if there are modifications in both the diagnostic and therapeutic techniques which consider both the special needs and the limitations of the elderly. Both of these suggestions are Pfeiffer's, as is the following list of modifications and special techniques to consider:

1. Important to reduce anxiety in initial treatment session
2. Attention to nonverbal communication
3. Need for multidimensional assessment
4. Need for interaction with family members
5. Slow pacing of history taking
6. Slow pacing of instructions to patient
7. Need for coordination of services

I would add the following considerations:

1. Importance of nurse role modeling for the staff on how a one-to-one relationship is conducted
2. Importance of excellent charting on the progress of the patient
3. Clear communication about the client to staff and relatives

4. Respect of the aged person's privacy during meetings; also observance of confidentiality regarding information revealed
5. Importance of activity, spontaneity of nurse therapist
6. Generous use of touch during interactions (unless intolerable to client)
7. Nurse therapist accepting "pseudofamily" role when appropriate
8. Accurate assessment of own feelings about aging and the aged client in the relationship

Butler (1973) recommends that, in this kind of relationship, "One must work compassionately and carefully to understand and encourage a realistic lowering of defenses rather than attacking them overtly." He also believes that efforts at restitution are crucial in psychotherapy with the elderly since one must deal with grief, loss, and physical decline. Lowenthal and Haven (1968) have explained the importance of a confidante for the elderly, and the nurse should consider this in finding and setting goals in one-to-one relationships.

REDUCING ANXIETY

Nurses who have been taught psychiatric concepts will be constantly aware of the need to decrease anxiety in interviews. However, the cues to anxiety in the aged and interventions have not been spelled out clearly in the literature. Suggestions on how to decrease anxiety (Kalkman and Davis, 1974) are applicable for aged clients; some of these are (1) serenity of the nurse, (2) nurse's physical presence and nonverbal reassurance, (3) detection of covert anxiety, (4) listening, (5) awareness of demands as expression of anxiety, (6) other measures to reduce anxiety such as performing some routine task, (7) supportive measures by the nurse, (8) facilitating desensitization, (9) planning a daily schedule, and (10) encouraging socialization.

Some very specific methods in addition to the above may be helpful: (1) share food and beverages (Burnside, 1970); (2) pace one's self to the aged; (3) make allowances for sensory deficit (sit closer to visually impaired and/or hard-of-hearing person); (4) use touch generously; (5) avoid asking many questions; (6) assign tasks which patient can successfully accomplish to avoid "catastrophic reactions"; and (7) constantly assess client's energy level during interview.

SOME PRACTICAL SUGGESTIONS

In both individual and group work with the aged person, the nurse-therapist has to be active; this is especially so in the beginning of the relationship. The client who is uncomfortable and seems ill should be made more comfortable and the anxiety level reduced.

There are physical comforts that should be taken care of during each interview. The room should be private so that others do not overhear the conversation. The surroundings should be quiet so the patient can hear and is not distracted by noises and activities of others. The temperature of the room should be comfortable. There should be no bright lights or glaring sunlight. Clients with eye problems, particularly, complain about this; therefore, they should not sit facing a window with a glare. Some patients prefer hard, straight-backed chairs to large, overstuffed ones.

It is sometimes important to begin the interview with superficial subjects and then move on to problem areas. Neophyte nurses often begin interviews with, "How are you?" and then are disappointed because the entire interview is spent on somatic complaints only. A more open-ended question permits the client who wishes to do so to discuss a variety of subjects. The client may have other problems besides physical complaints; old people usually do.

Be sure to take into account the sensory deficits. Check out immediately in the first interview how well the clients can see and hear. If they do not hear well, sit closer to them. If they do not see well, move in until they say you are within their range of vision. This might make nurses uncomfortable, and they may have to accustom themselves to such physical closeness in order to communicate. Speak as loud as is necessary to be heard, and speak slowly so that words are not missed.

If the client is depressed, acknowledge the fact by noticing. Comments such as, "That must be pretty rough," or "No wonder you are sad," or "You have had a lot of losses to contend with," convey empathy and concern.

Although nurses must listen closely to what clients are saying verbally, they must also be aware of nonverbal communication; e.g., observe the face for wincing, quivering of the lips, or tears forming in the eyes. Anxiety is often shown by movement of the extremities; observing hand, foot, and leg movements is also important. Smokers also indicate anxiety by the amount of smoking, the nervous gestures with

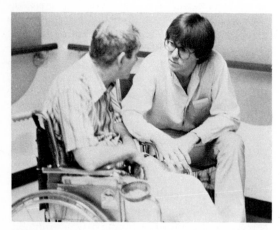

FIGURE 6-5 Physical closeness is important in reducing anxiety in an interaction. Note the attentive listening and also the proximity of the therapist in this photograph. (*Courtesy of Anthony J. Skirlick, Jr.*)

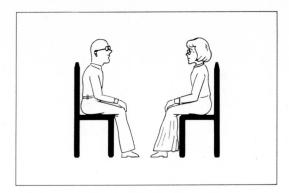

FIGURE 6-6 Ordinarily the interviewer should sit very close to and vis-à-vis a confused aged client. Seating as close as 1 to 2 feet is acceptable when there is loss of vision or hearing. The "bubble" can be greater at the beginning of the interview and then lessened as the interview progresses if the individual seems guarded or frightened. Closeness also permits the interviewer to easily reach out and touch the aged person. The interviewer should, of course, be seated, with head as near to client's eye level as possible.

the cigarette, cigar, or pipe, and, occasionally, chewing tobacco or snuff.

Instructions should be given slowly and clearly and should also be written down to be read at a later date when the anxiety level is lowered. Be sure the client knows what is to happen next; when, where, and how long you will meet the next time; also, anything you expect to be done in the interim. (See Table 6-1 regarding instructions for teaching the aged person.)

As much as possible, offer a ray of hope to the client. In a one-to-one relationship with a dying patient, saying "I will see you on Tuesday," gives him something to look forward to. One student working with withdrawn long-term hospitalized individuals asked what they would like brought to them and then brought the chocolate, the grapes, cigarettes, or whatever the special desire was. Meeting these needs is

TABLE 6-1
INSTRUCTIONAL IMPLICATIONS OF LABORATORY EXPERIMENTAL GERO-PSYCHOLOGICAL RESEARCH

Instructional Variable	Researcher(s)	Implications
Rate of presentation of information	Canestrari (1963) Monge and Hultsch (1971)	Present new information at a fairly slow rate Let adult learner proceed at his or her own rate whenever feasible Provide adult learner with ample time to respond to questions Present a limited amount of material in any single presentation to prevent swamping effects
Organization of information	Hultsch (1969, 1971) Lawrence (1967) Rabbitt (1968)	Present new information in a highly organized fashion Use section headings, handouts, summaries, etc., so that adult learner can get a "handle" on material If memory processes are taxed in a learning project, encourage adult learner to use retrieval plans Avoid introduction of irrelevant information in order to prevent confusion If visual displays are used, employ simple stimulus configurations
Mode of presenting information	Denney and Denney (1974) Taub (1972) Taub and Kline (1976)	Use auditory mode of presentation when presenting discrete bits of information to be used immediately Use visual mode when presenting textual materials to capitalize on opportunity for review during reading Utilize models to facilitate strategy development

TABLE 6-1

INSTRUCTIONAL IMPLICATIONS (*Continued*)

Instructional Variable	Researcher(s)	Implications
Covert strategies	Canestrari (1963) Hulicka and Grossman (1967)	Encourage adult learner to generate his or her own mediators
	Labouvie-Vief and Gonda (1976) Robertson-Tchabo et al. (1976) Treat and Reese (1976)	Supply adult learner with mediators when necessary With concrete material, imagery mediators are superior to verbal mediators and interacting images better than conjunctive images Whenever feasible, train adult learner in use of mnemonic devices Encourage adult learner to generate covert monitoring verbalizations and provide training when necessary
Meaningfulness of material	Arenberg (1968)	Present information which is meaningful to adult learner Assess cognitive structure of adult learner to ensure that material is introduced at appropriate level Use examples, illustrations, etc., which are concrete
Degree of learning	Hulicka and Weiss (1965)	Provide ample opportunity for adult learner to over-learn material before moving on to new material Remove time constraints from instructional and evaluation process
Introduction of new material	Christensen (1968) Heglin (1956) Lair et al. (1969) Sanders et al. (1976)	As initial step in learning, identify and eliminate inappropriate responses which may "compete" with appropriate response Organize instructional units so that potentially interfering materials are spaced far away from each other Stress differences between concepts before similarities Make instructional sequence parallel hierarchy of knowledge in any given area Instructional procedures should be premised on knowledge of conditions required for a type of learning based on task analysis Introduce a variety of techniques for solving problems
Transfer effects	Hultsch (1969)	Take advantage of experience the adult learner possesses Relate new information to what adult learner already knows Develop learning sets which maximize opportunity for positive transfer effects (i.e., learning to learn effects)
Feedback effects	Bellucci and Hoyer (1975) Hornblum and Overton (1976) Schultz and Hoyer (1976)	Provide verbal feedback concerning correctness of responses after each component of task is completed Do *not* assume that initially poor performance on a novel, complex task is indicative of low aptitude
Climate	Birkhill and Schaie (1975) Leech and Witte (1971) Ross (1968)	Establish a supportive climate Engage adult learner in information-oriented, collaborative evaluation Encourage adult learner to take educated guesses

SOURCE: Morris A. Okun, 1977.

perhaps more important than one realizes. Food can be an adjunct to therapy with the elderly (Burnside, 1971, 1970).

Pace yourself to the aged person; do not move quickly, rush, or jostle (Burnside, 1980). Simply getting out of the chair may be difficult. Even if the time together is brief, e.g., as in brief psychotherapy (Godbole and Verinis, 1974), take time, and make the quality, not the quantity, of the time spent together the main thing.

An important suggestion is this one: *Never underestimate the potential for growth and change in the elderly person.* The elderly are usually sold short. Expectations that they can change and treating them with that anticipation may well produce change faster than the nurse expects.

TERMINATION

To be able to handle the termination process well is a sign of sophistication in any nurse-client relationship. For some students, termination is a very difficult time. In a termination exercise in class, students were to write a good-bye message on a balloon, inflate it, and give it to a classmate. One student wrote, "Hello." Her explanation, "I can't handle good-byes." It can also be a difficult period for the elderly client; however, they are generally quite experienced in the "good-byes" of life. It is helpful to plan with the client what he or she will do after the relationship. I do not believe in final terminations with the elderly. If a student chooses to send a card or note, or visit again, or phone the client, it seems to ease the terminating; this offers some sort of future for the aged individual.

One distinct advantage in not terminating the relationship abruptly is that it gives the student a chance to watch the progress of the client and to assess how successful the intervention was during the relationship. It also serves as a preventive; if the elderly person changes suddenly, the student can advise or counsel the person to seek help.

If there is no sadness when the student terminates a relationship, one is inclined to wonder if there was much involvement in the first place. Involvement with the elderly is not a lack of professionalism; it is a necessity to be maximally therapeutic in the one-to-one relationship.

As an instructor, I have found I can teach some students more effectively by the use of poetry. These beautiful lines by Rilke (1957) are especially apropos when explaining the termination phase of the one-to-one relationship:

> Who has turned us about like this, that we, do what we may, forever assume the attitude of one about to depart? As he on the highest hill who sees his valley one last time will turn and linger—so do we live forever taking our leave.

FORCE-FIELD APPROACH

Egan (1975) has explained the force-field analysis approach to problem solving, which might be useful for the nurse-therapist in a one-to-one relationship. *Force-field analysis* is actually a sophisticated term for a process that involves problem solving. The client must perceive the goal to see what forces keep him or her moving toward it. Then it is up to the client to choose the practical means, and those in accord with personal values, to implement them and to evaluate progress. The field is the area in which the person struggles to live and function more effectively.

Some well-defined, concrete suggestions for the nurse are offered here as outlined by Egan (1975):

1. Identify and clarify the problems in the client's life.
2. Establish priorities as to which one needs immediate attention; do not work on too many problems at once.
3. Establish concrete, workable goals.
4. Take a census of the means available for achieving each concrete goal. List the facilitating forces and the restraining forces.
5. Choose means in keeping with the client's value system which will be most effective to achieve the goals.
6. Establish criteria by which the programs can be evaluated.
7. Implement; use chosen means to achieve established goals.
8. Review and evaluate the client's progress.

This summary of the steps can be explained by a simple and rather poignant case example:

1. The identified problem was that an old man in a nursing home was illiterate and desperately wanted to learn to write his name before he died.
2. That was the priority over other social and health problems he also described.
3. His concrete goal was to learn to write his signature.
4. The means available included a student nurse in a one-to-one relationship and a nurse's aide who was very fond of the gentleman and looked on him as a grandfather figure since he reminded her of her own grandfather.
5. The client at that time did not wish to learn to write anything else or to learn to read, so nothing else was undertaken.
6. The criteria to evaluate the outcome were: Would he be pleased with the way he learned to sign his name? Was it legible? Could he use his signature?
7. The means chosen to achieve the goal was the tutelage of the student nurse. She taught him all she knew about writing and penmanship, and she even learned some Palmer method penmanship to teach him more skillfully. She wrote his name down and had him write over it. She also had other people write his name so he could practice on the signatures and decide which one felt right for him. The nurse's aide incorporated the practice of the signature into his daily care routine. One was done each day which he could privately share with the student nurse when she came on her weekly interview.
8. The evaluation came when he signed his social security check for the first time with his name instead of an *X!* He had, indeed, learned to sign his name legibly, and it was legally acceptable.

TELEPHONE THERAPY

Butler and Lewis (1973) describe the importance of telephone psychotherapy with the aged. This should be considered by nurses in rural areas or by one with a large case load or clients who lack transportation, energy, finances, or all three.

In conducting a follow-up survey of persons in the community who had attempted suicide, I was surprised at the sharing and openness of all the interviewees on the first phone call, and most especially, the older people. Telephones are very important to housebound or bedridden aged persons.

Many older people living alone fear they will fall or be taken suddenly ill and be unable to call for help. The telephone reassurance call provides a daily contact for an older person who might otherwise have no outside contact for long periods of time because of having no friends or relatives close by, or none at all.

Telephone reassurance calls are made at a predetermined time each day. If the person does not answer, help is immediately sent—a neighbor, relative, or nearby police or fire station is asked to make a personal check.

Telephone reassurance generally costs little in money and can be provided by callers of any age from teen-agers to older people themselves. Such calls are sponsored by a variety of organizations ranging from women's clubs to health agencies. See "Other Resources" at the end of the chapter for available publications on this topic.

IMPORTANCE OF PETS

The importance of pets has received little attention by any of the disciplines. I think veterinarians probably have the most pragmatic information regarding pets and the elderly. The PBS TV show on the elderly, "Over Easy," frequently has a veterinarian on the program. Students working in therapeutic relationships need to be very much aware of the role a pet may play in an old person's life and include the pets in the nursing care plan because McGinnis (1978) says, "For some individuals, pets are an integral part of self-identity and self-esteem."

If clients have serious heart disease, pets may increase their chances of survival the first year after hospitalization. Erika Friedman (1978) reported that social isolation and lack of com-

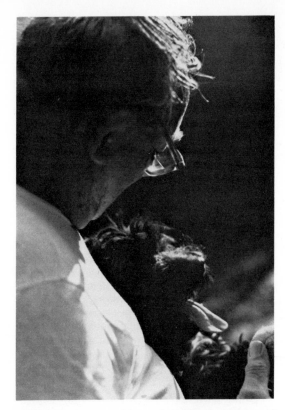

FIGURE 6-7 Pet ownership may be an important source of companionship with positive health benefits. The therapist should remember that for some individuals the pets they own may contribute to self-identity and self-esteem. (*Courtesy of Anthony J. Skirlick, Jr.*)

This relationship held up regardless of how serious the illness. All 92 subjects (64 men, 28 women) had been admitted to the hospital with a diagnosis of heart attack or severe chest pain. They were placed in coronary or medical intensive care units. Each person's illness was "graded": two points for heart attack, one for severe chest pain, one point if congestive heart failure was present, and a point for irregular cardiac rhythm. Each previous heart attack added one-half point. This score, called the *physiological index,* or *PI,* and pet ownership were singled out among the many factors influencing patient recovery.

Subtracting 43 subjects who were dog owners from the group (on the assumption that the need to walk dogs added a possibly confusing variable) made no difference. The owners of other pets—including cats, birds, gerbils, even iguanas—were more likely to be alive after 1 year.

Friedman suggested that pet ownership may be an important source of companionship with positive health benefits. Although it is not known how the process works, perhaps the specific kind of person who owns a pet is more likely to survive. She recommended that pet ownership be investigated as a therapeutic tool for discharged patients, especially those who lead relatively isolated lives.

This is apparently one of the first research studies to consider pets as "significant others" and to consider pet ownership as affecting physical health. It may well be a pioneer study.

panionship have been shown to increase the likelihood of developing coronary heart disease (CHD).

One measure of companionship—pet ownership—turned out to have a strong positive correlation with 1-year survival! In a study of 92 CHD patients, 39 did not own pets. Of these subjects, 11 died within 1 year of admission to the hospital; in contrast, all but 3 of the 53 pet owners were alive at the end of a year.

The figures Friedman collected were part of a much larger profile of social and psychological data on CHD patients, including whether the person lived alone. When all the variables were compared statistically, pet ownership definitely seemed associated with a better posthospital outcome.

GUIDELINES AND SUGGESTIONS

The rest of this chapter will offer in a schematic way guidelines and suggestions for interviewing and forming a therapeutic one-to-one relationship with an elderly client. Many, not all, of them have been mentioned or explained earlier in the chapter, but I hope students will find these lists handy for refreshing the memory and quick reference. At the end, I have added a list of questions which I have found useful to ask myself to increase my own sensitivity to the needs of aged clients and to ensure that I am meeting these needs in my relationship with clients.

AIMS OF THE INTERVIEW

It is sometimes difficult to sort out from the information gained in an interview what is relevant and important. In order to do so, it is usually useful to keep in mind the aims of the interview, which in this case might be stated as follows (McLeod, 1978):

1. To establish a therapeutic alliance between the interviewer and interviewee.
2. To arrange the history in a linear fashion.
3. To abstract the significant life events.
4. To focus on the current crisis.
5. To integrate these factors with the response of the client.
6. To assess the mental and physical status before speculation as to the "why" of the patient's presentation.
7. To establish the problem areas to be attended to which can be settled by medical, psychological, social, group, or one-to-one psychotherapeutic intervention.

Hear the needs. Devising a plan of management provides the person with someone who really listens; this may be alien to the client's experience (McLeod, 1978).

SPECIFIC GUIDELINES IN ONE-TO-ONE INTERVIEWS

1. Be sure the client is comfortable in regard to chair (or bed) and that pain is under control. Try not to interview someone who is obviously in pain.
2. Select appropriate milieu for interview; privacy is important. Try to have the correct temperature for the aged client, not the interviewer, and no bright lights or glares. Do not have the client face a window with a glare. Some old persons prefer hard, straight-backed chairs to large, overstuffed ones.
3. Check sensory losses early in the first interview. See "Interviewing the Aged" (Burnside, 1980).
4. Sit close to clients with sensory loss and/or those experiencing confusion or disorientation. See Figure 6-6.
5. Use eye contact.
6. Establish rapport rapidly.

7. Show respect; be attentive.
8. Recognize the client as a person.
9. Know the person's correct name; use it often.
10. Give options and explain them (there are fewer and fewer choices as one ages).
11. Use reminiscing strategies when possible to gain information. Show that clients are in control of their lives.
12. If possible, use a conversational style instead of a structured outline to fill in.
13. If low self-esteem is observed and negative views of society internalized, intervene, e.g., point out client's strengths.
14. Be an advocate.
15. Watch for fatigue; take interest in physical complaints. Keep interviews brief; however, gauge the client's attention span.
16. Slow your pace if necessary to match client's needs; develop unhurried style.
17. Assess your own anxiety as well as client's.
18. Allow enough time for client to think and to respond.
19. Explain why information is needed.
20. Be honest.
21. Stimulate memory chains; attempt to stimulate patterns of association that will improve the client's recall.
22. Aid in reality testing.
23. Include the client in everything.
24. Give instructions slowly and clearly and write them down to be read later when the anxiety level is lowered. Be sure the patient knows what is to happen next, i.e., when, where, and how long you will meet the next time and also anything you expect the client to do in the interim.
25. If clients are depressed, acknowledge the fact by commenting on the way they feel. Statements such as, "That must be pretty rough," or "No wonder you are sad," or "You have had a lot of losses to contend with," convey empathy and concern.
26. Be aware of nonverbal communication; e.g., observe the face for wincing, quivering of the lips, or tears forming in the eyes. Anxiety is often shown by movement of the extremities; observing hand, foot, and leg movements is also important. Smokers indicate anxiety by amount of smoking, nervous gestures with the cigarette, cigar, or pipe, and, occasionally, chewing tobacco or snuff.

27. The need to be needed is often overlooked in working with the elderly client. The interviewer should try to assess this need.
28. Help the client to leave the interview feeling that someone cares.
29. Remember that the old person has something to teach you and probably would be happy to do so.
30. Always look at your own behavior and its impact on the interview.
31. Take care of yourself; i.e., watch for overscheduling, overcommitment, depression, overextension, weariness, frustration, etc.

While I have given general guidelines for nurse-therapists, a social worker, Mary Gwynne Schmidt (1975), has sensitively selected points to remember when working with the old-old.

GUIDELINES FOR INTERVIEWING THE OLD-OLD[2]

1. The interviewer should be alert to special challenges, e.g., intermittent confusion, chronic confusion, dysphagia, problems of vision and hearing, unwillingness, and overprotective nurses and/or relatives.
2. *Go slowly* is the overarching rule.
3. Reduce suspicion and mistrust.
4. Let the respondent observe the interviewer for awhile, for instance. In institutional settings, the interviewer may appear first as a participant observer on the ward rather than as interviewer.
5. Interact with staff on a friendly basis in front of the interviewee.
6. In community setting, let the respondent examine interviewer; talk with other members of household first, then aged person.
7. Do not be pressing or pushy; maintain a low-key manner.
8. Use terms which are familiar to the aged client.
9. Endeavor to leave respondent with a sense of accomplishment.
10. Be aware that appropriate affect may be independent of articulate speech.

---

[2] Adapted from Mary Gwynne Schmidt, 1975.

11. Watch for relatives and nurses who want to censor your content.
12. Do not compete with the visitor's time.

QUESTIONS FOR SELF-EVALUATION

The following questions should help heighten a nurse's self-awareness and also be a guide to special areas of concern in one-to-one relationships with the elderly. Process recordings will help students analyze abilities and behavior; however, the students need immediate feedback from the instructor in order to improve interviewing skills and, if necessary, to change their behavior.

1. Do I handle denial without completely stripping him or her of this defense mechanism?
2. Do I reality-test well and consistently?
3. Do I differentiate between acute and chronic brain syndromes?
4. Do I alert staff members to the changes I see?
5. Do I know techniques to increase self-esteem?
6. Do I recognize cues to anxiety and seek ways to reduce the anxiety?
7. Do I know the drug regimen of the patient and observe for reactions?
8. Do I know "cries for help" in the potential suicidal person?
9. Do I check out suicidal ideation in deeply depressed aged individuals?
10. Do I handle my own losses, grief, anxiety, anger, and depression effectively?
11. Do I try to manipulate the environment of the aged when it would improve their lot?
12. Do I encourage the uniqueness and individuality of the aged client?

This chapter has not thus far mentioned the importance of the warmth and closeness in the relationship. With the loss of so many significant others, the nurse may need to make a special effort to show concern about the aged individual. Caring may be more important than the nurse realizes. One poet, in her succinct imagery, has described the loss of significant others for an elderly woman (Swenson, 1970):

Midnight on the subway I watch
an old woman fall asleep
against the handle of her new rake.
But it is mid-summer.
Whom does she have for leaves?

REFERENCES

Bancroft, Anne Vandermay: Now she's a disposition problem, *Perspectives in Psychiatric Care,* **9**(3):96–102, 1971.

Brammer, Lawrence M.: *The Helping Relationship: Process and Skills,* Prentice-Hall, New York, 1973.

Brown, Lucille, and Jennie Ritter: Reality therapy for the geriatric psychiatric patient, *Perspectives in Psychiatric Care,* **10**(3):135–138, July/August 1972.

Burnside, Irene M.: Crisis intervention with hospitalized geriatric patients, *Journal of Psychiatric Nursing,* **8**(2):17–20, March/April 1970.

——————: Gerontion: A case study, *Perspectives in Psychiatric Care,* **9**(3):103–109, 1971.

——————: Interviewing the aged, in Irene Mortenson Burnside (ed.), *Psychosocial Nursing Care of the Aged,* 2d ed., McGraw-Hill, New York, 1980.

Butler, Robert N., and Myrna I. Lewis: *Aging and Mental Health: Positive Psychosocial Approach,* Mosby, St. Louis, 1973, p. 235.

Cumulative Index to Nursing and Allied Health Literature, The Seventh Day Adventist Hospital Association, Glendale, Calif., 1956, October 1978.

Dominick, Joan: Nursing care factors in psychotic depressive reactions in elderly patients, *Perspectives in Psychiatric Care* **6**(1):28–32, January/February 1968.

Egan, Gerard: *The Skilled Helper: A Model for Systematic Helping and Interpersonal Relating,* Brooks/Cole, Belmont, Calif., 1975.

Friedman, Erika: Your pet may be your best friend, *American Heart News,* Annual Meeting Editions, Dallas, Texas, Nov. 17, 1978, p. 2.

Gedan, Sharon, Lei Honda, and Joan Marks: The nurse therapist: A staff nurse position which emphasizes clinical practice, *Journal of Psychiatric Nursing,* **11**(1):18–23, 1973.

Godbole, Anil, and S. Scott Verinis: Brief psychotherapy in the treatment of emotional disorders in physically ill geriatric patients, *Gerontologist,* **14**(2):143–148, April 1974.

Gollicker, Jacqueline: A new life at 77, *Nursing Mirror,* **137**(2):34–37, July 13, 1973.

Kalkman, Marion E., and Anne J. Davis (eds.): *New Dimensions in Mental Health: Psychiatric Nursing,* McGraw-Hill, New York, 1974.

Lowenthal, M., and C. Haven: Interaction and adaptation: Intimacy as a crucial variable, *American Sociological Review,* **33**(1):20–30, February 1968.

McGinnis, Terri: Why people own pets, *Family Health,* **110**(10):14, October 1978.

McLeod, W. R.: Making the most of the interview: Psychological and psychiatric aspects, *Patient Management,* **2**(7):9–16, July 1978.

Marram, Gwen D.: Toward a greater understanding of mutual withdrawal in a psychiatric setting, *Journal of Psychiatric Nursing,* **7**(4):160–163, July/August 1969.

Okun, Morris A.: Implications of geropsychological research, for the instruction of older adults, *Adult Education,* **XXVII**(3):139–155, 1977.

Pfeiffer, Eric: Interacting with older patients, in Ewald Busse and Eric Pfeiffer (eds.), *Mental Illness in Later Life,* American Psychiatric Association, Washington, 1973.

Rilke, Rainer Maria: *The Duino Elegies,* Harry Behn (translator), Peter Pauper, Mount Vernon, N.Y., 1957.

Rynerson, Barbara C.: Need for self-esteem in the aged: A literature review, *Journal of Psychiatric Nursing,* **10**(1):22–25, January/February 1972.

Schmidt, Mary Gwynne: Interviewing the old-old, *The Gerontologist,* **15**(6):544–547, December 1975.

Sullivan, Harry Stack: *The Interpersonal Theory of Psychiatry,* Norton, New York, 1953, p. xviii.

Swenson, Karen: *The New York Times Book of Verse,* Thomas Lask (ed.), Macmillan, New York, 1970, p. 11.

Travelbee, Joyce: Aspects of the one-to-one relationship, in Joyce Travelbee (ed.), *Intervention in Psychiatric Nursing Process in the 1:1 Relationship,* Davis, Philadelphia, 1969.

Tudor, Gwen: A sociopsychiatric nursing intervention in a problem of mutual withdrawal in a mental hospital, *Psychiatry,* **15**(2):193–217, 1952.

Tyler, Carol Ruth: The nurse's influence on Mr. Brown's orientation, in *ANA Clinical Conferences,* Appleton Century Crofts, New York, 1969.

TELEPHONE REASSURANCE RESOURCES

Guidelines for a Telephone Reassurance Program, Report on the Michigan program, available from AoA, DHEW Publication no. (OHD) 73-20200, Washington.

Suggestions for Operating a Ring-A-Day Telephone Reassurance Program, Nassau County Dept. of Senior Citizen Affairs, One Old County Road, Carle Place, N.Y. 11514.

Telephone Reassurance, a People-to-People Program, Public Information Office, State of Nebraska Advisory Committee on Aging, State House Station 94784, Lincoln, NE 68509.

SEVEN

ESTABLISHING NEWCOMERS' GROUPS

David I. Berland
Raymond G. Poggi

When I was a child my mother read to me a sentimental ballad by Will Carelton, who was a very popular poet in those days. One I remember clearly was entitled, "Over the Hill to the Poorhouse," and portrayed the dismal end of a poor but proud couple when friends and jobs and their childrens' largess had run out, and there was nothing left for them but a weary trail to the awful place "over the hill"—the poorhouse. I grew up with the horror of something I had never seen, the "poorhouse," along with the "orphans' home" and the "insane asylum," and the "pest house."

Karl Menninger, 1979

LEARNING OBJECTIVES

- Describe why newcomers' groups are helpful and necessary for the elderly who move into a retirement home.
- Describe how to establish a newcomers' group.
- List three phases of newcomers' groups.
- Describe three problems of conducting a newcomers' group that a leader may expect.
- List three stages in the process of moving into a retirement home.
- Describe how other authors link the concepts of stress and psychological illness.
- List two areas for further research.

The authors wish to express their gratitude to the staff and members of the United Methodist Home for the Aged, Inc., for their warmth and cooperation during the time of this study.

While there is a significant stress in any move (Holmes and Rahe, 1967), no one has systematically studied the stress of the final move into a retirement home. We first became aware of the severity of that stress while conducting long-term expressive group psychotherapy with residents of a retirement home (Poggi and Berland, 1978). To assist the elderly in making this transition, we designed a second group, composed of newcomers to the home, which met to discuss this move. We learned from the previous group that elderly could benefit from expressive techniques (Berland and Poggi, 1979). We utilized elements of expressive technique in this new, more focused, group. This chapter describes how we mobilized dormant, existing competencies in members of the group which subsequently aided them in adjusting to their new living situation.

REVIEW OF THE LITERATURE

Our chapter concerns establishment of a group designed to help the elderly cope with the stress of their final move. The issue of stress has been a matter of increasing controversy (Dohrenwend and Dohrenwend, 1978). Research devoted to the concept of stress has demonstrated the psychological and physiological effects only in certain circumstances. Laboratory studies with animals, as well as studies of the aftermath of holocausts, have shown the connection between stress and illness. However, major controversy surrounds the subject of the stress of normal life events and disability. Do marriage, divorce, relocation, and retirement produce sufficient stress to cause illness (Holmes and Rahe, 1967; Dohrenwend and Dohrenwend, 1978; Wolff, 1968; Rahe and Arthor, 1979)?

Current literature tends to support the notion if certain conditions exist. A demand for adaptation to a novel event can be stressful, particularly if the novelty eliminates the opportunity for repetition and practice and, consequently, for habituation and attenuation of the stress. Lack of social bonds will cause an event to be more stressful (Wolff, 1968; Rahe and Arthor, 1979; Andrews et al., 1978a). Adverse

childhood experiences and the distress component of a life event also increase the probability of psychiatric illness in response to life events (Tennant and Andrews, 1978; Andrews et al., 1978b). Suddenness of an event, which prevents the opportunity for anticipation, increases the stressfulness of the event; similarly, control over the event can reduce its inherent stressfulness.

Yet individuals, because of personal and idiosyncratic problems, can perceive themselves as having less control than is in fact possible. Thus, the individual's personality can influence the degree to which the stress results in disability. Most authors conclude that the aforementioned factors determine the effects of stress derived from everyday life events.

Authors studying stress in the elderly generally assume that life events can be stressful. They focus attention on the reaction among the elderly to stress. Is it different from other age groups, and, if so, how is it different?

In general, authors conclude that the elderly are more likely to react both psychologically and physically to stress than other age groups. Depression and acute organic brain syndromes seem to be the most prevalent responses to change and stress among the elderly. The earliest response to such stress involves memory problems. In fact, some authors define two distinct responses to stress: a reversible, benign memory impairment and a more ominous, permanent memory difficulty. The more benign memory deficiency entails the loss of immediate and recent recall with remote memory remaining intact. If a clear precipitating life circumstance is evident, this memory problem may be reversible if the situation is handled expeditiously (Kral 1967; Kral, Brad, and Berenson, 1968).

Death of a spouse and the final move are particularly stressful for the elderly. K. F. Rowland (1977) has examined the relevant literature from 1955 through 1975. We have reviewed the relevant literature from 1975 through 1978 on the impact of retirement, relocation, and the death of a spouse on the elderly. From the research regarding the impact of death of a spouse on the elderly, the author draws two main conclusions. (1) The risk of one's own death, following the death of one's spouse, may be significantly increased, especially for surviving males. (2) This risk of death is greatest during the first year of bereavement. It returns to normal if the spouse survives the first year. While reasons for this impact remain unclear, Rowland suggests several possibilities: contagion (the spouses or relative shared the same environment); unhealthy people tend to marry unhealthy people and may have the same life expectancy; widowhood itself may produce sufficient psychological and emotional stress to increase the risk of death.

Regarding the effects of relocation on the elderly, Rowland (1977) and others (McIvor and Sorgen, 1978; Wolanin, 1978; Mullen, 1977) found that relocation may result in the elderly's death particularly if the person is in poor health. One study is reported to have shown that these effects are most likely to occur within the first 3 months after a move. At the same time, it is difficult to interpret some of these studies. For instance, one reported a move from a more rundown to a more comfortable environment. Happily, mortality decreased with this move. The decreases probably resulted from the improved environment to which these people moved. Other compounding problems involved the natural selection of people who move. Some may be in particularly poor health which necessitates their institutionalization. These people may die with or without institutionalization, and there are no control studies to explore that possibility.

Rowland (1977) reports on a group of articles particularly relevant to our study. These suggest that mortality rates associated with moves are directly related to the elderly's preparation for the move (Wolanin, 1978). Those who make the move "voluntarily" do much better in relocation than those who experience it as an "involuntary choice."

The final death-predicting event that Rowland explores is retirement. Here the author concludes that the research has not been well-enough designed to draw conclusions whether retirement actually does or does not predict death. Some existing problems involve people's motives for retirement. Certainly those who retire because of poor health are likely to die shortly after retirement. Those whose self-esteem and identity are intimately tied with their work may suffer upon retirement. Rowland notes, however, that as retirement becomes more accepted as a way of life, its psychological impact will decrease.

In summary, after surveying the 20 years of literature on the subject, Rowland found that death of a spouse (or, at times, sibling or parent) may increase the chances for death of the survivor, particularly if the survivor is a man. The period of greatest risk is the first year after the loss. Relocation can also predict death in the elderly, particularly those in poor health. There is debated evidence in the literature to suggest that retirement per se predicts death in the elderly.

Although others have examined the topic of relocation, there is little in the literature concerning the use of groups to study further and intervene in the effects of relocation. The group that we are describing in this chapter allows investigators to focus their attention on the impact of a particular kind of stress on a particular group of people. The possibilities for more accurately studying the concept and effects of stress are evident. In addition, the use of expressive techniques in the conduct of the newcomers' group allows study of one of the least studied aspects of stress, namely, the very personal perception the individual has of the event and how that perception effects adaptation.

ESTABLISHING THE GROUP

The setting was a private, nonprofit, church-related institution, which has 138 single- and 15 double-room apartments. It was built in 1914 with additions in the 1920s and 1950s. The home also has a 72-bed health unit with 14 nurses and 40 aides to care for debilitated residents. The age range for the retirees usually is 65 to 102 with an average age of 85.

THE ENTREE

Because of our previous work in the home, we had a well-established relationship with the administration. We were also fortunate in that the administrators of the home were sensitive to the psychological needs of the residents and willing to cooperate with us to meet those needs. We met with them and the other administrators for approximately 3 to 4 months prior to the beginning of the group. These meetings with the head nurse, chaplain, director of residents, and chief social worker provided us with valuable insights into the problems which the residents faced as they moved into the home. The residents' director used this time to tell us about new admissions as they prepared to move into the home. The social worker and chaplain were able to provide us with more detailed information regarding an individual's struggles with family and friends. The head nurse provided us with accurate appraisals of the physical limitations of the various residents. This information and support were particularly important to us in assessing whether a member's complaints were more psychologically or organically determined. Her attendance at these meetings also supported participation of residents in the group who were temporarily housed on the health unit.

We continued to meet with this group of personnel monthly after beginning the newcomers' group. We discussed recent events in the home, their impact on the group, and the effects of the group on the home. It is important to point out that in order to maintain confidentiality, we did not discuss the content of group meetings with the staff. We told group members about our meetings with the staff; we shared the content of these meetings with the group members if they expressed interest. As a consequence of our meetings with the staff and our willingness to discuss these meetings in the group, the administration did not feel we were unsympathetic outsiders nor did the group believe us to be agents of the administration.

PARAMETERS OF THE GROUP

The newcomers' group was time-limited and composed of people who had recently moved into the home. All newly admitted persons without severe organic pathology that precluded their participation (for example, total deafness, severe memory impairment) joined the group after 1 or 2 weeks in an existing staff-run orientation program. They stayed in our group for 12 weeks. Hence this group experience was particularly rich because people were at different stages of coming and going in the group and the home and, therefore, had different experiences and understanding of what was happening to them. Members were able to share this knowledge with each other. A group of 8 or 10 members met with us for 1 hour weekly.

INITIAL INTERVIEW

After the administrators gave us a list of newcomers, we divided the list in half, and one of us interviewed each prospective member privately. We held these private interviews to introduce the idea of the newcomers' group to the new residents and to enable the new resident to meet one of the leaders of the group. We wanted to assess not only physical limitations to participation in the group but also individual objections and anxieties to talking in a group about personal issues. To accomplish these goals, we followed a general outline as follows.

INTERVIEW FORMAT

We introduced ourselves and stated the purpose of the group: for newcomers to get together for an hour a week and discuss moving into the home. The interviews were $\frac{1}{2}$ to 1 hour long and conducted in the resident's room. We also told prospective members why we thought the group was important. At times, interviewees became anxious and told us they had no problems whatsoever. We might respond that we could appreciate that and asked if they were interested in helping others who did have problems. We did not argue with them. Instead, we returned at a later date to talk with them again about the group. We recognized that the move was stressful and we did not want to add to that stress. At other times, residents became anxious after we introduced ourselves as psychiatrists. We had to spend extra time explaining to these residents that even though we were members of the mental health profession, we did not view everyone as disturbed and crazy. Rather, we recognized they were going through a difficult time in their life and simply wanted to talk with them about it. We tried, at the conclusion of the initial interview, to arrive at an agreement with the resident to attend the next twelve 1-hour sessions of the group.

MENTAL STATUS EXAMINATION

We also performed a modified mental status examination. At times, we asked the residents if they remembered who we were or if they remembered how often and when the group met. If they were unable to remember, we would suggest that they make written notes to aid their memory. At times, we encountered severe organic impairment and had to exclude those people from the group. As the staff became more familiar with our selection criteria, we no longer encountered unsuitable prospective members.

We also talked to members of the group about their move, some of the circumstances surrounding it, and their immediate adjustment to the new home. Such discussions served as a preview for the resident of the discussions in the group. These talks also provided a foundation for a personal relationship with one of the leaders which was useful for the members during the initial anxieties of the group; not everyone in the group was a stranger.

CONDUCT OF THE GROUP

As noted above, we employed modified expressive psychotherapeutic techniques in our group. Traditionally, expressive psychotherapy has had several characteristics. It is not didactic, it is not heavily structured, and it is not a social gathering where food and drinks are served. The boundaries of the group are maintained so that new members are added in a systematic as opposed to random fashion. The therapists assume a nontransparent stance, implying minimal social contact with members of the group outside the session. They also engage in self-analysis to understand their countertransference. Such a

stance encourages transference among the members of the group and between the members and the therapist. The therapists interpret these transference phenomena, providing insight for the group members which help them achieve an understanding of their thoughts and feelings about current and past experiences. They can use this new understanding to change present behavior and can achieve greater freedom from instinctual pressures.

Expressive techniques are most useful to explore a person's general personality and character makeup as well as symptomatic behavior. We modified the expressive technique. We confined our intervention to drawing members' attention to the stresses they experienced resulting from the move and how they dealt with those stresses. Specifically, we did not engage in advice giving or counseling. We minimized dependency on the leaders by: (1) adopting a more transparent position, (2) avoiding transference interpretation, and (3) avoiding direct advice giving. At times, when links to genetic material or transference issues were obvious and clearly related to current difficulties, we made them explicit. A vignette explains one intervention in the group.

VIGNETTE 1

Mrs. C., an 88-year-old member of the group, was the youngest of seven children. Her parents, siblings, and later her husband and her own children perpetuated the myth that she was the helpless baby in her family. After her husband's death 1 year before her final move, she was alone for the first time in her life. Her incessant demands on her children resulted in their placing her in the home. Once there, anxiety about spending nights alone forced her into unceasing activity and talk. Further, she refused to acknowledge her age and relation to other members of the home. In the group, this anxiety was also apparent, isolating her from other newcomers.

In order to intervene, we offered her the following interpretation given over several group sessions: "As you have told us, all your life you have been treated as 'a helpless baby.' People have always taken care of you. Now you're faced with doing things on your own and you're scared. So scared that you're anxiously running around trying to prove to yourself that you don't need anybody. You have a choice of remaining a 'helpless baby' or for the first time, learning to rely on yourself."

These comments precipitated a reactive depression from which Mrs. C. is emerging. She is also showing signs of improved adaptation to life in the home. It is important to note that our continued meetings with the staff in the home were essential support for our interpretive work. We all agreed that the staff should treat her like any other member of the home and thus avoid a repetition of previous family experience.

Sometimes it is useful to remain in the metaphor that the group raises. At times leaders may find themselves translating the metaphor and then returning to the metaphor in order to respond. For example, members of the group were discussing the small towns from which they had come. They talked of the value and riches of small town life. Many people now had forgotten these towns. In fact, some towns had lost their post offices and were on the verge of becoming extinct. One of the greatest blows to the old towns involved the new superhighways which often did not go through them, steering traffic and interest away from them. The leaders responded to this talk by exploring the rich values of old towns and how much they still can contribute to our way of life.

Clearly the discussion of the old towns was the members' way of talking about themselves. Staying in the metaphor can produce change in the members of the group. They spoke more freely about the riches and values of the old towns and seemed to light up and feel proud of themselves and their accomplishments. Only when the discussion in metaphor has served as a way of avoiding other topics do we interpret its underlying meaning to the group.

Gordon (1970) labels these expressive techniques as "active listening." This technique involves the listeners' assiduously avoiding the "typical 12" obstacles to communication. These obstacles are:

1. Ordering, directing, commanding
2. Warning, admonishing, threatening
3. Exhorting, moralizing, preaching
4. Advising, giving solutions or suggestions
5. Lecturing, teaching, giving logical arguments
6. Judging, criticizing, disagreeing, blaming
7. Praising, agreeing
8. Name calling, ridiculing, shaming.
9. Interpreting, analyzing, diagnosing
10. Reassuring, sympathizing, consoling, supporting
11. Probing, questioning, interrogating
12. Withdrawing, distracting, or humoring

He notes that ordinary communication is filled with these roadblocks. Hence, he proposes listening for the feelings behind the statement and commenting on the feelings to the individual. For example, when a member of the group said that "losses are better left behind," one of the leaders said, "Talking about losses is very painful and difficult." The member of the group then began to talk about her very difficult marriage. This response avoids the trap of reassuring the member that it was safe to talk about such things, colluding with her to forget such emotional material, or pressing her to talk.

INITIAL SESSION

During the initial session there is much anxiety in both the leaders and the members of the group. The therapist's anxiety may arise from many sources. One obvious concern is that the group will fail. He or she has already invested a great deal of time in the individual interviews and the work with the administration of the home. Now, the leader is faced with the group. Will they think it is a good idea? Will they talk? If there is silence, what can the leader do? What if a member asks a question and the leader does not know the answer?

COLEADERSHIP

Coleadership raises additional anxieties, among them competition and exposing one's work to a colleague. With these additional anxieties about coleadership, why is it useful to have two leaders? First, with two leaders the group is likely to continue uninterrupted when one leader misses because of illness or vacation. Second, the model is useful for training where an experienced leader can train a less experienced one. Third, coleaders have an opportunity to discuss the group process with each other to sort out more effectively their own feelings.

A DEEPER UNEASINESS

In addition to the anxieties concerning the setting, therapists may experience a deeper uneasiness. The leader may question, "Who am I to help someone two or three times my age?" The leader may wonder whether the group members will experience him or her as a young inexperienced "kid." Will they accept what the leader says? If unrecognized, these feelings may be expressed as anger toward the members, taking the form of overaggressive intervention or feelings that the work is useless; after all, these old people will die soon anyway. In general, these tensions relate to experiences the leader may have had with his or her own parents or grandparents and/or people in authority, which can become intensely reactivated in work with the elderly.

ANXIETIES OF RESIDENTS

The residents also have their anxieties. As newcomers to the home, they are strangers to one another. Many have never had any contact with the mental health profession and, in spite of the individual pregroup interview, may hold biases against mental health professionals. They, too, wonder whether others will accept them. They wonder whether their memory of the description of the group from the individual interview is accurate. Most importantly, they are still tense about the recent move, the reason for the group. On a different level, they can carry resentment into the group toward younger people who have more mobility and more respect in the community than they do. Younger people also may have

forced them into this move. They may displace this anger onto the leaders of the group. We do not believe it is possible to trace all the roots of such displacements or work through all the anger in 12 group sessions. Hence, we assume the more transparent stance to highlight the difference between us and other real people in their lives.

These anxieties will affect behavior; some residents may not come to the group. We found it useful to visit these residents again and to talk with them about coming to the next session. Other residents may come and sit silently.

FIRST SESSION

With all this anxiety, how does one begin the initial session? The first session of our newcomers' group began with one of the leaders making the preliminary introductions. After making certain that all the members had been introduced to one another, the leader restated the purpose of the group, to talk about the stresses, strains, and events that led to entry into the home. In addition, we clarified details about the meeting, reaffirming the time, place, and total number of sessions. After this initial few minutes, the group fell silent. We allowed the silence to continue. One of the coleaders then said, "It's going to be difficult for the first person to speak in the group." There was more silence and one of the leaders said further, "Despite the difficulty in breaking the ice, there are many things to talk about." At this point one of the members of the group began talking and described very vividly the difficulties he was having in moving into the home. Each person in turn then gave a brief résumé of who they were and why they were there.

Silence need not be broken immediately, and, above all, the coleaders should not anxiously fill the silence with chatter. We chose to speak of the feelings that might make talking difficult. This intervention was sufficient to aid that first person in starting the session of that particular newcomers' group. We kept the focus on the anxiety present in the session, noting, when appropriate, its various manifestations. It is particularly important to prevent one member of the group from attempting to reduce the tension by going into a long personal, perhaps even tragic, story of his or her move to the home. The talker is usually left feeling alone and unsupported. We will have more to say about this problem later.

MIDDLE SESSIONS

While both leaders and members of the group will still have anxiety after the initial session, their return to the group indicates a willingness to meet and talk in spite of the anxiety. During this phase, various themes will emerge as the leaders utilize the techniques previously described. We will discuss the themes specifically in another section of this chapter. We would like now to illustrate the use of our techniques in eliciting material from group members with this vignette.

VIGNETTE 2

Mrs. D. took the floor and indicated that she was distressed about her memory problem. She then demonstrated her problem by stating that she had only been in the home a week. Other members of the group indicated by looks and nods that she had been there much longer. Dr. Berland pursued the subject further and said to Mrs. D. that she could not possibly have been in the home only a week since he had seen her himself over 2 weeks ago. Other members of the group then mentioned that she had been in the home 4 months. Mrs. D. became extremely angry when confronted with this information and refused to believe it. The situation was diffused when Dr. Poggi then pointed out to Mrs. D. that her memory problem obviously distressed her and she was even distressed at being reminded that such a problem existed. She agreed, calmed down, and became more of a participant in the group discussion. The people in the group then began talking about age. There was a lot of good-natured joking and humor about how "old people are."

This vignette illustrates the importance of responding to the feelings behind Mrs. D.'s protests and her refusal to listen to the other members of the group. In so doing, we were able to bring the feelings to awareness and helped Mrs. D. overcome her denial of her difficulty, which enabled her to enter into a good-natured helping relationship with other members of the group for the remainder of the sessions.

FOCUS ON BEHAVIOR

The following clinical vignette illustrates the usefulness of focusing attention on people's behavior within the group. One member noticed that some members were missing and wondered, "Why don't some people come?" Following this question, Dr. Berland reminded members of the group that during the last session we had been talking about how hard it was to become a group. Some people did not come, some people could not hear, some did not remember, some were simply distracted or preoccupied by the past and did not pay attention to what was going on now. Discussion followed during which the members of the group attempted to avoid this troublesome question by saying, "Well, that's the way it always is; there are only a few dependable responsible people who do the work." At that point, Dr. Poggi noted, "That only raises another and perhaps, more important question: What does it feel like for all of the people who come and are left to do all the work?" People then started talking about their personal need to remain active. They found people who were inactive impossible to understand and somehow irritating. As we talked further about the importance of keeping busy, a concern surfaced that "if we don't keep busy, we are going to deteriorate physically and mentally."

The focusing of attention on the life of the group allowed members to reveal issues that were of immediate concern to them. The leaders, by redirecting attention to the ongoing concerns in the group, helped diminish members' reluctance to discuss their concerns about physical and mental deterioration.

The following vignette again illustrates how

useful it is to understand feelings and concerns which may lie just behind a member's ongoing behavior.

VIGNETTE 3

Mrs. E. was a 75-year-old childless widow who was preoccupied with her family's genealogy and was consumed with the need to complete it quickly. This genealogy was all that she would talk about in the group. The discussion isolated her from other members of the group and caused some to say, "Here we go again" whenever she would talk. During the third session of the group, Mrs. E. said once again, "What if I can't finish it?" Leaders of the group responded to her by acknowledging how important the genealogy was to her and added that they thought she was avoiding her concern about dying through all this talk about her family tree. Mrs. E. agreed that she was concerned about dying and began to discuss that issue.

The concern about death was, of course, the concern common to all members of the group who joined in this discussion with Mrs. E. Hence, our speaking to the concerns behind the expressed topic allowed Mrs. E. to talk about these concerns and become a more accepted member of the group. This maneuver was also very important in redirecting her interest from her own, private world outward into the world of others.

SAYING GOOD-BYE

With the time-limited contract to participate in the group, everyone knows when each member's last session will be. When a member has three sessions remaining, the leaders make the fact explicit at the beginning of each of the last three sessions. This newcomer is by then a seasoned veteran who has helped other people in the process of joining the group and provided them with information about the home. And it is time to say good-bye. During the second to last session for five "old-timers," members of the group talked about the importance of preserving relics of the past. One talked about a 65-year-old

rug that belonged to her mother, another talked about her genealogy. There was then talk about how old they were and that a new home being built by the same organization which ran their retirement home would not be ready in time for their use. The leaders acknowledged the relative peace with which members of the group were accepting the fact they were old and would die. There was no bitterness. Members then began to give the leaders advice: "To live a long life you must eat a good breakfast. You must avoid coffee and avoid fried foods." At that point, the leaders acknowledged to each other that the advice was a touching gift. They went on to say, "It seems that one of the things being addressed only indirectly involves saying good-bye to five old members of the group." These members then asked whether they would get a diploma at the conclusion of the group. One of the leaders responded that perhaps they were trying to find ways to maintain their memories of the group. The members agreed and adjourned for their final session.

ISSUES ABOUT TERMINATION

Termination raises many issues. Among these is a desire to have a chance to say what has been left unsaid, words of both praise and criticism. Many of these are expressed most vividly to the leaders because the other members of the group will continue to see each other daily. In addition, the parting members want to hear things from the leaders. Did they like knowing them? Did they learn something from them? One of the members of the group indicated her wish to hear from the leaders what they thought of her contribution in the group by bringing up in a joking fashion, her impending graduation from the group. She said in a joking way, "The two of us who have not missed a single session should be designated by you the valedictorian and salutatorian of the group." She then went on quickly to note an article she had read in the paper about some psychiatrists who appeared on a television show. They received calls from viewers and talked with them about their problems. At that point, a leader said that although they were not on television, they were psychiatrists with whom they had been talking for 12 weeks and that perhaps there was something more they wanted to discuss. The departing group members then began to evaluate their experiences in the group. They noted that they had not been in treatment but had been in a newcomers' group with psychiatrists who helped them adjust to the changes in their lives. One member of the group noted that an important benefit for her was her association with the other members of the group.

Criticism of the group surfaced in more indirect ways. For instance, still another member mentioned obliquely that she still was having some problems and anxieties, indicating that she was disappointed that 12 weeks in the group had not answered all the questions on her mind. We chose to respond to direct questions from members of the group concerning our opinions of them and, in fact, told the departing members of the group very directly what we had been fortunate enough to learn from them that would be useful to us in the future.

The other problem in the termination phase of this type of group is that although some members are leaving, others are staying; it is a task of the therapists or leaders to acknowledge the sense of loss that those remaining members will experience. Such feelings, if left unacknowledged, might make it very difficult for members to continue with their participation in the group.

For instance, during the session in which several members are terminating, one of the leaders said that it was very appropriate to be dealing with the ending of the group for those people who were leaving, but he felt the need to acknowledge that there were others in the group who would be continuing and that also was going to be difficult. The other leader then mentioned that it was going to be a strange experience to be in the group the following week. For all practical purposes, it would be a new group, strange people would be joining, and familiar faces would be missed. As a consequence of these remarks, those members who were continuing with the group spoke up at the end of the session. They mentioned that they were still gaining from the group, that they were still having trouble adjusting to life in the home, and that there were needs to be met even though the group would be different next time.

PROBLEMS

ADDING MEMBERS

Adding members to existing groups is a difficult process. In a topic-focused, time-limited group such as ours, we did not always prepare members for the addition of a new member before the actual meeting. However, we made it clear during our individual interviews with prospective members that people would be added to the group as they came into the retirement home.

It is important that the new member be added "gradually." Failure to do so can result in unwarranted invasion of privacy and/or of self-esteem in the newcomer. For example, one newcomer was brought by a member of the group before we had interviewed her. Other members of the group encouraged her to talk to them. We did not intervene soon enough to prevent her from anxiously divulging deeply personal material. That new member did not return the following week. We visited her after she missed the meeting, and she subsequently returned to the group and participated actively. We believe that our visit to her reassured her that we were not frightened or offended by her divulging so much personal material so quickly and that we would be in control of the group.

What we failed to recognize in that session involved the fantasy of the new member entering an established group. The new member may believe that all the other members of the group have known each other for a long time and are the best of friends. He or she will want to join that group and may believe that the best way to do that is by revealing a great deal about himself or herself. In retrospect, however, the new member will recognize that he or she has exposed himself or herself to many and will wonder what these unknown people will think. Other members of the group who are reluctant to talk about themselves will confound this problem. Their willingness to remain silent seems like pressure to divulge to a newcomer. In this particular setting, when a member's self-esteem is lower as a result of the move to the home with its attendant losses, that new member's dependency needs are acutely stimulated. Hence, the members will want the other members of the group to accept him or her almost at any cost.

A more effective way to add new members would involve more superficial conversation among the members including such topics as where they are from, where they live in the home, and what hobbies they have. When members talk about some of their losses, the leaders of the group should respect that discussion but lateralize it to include other members. By saying such things as, "Mrs. A., didn't you have a similar experience when you had to give up your car?" the leaders can encourage a feeling of universality among the members of the group. Another effective intervention involves the leaders' acknowledging openly how difficult it is to move into the group. The leaders can then invite other members to talk about their experiences moving into the group. This maneuver has the advantage of leading one member of the group to teach another member the process. Thus, the newcomer becomes the healer (Almond, 1974).

DROPOUTS

In this group, a member's capacity to adjust to the group reflects the capacity of that member to adjust to communal living in the retirement home. Some will have more trouble adjusting to the home and the group than others. Some will drop out of the group. Our requirements for dropping out include the member's talking about his or her decision in the presence of the group. This discussion is important so that other members will have a chance to deal with their feelings about a member's leaving. A common fantasy among the members involves their feeling that the dropout left because he or she did not like other members. The public discussion also gives the leaders a chance to comment on what they feel is important in the decision to drop out. Sometimes the decision reflects more serious maladaptation. The public discussion also underlines the capacity of the members to talk about their decision and the leaders' respect for them for making a choice.

VIGNETTE 4

A male member expressed openly his wish not to participate further in the group. His reason was that he was a businessman and used to more task-oriented things. He did not want to get involved in this kind of work. He went on further to say that he really wanted to talk to men (other members of the group were women) and there were not any men in the group. Another member of the group became quite irritated because of Mr. R.'s remarks. She stated that she was a businesswoman as much as he was a businessman and she was here in the group and in the home. Dr. F., another professional woman in the group, said that she had been a professional person for 59 years and she was there. She added that if he was going to make it in the home, he was going to have to give a little rather than just stating what he wanted. "You're going to have to change your way of thinking." The leaders in the group noted that Mr. R. was having difficulty facing a very lonely fact of life, that there were not many men in his age group. That fact was not going to change in the group, and it was not going to change in the home. Somehow or other he was going to have to find a way to change his view about women. If he did not, he was going to continue to be frustrated and become very lonely. Mr. R. became very angry, saying that it sounded like the leader was telling him that he was forced into doing something. We pointed out to him that he did not have to do anything, except be aware of the consequences of his choice, namely, the animosity of the women with whom he was living in the home and continued frustration and loneliness. At the conclusion of the group everyone had an opportunity, including Mr. R., to say good-bye and to express hope that he found a solution to his difficulties.

NO-SHOWS

At times members of the group will not show up for appointments. We discussed the absentees to determine whether they had left messages with other members regarding their missing the session. If there were no such messages, one of the leaders would go and get the absentee while the other would remain in the group. At times the "forgetting" of the meeting time served as a way for members of the group to have "individual" time with one of the leaders. One member, in particular, appreciated this individual time. However, she began to remember the group when one of the leaders simply interpreted that fact to her in a jocular way: "I know you can remember these groups and my guess is that you simply want to meet alone with me. If you do, that's alright, but perhaps we could find another way to do it than have you forget the group." The member became a little annoyed and appeared for the remaining sessions on time.

WHAT WE HAVE LEARNED

We have learned that there are three stages of preparation before the move into the retirement home: (1) the last real choice, (2) the investigation, (3) the final event.

Members of the group emphasized that coming to this retirement home would be their last real choice to move. They would die in the home, and they discussed death freely. Significantly, they wished this move to be free of coercion from their family or friends. Some members of the group, however, noted a certain subtle concern (or was it pressure?) that they come into the home. This concern from their social network represented an external pressure contrasted with the internal pressure from the member's fear of becoming a burden to his or her family. Many felt they had nothing more to give to family or friends. Fear of becoming invalids provided further internal motivation for the move. Members were afraid that once they were invalids, they could no longer make a real choice to move into the home.

Having once confronted the decision to move into the home, the members of the group entered the second stage—investigation. Depending on the results of this stage, they would decide whether to move into the home. This phase of the moving process impressed us because of its length, 1 to 3 years. The initial phase of this stage involved making the decision of which retirement home to investigate. Members based their choice on a previous connection to the institution. In the case of our retirement home, this link may have been provided through church, relatives, or friends who lived there. Another influence on the choice of the home involved the feeling of prior ownership. Many of the members had contributed to the home throughout their lives and believed they partially owned it. It was not a faceless, charitable institution. The second phase was active and involved actual examination of the facility. Nearly all members of the group examined the home before the move. Yet, the investigation at times was quite subtle. One member of the group visited a relative in the home to see if it was good enough for her.

The third phase of the move involved the final event. While that event took many forms, one theme was common to all—loss. All members of the group had to part with many possessions. They prepared to move from home or apartments to a single-room apartment with a bathroom. The selling of possessions is a point of no return; once they are gone, they are impossible to reclaim. Several members of our group lost lifelong companions (spouses and siblings) after the sale of possessions, immediately before the move into the home. Another member lost a spouse several months before the final event. Still another member deteriorated rapidly after the move into the home as she continued to talk about all her losses. While relatives may greet the sale of possessions and preparations happily as meaning that the move will occur at last, our experience strongly suggests that the actual sale is a dangerous time for the retiree. Long-time companions of the retiree became ill and died in close temporal sequence to that sale.

Once in the retirement home, the resident faces a new series of stresses: orienting himself or herself to the home, living in a group, and coming to grips with loneliness and dependency. One particular detail the members of the group found useful involved the placement of their possessions in the home. Indeed this placement occupied almost all the members' attention during the first week or two there. Members of our group agreed that only after they had organized their living space and found a place for all their goods could they redirect their attention to the new people and new places in their environment. One member found it was useful to have a floor plan of the room so that she could plan the exact location for all her things.

Living in a group home created new problems. Members of the group had problems with people living next door whom they simply did not like. No longer did they have physical space to separate them from their neighbors. Although having people around could decrease the loneliness and fear of being alone when in need of help, the liability was feeling crowded and unable to find any private time or space. An additional problem of the close living quarters involved confronting members of the group with debilitated dependent neighbors. That confrontation awakened considerable anxiety within them about their own future.

The personal loss that led to the sense of loneliness in each of the members also acted as a barrier against forming new bonds. The fear of future loss was so great that some residents preferred to remain isolated.

UNANSWERED QUESTIONS

Other material which has arisen in the group through the use of these techniques has been equally exciting. It has raised questions in our minds regarding the role of the superego in the elderly as well as that of role models. When a person reaches 90 or 95 years of age, how many people are there left to serve as role models? Why do the elderly turn to younger people for approval? This intriguing question cannot be answered here, but we hope that our work will provide material with which to attempt an answer in the future.

REFERENCES

Almond, Richard: *The Healing Community: Dynamics of the Therapeutic Milieu*, J. Aronson, New York, 1974.

Andrews, G., et al.: Life event stress, social support, coping style, and the risk of psychological impairment, *Journal of Nervous and Mental Disease*, **166**(5):307–316, May 1978a.

———: The relation of social factors to physical and psychiatric illness, *American Journal of Epidemiology*, **108**(1):27–35, July 1978b.

Berland, David I., and Raymond Poggi: Expressive group psychotherapy with the aging, *International Journal of Group Psychotherapy*, **29**(1):87–108, January 1979.

Dohrenwend, Barbara Snell, and Bruce P. Dohrenwend: Some issues in research on stressful life events, *Journal of Nervous and Mental Disease*, **166**(1):7–15, January 1978.

Gordon, Thomas: *Parent Effectiveness Training: The Tested Way to Raise Responsible Children*, Wyden, New York, 1970.

Holmes, Thomas H., and Richard R. Rahe: The social readjustment rating scale, *Journal of Psychosomatic Research*, **11**(2):213–218, August 1967.

Kral, V. A.: Stress reactions in old age, *Laval Medicine*, **38**:561–566, June 1967.

———, B. Brad, and J. Berenson: Stress reactions resulting from the relocation of an aged population, *Canadian Psychiatric Association Journal*, **13**(3):201–209, June 1968.

McIvor, Janet, and Lewis Sorgen: One day the door closes, *Canadian Nurse*, **74**(3):30–33, March 1978.

Menninger, Karl: Address to the governor's first gerontological congress, Kansas State University, Manhattan, Kan., Jan. 19, 1979.

Mullen, Elaine: Relocation of the elderly: Implications for nursing, *Journal of Gerontological Nursing*, **3**(4):13–16, July/August 1977.

Poggi, Raymond G., and David Berland: Newcomers' groups: A preliminary report, *Journal of NAPPH*, **10**(1):47–51, Fall 1978.

Rahe, R. H., and R. J. Arthor: Life changes and illness studies, *Journal of Human Stress*, **4**(1):3–15, March 1979.

Rowland, K. F.: Environmental events predicting death for the elderly, *Psychological Bulletin*, **84**(2):349–372, March 1977.

Tennant, C., and G. Andrews: The pathogenic quality of life event stress in neurotic impairment, *Archives of General Psychiatry*, **35**(7):859–863, July 1978.

Wolanin, Mary Opal: Relocation of the elderly, *Journal of Gerontological Nursing*, **4**(2):47–50, May/June 1978.

Wolff, H. G.: The nature of stress for man: Hazards in his environment, *Stress & Disease*, 2d ed., Charles C Thomas Publishers, Springfield, Ill., 1968, pp. 3–12.

EIGHT

REMINISCING AS THERAPY: AN OVERVIEW

Irene Mortenson Burnside

An experience, specially in youth, is quickly over-laid by others, and is not at the moment fully com-prehended. But it is overlaid, not lost. Time hurries it from us, but also keeps it in store, and it can later be recaptured and amplified by memory so that at leisure we can interpret its meaning and enjoy its savor.
John Buchan, 1940

LEARNING OBJECTIVES

- Define life review.
- Define reminiscing.
- Identify two theoretical frameworks which serve as the foundation for reminiscing therapy.
- Describe problems of the leader in conducting a reminiscing group.
- Compare and contrast free-flowing reminiscing vs. structured reminiscing.

This chapter provides an overview of the literature on reminiscing with the aged client (or clients) and draws from the literature some ways in which nurses can use reminiscing in day-to-day contacts with old people, whether the client is well, sick, or in between, whether the person is a "young old" or a centenarian, competent or regressed. The logistics and operational aspects of reminiscing are not discussed in depth in this chapter since they are covered in another text (Ebersole, 1978).

DEFINITION

Webster's dictionary (1975) defines *reminiscing* as "to call past events or experiences to mind" and to "talk or write about remembered events or experiences"; the word is derived from the Latin *reminiscere,* meaning "to remember." In fact, the second Sunday of Lent is called Reminiscence Sunday because it is a time set apart for a review of a person's life in the past year.

Coleman (1974, p. 294) defined reminiscence in his study as "linguistic acts of referring to the remote past," though he noted some difficulty in the definition and the use of the word *remote.* The word *reminiscent* describes one who engages in reminiscing.

EARLIEST WRITINGS

The first article in the literature about reminiscence dates back to a United Kingdom article in 1913 (Ballard, 1913). Then nothing appeared until 1926 when Williams published "A Study of the Phenomenon of Reminiscence" (Williams, 1926). Two articles appeared in the thirties (McGeoch, 1935; Bunch, 1938). Thumin (1956, 1957) is the first to write a master's thesis and a doctoral dissertation on reminiscence. See Table 8-2 for articles published.

BUTLER'S CONTRIBUTIONS

The theoretical framework for reminiscing in both one-to-one relationships and group work with the elderly has its roots in Robert Butler's now classic article, "The Life Review: An In-

TABLE 8-1
QUOTATIONS ON REMINISCING

What makes old age hard to bear is not a failing of one's faculties, mental and physical, but the burden of one's memories.

Maugham, *Points of View,* 1959

> It's no fun going deaf,
> But there are worse things,
> And I do have a lot of good memories
> To listen to.

"I Don't Hear As Well As I Used To," *Green Winter: Celebrations of Old Age,* Elise Maclay, 1977

Well, this is a time for introspection, to take inventory of himself, to evaluate the mistakes made and opportunities lost, to recognize and appreciate the many virtues of others that had been overlooked. It is also a time for retrospection, and here begins the real second childhood. To many this is a comforting and rewarding period. He now begins to relive his life backward. He is astonished to see so much beauty in nature, and also in people, he has by-passed. He finds it more difficult to recall quite recent incidents than those which occurred further back, that the farther he goes the better his memory becomes until he reaches early childhood when everything becomes clearly bright.

The unedited passage above is from the essay "Second Childhood" written by Mr. Albert Davis, age 100, in August, 1959. He died in March, 1963, at the age of 104.

Memory is the thing I forget with.

Five-year-old

This set of sagas, memory. Over and over self-told, as if the mind must have a way to pass its time, docket all the promptings for itself, within its narrow bone care. A final flame-lit prism of remembering . . . .

Ivan Doig, *The House of Sky: Landscapes of a Western Mind,* Harcourt Brace Jovanovich

In our arrogant worship of the new forms we sometimes forget that the treasures of memory and the linkage of the young with the old are the ingredients of saga.

Kirsch, The Book Report, *San Jose Mercury*

TABLE 8-2
DISSERTATIONS ON REMINISCING

Year	Author	Title	University
1957	Thumin, Frederick	Reminiscence as a function of mental and chronological age	Washington University
1960	Getoff, Louis	The earliest memories of three age groups	Columbia University
1968	Gorney, J. E.	Experience and age patterns of reminiscences among the elderly	University of Chicago
1969	Falk, J. M.	The organization of remembered life experience of older people: Its relation to anticipated stress, to subsequent adaptation, and to age	University of Chicago
1970	Lewis, C. N.	Reminiscence and self-concept in old age	Boston University
1970	Postems, L. J.	Reminiscing time orientation and self-concept in aged	Michigan State University
1972	Coleman, Peter G.	The role of the past in adaptation to old age	University of London
1975	Runyan, William McKinley	Life histories: A field of inquiry and a framework for intervention	Harvard University
1976	Fallot, Roger Dale	The life story through reminiscence in adulthood	Yale University
1977	McCarthy, Henry Francis	Reminiscence and old age: An attributional analysis	University of Kansas
1978	Romaniuk, Michael	Reminiscence and the elderly: An exploration of its content, function, press and product	University of Wisconsin, Madison
1978	Hendricks, Laura Ann	The relationship between life satisfaction and life review process among older persons	Florida State University

terpretation of Reminiscence in the Aged" (Butler, 1963a). One other classic article by McMahon and Rhudick (1964) and the writings of Erik Erikson (1950, 1957) have also provided a theoretical basis for the framework of reminiscing.

Butler (1963a) postulated that the life review was "a universal occurrence in older people of an inner experience or mental process. A life review is characterized by the progressive return to consciousness of past experiences and particularly the resurgence of unresolved conflicts which can be looked at again and reintegrated. . . . [A successful review] can give new significance and meaning to one's life and prepare one for death, by mitigating fear and anxiety."

Butler's writings on the life review are highly recommended to all those undertaking reminiscing in their own clinical practice.

Qualitative aspects of memory in older persons were discussed in detail by Butler (1963b) in one of his early articles. He discussed the content and meaning of memories and some of the interpersonal contexts. Table 8-3 is taken from that particular article in which he categorized and summarized some of the aspects of the life review. His observations indicated that "inner experience occurs even in the most idealized, crisis-free situation, but that in its more severe form it may itself lead to crises of great proportion. Thus one may see obsessive rumination and guilt concerning times past, which may be followed by despair and suicide" (Butler, 1963b, p. 524).

TABLE 8-3
THE LIFE REVIEW

1. Reminiscence: Nostalgia, regret, pleasure, idealization of past.
2. Complications: Pain, guilt, obsessive rumination over the past, despair, depression, "torschlusspanik," suicide.
3. Resolution: Constructive reorganization, creativity, wisdom, atonement, philanthropy, serenity, contentment, summarization (memoirs, treatise, history, biography), maturity, autonomy, honesty, judgment, philosophical development, living in the present.

SOURCE: Butler, 1963b.

UNIVERSALITY OF REMINISCENCE

Havighurst and Glasser (1972, p. 245) agree with Butler when they state, "Reminiscence appears to be universal at all ages . . . ." According to these researchers, reminiscence is not identical with memory. It is one aspect of memory, and they consider both purposeful and spontaneous retrospection to be reminiscence. They also re-

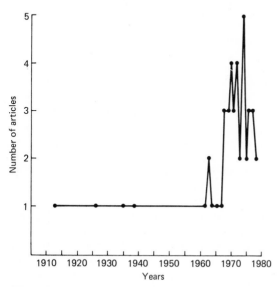

FIGURE 8-1 Journal articles on reminiscing, from 1913 to 1978.

mind their readers that, although much of the work in reminiscing has concentrated on oral reminiscence, much more reminiscence is silent and without an audience.

Five groups of subjects, both men and women, between the ages of 62 and 89 answered questions about their past and present reminiscing. Some of the conclusions drawn by the researchers of this study were the following:

1. Sexes do not differ as significantly in the frequency as in the affective quality of reminiscence. The variance in reminiscence affect was more than three times greater for women than for men.
2. People for whom reminiscence produced a pleasant affect tended to have a higher frequency of reminiscence.
3. Pleasant reminiscences or those with a positive mood were also associated with the individual's good adjustment and morale.
4. A positive mood or affect correlated with a positive evaluation by the reminiscent in relation to others who were of the same age.

Havighurst and Glasser (1972) conclude, "Reminiscence is a phenomenon caused by a multiplicity of factors in the personality and the life experience of a person."

ADAPTIVE FUNCTION OF REMINISCENCE

In another classic study, McMahon and Rhudick (1964) found an adaptational significance of reminiscing for the aged. They studied 25 noninstitutionalized Spanish-American War Veterans and concluded that reminiscing was ". . . a complex organized mental activity under ego control and varying into personality structure . . . positively correlated with successful adaptation to old age through the maintenance of self-esteem, reaffirming a sense of identity, working through and mastery of personal losses and means of contributing positively to society" (p. 297).

Another researcher, J. M. Falk (1969), has reported that his findings did not confirm the view of McMahon and Rhudick and others that reminiscence has adaptive value and that reviewing one's life is a universal task among those faced with imminent death.

Falk (1969) delineated some factors which influence the style of reminiscence upon life experience in old age. Three sample groups included: (1) 35 elderly persons who were active members of an urban community, (2) 84 elderly persons accepted for placement at homes for the aged, and (3) 23 long-term residents of old-age homes. The mean age of subjects was 79. Life histories of subjects were recorded in running narrative form.

The major findings of this study included the following:

1. The childhood portion of the life review appeared to be a more sensitive reflection of the current situation than did the adulthood segment; the two segments showed independence of organization.
2. Old people in a situation of stress (e.g., imminent institutionalization) organize their life histories somewhat differently from persons who are in stable situations.
3. There is a decrease in older subjects' reports of trivial unhappinesses of the remote past, and also there is a lack of negative affect when describing childhood deprivation.
4. Old people close to death talk less about their lives than persons who are distant from death.

ADAPTATION TO STRESS

Lieberman and Falk (1971) studied aged respondents during an investigation of adaptation to stress. These researchers considered four general areas: (1) the importance of reminiscing to the subject, (2) the restructuring of memories, (3) the selection processes the subject used to report his or her life history, and (4) the role of recollections in the subject's current psychological economy. The researchers suggest that their findings are "still crude" and reveal the need to examine other influences, such as "the effect of the individual's current level of social interaction on the degree to which he is involved in remembering past activities (and the degree to which the) individual's personal reflections are impor-

tant to him" (p. 140). Their findings did show the value of reminiscence information for a better understanding of psychology of old age.

Tobin and Etigson (1968) in their study found that the present level of stress and the affective state of an individual can be discovered through readily shared memories.

Lewis (1970) studied reminiscents to determine whether, when an individual was under a social threat, there were cognitive differences in the consistency of the self-concept when compared with nonreminiscents. Twenty-four males over 65 were subjects in two 1-hour nondirective interviews which were taped. Tapes were then reviewed, and subjects were classified as reminiscents or nonreminiscents on the basis of the percentage of sentences referring to the past. The subjects then participated in two sessions, one describing their present self and one describing their past self.

Reminiscing was consistent between sessions, which indicated that the classifications were not based on simply random behavior. Reminiscents and nonreminiscents showed no differences in self-concept in a conversation situation. However, under threat, reminiscents shifted their self-concepts to make the present self-concept more consistent with the past self-concept. This switch was interpreted as a strategy to enable reminiscents to identify with their pasts. Thus, they could avoid the full impact of present ego stresses which invariably accompany old age.

IMPORTANCE OF STUDYING MEMORIES

Tobin (1972) felt that studying the earliest memory not only provided useful data for research in gerontology, but it also had "potential in revealing current concerns of the aged respondent." A pool of 120 earliest memories were analyzed for the dominant themes. The data were gathered from three samples of community ($N = 40$), waiting list for an institution ($N = 100$), and institutionalized ($N = 100$) aged. The mean age was 78. Memories when shared can give clues to present concerns of the reminiscent. See Figure 8-2 for a group discussing drawings they made of an early memory.

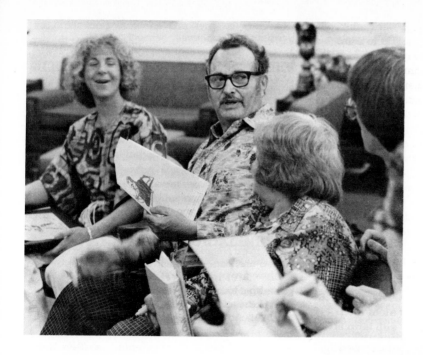

FIGURE 8-2 Drawing early memories was the theme of this inservice class on reminiscing therapy. Jim Kelly, the instructor, is asking members of the class to describe the memory and why it has been so important to them. (*Courtesy of Anthony J. Skirlick, Jr.*)

Schachtel (1947, p. 3) has concluded that "memory as a function of the living personality can be understood only as a capacity for the organization and reconstruction of past experiences and impressions in the service of present needs, fears and interest."

Cameron (1972) performed three studies of subjects of various ages in a variety of settings. The subjects' reminiscences were interrupted, and they were either asked what they were thinking about or given a questionnaire asking the questions. No sex differences were found. Adults think most frequently about the present and think next most about the future. They think about the past least of all. Cameron found a tendency for the older adult to think less frequently about the future and more frequently about the present, although evidence did not support the notion that the older person thinks more often about the past than do people in other age groups. He also stated, "Thinking about the past is not the same thing as reminiscing. The concept 'reminiscing' refers to thinking about relatively remote events rather than immediately past events" (Cameron, 1972, p. 119).

Lewis (1973) agrees with Tobin that the memories of an aged client can be useful to a

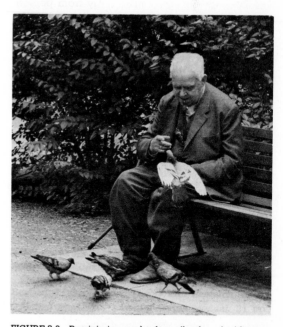

FIGURE 8-3 Reminiscing can be done silently and without an audience, although the man in the above photograph seems to have found a particular kind of audience. (Notice how baggy the pants, how big the suit jacket—caretakers need to help the aged client's self-esteem by clothes that are comfortable and that fit decently.) (*World Health Organization, Courtesy of E. Mandelmann.*)

therapist working with a client. He observes that the therapist who considers only the symbolic value of the client's memories may not notice that the significance of time is one way an old person copes with stress. While the proclivity to reminisce is widespread in old age, it may also be evidenced in other very stressful, even life-threatening, situations, as shown, for example, in Frankl's (1959) accounts of concentration camp life during the Nazi regime.

Weinberg (1974) encourages aged parents to reminisce about their lives so that if the adult children really listen, they can learn about their origins and identity. He suggests ways to improve communication and get "the hidden meaning," and argues that listening is a creative process. Early photographs of parents and grandparents may be found to use as a catalyst for stimulating memory and also to stimulate the aged client. See Figure 8-4.

Charles Lewis (1973) says that ". . . reminiscing may be a general way, not limited to old age, for coping with the loss of cherished physical objects, or life-long social roles" (p. 118). Old people may also feel stripped of their past identity when they are moved about and are often alone in strange environs with new people.

COGNITIVE DISSONANCE

Lewis (1973) also relates the cognitive dissonance theory to reminiscence in a discussion of using reminiscing to reduce dissonance between the old persons' self-expectations from the past and their present behavior. Simply maintaining a sense of worthiness may not be adequate to the client's needs; it may be helpful to reconstruct attitudes which change a potential dissonant evaluation into a more consonant one. Many old people lack formal education and rue the fact that they did not complete their schooling; yet in reminiscing groups they and others can discover how intelligent they are and what they have learned in a lifetime. (See Chapter 4 for a description of fluid and crystal intelligence.)

Dissonance theory (Festinger, 1957) does emphasize the importance of having a social support to reinforce one's internal beliefs, and, therefore, it is well to remember that reminiscing might require the involvement of another person. Repetition, says Lewis, may be necessary until the dissonance is reduced. Reminiscing should be viewed as ego-building and encouraged for its therapeutic value, rather than being considered as garrulous behavior with little meaning (Lewis, 1973). (Unfortunately, many health professionals still regard reminiscing as repetitive storytelling or garrulousness.)

GENERAL CHARACTERISTICS OF REMINISCENCE

Coleman (1974) measured reminiscing characteristics and life reviewing as elicited from the "spontaneous conversation" of elderly people living in sheltered housing in London. The sample was a small one, 38 women and 32 men. Only old people living alone were visited for the study. Three women and three men died during the data collection period of 2 years, and another

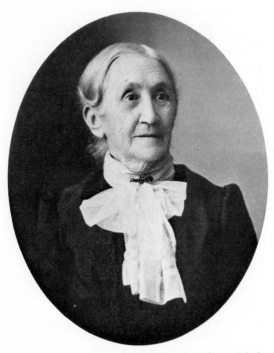

FIGURE 8-4 Old photographs provide a basis for reminiscing by the old person. They can give a child a sense of connectedness and show the styles and fashions of another era. (*Courtesy of Miriam Hawkins.*)

10 women and 6 men were not cooperative in providing tape recordings and completing questionnaires. Of the remainder, 19 of the women and 18 of the men were widowed; the women were more disabled than the men. Eight women and four men were homebound. The average number of visits per person was six, spread over the period of $1\frac{1}{2}$ to 2 years.

The study showed that the psychological processes which occur in the consciousness during the life review can be studied by using a conversational approach, and although the researcher cannot observe or classify thoughts themselves, it is possible to classify the natural speech, which does mirror the psychological processes.

Boylin et al. (1976) administered a questionnaire to 41 elderly institutionalized veterans in a Veterans' Administration hospital in New York. *The mean age was 64.37* (a much younger sample than that of McMahon and Rhudick's study). This article carefully and critically examines the empirical studies on reminiscing and suggests that a major problem in developing scales which correspond to Erikson's stages is to select items that will be characteristic of only one stage, and will at the same time follow Erikson's theoretical assumptions (Erikson, 1950). These researchers found "a significant correlation between frequency of reminiscing and . . . ego adjustment. . . . in a sample of elderly institutionalized males." The researchers also suggest, as did McMahon and Rhudick, that reminiscing does serve as an adaptive function for the older person.

In 1957 and 1962 Thumin investigated the amount of reminiscence as a function of chronological age, mental age, sex, and the rest interval prior to recall. The subjects were equally divided among male and female and included older adults, adults, adolescents, and children. One group was labeled "advanced adults" and ranged from age 49 to 72. This group had the highest mean chronological age of any group; *it was 58.*

Results showed that (1) reminiscence increased between late childhood and early adulthood and decreased between early adulthood and advanced adulthood; (2) the amount of reminiscence did not vary as a function of chronological age but did vary as a function of mental age; (3) the rest intervals, which were between 3 and 6 minutes, did not predict any significantly different amounts of reminiscence for any subject classification; (4) males and females did not show significantly different amounts of reminiscence.

Gorney (1968) is another early researcher in the study of reminiscing. He studied 175 aged subjects to examine the process of older persons introspectively examining their feelings. Three subgroups were used with these aged subjects: (1) those on a waiting list for old-age homes, 78.8; (2) community residents, 78.9; and (3) institutionalized residents, 80.8. There were three styles of organizing and evaluating their past life experiences: (1) flight from past, (2) manifestation of conflict (active life review), and (3) resolution.

MEMORIES OF CENTENARIANS

Costa and Kastenbaum (1967) studied aspects of the memories and ambitions of centenarians. The subjects of the study were centenarians registered with the Social Security Administration, and the interviews were conducted from 1958 to 1960. The sample was 276; 90 percent were between 100 and 103 years of age when interviewed; 70 percent were men. One measure of the centenarians' perspectives is the time period in their lives in which they locate their memories. Three memory-recall items included: (1) earliest memory, (2) most salient historical event, and (3) most exciting event. The findings revealed that centenarians tended to put their memories into perspective rather than show a gross ignorance in their recollections.

Beard (1968) stated that the centenarians she studied accepted the popular attitude toward memory loss in the aged and that few felt embarrassed by it; some, however, considered it a nuisance, and others worked assiduously to retain their memory powers.

FREE-FLOWING REMINISCING

One form of reminiscing, free-flowing, without purposeful direction, may involve talking at length without referring to one's self or one's own problems. Another form of reminiscing takes a definite direction and is used to enable the worker to see clients in a different setting where they were competent people and in relationship to others, particularly significant others. Reminiscing about this aspect of their lives can awaken emotional faculties, delay further deterioration, and sustain that part of the individual which is still functioning.

REGRESSED OLDSTERS

Lewis and Butler (1974, p. 169) state that "life-review therapy need not be ruled out because of brain damage." They do advise, however, that one should prevent catastrophic reactions. (See Chapter 14 for discussion of such reactions which can be triggered in brain-damaged individuals.) These authors suggest that although the brain damage is irreversible, the depression can be alleviated and also that adaptation can be encouraged.

Liton and Olstein (1969) state that regressed oldsters, who fail to respond to conventional approaches, are more involved in telling memories which were dated in the remote past as compared with recent past. "Reminiscing can enable such clients to regain that part of their identity . . . and may even bring about a further development of their identity" (p. 263). The older person's reminiscing may serve as a substitute for actual experience, and also the old person's present situation may color the memories shared.

REMINISCING: AN ANTIDOTE TO BOREDOM

In a classic article on boredom, Heron (1957) described subjects' reactions to the isolation they were experiencing. At first the subjects thought about the studies and the experiment they were involved in, then about their personal problems, later they began to reminisce about past incidents, their families, and peers. If it is important for young people to reminisce in their moments of isolation and when experiencing extreme lack of stimuli, then how much importance must rem-

iniscing have for the elderly person who is institutionalized in a dull and sterile environment! Often severe sensory loss accompanies the isolation from the mainstream of life.

NURSES' CONTRIBUTIONS

Nurses have published a number of useful articles primarily concerned with problems and methods of implementing reminiscence therapy in groups. Burnside discussed the cultivation of "memory gardens" with the aged and emphasized the importance of discussion of the "there and then" as well as the "here and now" with group members (Burnside, 1969, 1971).

Wichita (1974) studied three groups of elderly residents in a 200-bed long-term care facility. Here groups consisted of "nonapathetic residents," "depressed residents," and "nondepressed residents." She noted several positive behavioral changes among the members of a reminiscing group which met at breakfast three times. Those changes included: increased eye contact, increased spoken response, increased movement of head and shoulders and use of hands. Wichita also noted that all residents in the experimental group showed positive behavior in the breakfast reminiscing group, but "some of those same residents when returned to the dining room for the noon and evening meal returned to their apathetic states."

Hala (1975) initiated a pilot project with two different groups of people who met each week to reminisce. Her objectives were (1) to give residents a chance to meet together 1 hour weekly, (2) to review their lives and prepare for death, (3) to encourage physical closeness by seating arrangements, and (4) to provide the mechanism for the displaying of interest and recognition by the leader and the other group members. In a step-by-step observation, Hala identified a process of increasing socialization for one resident who did join the group and was not accustomed to socializing.

She pointed out that there had been some initial need to explain the reminiscing group because reminiscing had some of the negative connotations for staff members which were mentioned earlier. Some staff members, for example, thought that "talking of the past was inappropriate for remotivation."

In the role of leader, Hala discovered that she became more methodical in the implementation of nursing interventions and saw the value of looking at the results with objectivity. She was "not so concerned that all results be positive."

In the following year, Ebersole (1976) wrote about the problems of group reminiscing with the institutionalized aged. Reminiscing as a group modality was described along with problems which occur in groupings: (1) helplessness and hopelessness of members, (2) repetitive reminiscing, (3) monologues concurrently, (4) confrontation, (5) crying in groups, (6) physical discomfort, (7) time factor, (8) interpersonal timing, (9) obsession of language, (10) the "good" group member, (11) sensory deprivation, and (12) guilt of members.

Blackman (1980) conducted a reminiscing group in the community; the three components basic to her group were resocialization, reminiscence, and the life review. She wrote, "If resocialization and reminiscence were cultivated, I postulated that the climate for the life review in group members would then be positively influenced. . . . I felt confident of the innate value in resocialization and reminiscence; they could stand alone as therapeutic tools" (p. 134). Later in the same chapter Blackman adds a very important statement: "I feel that it is important to be aware of the lack of understanding for or experience with the small group modality, because reading the literature does not prepare one for that" (p. 140).

The following excerpt from a nursing instructor in Australia describes how one reminiscing experience was initiated by a student nurse:

One of my students decided that week after a lecture on reminiscing that she would try out some reminiscing group work on the ward to which she was assigned. She collected six people (and two more joined the group themselves) and introduced herself, saying where she lived and where she was born. One elderly lady who is slightly dysphasic chimed in saying, "My father was the first glassblower in Victoria, and I was born at Zuchworth." (This is an old Australian gold-mining town from the last century.)

One of the gentlemen stated his name and proceeded to say how glassblowers used to visit his school when he was a child, making little animals for the children, upon which a lady who had joined the group of her own volition said, "I collect old bottles, and I have one with a Dawson seal." (This must be quite something to the collector, I guess!) Amazingly, the first lady then exclaimed, "My maiden name was Dawson, so you must have one of my father's bottles!"

Isn't that great? And so fortunate to have all that happen on the first attempt! That ward now runs such a group on a weekly basis, and the Charge Sister tells me that she has noticed a change of attitude among the nursing aides; no longer are their patients simply "so many old men and women," but they now are able to view them and relate to them as people who have lived an interesting life, loved and lost—just as they themselves are doing. (Jones, 1978)

PROFESSIONALS FROM MANY DISCIPLINES LEAD REMINISCING GROUPS

Zeiger (1976) used life review in her art therapy groups with aged members. She concluded that it is normal for old people to talk about their past, that the therapist needs to be a sympathetic listener, and that sensitivity is important. Activities combined with reminiscing can help people recall what they have forgotten or comprehend material they had not previously understood.

Weisman and Shusterman (1977) describe ways they combine reminiscing, remembering, and the life review in their activity programs at a Hebrew home, a 265-bed, long-term care facility. Eight activities are regularly scheduled daily from 9:00 A.M. to 9:00 P.M., 7 days a week. The most extensive activity at the home was an oral history project in which more than 50 residents were interviewed. Case examples offered in-

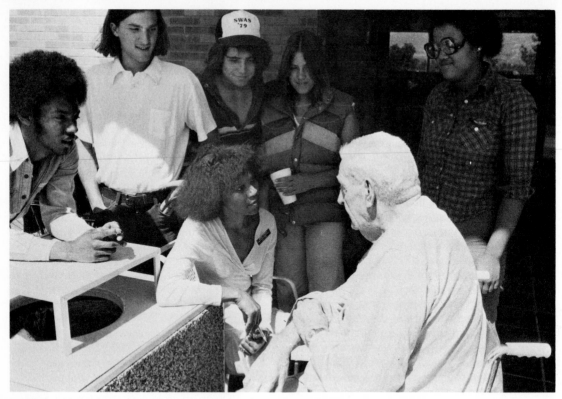

FIGURE 8-5 "In our arrogant worship of the new forms, we sometimes forget that the treasure of memory and the linkage of the young with the old are the ingredients of saga" (Kirsch, 1978). (*Courtesy of Anthony J. Skirlick, Jr.*)

clude discussion of depression and the use of music, poetry, antiques, night school, and trigger films as catalysts for reminiscing in activities.

Pincus (1970) wrote an article for social workers on the use of reminiscence with aged clients and the implications for social work practice. He stated that "both the amount and content of the elderly client's reminiscence provide diagnostic clues to the worker." He suggested that an absence of reminiscing might be indicative of depression, although that would have to be checked out carefully by the nurse. The content of the reminiscing, he noted, might reflect some of the internal struggles of the individual.

Butler (1974) feels that nonprofessionals can also function as therapists if they become skilled in their listening abilities when older people are telling about their lives. And old people also can be helped to handle their own life reviews.

CHRONICLES OF LIVES OF OLD PEOPLE

English teachers are also involved in positive production about reminiscing. High school magazines have now become popular as an effective way to teach English. *Foxfire* was in the vanguard of this trend in Rabun Gap–Nacoochee School in Georgia. High school students interview and photograph old people and their lives and accomplishments. The students are taught interviewing techniques, and they then become chroniclers of the lives of old people and the contributions they have made in their environment. Other high school magazines in other states include *Salt*, Kennebunkport, Maine; *Three Wire Winter*, Steamboat Springs, Colorado; *Mo'Olelo*, Kapaa and Kauai High Schools, Kauai, Hawaii. One book advises students about the details of film processing, maintaining sub-scriptions lists, and courteous interviewing techniques (Wood, 1975).

The yield from these student publications is threefold: (1) the high school student learns to write English more readily when there are real events and the interesting perspective of old people to write about, (2) the old people benefit when they are interviewed and encouraged to reminisce for publication, and (3) current readers and posterity can benefit from the experiences of the old people.

Kirsch (1978) said, "In our arrogant worship of the new forms, we sometimes forget that the treasure of memory and the linkage of the young with the old are the ingredients of saga."

STATEMENTS ABOUT REMINISCING FROM THE LITERATURE

MECHANICS OF REMINISCING

- Reminiscing can be verbal (Webster's, 1975).
- Reminiscing can be written (Webster's, 1975).
- Reminiscing can be conversational (Coleman, 1974).
- Reminiscing is a linguistic act which refers to the remote past (Coleman, 1974).
- Reminiscing provides a set of sagas (Kirsch, 1978).
- Life reminiscing is an inner experience or mental process (Havighurst and Glasser, 1972; Butler, 1963a).
- Reminiscing can be free-flowing with no direction (Liton and Olstein, 1969).
- Reminiscing can be structured with direction (Liton and Olstein, 1969).

REMINISCING AS A BASIS FOR ESTABLISHING COMMUNICATION

- Reminiscing can include:
  Earliest memory
  Most salient historical event
  Most exciting event in one's lifetime (Costa and Kastenbaum, 1967)

- Reminiscing is adaptive for the aged (McMahon and Rhudick, 1964).
- Reminiscing helps regain identity (Liton and Olstein, 1969; McMahon and Rhudick, 1964).
- Individual's personal reflections are important to the reminiscer (Lieberman and Falk, 1971).
- Studying the earliest memory is useful (Tobin, 1972).
- Memories by centenarians can be put into perspective (Costa and Kastenbaum, 1967).
- Regressing aged can benefit from reminiscing (Lewis and Butler, 1974; Liton and Olstein, 1969).
- Sexes do not differ significantly on frequency or affective tone of reminiscing (Havighurst and Glasser, 1972).
- High frequency of reminiscing is associated positively with a pleasant affect (Havighurst and Glasser, 1972).
- Photographs may be catalysts for stimulating memories (Weinberg, 1974).

REMINISCING IN NURSING PRACTICE

Reminiscing is an integral component of geron-tological nursing and should be encouraged in the care of and interaction with the older client, in both individual and group modalities. The use of reminiscing in a client's problems of social iso-lation, rejection, and loss of identity is an impor-tant therapeutic approach.

Oral history is another term used and is de-fined by Hoopes (1979, p. 7) as "the collecting of any individual's spoken memories of his life, of people he has known, and events he has wit-nessed or participated in."

SPECIFIC RECOMMENDATIONS BY LEWIS AND BUTLER

Lewis and Butler (1974) describe ways to put memories to work in the individual or group therapy session. In individual psychotherapy, they recommend (1) written or taped autobiog-raphies; (2) pilgrimages; (3) reunions; (4) genealogy; (5) scrapbooks, photo albums, old letters, memorabilia; (6) summation of life work; (7) preserving ethnic identity. In group psychotherapy, they recommend age-integrated groups, so that the elderly can assume an active learning role concurrently with their teaching stance in the group. Such groups can decrease the older person's feelings of uselessness and isolation. They may hear familiar themes of their own life from younger group members; they do contribute meaning for perspective to such groups.

Memories are also the stuff of autobiographies and fiction; the literature is replete with stories and sagas based on memory told by skilled storytellers. Nurses can encourage clients to write or tape memoirs.

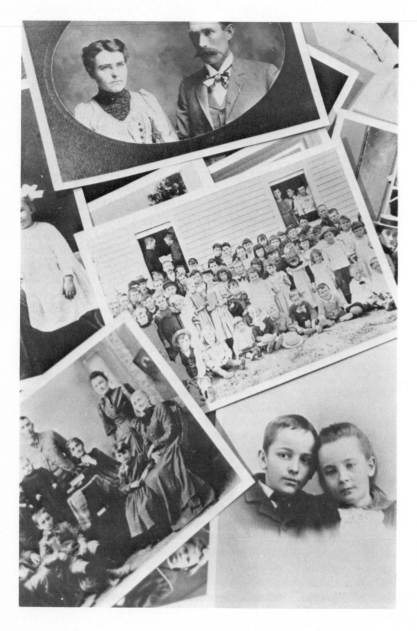

FIGURE 8-6 An important prop in reminiscing with aged group members is a photograph that helps them cultivate memory gardens. Photos also serve as catalysts for triggering memories, and the group members often get ideas from the person describing the memory. (*Courtesy of Anthony J. Skirlick, Jr.*)

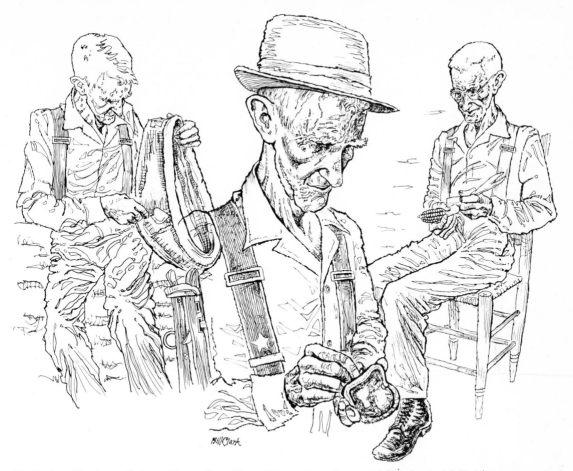

FIGURE 8-7 "Jack's grandfather is 96. . . . Sit awhile and hear a story of long ago." (*Drawing by Bill Clark.*)

OTHER RECOMMENDATIONS

1. Use in-service classes to teach reminiscing therapy (see Figure 8-3).
2. Encourage reminiscing through the verbal or written mode. Drawings of memories can be powerful and effective.
3. Learn both the free-flowing approach and also ways to structure reminiscing therapy, for example, when working with chronic brain-syndrome individuals.
4. Use easy approaches in the beginning; e.g., use earliest memory, an exciting moment in history, or an exciting event out of a person's life (Costa and Kastenbaum, 1967).
5. Encourage reminiscing that restores identity; e.g., consider the past jobs and accomplishments of the individual.
6. Try to put the memories of 90-year-olds and centenarians into chronological perspective to better grasp the significance and the span of their lives.
7. Go slowly when pressing chronic brain-syndrome individuals for memories—do not create catastrophic reactions in your therapeutic wake.
8. Listen for tone of voice and pitch and watch facial expression during telling of memory to ascertain importance and power of that particular memory.
9. Use photographs and memorabilia as catalysts (Weinberg, 1974).

10. Students should experience a reminiscing group before they lead one or do their own life review.
11. When beginning, do not press for more information in the painful areas recounted. Allow time and increased trust. Later, aged persons will often return and finish describing the painful memory.
12. Use much sensory stimulation and a variety of props in reminiscing groups with the regressed aged.

In the preface of a book is this descriptive passage:

> As we age, the mystery of Time more and more dominates the mind. We live less in the present, which no longer has the solidity that it had in youth; less in the future, for the future every day narrows its span. The abiding things lie in the past, and the mind busies itself. . . . (Buchan, 1940, p. 7)

As professionals, can we more often help memory hold open the door to the abiding things of the past for those aged in our care?

REFERENCES

Ballard, P. B.: Oblivescence and reminiscing, *British Journal of Psychology Monograph Supplement,* **1**(2), 1913.

Beard, Belle Boone: Some characteristics of recent memory of centenarians, *Journal of Gerontology,* **23**(1):23–30, 1968.

Blackman, Janet C.: Group work in the community: Experiences with reminiscence, in Irene Mortenson Burnside (ed.), *Psychosocial Nursing Care of the Aged,* 2d ed., McGraw-Hill, New York, 1980, pp. 134, 140.

Boylin, William, Susan K. Gordon, and Milton F. Nehrke: Reminiscing and ego integrity in institutionalized elderly males, *Gerontologist,* **16**(2):118–124, April 1976.

Buchan, John: *Memory Hold the Door,* Hodder, London, 1940, p. 7.

Bunch, M. E.: The measure of reminiscence, *Psychological Review,* **45**:525–531, 1938.

Burnside, Irene Mortenson: Group work among the aged, *Nursing Outlook,* **17**(6):68–72, June 1969.

————: Long-term group work with hospitalized aged, pt. I, *Gerontologist,* **11**(3):213–218, Autumn 1971.

Butler, Robert N.: The life review: An interpretation of reminiscence in the aged, *Psychiatry,* **26**(1):65–76, February 1963a.

————: Recall in retrospections, *Journal of American Geriatric Society,* **11**(6):523–529, June 1963b.

————: Successful aging and the role of the life review, *Journal of the American Geriatrics Society,* **22**(12):529–535, December 1974.

Cameron, Paul: The generation gap: Time orientation, *Gerontologist,* pt. I, **12**(2):117–119, Summer 1972.

Coleman, P. G.: Measuring reminiscence characteristics from conversations as adaptive features of old age, *International Journal of Aging and Human Development,* **5**(3):281–294, Summer 1974.

————: The role of the past in adaptation to old age, Ph.D. thesis, University of London, 1972.

Costa, Paul, and Robert Kastenbaum: Some aspects of memories and ambition in centenarians, *Journal of Genetic Psychology,* **110**:3–6, March 1967.

Ebersole, Priscilla: Establishing reminiscing groups, in Irene M. Burnside (ed.), *Working with the Elderly: Group Process and Techniques,* Duxbury, North Scituate, Mass., 1978.

————: Problems of group reminiscing with the institutionalized aged, *Journal of Gerontological Nursing,* **2**(6):23–27, November–December 1976.

Erikson, E. H.: *Childhood and Society,* Norton, New York, 1950.

————: Identity and the life cycle, *Psychological Issues,* I. Monograph, (1): International Universities, New York, 1957.

Falk, J. M.: The organization of remembered life experience of older people: Its relation to anticipated stress, to subsequent adaptation and to age, Unpublished doctoral dissertation, University of Chicago, 1969.

Festinger, L.: *A Theory of Cognitive Dissonance,* Stanford University, Stanford, Calif., 1957.

Frankl, Viktor: *From Death Camp to Existentialism,* Beacon Press, Boston, 1959.

Gorney, J. E.: Experiencing and age: Patterns of reminiscence among the elderly, Ph.D. abstract, The Committee on Human Development, University of Chicago, 1968.

Hala, Michele P.: Reminiscence group therapy project, *Journal of Gerontological Nursing,* **1**(3):34–41, July/August 1975.

Havighurst, R. J., and G. Glasser: An exploratory study of reminiscence, *Journal of Gerontology,* **27**(2):245–253, 1972.

Heron, Woodburn: The pathology of boredom, *Scientific American* **196**(1):52–56, January 1957.

Hoopes, James: *Oral History: Introduction for Student,* University of North Carolina, Chapel Hill, N.C., 1979.

Jones, Gail: Personal communication, 1978.

Kirsch, Robert: Ivan Doig: Hewn from Montana (a

book report), *San Jose Mercury News*, September 1978.

Lewis, Charles: The adaptive value of reminiscing in old age, *Journal of Geriatric Psychiatry*, **6**(1):117–121, 1973.

————— : Reminiscence and self-concept in old age, doctoral dissertation, Boston University, 1970.

Lewis, Myrna I., and Robert N. Butler: Life-review therapy: Putting memories to work in individual and group psychotherapy, *Geriatrics*, **22**(11):166–173, November 1974.

Lieberman, M. A., and J. M. Falk: The remembered past as a source of data for research on the life cycle, *Human Development*, **14**(2):132–141, 1971.

Liton, J., and S. C. Olstein: Therapeutic aspects of reminiscence, *Social Casework*, **50**:263–268, 1969.

McGeoch, G. O.: The condition of reminiscence, *American Journal of Psychology*, **47**:65–87, 1935.

McMahon, A., and P. Rhudick: Reminiscing: Adaptational significance for the aged, *Archives of General Psychiatry*, **10**(3):292–298, March 1964.

Pincus, Allen: Reminiscence in aging and its implications for social work practice, *Social Work*, **15**(4):42–51, October 1970.

Schachtel, E.: On memory and childhood amnesia, *Psychiatry*, **10**:1–26, 1947.

Thumin, Frederick: Reminiscence as a function of chronological and mental age, *Journal of Gerontology*, **17**(4):392–396, October 1962.

————— : Reminiscence as a function of mental age and chronological age, unpublished doctoral dissertation, Washington University, 1957.

————— : Unpublished master's thesis, 1956.

Tobin, Sheldon S.: The earliest memory as data for research in aging, in Donald P. Kent, Robert Kastenbaum, and Sylvia Therwood (eds.), *Research Planning and Action for the Elderly*, Behavioral Publications, New York, 1972.

—————, **and E. Etigson:** Effect of stress on the earliest memory, *Archives of General Psychiatry*, **19**:435–444, October 1968.

Webster's New Twentieth Century Dictionary: William, Collins and World, 1975.

Weinberg, Jack: What do I say to my mother when I have nothing to say?, *Geriatrics*, **22**(11):155–159, November 1974.

Weisman, Shulmatia, and Rochelle Shusterman: Remembering, reminiscing and life reviewing in an activity program for the elderly, *Concern*, December–January 1977, pp. 22–26.

Wichita, Carol: Reminiscing as a therapy for apathetic and confused residents of nursing homes, unpublished master's thesis, University of Arizona, Tucson, 1974.

Wigginton, Eliot: *The Foxfire Book*, Anchor Press, Garden City, N.J., 1972.

Williams, O. A.: A study of the phenomenon of reminiscence, *Journal of Experimental Psychology*, **9**:368–387, 1926.

Wood, Pamela: *You and Aunt Aries*, Ideas, Dept. R., Magnolia Star Route, Nederland, Colorado, 1975.

Zeiger, Betty L.: Life review in art therapy with the aged, *American Journal of Art Therapy*, **15**(2):47–50, January 1976.

OTHER RESOURCE

Past Present: Recording Life Stories of Older People. This report by Sara Jenkins describes a "listening project" using older volunteers trained in interviewing to record the memories of their peers. 150 pages. NCOA Publications Department, 1828 L Street, N.W., Washington, DC 20036.

NINE

FAMILY THERAPY

John J. Herr
John H. Weakland

Probably the hardest thing to do is to relate to older family members *as they are now* rather than as they were in the past.
Lillian Troll, Sheila Miller, Robert Atchley
Families in Later Life, **1979, p. 128**

LEARNING OBJECTIVES

- Identify the source of knowledge about family systems.
- Define an "identified patient."
- Discuss the reasons an elder is cast in a medical role of "patient."
- Discuss how one symptom, hypochondriasis in an elder, might increase and become a problem within a family.
- List interventions in the problem of hypochondriasis that might help to de-escalate the symptoms.
- List data that will be needed during interviews if a family describes an elder member as having "the problem."
- Describe in detail three typical problems a nurse could expect to find in a family that presents complaints about an older member.

As a nurse and a health professional what you say to your clients and their families has a significant impact, for better or worse. Frequently the impact will not be as you intended—for instance, a client or family fails to take your direct advice—but an impact, even if negative, will still be there. In a similar way, as a result of their interactions, family members exert an enormous amount of influence on other family members: on how they think, how they feel, and how they act with one another. The purpose of this chapter is to consider how interactions, within families in contact with health professionals, can clarify and explain some kinds of behavioral problems of elder family members. These problems are not to any appreciable degree related to age changes (deficits) in brain or other body tissue—though such a physiological basis might often be ascribed to such problems.

FAMILY INTERACTION AND BEHAVIOR PROBLEMS

It has been known for some time that the way family members relate to one another can create behavioral problems in one or more of the members of the family (Bateson et al., 1956; Bell, 1961). By *behavioral problems* we mean persistent (or recurrent) behavior on the part of an individual which is seriously distressing either to the individual or to other members of the family or society who are concerned about the individual's behavior.

Much knowledge about how family systems can create and perpetuate problematic behavior comes from work done in the fields of child psychiatry and the treatment of young adult schizophrenics. For example, it was clearly observed that children and young adults could be removed from their home, successfully treated for their psychiatric symptoms, only to relapse when they returned to their family settings. The family therapy movement of the early 1950s arose in response to recognition of this unfortunate pattern of events and other indications of the powerful influence of family interaction (Guerin, 1976). Family therapists attempted to intervene on the family level so that the entire family changed instead of only the identified pa-

tient (i.e., the child who was identified by the parents as having "the problem"). In this model, behavioral problems of young people were seen as inseparable from the interactional patterns of their families.

The family therapy movement was so successful that today few therapists would be willing to provide therapy for a child without significant involvement of at least the parents and often the entire family. Unhappily, in the field of aging there has not been equal progress.

It was not until the mid-1960s that the success of the family therapy movement with families where young people were the identified patients (IPs) was recognized in the gerontological literature as having relevance for dealing with elders exhibiting problematic behavior (Brody, 1966). In some ways, this fact is rather peculiar, since elders and young people, particularly adolescents, face similar developmental challenges: both groups must deal with physical changes and changes within the family power structure (teen-agers becoming more powerful and elders less powerful). In other ways, this is not so surprising: For practicing gerontologists, probably the greatest single impediment to seeing the value of working with family systems as opposed to isolated individuals is the fact that most elders have at least some chronic *physical* problems unique to them and associated with the aging process. Thus, the elder is already cast in the medical role of "patient." Given the cultural stereotype that "everyone eventually gets senile," it is not difficult to understand how the behavioral problems of elders were readily, almost automatically, interpreted as the simple sequelae of age-related deficits within that individual—usually attributed to brain impairment—such that the elder presenting behavioral problems could be rather easily reclassified from "patient" in the general medical sense of the word to "identified patient" in the mental health sense of the word.

Despite the handicap of a late start and the constant temptation to refer problematic behavior uncritically to chronic physiological problems, viewing the problems of elders from a family systems point of view has gained increasing recognition as a useful tool for designing therapeutic interventions intended to change the family system to end (or ameliorate) the problematic behavior (Brody, 1977; Herr and Weak-land, 1978).

UNAVOIDABILITY OF INTERACTIONS BETWEEN FAMILY SYSTEMS AND HEALTH PROFESSIONALS

Whether you wish it or not, when working with elders, you are also working with their family system. Only 5 percent of all people over 65 are without either a living spouse, child, or sibling (Harris et al., 1975). *In other words, few elders are true isolates.* Most families are so involved with their elders that the old stereotype that "families dump their old people" is universally recognized by gerontologists to be only mythology.

Aside from the mere existence of family members, as a health professional you will find them unavoidable for an additional reason: Traditionally, when elders develop mental health problems, family members are most likely to take the initiative for treatment by contacting the general medical community, as opposed to the mental health community (Gurian, 1975). As a consequence, elders with behavioral problems are most likely to be presented through younger relatives (usually the oldest daughter or daughter-in-law) to their family physician, nurse practitioner, or other professionals. In the role of a health professional, you may be called upon to evaluate the presenting behavioral problems and recommend treatment or referral. Yet this process may begin outside the presence of the elder. A typical example might be:

Clinic nurse: What you've told me [about a parent's forgetfulness, for example] is very interesting. I wonder if you have talked to your mother about what you've just told me.

Middle-aged child: Oh, I've touched on it. But it is awfully sensitive, you know. Mother doesn't know I've come here to talk to you about it.

Consider the position in which you are placed. You have been told about a problem, asked for a professional opinion, yet have not even seen the person who is supposed to have the problem. Even if you make the referral to a mental health center, the likelihood is that again the initial contact will be made by the same concerned family member. If you are on the other end of such a referral, you will begin where the referring source left off: in the middle of the family even before you have met the IP. Certainly you might wonder, "Can the initiating family member really give an objective report about the behavior of the elder?" The answer is, "Probably not." When people get caught up in a problem—and you know family members are "caught up" if they initiate the call for help—they frequently lose their perspective as to the scope and nature of the problem.

As if the unreliability of the relative describing the behavioral problems of the elder were not enough, there are other factors that should compel a nurse working in either a traditional physical or mental health setting to consider the family situation. Often, particularly in a mental health setting, the initial contact will be made during a crisis situation. "Something has to be done *now*," probably characterizes this situation best. Yet, to help resolve the crisis, you will need to know who has decided that something has to be done. Is it a neighbor ("You just have to do something about your mother, she is gardening at three o'clock in the morning")? Is it an out-of-town relative ("I just got a crazy call from Dad, you have to do something about him, you live closest")? Or is it the relative initiating contact? Also, you will need to know, "Why now? Why not last week or next week?"

The problem can be overwhelming. There is almost no group more difficult to work with than a family in crisis looking for an instant solution to a problem that may have been slowly building over a period of several years. Yet to fail to grasp the significance of your involvement with the family system is to proceed blindly on the assumption that middle-aged children give objective data and reach reliable conclusions in dealing with their parents. Actions based on such an assumption are rarely useful for either elders or their families; the only alternative is to admit the significance of the family interaction and to systematically learn more about it.

LOOKING AT PROBLEMATIC BEHAVIOR THROUGH A FAMILY SYSTEM LENS

To examine the family systems view as applied specifically to a problematic behavior on the part of an elder, consider the case of an elder who habitually and consistently presents a plethora of symptoms, although upon examination yields no objective, physical signs of illness. Commonly and professionally such people are called *hypochondriacs.* Under some conditions they are so well known to members of the medical community that they become legends in their own time. The label *hypochondriac* implies that the source of the problem resides within the person. Presumably, if the source could be treated, then the person's psyche could be repaired, and the hypochondria would disappear.

If we accept the model in which hypochondriasis represents a deficit within the individual, then we account for the "symptoms" of the "disease" by saying that the elder patient develops hypochondriasis in response to increasing age-related deficits, in both physical and mental activities. Eventually these cumulative deficits of aging overwhelm the elder's ability to successfully function in the social milieu.

From a family systems point of view, however, we would take a different view of the problem. A family therapist might say, "I wonder under what conditions this hypochondriacal behavior would make sense?" Consequently, a family therapist might look for a family or social situation similar to the following: The elder typically feels slightly lonely and ignored. The elder takes a physical complaint to a physician. After a cursory examination, the physician tells the elder that the physical complaint "doesn't really exist." Already slightly ignored, the elder then feels more ignored since the physician seems to refuse to take him or her seriously. At this point, the elder very likely takes up the complaint with members of the family.

So as not to be ignored, the elder exaggerates the distress of the symptoms. Family members listen or come when called, yet are likely to feel manipulated and resentful. The elder detects their resentment and interprets it as rejec-

tion, disapproval—yet another example of how difficult it is to be taken seriously. To prove the reality and perhaps gravity of the illness, the elder redoubles efforts to convince the medical community of the legitimacy of the symptoms—again exaggerating in an ill-fated attempt to avoid being ignored or taken lightly. In response, members of the medical community become frustrated—like family members, they frequently feel manipulated. In anger, physicians, nurses, or aides are apt to say, "There is nothing wrong with you; it's all in your head." To hypochondriacal elders, such a statement is even more proof that no one understands their physical *condition* or will even *take them seriously.* So the elders redouble their efforts again, either with other physicians, clinics, or hospitals, or with their families.

FAMILY MEMBERS FEEL CONCERN AND ANNOYANCE

In such a situation, most family members will have growing feelings of both concern and annoyance. They feel concern that if they ignore their elders' complaints, they might erroneously dismiss a developing and life-threatening or terminal physical condition. They feel annoyed since they feel blackmailed into taking telephone calls and making visits which are "required" rather than desired. The elder, during all this uproar, is unfortunately feeling miserable. First, the elder either feels guilty for exaggerating the symptoms or, worse still, actually experiences severe symptoms to avoid feeling guilty. Second, the elder's original feelings of loneliness and unimportance have grown stronger, since family members now *initiate* contact less frequently than before the hypochondriasis began. The elder fails to see that the total amount of contact may be the same—frequently even more—but the pattern of initiation has changed such that the elder does all the initiating. If you ask a middle-aged daughter why she does not call her hypochondriacal father more often, she would be likely to answer, "What? I already listen to enough of his 'organ recitals.' To call him more I'd have to be a masochist!"

Third, the elder's feelings of being considered insignificant by the medical community are fostered by the fact that because of such a history, his or her symptoms actually are taken less seriously. In fact, physicians and nurses are less likely to return the elder's first call promptly, if at all. If you were to ask them to explain, they might tell you the same thing, "We only know it's important if he calls three times in the same day." The elder is getting more attention than in the past, but feeling less attended.

From a family systems point of view, then, hypochondriasis is not the simple result of a deficit within an older individual. Instead, it is problematic behavior being expressed by one person (the symptomatic elder) which is the result of many interactions of different people within the system: this system includes the elder, family members, and health professionals. The vicious cycle of hypochondriasis continues because each member of the system believes that what he or she is doing is helping to solve the problem, when in fact the opposite is true: It is the ineffective solution system members continue to apply that is perpetuating the vicious cycle, which in this case has been named *hypochondriasis*.

The concept of the solution being the problem is worth further exploration since it is the crux of much of the family systems view. Again referring to the example, the health professionals believe the solution to the problem is eventually to logically convince the elder not to feel the way he or she feels. ("It's all in your head.") Instead of helping, this approach hurts, since it only convinces the elder that he or she has still not been heard. Instead of relieving worry, the health professionals' lack of worry becomes worrisome in itself to the elder. Think about it: how would you like to be experiencing a bellyache that no one will take seriously? How would you like to be told that the pain you experience in your abdomen is really only in your head? Would you feel reassured?

ONE SOLUTION: IGNORE THE SITUATION

For family members, the solution seems to be to try to ignore the situation as long as possible until a major problem develops. Frequently, family members may take the side of the health professionals ("Oh, Dad, you know the doctor said it was all in your head; you're making too much out of all this!"). Again, by not taking the symptoms of the elder seriously and *only attending to the elder during an impending or actual medical crisis,* the family is inviting a medical problem. How else will the elder get to see them? What other reason is there to call?

For elders, the solution is also the problem: The more they escalate the severity of their symptoms, the less seriously they are taken. Yet escalating the symptoms does have one positive outcome, even if it is not the desired outcome: It keeps elders in contact with friends, family, and many health professionals. To give up the symptoms seems to elders as if to give up everything, just as calling elders seems to family members to be inviting an "organ recital," or as sympathizing with the pain seems to the physician to invite even more visits by the elder.

Looking at this problematic behavior from the family systems view, what is important is to help all members of the system—elders, family, and health professionals—to discontinue behavior they already can observe as ineffective in solving the problem. The necessary task, stated plainly, is to get them to stop doing what, in their own experience, has not worked. Interestingly enough, a change by any one member of the system will probably result in a change in the behavior of all. That is, if the hypochondriacal elders stop exaggerating how they feel, there is a much greater likelihood that their families—and health professionals—will take them more seriously in the future. Should family members change the way they are dealing with the situation, say, by calling elders on a daily basis for 5 minutes every evening ("just called to see how you are doing"), there is a great likelihood that elders will stop feeling ignored and not need to escalate their symptoms. Similarly, should the health professionals sympathize with elders rather than tell them they should not feel as they do, say, by taking the position "I'm sorry you are feeling so poorly; it must be terrible to have such a pain in your stomach and not be able to get any kind of definite answer from us," elders may be able to set aside the need to exaggerate their symptoms. This will also make them better patients—at least far more believable—in the event of serious illness in the future.

PUTTING FAMILY SYSTEMS THEORY TO WORK IN A CLINICAL SETTING

While this chapter is certainly far too brief to give you all the tools necessary to become a competent family therapist for elders, it is possible to cover the basics of working from a family systems model. For those interested in developing greater skills, the subject is covered elsewhere in considerable depth (Herr and Weakland, 1979).

For a start, in any series of interviews in which an elder has been identified as having "the problem," there are some things you should want to know. First, you will want to know the *nature* of the problem; that is, what specific behaviors by the elder are seen as constituting problems. Even more important, you will want to determine who is being affected by these behaviors. In other words, what is the elder actually doing that is causing a problem and for what other members of the family? Are family members losing sleep over worry? Are their marriages suffering? Are they embarrassed in front of their friends by their elder relative's behavior? How exactly is the problematic behavior of the elder becoming a problem for others? When you know this information, you will have a better grasp (as will the family) of how the problem belongs to the whole family system instead of just the elder.

Second, you will want to know *how family members*—including the elder—*have been trying to solve the problem.* What have they been doing that has been successful? What have they been doing that has not been successful? As you and the family broaden your base of information about the family system, you will begin to see how the family, including the elder, is creating a vicious cycle in which most, if not all, of their attempted solutions are turning out to intensify and sustain the problem rather than solve it.

Third, you will want to *determine a realistic* (concrete and measurable) *goal* which family members can agree represents the least amount of change in the situation that would give them a sense of progress. All too often, families with elders are seeking giant, final solutions overnight. Of course, they fail at achieving these solutions and fall into even greater despair. By specifying a measurable, realistic goal, families can frequently gain some sense of progress even if the progress is quite small. Certainly this is better than a sense of failure. Often, setting a realistic goal means making progress toward learning how to minimize the impact of a tragic situation (stroke, terminal cancer) rather than to overcome it. Only by realistic, measurable goal setting can such a positive experience come from an essentially negative event.

Fourth and finally, you will want to evaluate the outcome of your interaction with the family. Do things seem to be getting better? Has the family gotten back "on track" after some self-examination? If the answer is "yes," then there may be no need for you to continue your work with the family. If the answer is "no," then you will need to consider some other possibilities. Perhaps the family should be referred to someone who specializes in family therapy. Alternatively, some other kind of intervention may be indicated. Such an intervention may be psychological or medical, but the referral to that resource will at least be based on your firsthand knowledge of the elder's psychosocial milieu rather than on a cursory, subjective description by the elder's distressed younger relative.

TYPICAL PRESENTING PROBLEMS WITH A FAMILY COMPONENT

CONFUSION

Frequently family members will complain that an elder is "getting senile" on the basis of a conflict of interest or disagreement between one or more family members and the elder. In such a case, instead of labeling the elder "stupid" or "stubborn" or "just acting like a fool," the elder is labeled with the pejorative term "senile." In some ways, it is as if the elders lose their rights to make human errors, except at the risk of the label "senile" and creating considerable demand on the part of a relative to have the courts appoint a legal conservator or guardian. The problem would not be so acute if younger members did not really believe the elder was, in fact, becoming "senile." It is their good intentions that do the damage. They see themselves as acting benignly instead of hastily or selfishly. Particularly in the case of an economic conflict of interest—say, how to invest retirement funds or changing the terms of a will—family members may use the label "senile" as a power play to bolster their own position. Ironically, in these situations, the more competent and persuasive the elder can be, the more insistent the younger relative can become that the problem is "senility" rather than a legitimate difference of opinion.

Almost always, when a family member is insistent about the "senility" of a family elder in spite of rather clear evidence to the contrary, you should suspect that the issue is really power, not failing cognitive abilities. See Chapters 14 through 17 for further information on confusion.

DEPRESSION

All too often, particularly during a mourning period, elders are apt to be understandably depressed, yet this causes panic among their younger relatives. The family attempts to cheer the elder by pushing activities, denying there is anything to be depressed about ("Mother, you have so much to live for") or, in the worst case, relocating the independently living elder to the home of a middle-aged child. The more the family discounts the elder's depression, the more depressed the elder becomes. Such a response is quite natural for the elder, since the elder feels more alienated and alone *because* of the actions of the family. Such messages as "What you need are more activities" and "You must stop dwelling in the past" may be very well intended, but they only serve to ignore the sincere psychological and spiritual pain the elder is experiencing. The family becomes convinced that should they discontinue their efforts of assuring their elder relative that "You really don't feel as bad as you say," the elder might even commit suicide. In

fact, usually the opposite is true: If only the family would back off by accepting the loneliness and temporary total despair of the elder, the possibility of the elder reengaging friends and society and making an adequate adjustment to recent life tragedies would be greatly increased. Usually getting such a family to "back off" is far more effective—although probably more difficult—than loading the elder with tricyclic antidepressant medication for what is really reactive depression sustained by well-intended, but nonetheless pathogenic, family interaction. See Chapter 10 for a discussion of depression.

INTERGENERATIONAL CONFLICT

Whenever family members are fighting, it is because the members involved in the fights chose to fight instead of withdraw; it is obviously impossible to fight alone. Generally, when elders are drawn into protracted situations of intergenerational conflict, it is because forms of more peaceful communication might prove more painful immediately—though eventually more productive. For example, if family fighting stopped, unpleasant yet realistic topics such as health, finances, or living arrangements might surface. Likewise, should the fighting between generations reach reasonable proportions, middle-aged children might have to confront problems in their own nuclear family: alcoholism, emptying nest, sexual dysfunction, or any number of other woes. To know that protracted quarrels require collaboration is not necessarily sufficient to convince family members that the statement "If only mother were easier to get along with, then we'd all be so happy," is *not* true.

Many times family fighting is used as an excuse by middle-aged children to move a parent from the children's home to alternative living arrangements. Frequently, in these cases, it is obvious to a counselor that the conditions under which the parent was to move in with the children were not clear, nor were the terms or conditions under which the elder might or should move on. Often in such families, members "need" a fight so they can say good-bye.

If the death of a spouse precipitated the move, frequently it is the elder who becomes impatient to resume his or her own life in a different setting but fears broaching the subject with the middle-aged children for fear of seeming ungrateful. Again, the fighting serves as a method to make sense out of saying good-bye if direct communication seems too difficult. See Chapter 39 regarding the dying aged person.

SUMMARY

From the above it should be clear that the family systems model applied to elders and their families is really a way of looking at problematic behavior rather than an ironclad set of rules with which to intervene in every case. While considering problematic behavior in the light of the family system is often more complex than using other models, it provides an encouraging view for mental and physical health professionals who have grown weary of repeatedly applying unsuccessful solutions to the "problems" of elders.

REFERENCES

Bateson, G., et al.: Toward a theory of schizophrenia, *Behavioral Science,* **1**:251–264, 1956.

Bell, J. E.: *Family Group Therapy,* Public Health Monograph no. 64, Government Printing Office, Washington, 1961.

Brody, E. M.: The aging family, *Gerontologist,* **6**:201–206, Autumn 1966.

———— : *Long-Term Care of Older People: A Practical Guide,* Human Sciences, New York, 1977.

Guerin, P. J.: Family therapy: The first twenty-five years, in P. J. Guerin (ed.), *Family Therapy: Theory and Practice,* Gardner, New York, 1976.

Gurian, Bennett S.: Psychogeriatrics and family medicine, *Gerontologist,* **15**(4):308–310, August 1975.

Harris, L., et al.: *The Myth and Reality of Aging in America,* National Council on the Aging, Washington, 1975.

Herr, J. J., and J. H. Weakland: *Counseling Elders and Their Families, Practical Techniques for Applied Gerontology,* Springer, New York, 1979.

———— and ———— : The family as a group, in I. M. Burnside (ed.), *Working with the Elderly, Group Process and Techniques,* Duxbury, North Scituate, Mass., 1978.

TEN

DEPRESSION AND GRIEF IN THE AGED PERSON

Irene Mortenson Burnside

. . . a sickness of the soul without any hope.
Robert Burton, 1576– 1640
The Anatomy of Melancholy

LEARNING OBJECTIVES

- Define depression.
- List 10 terms which could be used to diagnose a depressive state.
- List the three types of depression which can occur in the aged client.
- List four atypical presentations of depression.
- Define underbonding.
- Define masked depression.
- Cite an example of masked depression.
- Define reactive depression.
- List seven physiological signs of depressive disorders.
- List two psychomotor disturbances of depressive disorders.
- List six psychological symptoms of depressive disorders.
- Compare and contrast endogenous and reactive depression.
- Compare and describe the three types of depressive states in the aged.

- List six important behaviors of the nurse who is communicating with the depressed aged person.
- List six interventions that can increase feelings of self-esteem of the aged client.
- List six diagnostic issues to consider in the depressed client.
- Define four types of grief reactions.
- Describe the classic symptoms of grief from Lindemann's research.
- Describe the six tasks in the management of grief.
- Describe the normal course of grief reactions.
- Describe four needs of a grieving spouse during acute grief.

Depression and grief are ubiquitous in the aged population, and nurses find depressed and/or grieving older persons in any setting—in a hospital ward for acutely ill persons, in a nursing home, in the community, and, of course, in psychiatric units. This chapter is about depression and grief in later life and is divided into two parts; the first discusses depression, the second discusses grief.

DEPRESSION

Parker (1978) quotes statistics from the World Health Organization (WHO) to indicate that the prevalence of depression is worldwide; WHO has estimated that depression significantly affects 100 million people. Not only is it the most common disorder for which clients seek professional help, it also drives a significant number to suicide (Parker, 1978). (See Chapter 12 for a discussion of suicide among the elderly.)

Depression affects from 10 to 30 percent of older people in the community, and there is a close association between depression and physical disease (Stenbäch, 1975).

MULTIPLICITY OF TERMS

The fact that such a multiplicity of terms is used in the diagnosis of depression says something about the elusiveness of the condition. Some of those terms are: (1) neurotic depression, (2) psychotic depression, (3) reactive depression, (4) exogenous depression, (5) endogenous depression, (6) unipolar depression, (7) bipolar depression, (8) involuntary melancholia, (9) agitated depression, (10) retarded depression, (11) manic-depressive psychosis, (12) affective disorder, (13) masked depression, (14) atypical depression, and (15) depressive equivalent (Parker, 1978).

This chapter will include explanations of the types, and terminology, of depression most relevant to the care of the aged.

DEFINITION

The definition of depression used in this chapter is as follows: "Depression is, most usually, a state of lowered self-esteem, with associated feelings of hopelessness and helplessness, which may be experienced by an individual and/or which may be evident to an observer. Thus it may be a symptom (reported by the sufferer) or a sign (observable to an examiner)" (Parker, 1978, p. 7).

This chapter will cover the three most common types of depression a nurse is likely to uncover in working with the elderly in practice: (1) masked depressions, (2) reactive depressions, and (3) the depressive states associated with chronic brain syndrome. It is true that the severely depressed person may require hospitalization and may have electric shock therapy, or may be under constant surveillance because of suicidal ideation. This chapter does not cover that severely depressed condition (known as endogenous depression); the reader is referred to geropsychiatric literature for further elaboration, e.g., Busse and Pfeiffer (1973), Butler and Lewis (1977), and Verwoerdt (1976). All are suggested readings. Also see Chapter 14 for the work of Kral.

CARDINAL FEATURES

The cardinal features of depression in the aged person are a lowered mood and a lack of psychic energy. There is a tense expression on the face, and there are deep central furrows in the forehead which might even reveal the diagnosis before the client begins to speak, says Williamson (1974). Other constant features are early awakening, the morbid quality of thoughts, and the loss of enjoyment of food and other pleasures which can continue into old age. There are not the elaborate delusions about unworthiness which the younger people suffer, but expressions of low self-esteem are expressed as, "I am no good," and "I am wasting your time."

The depression may be substantially or completely submerged in a preexisting disability. For example, the stroke patient may make satisfactory progress but then begin to fail further rehabilitation efforts. Or another patient may present a long list of hypochondriacal complaints. Constipation is common, and there may be a marked preoccupation with this problem.

Williamson (1974) points out that he has seen cases in which nocturia, unaccompanied by urinary frequency during the day, occurred in a depressive state. If there is no other explanation for this complaint, then one might consider depression as a possible cause. (This observation has not previously been pointed out in the literature on depression.)

A continued follow-up of any older person is a must for one who has been treated for a depression. The chance of a relapse is always present. Also old people are not always prompt about reporting illness, and the very nature of depression makes it probable that it will not be reported (i.e., lowered energy, a desire not to be intrusive or a nuisance). Every old person who has had a depression should be seen on a regular basis after that by a caretaker who is knowledgeable about the illness (Williamson, 1974).

Caretakers should be aware of the type of old person most prone to depression (see Table 10-1).

Parker (1978) has written an excellent book on depression; however, all the case examples depict younger individuals. Parker says that even though *underbonding* is accepted by most psychiatrists as parental deprivation of care, it is also associated with reactive depression in later life. In the clinical area, Parker describes underbonded depressive individuals as being divided into two contrasting groups. He describes them as having a "stunted self-esteem" or a "sensitized self-esteem." The ones with stunted self-esteem are seen as habitual depressives; they are full of

TABLE 10-1
THE PROFILE OF THE ELDERLY PERSON PRONE TO BE DEPRESSED

1. More likely to be female.
2. More likely to be lonely or isolated.
3. More likely to have painful, limiting, and distressing illness (rheumatoid arthritis, Parkinson's disease, stroke, or illnesses associated with dyspnea).
4. More likely to have recently been widowed, especially after a prolonged period of stress in caring for a dying spouse. (The sudden loss of a sense of purpose, and personal loss and exhaustion may be overwhelming.)
5. More likely to have a bereavement of the loss of a child.
6. More likely to have recently experienced relocation.

SOURCE: Adapted from James Williamson, *Geriatric Medicine,* Academic, London, 1974. Copyright by Academic Press Inc. (London) Ltd. Reprinted by permission.

negative assumptions about themselves, their abilities, and their future life and tend to be inhibited, unassertive, rigid, and inflexible.

The group with sensitized self-esteems manage better in the world and decompensate into depressive states only when there are precipitating events. These are often in comparison with earlier traumas in the earlier underbonded relationships; one example is rejection. These persons do have a greater flexibility and variation in personality and ways of coping. They also basically have less anxiety. There is, however, overlap between the two groups. One aspect of Parker's analysis of depression that might be relevant for nurses working with older persons to consider is the bonding quality of their earlier life. Nurses should take a careful history to elicit such information.

DENIAL AND DEPRESSION

In a study of older men to determine what effects certain personality traits and also critical experiences had upon survival and adaptation, Butler (1967) found "active denial of age and change appeared somewhat more frequently in individuals with evidence of depressive manifestations. Such denial might be reparative in the face of depression." He suggests that denial could be viewed as an "active, optimistic striving or affirmation," and that "denial is useful as a first step in rapid adaptation to changes in taking aging 'in stride.'" Levin (1967), however, states that the use of the mechanism of denial may help the aged person by protecting him from depression. Denial, however, could also be a poor way to cope because the person may take such risks as driving at night because of not being able to admit to night blindness or decreased vision. A person's tendency to push himself or herself beyond the limits of a waning energy can also be caused by a denial of a physical problem or deterioration.

UNRECOGNIZED DEPRESSION IN THE AGED: MASKED DEPRESSION

Depressed states in the elderly are often unnoticed. Some have suggested that the term *masked* should be replaced by the term *missed* since the diagnostician has failed to detect the symptoms indicative of a depressive state. Carter (1974) calls it "hidden depression" in an excellent article about recognizing this psychiatric symptom in black Americans.

Careful observation is required if a nurse is to detect depression in an older adult. Because a depressive state can mimic an organic brain syndrome, it may be mistakenly diagnosed as a brain syndrome (organic brain syndromes are covered in Chapters 14 to 17). When an older person commits suicide, it is not uncommon to hear close friends and relatives comment that they were unaware that the individual was depressed. (Suicide is discussed in Chapter 12.) One reason that a depression in an older person may go unrecognized, explains Levin (1967), is that depression in the aged tends to be somewhat different from that found in younger persons. Apathy is much more characteristic of depression in later life than in earlier years. Older persons may appear to lack interest in their environment and may sit staring off into space, seeming preoccupied. This is particularly true of residents in long-term care facilities. Staff reaction to depressed elderly can be one of extreme

annoyance ("I can't get her to do anything; she just sits"). This reaction can lead staff members to absolutely ignore the withdrawn persons or force them to do things against their will. I recall one elderly withdrawn woman repeatedly saying, "No, no, no" as the nurse's aide, with grim determination, pushed her down the hall to play bingo, chanting all the way, "You'll just love playing bingo."

Although irritability is a common symptom of depression in a person of any age, it can be written off as cantankerousness when it appears in an older person; people often comment that "He is just getting old."

REACTIVE DEPRESSION

A reactive depression is "made up of a combination of symptoms which are abnormal in intensity and may be looked on as the response of any individual to a particular stressful situation" (Parker, 1978). The term *reactive,* which is preferable to the term *neurotic depression,* is a useful one because it suggests that the depression is a response to a stimulus. There are many theories which attempt to explain reactive depressions, but they will not be covered here. The reader is referred to Becker (1974) who did a comprehensive review of these theories.

The precipitants to reactive depression can involve an acute need, deprivation in the form of a physical illness, a disruption of significant relationships, or a community tragedy. The loss of a significant other is a frequent precipitating cause of depression, but the most frequent precipitant that the psychiatrist sees in clinical practice is the breakup of a relationship (Parker, 1978). Van Tiggelen (1978) uses the term *lack syndrome* to cover the many losses and also the lack of meaning and lack of positive reinforcement given to the elderly, all of which can help bring about depression.

Awareness of the following qualities of reactive depression can be helpful for the nurse assessing depressed individuals:

1. The quality of the depressive state matches "normal" depression or grief.
2. Rather than a definite retardation, there is usually avoidance behavior, for example, staying in bed or not socializing. Anxiety is

also associated with this type of depression and appears more often as a verbal statement than in agitative behavior.

3. Sleep is usually in the form of initial insomnia; the depressed individual usually wakes at the normal hour.
4. The depressed mood worsens as the day goes on, and it may be worsened by the day's events.
5. The client is likely to be affected by the surroundings.
6. Onset is often abrupt and may follow the ending of an important relationship. Usually an appropriate precipitating event can be described.
7. Weight loss is slight; sometimes there is weight gain because of eating for comfort.
8. Body functions are not usually disturbed.
9. There is no apparent age predilection.
10. Disturbances of attention, concentration, and memory are slight (Parker, 1978).

To differentiate between endogenous depression and reactive depression, see Table 10-2.

TABLE 10-2

Endogenous Depression	Reactive Depression
Quality: despair, self-blame, guilt	Quality: sadness, sorrow, blame others
Agitation or retardation of activity and thought	Anxiety or avoidance behavior
Early morning awakening	Difficulty in getting to sleep
Depression worse in morning	Depression worse in evening
Mood not reactive to environment	Mood reactive to environment
Precipitating events rare	Precipitating events usually apparent
Significant weight loss	Slight weight loss or gain
Disturbances of body function	Body function rarely affected
Usually older than 40 years	No age predilection

SOURCE: Parker, 1978.

Reactive depressions involve losses, and researchers noted on both cross-sectional and longitudinal studies that *older people could better tolerate the loss of love objects and also of prestige than they could losses in their physical health* (Busse and Pfeiffer, 1973). *This means that prevention of physical health problems could also ultimately help prevent depression.* Nurses are in key positions to educate others and work on the preventive aspects of health care. (See Table 10-3 for diagnostic criteria to study.)

DEPRESSION AND DEMENTIA

In writing about depression in cases of brain disease and dementia, Kral states that a special kind of depressive reaction can be found in patients with incipient cerebral arteriosclerosis and Parkinson's disease. Older people feel that their mental capacities are waning and their reactions are much slower, and often express hopelessness and fear of the future. They do not usually present hypochondriacal ideas nor hostility; however they do seek reassurance. The depressive episode can occur in the course of an advanced presenile, or senile dementia. In these cases the symptoms of depression are modified and, in fact, are overshadowed by the classic picture of the chronic brain syndrome (forgetfulness, poor judgment, confusions, and disorientation). There may also be signs of neocortical deficit such as aphasia or apraxia (Kral, 1972).

Wells (1977) states that depression as one of the early features of dementia has been observed so frequently that at one time it was thought that, in the elderly, depression actually progressed to the demented condition.

Men suffering from Alzheimer's disease frequently express to their physicians significant awareness of and insight into the severity of their condition (Storrie, 1978).

Wells (1977) points out that when a client's symptoms center on emotional experiences, there are two tendencies which must be avoided. One is to consider mental dysfunction in the young as nonorganic in origin and to neglect considering organic cerebral disease. The converse tendency is to regard all mental symptomatology which occurs in old age as due to

TABLE 10-3
Depression (the withdrawn, apathetic patient)

1. Diagnostic issues
   a. Depressed mood
   b. Apathy and withdrawal
   c. Sleep disturbance (especially early morning awakening)
   d. Eating disturbance (usually decreased appetite)
   e. Fatigue
   f. Constipation
   g. Slowed movements and speech
   h. Reduced eye contact
   i. Occasionally agitation, paranoid ideas, and somatic delusions
   j. Avoidance of social and recreational activities
   k. Afraid to try anything new; hopeless that anything will help
2. Rehabilitation issues and suggestions
   a. Frequent staff contact, with reaching out by the staff (and without an immediate expectation that the patient will respond). This reaching out can often occur during daily chores (e.g., making the bed) and do not have to be confined to planned interviews.
   b. Attention by staff to personal and physical needs of patient (e.g., grooming). Depressed and withdrawn elderly patients often respond first to touch and to someone expressing a caring attitude nonverbally rather than verbally.
   c. Contact with familiar care-giving persons.
   d. Using and keeping familiar objects (clothes, pictures, personal mementos); maintaining and keeping alive the memories and symbols of life outside the nursing home as much as possible.
   e. Assess the impact of racial, religious, or cultural differences between the patient and the other residents and staff (does the patient feel depressed because of cultural isolation?).
   f. Antidepressant medication (usually tricyclic antidepressants) will often be the drugs of choice; cardiac status must be carefully assessed because of the capacity of these drugs to produce abnormal heart rhythms.
   g. Assessment to rule out a medical disorder creating depression. At times, some medicines themselves produce a profound depression (for example, reserpine).
   h. Gradual reentry into social activities and recreational activities.
   i. Establishing increasing amounts of useful activities which the patient can do and experience success at.
   j. Reestablishing contact with family and friends as much as possible.
   k. Using depressed patients as helpers of other patients, as a way to feel useful and needed again.
   l. A patient who is experiencing a grief reaction (mourning the loss of a friend or relative) needs to have enough time talking with an empathic person to gradually bring out pent-up feelings. With such patients medications tend to prevent the resolution of the grief.
   m. An accurate assessment of the depressed patient's capacities should be made, and a program tailored to the patient to reinforce accomplishment. An unrealistic program will lead to failure and more depression.
   n. Does the physical layout of the facility encourage patient contact or patient isolation? (Are chairs lined up against the wall, or grouped in more sociable arrangements?)
   o. Are depressed patients being ignored because such patients make the staff feel uncomfortable, guilty, or inadequate?

SOURCE: From the discussion guide for the film *The Disturbed Nursing Home Patient,* produced by Hugh James Lurie, University of Washington, Seattle. Funded by an NIMH-PS grant to the Bureau of Mental Health, DSHS, Olympia, Wash.

cerebral deterioration. Caretakers should always remember the danger that the depressive illness of an elderly person may be masked by pseudodementia.

Because nurses work so closely with elderly clients and patients, they should discipline themselves to always look for the signs and symptoms of depression. It is also necessary to determine carefully the severity of an individual's dementia, because it is very easy to treat dementia patients as nonhumans who do not understand anything at anytime. A depressed individual who is incorrectly diagnosed could receive treatment intended for a demented person; regardless of how earnestly or sincerely such treatment is provided, it may be a nontherapeutic approach for a depressed individual already struggling with a low self-esteem. Low self-esteem is the most common underlying psychogenic factor in depression among the elderly (Wells, 1977).

ATYPICAL PRESENTATION OF DEPRESSION

1. Depressive pseudodementia: The patient may appear perplexed. Forgetfulness and disorientation mimic an organic mental syndrome. Differentiation from genuine organic syndromes may be difficult, but the onset is often sudden, premorbid intelligence is often low, and the patient at interview tends to show apathy and disinterestedness rather than give wrong or confabulated replies.
2. Hypochondriasis shows in the form of unjustified complaints or an unwarranted conviction of physical disease, especially if found in a previously uncomplaining patient. Alternatively, it may present with demands for an indulgence in polypharmacy, often with severe intolerance of the drugs prescribed.
3. Concurrent long-standing physical or neurotic illness may be present and may mask a superimposed depression.
4. Cases may also present with unexplained subnutrition and self-neglect, especially in patients living alone.
5. The quiet uncomplaining patient, perhaps unheeded from the psychiatric viewpoint, in the corner of a general ward, i.e., the too patient patient, may also be depressed.
6. The histrionic or predominantly anxious patient (including those with phobias) without a previous history of neurosis who presents for the first time over the age of 60 years should be suspect.
7. Unwarranted and premature retirement blamed on overwork may be an early symptom.
8. Unreasonable and sometimes repetitive changes of residence or routine can also be motivated by depressive thinking (Langley, 1975).

SADNESS VERSUS DEPRESSION

It is important to distinguish between sadness and depression. "Existential depression" should be viewed as a normal response to some of the very real problems in life. The guidelines which indicate that a person is suffering from depression rather than sadness are these: (1) the symptoms continue beyond 6 weeks, (2) significant weight loss has occurred and continues to occur, (3) the depth of the depressed mood seems to far exceed the amount of the individual's situational stresses (Eisdorfer and Epstein, 1977).

Since sadness could well be a nursing diagnosis, the above information is pertinent.

DEPRESSION IS CONTAGIOUS

Poskanzer (1975) described a depressed patient as one who "looks depressed, sounds depressed and makes you depressed."

The difficulties of working with a depressed person are well expressed in the Schulz cartoon (see Figure 10-1). Depressed people can make those around them sad, depressed, or uncomfortable; therefore, people tend to avoid the depressed person (Eisdorfer and Epstein, 1977). The institutionalized person who is depressed may be seen as a model patient, a "good" pa-

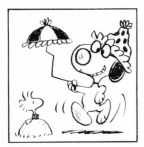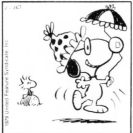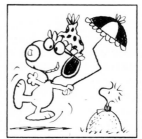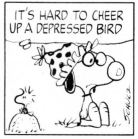

FIGURE 10-1 © 1979, United Feature Syndicate, Inc.

tient, because she or he is quiet, asks for little, and often is not even observed as manifesting depressed behavior.

Nurses must try not to absorb the depressed feelings of their patients. Nursing intervention should be geared to help the aged person feel less helpless and inept and to reward, encourage, or support behaviors that are effective for the individual.

Since organic problems, either physical ill health or stress, may be the most common precipitators of depression in older persons, the nurse is in an advantageous position to be helpful. Reserpine is noted for the severe depressions it can cause. There can be many stresses of the environment, such as living with relatives or moving often, and so constant assessment of the elderly person's real and imagined losses is important. (Alcoholism and drug misuse can also be causes of depression.)

COMMUNICATION WITH THE DEPRESSED PERSON

Kalkman and Davis (1974) advise giving simple, direct information regarding the practical aspects of the illness which may be causing the client great concern; caretakers should carefully explain: (1) drugs and their effects, (2) any electric shock program to be initiated, (3) the cost of the treatments, (4) the sick leave available if the person is employed, and (5) the home responsibilities. Such explanations may help reduce the anxiety. Depressed patients need to be given simple and repeated words of reassurance and comfort (Ayd, 1961). It is advisable not to allow the client to lapse into long silences during an interview, because they may increase the anxiety. One should not speak too rapidly or too emphatically (Ayd, 1961).

Sometimes depressed individuals have great difficulty in making decisions or starting actions simply because their depression slows their mental processes. Decision making should not be stressed during depressive states, and Ruesch (1961) recommends that depressed individuals be protected from making decisions. Kalkman and Davis (1974) advise that only those whom clients trust should be able to decide what is best for them. However, caretakers

should carefully consider the decisions which must be made by depressed elderly clients and encourage them to make as many for themselves as they can in order to bolster their self-esteem and self-confidence. In this matter of decision making, caretakers must delicately walk a fine line between giving the help necessary to avoid putting too much pressure on depressed clients and protecting them so much as to reinforce low self-esteem and lack of self-confidence.

HOPE

Stotland (1969) has written an entire book on hope, but unfortunately there is no mention of hope and the aged. In it he explains (p. 206) that schizophrenic patients "can become hopeful through a total push in which all aspects of the patient's life are directed to communicating hopefulness." He describes hopeful communications from staff and actions which signify respect for the patient and a "hopeful catering to his strengths rather than his pathology." Encouraging a person to play a musical instrument or describe a successful part of her or his life might be ways to cater to strengths. The same can be said for the use of hope with the aged, because therapy of hope is crucial in the care and treatment of the older adult. Health professionals have failed the aged in this area because unfortunately helpers often get bogged down in "therapeutic nihilism" and forget about "total pushes."

The element of hope is important for nurses to remember, and yet how does one teach the ability to radiate an air of hope to neophyte nurses? And there is always the danger of becoming overly hopeful or cheerful so that one does not acknowledge the despair and sorrow the older person may be experiencing. The "cheer up, tomorrow will be better" admonitions fall flat. One practitioner who was seeing a depressed terminal patient prescribed a program of the patient's favorite broadcasting station. That act alone, she said, gave the patient renewed hope, even though she knew her time was limited (Eissler, 1955). Peguy (1973) wrote that "hope sees what is not but yet will be." Elderly persons at times have difficulty in seeing anything positive in what "yet will be" in their lives. And that is understandable sometimes, when one lists possible causes of depression.

TREATMENT

Dominick (1968) recommends these aspects of nursing care of depressed elderly: (1) increase individualization of care, (2) increase instructions and information about nurses' role and plan for treatment, (3) increase socialization, (4) increase participation in activities, (5) sustain hope, and (6) reassure the patient that help is in the offing. Further suggestions I have found helpful include:

1. Establish a one-to-one relationship.
2. Provide for group membership.
3. Offer sincere compliments to the aged individual.
4. Display sincere interest in the aged person and in his or her interests.
5. Seek the aged person's counsel or advice, or request teaching assistance. (See vignette below.)
6. Comment on performances (past ones if the present ones are slipping). (For example, a hospital administrator was once heard to say to a frowsy old woman in the hall, "Mrs. J., you looked so nice yesterday.")
7. Assist in the expression of anger if it exists.
8. Share guilt feelings.

Pfeiffer (1978, p. 43) states,

Group psychotherapy is of exceptional value for persons with depressive syndromes precipitated by significant object loss. A single therapist can treat more than one patient in a given amount of time (between six to ten patients are ideal for group therapy with older patients; . . . other patients often provide excellent models of coping behaviors and replacement strategies. Furthermore, the fact of belonging to a group is of itself an important therapeutic tool. Relationships to groups, not only to individuals, have often been lost, and the capacity to reestablish membership in a group is itself of therapeutic value.

Table 10-4 should provide some ideas for nurses to put into operation since these are reasons for depressions listed by institutionalized

TABLE 10-4
SOME REASONS FOR THE RELIEF OF DEPRESSION IN HOSPITAL

	Cases
Relief of loneliness and provision of companionship	15
Implicit rejection of self-pity and invalidism by physical rehabilitation: assumption of erect posture; walking; wearing of clothes; self-care	15
Translation to a comfortable environment	11
Provision of hopeful, therapeutic atmosphere	11
Treatment of physical illness and relief of somatic symptoms	9
Provision of guidance and sense of being organized to mildly demented patient	7
From hostile environment to one of acceptance	7
Reassurance about physical health	7
Restoration of lost sublimation and self-esteem	6
Withdrawal of hypnotic drugs	6
Containment of aggressive impulses by ward disciplines	5
Nourishment	3
Relief from responsibilities	3
Compensation for poor vision and hearing	2
Away from pessimistic community attitudes	2
Withdrawal of alcohol	1

SOURCE: Reprinted with permission from L. A. Wilson and I. R. Lawson, Situational depression in the elderly: A study of 23 cases, *Gerontologica Clinica Additamentum*, Karger, Basel, pp. 59–71, 1962.

aged people. The same reasons could apply at home.

VIGNETTE[1]
Miss S. was a 90-year-old spinster living in a county hospital, a former elementary

[1] I am grateful to Carol Brink and Thelma Wells for facilitating this teaching experience, and to Carol for continued follow-up visits on this woman. She subsequently fractured a hip, was sent to an acute hospital, and remained clear and oriented during Carol's visitings.

school principal. She was presented in clinical nursing rounds for a class of master's degree students in gerontological nursing. She was chosen because her chart said, "Over the past months she has slipped from an independent, proud and outspoken woman to one who is losing her independence, is no longer motivated to care for herself or voice her needs—either physical or emotional. Recent vaginitis and bleeding have increased her depression." It is worth noting that in 1975 she had been referred to the psychiatric clinic because, as the psychiatrist paraphrased the staff on her chart, "she refused glucose tolerance tests and . . . she had been hard to get along with recently." At that time she was diagnosed by him as experiencing "mild dementia secondary to cerebrovascular disease and adjustment reaction of late life with mild depression." Incidentally, I might add that her other "lack syndromes" included: loss of sister, loss of home, and diagnoses of vaginitis with bleeding, arteriosclerotic cardiovascular disease (ASCVD), otitis media, allergy, macular degeneration of one eye and retinopathy of the other, mild dementia secondary to ASCVD, mild depression, cholelithiasis, diabetes mellitus, and head trauma (in 1970).

Instructors from the university asked her to assist in teaching a class and to share her feelings about being 90 years old. With great poise and apparent ease in front of the class, she told them what it was like to be living in a worn out body with a mind that still raced on. At the close of the class, she stood up, leaned on her three-pronged walker, and thanked each of the students for coming. One nursing instructor did a follow-up for 2 months, once with a check to pay her for the teaching (tears came to the eyes of Miss S. as she accepted it) and later to bring her spring flowers as another positive reinforcement for her excellent teaching.

The instructor wrote, "The staff is amazed at the change. She is coming out of her room, she is interacting with others, and there is a smile on her face. She remembered the instructor's name" (Brink, 1979).

HANDLING ONE'S OWN DEPRESSION

It is helpful for student nurses to learn to deal with their own depressions effectively. They will have to intervene not only with the depressed elderly, but often with depressed relatives of an aged client or with depressed staff members. *It is not uncommon for students to experience depressed feelings when they begin clinical experience with the aged.* This also can happen to a seasoned and experienced nurse, as well as to a student (Burnside, 1969). Instructors can be helpful and supportive to students by sharing the aging process of friends or families or both. Students sometimes return from a vacation with their parents quite depressed. They say, "I just realized how old my parents are getting," or "It hurts to see my grandparents failing so fast."

Butler and Lewis (1977) have phrased this need for self-awareness by health professionals very well. "A mental health specialist must know where he is coming from emotionally, before he can effectively use himself to help others."

PRIMARY PREVENTION

Primary prevention of depression should be aimed at alleviating the loneliness of the elderly, and it can be augmented by improved education, improved social services, and more decent and humane housing policies. New experiments in producing purposeful activity and recreation for the aged are also needed (see Chapter 45).

It is necessary to secure an early diagnosis so that treatment can be more effective and the effects of prolonged immobility and/or malnutrition be reduced. It is also most important to reduce the exhaustion and demoralization of the relatives of the depressed oldster.

Gurland (1972) believes that depression in the aged will be increasingly diagnosed in the future because of caretakers' increased sensitivity in interviewing the aged and in making physical assessments. They will be able to pick up depressions which are masked by complaints of anxiety, insomnia, lowering of energy level, subnutrition, and, of course, ill health. As stated before, poor physical health often causes depression in the aged, and since some old people present such multiple diagnoses and problems, it will be necessary to maintain a holistic approach to elderly patients. Nurses need to be "detectives," ever alert for a new or different clue in the aged client.

Regarding depression in old age, Williamson (1974) states that there are "few conditions which have given me personally more satisfaction in diagnosis and treatment."

GRIEF WORK IN THE ELDERLY

For me who goes
For you who stay—
Two autumns.

Buson (1716–1784)

DEFINITIONS

Several terms are used when discussing grief; most of them come from Lindemann's (1944) pioneering work. The process of handling the grief is usually called *grief work.* I use *acute grief* to mean the grief which follows a sudden unanticipated loss (as Lindemann used it in describing the victims of the Coconut Grove fire). *Chronic grief,* according to Butler and Lewis (1977), is "prolonged intense grief over an extended or limited time period." I think that the definition of chronic grief should include the feelings of a mourner who has to endure the constant observation of a deteriorating process in a loved one. Perhaps the children of deteriorating parents experience chronic grief over such conditions as Parkinson's disease, organic brain syndrome, multiple or lateral sclerosis, and stroke consequences.

Anticipating grief is a term also coined by Lindemann. Other terms for this phenomenon, *preparatory grief, premourning behavior,* and *anticipatory grief,* appeared in the literature in the 1940s and focused on wartime separations and war-related deaths. [See "Loneliness and Grief in Senescence" for an expansion of anticipatory grief (Burnside, 1979).] A *morbid grief reaction* is a distortion of the grief process by prolongation and excessive preoccupation with the grief. *Delayed grief reaction* is one which may be delayed for days, months, or years and includes hostility or ambivalence toward the deceased. The following poem poignantly describes continued grieving and hostile behavior.

PORTRAIT OF A LADY[2]

Evenings, alone,
  she counts off her beads
    invoking not so much Mary
in our kitchen
  as my father,
    now death's removed him.
That agony gone,
  she no longer rails against him
    but mounts to his name
instead, tiny altars
  all over the house—
    snapshots from
his last terrible months—
  backed by sprigs of flowers
    stuck in tumblers.
The first year
  she lingered in dark
    corners of the house,
sobbed for her lover gone,
  sighed like the wind
    at winter's desolation,
hated us all for not having loved him enough.

Thomas Cole

Inhibited grief reaction is one with a minimal amount of mourning. The mourner may develop somatic complaints, resort to overactivity, or display disturbed social interactions (Butler and Lewis, 1977).

An *involutional grief reaction* occurs in early midlife and may be a part of a middle-age crisis (Verwoerdt, 1976). The contributory factors include: (1) failure to attain ideals, (2) an awareness of one's mortality, (3) seeing lack of yearly progress, (4) other disillusionments, (5) biological stresses, and (6) social stresses.

Bereavement overload occurs when multiple grief reactions are superimposed (Kastenbaum, 1969).

Lindemann's classic work on grief was published in 1944. He did not state the ages of the

---

[2] "Portrait of a Lady" in *The Various Light,* Dr. C. Muses (ed.), Lausanne, 1958.

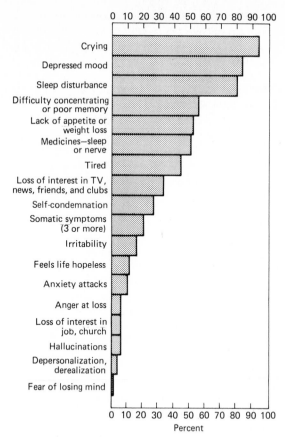

	0 10 20 30 40 50 60 70 80 90 100
Crying	
Depressed mood	
Sleep disturbance	
Difficulty concentrating or poor memory	
Lack of appetite or weight loss	
Medicines—sleep or nerve	
Tired	
Loss of interest in TV, news, friends, and clubs	
Self-condemnation	
Somatic symptoms (3 or more)	
Irritability	
Feels life hopeless	
Anxiety attacks	
Anger at loss	
Loss of interest in job, church	
Hallucinations	
Depersonalization, derealization	
Fear of losing mind	

0 10 20 30 40 50 60 70 80 90 100
Percent

FIGURE 10-2 Percentage of 109 recently widowed persons reporting symptoms of bereavement. [*P. J. Clayton, J. A. Halikes, and W. L. Maurice, The bereavement of the widowed, Diseases of the Nervous System, 32(9):597–604, 1971.*]

has difficulty maintaining organized forms of activity. Usually, 4 to 6 weeks are necessary to move through the acute stage of grief. (I believe this period is longer for the aged who may do tasks more slowly and whose relationship with the deceased may have been a very long one.) Frequently, I have heard a surviving spouse ruefully say, "I don't think I will ever get over it." This feeling is well expressed in the poem, "How It Is with Me Now." See Figure 10-2 for common symptoms of bereavement.

HOW IT IS WITH ME NOW

From my beginning
I changed one hood
for another, design
and pattern shifting slowly
so that sometimes
I was unaware my hood
had slipped into different
style and texture—
batiste, soft wool, crisp cotton,
linen, and silk.

It is true I had to learn
to rearrange a fold or two
and some hoods were more
cumbersome than others.
When I learned to wear it,
I glorified in my wifehood,
cloth of gold with changing flecks
of color, sheer as a sari.

Ripping off my precious hood
the Hatter gone mad surely
clamped on a helmet
iron black and heavy
so heavy
I could not hold my head up. Tight
so tight
I could not breathe or hear or speak.

I was a long time
learning to wear
the most alien of all my hoods.
It sits lighter
on my shoulders now,
fabric softened and thinned
by tears and time,
blackness bleached
by sun and love of friends.

101 grievers studied, and so we do not know how many old people were in his sample.

Lindemann found definite psychological and somatic symptoms. The pattern shown by persons in acute grief is remarkably uniform. Here are some of his findings: somatic distress (lasting 20 minutes to 1 hour), tightness of throat, choking, sobbing, and a need for sighing; this was most obvious when the patient was discussing the grief. The griever suffers from a lack of strength, from exhaustion, and from digestive symptoms. The sensorium is somewhat altered. There is a slight sense of unreality and the feeling of increased distance from other people, along with an intense preoccupation with the image of the dead person. The griever feels intense guilt, is disturbed by hostile feelings, and

I thought
you would like to know
how it is with me now
after four years of wearing
this hood, which though easier
to bear, still
I hate.

Alice J. Davis

MANAGEMENT OF GRIEF

Suggestions for management of grief (Lindemann, 1944) include:

1. Accept the pain of bereavement.
2. Review the relation to the deceased.
3. Work through the overflow of hostility.
4. Express sorrow and sense of loss.
5. Formulate the future relationship to the deceased (how will he or she be remembered?).
6. Verbalize feelings of guilt.

NORMAL COURSE OF GRIEF REACTION

In the normal grief reaction as described by Lindemann (1944), the griever:

1. Begins to emancipate himself or herself from the bondage of the deceased
2. Readjusts to the environment in which the deceased is missing
3. Forms new relationships which bring rewards and satisfaction

Gramlich (1968), in a classic article, wrote that he encourages elderly grieving patients to cry. He suggested telling them they are in the process of grief and mourning; many do not connect their pain and misery to their loss. Help them share the guilt, so that it can be forgiven. The aged person who is grieving should also be encouraged to talk about his anger. Caretakers should not react with counterhostility (Gramlich, 1968). Preventing suicide of the bereaved elderly is extremely important and will be discussed further in Chapter 12. There are persons who do not grieve until a long time after the loss; then grief seems to catch up with them, and they have a delayed grief reaction. One should be particularly aware of late grief in the elderly and check anniversaries of previous deaths of sig-

nificant others, which are likely occasions of delayed grief. Gramlich (1968) notes that they are often not aware of their grief or that it is associated with an anniversary.

Old people also grieve over the loss of a pet and over the loss of something very dear to them, like their home (Burnside, 1973). They also grieve over loss of limb, eyes, vision. As we age, we have to deal constantly with a changing body image. Some of the bodies of the elderly have suffered many "insults" or traumas, and so the elderly may also grieve over changes in body image. Janis (1953) has done studies on surgical patients which deal with the anxiety over the severe restrictions placed on their movement, both physical and cognitive, by surgical necessity. Since many of the elderly experience amputations, loss of a breast, operations for cancer, colostomies, broken hips, and similar traumas, his work bears consideration by gerontological nurses.

Care givers should concentrate on being able to handle their own grief in order to assist aged clients in working through their grief. The staff should also be encouraged to express its feelings of sadness. One director of nurses told about having nine deaths within a short period of time in her facility and about the tremendous impact it had on the staff. Staff members need considerable support when death rates increase among their clients. Suggestions for intervention in grief of the elderly have been given by a nurse (Burnside, 1969).

GRIEF THERAPY GROUPS

Grief therapy groups have been started and run by the Minneapolis Age and Opportunity Center, Inc., a nonprofit organization run by the elderly. The first group began in 1975, when 12 people talked about their feelings and problems with a counselor-leader. As the group grew and became more adroit in its work, there was less need for the counselor. At one time this organization had five grief therapy groups in progress.

McWhorter (1980) has described grief therapy groups for an outpatient group of women who were high utilizers of clinic facilities. She used a directive-verbal approach dealing with the here and now, and an effort was made for them to decrease their psychosomatic complaints as the way of communicating their stress.

ROLE OF AMBIVALENCE IN GRIEF WORK

One author describes well the role of ambivalent feelings. "If the individuals used to have ambivalent feelings about the lost object, the grief reaction comes to an impasse. If a person had mixed feelings about having something, he will also have mixed feelings about not having it. Thus the working through of the loss tends to get into a deadlock" (Verwoerdt, 1976, p. 75).

NEEDS AND SOME GUIDELINES: ACUTE GRIEF

1. These are identified needs of grieving spouses (Hampe, 1975):
   a. To be with the dying person
   b. To be helpful to the dying person
   c. To be reassured as to the comfort of the dying person
   d. To be informed of the mate's condition
   e. To be informed of the impending death
2. Other needs include:
   a. To ventilate feelings
   b. Comfort and support of family members
   c. Support of the health professionals
3. Be honest.
4. Give a clear explanation of what is being done and why it is being done.
5. Keep relatives informed of the dying person's condition; try to make relatives comfortable and show interest in answering their questions (Hampe, 1975).
6. The technique of "cry with me," that is, crying with the grieving person, is not for every professional. Sometimes it can be therapeutic for survivors, however. Carefully analyze your own emotions and their impact on present grief of the family.
7. Ambivalence may cause a deadlock in grief-work (Verwoerdt, 1976).

CHRONIC GRIEF

1. The chronic griever may be physically exhausted from the burden of care.
2. The chronic griever may be neglecting self.

3. Some may choose to cheer up by spinning tales of others much worse off.
4. People who are experiencing or have experienced similar loss may add to the heaviness of a discussion by relating sad tales.

Kastenbaum (1977, p. 42) reminds us that "greater sensitivity to the burden of sorrow carried by many old people would be an improvement over the present tendency to dismiss all the problems as inevitable consequences of advanced age."

ISSUES FOR NURSING DIAGNOSIS OF GRIEF

1. How long since the loss?
2. Was the dying process long and drawn out?
3. Is bereavement overload present, i.e., was there more than one loss?
4. Is grief due to change? Was the change sudden or unexpected?
5. Was the person permitted to be with the dying spouse?
6. Is the grief acute or chronic?
7. Are there covert and overt reactions (e.g., is there denial, anger, sadness, guilt, ambivalence)?

A lovely haiku seems to capture the final solitude of grief.

> *How will you*
> *alone cross the mountain*
> *we could not cross*
> *together?*

REFERENCES

Ayd, Frank J., Jr.: *Recognizing the Depressed Patient,* Grune & Stratton, New York, 1961, p. 118.

Becker, J.: *Depression: Theory and Research,* Wiley, New York, 1974.

Brink, Carol: Personal letter, 1979.

Burnside, Irene M.: Grief work in the aged patient, *Nursing Forum,* 8(4):417–427, 1969.

———— : Loneliness and grief in senescence, in *Psychosocial Caring throughout the Life Span,* I. Burnside, P. Ebersole, H. Monea (eds.), McGraw-Hill, New York, 1979.

_____: Multiple losses in the aged, *Gerontologist,* **13**(2):157–162, Summer 1973.

Busse, Ewald, and Eric Pfeiffer (eds.): *Mental Illness in Later Life,* American Psychiatric Association, Washington, 1973.

Butler, Robert N.: Aspects of survival and adaptation in human aging, *American Journal of Psychiatry,* **123**:1233–1243, April 1967.

_____, and Myrna I. Lewis: *Aging and Mental Health,* 2d ed., Mosby, St. Louis, 1977.

Carter, James H.: Recognizing psychiatric symptoms in black Americans, *Geriatrics,* **29**(11):95–99, November 1974.

Dominick, Joan: Nursing care factors in psychotic depressive reactions in elderly patients, *Perspectives in Psychiatric Care,* **6**(1):28–32, 1968.

Eisdorfer, Carl, and Leon Epstein: *Depression I, Workshop on Aging,* Sandoz Pharmaceutical, East Hanover, N.J., 1977.

Eissler, K. R.: *The Psychiatrist and the Dying Patient,* International Universities Press, New York, 1955.

Gramlich, E.: Recognition and management of grief in elderly patients, *Geriatrics,* **23**:87–92, July 1968.

Gurland, Barry: Depression: Differential diagnoses, paper presented at Gerontology Society Meeting, San Juan, Puerto Rico, December 1972.

Hampe, S. O.: Needs of the grieving spouse in a hospital setting, *Nursing Research,* **24**(2):113–120, March/April 1975.

Janis, I. L.: *Psychoanalytic and Behavioral Studies of Surgical Patients,* Wiley, New York, 1953.

Kalkman, Marion E., and Anne J. Davis: *New Dimensions in Mental Health—Psychiatric Nursing,* McGraw-Hill, New York, 1974.

Kastenbaum, Robert: Death and bereavement in later life, in A. H. Kutscher (ed.), *Death and Bereavement,* Charles C Thomas, Springfield, Ill., 1969, pp. 28–54.

_____: Death and development through the life span, in Herman Feifel (ed.), *New Meanings of Death,* McGraw-Hill, New York, 1977.

Kral, V. A.: Depressions in the aged and their treatment, *Psychiatry Digest,* (12):49–56, December 1972.

Langley, G. E.: Functional psychoses, in John G. Howells (ed.), *Modern Perspectives in the Psychiatry of Old Age,* Brunner/Mazel, New York, 1975, pp. 326–355.

Levin, Sidney: Depression in the aged, in Martin A. Berezin and Stanley H. Cath (eds.), *Geriatric Psychiatry,* International Universities Press, New York, 1967, p. 205.

Lindemann, Erich: Symptomatology and management of acute grief, *American Journal of Psychiatry,* **101**:141–148, September 1944.

McWhorter, Julianne: Group therapy for high utilizers of clinic facilities, in Irene M. Burnside (ed.), *Psychosocial Nursing Care of the Aged,* 2d ed., McGraw-Hill, New York, 1980.

Parker, Gordon: *The Bond of Depression,* Angus & Robertson, Sydney, Australia, 1978.

Peguy, Charles: *The Year 1974,* Conception Abbey, Conception, Missouri, 1973.

Pfeiffer, Eric: Psychotherapy of the elderly, *Journal of the National Association of Private Psychiatric Hospitals,* **10**(1):41–46, Fall 1978.

Poskanzer, David: (quoted by A. Osfeld) in *Epidemiology of Aging,* DHEW Publication no. (NIH) 77-7111, Washington, 1975, p. 131.

Ruesch, Jurgen: *Therapeutic Communication,* Norton, New York, 1961.

Stenbäch, A.: Psychosomatic states, in John G. Howells (ed.), *Modern Perspectives in the Psychiatry of Old Age,* Brunner/Mazel, New York, 1975.

Storrie, Michael: Personal communication, 1978.

Stotland, Ezra: *The Psychology of Hope,* Jossey-Basse, San Francisco, 1969, p. 206.

Toffler, Alvin: *Future Shock,* Bantam, New York, 1970.

Van Tiggelen, Cees: Depression, unpublished manuscript, Melbourne, Australia, 1978.

Verwoerdt, Adrian: *Clinical Geropsychiatry,* Williams & Wilkins, Baltimore, Maryland, 1976.

Wells, Charles E.: *Dementia,* 2d ed., Davis, Philadelphia, 1977.

Williamson, James: Depression, in W. Ferguson Anderson and T. G. Judge (eds.), *Geriatric Medicine,* Harcourt Brace Jovanovich, New York, 1974.

Wilson, L. A., and I. R. Lawson: Situational depression in the elderly: A study of 23 cases, *Gerontologica Clinica Additamentum,* Karger, Basel, pp. 59–71, 1962.

OTHER RESOURCES

NRTA Widowed Persons Service, NRTA, 1909 "K" Street, N.W. Washington, D.C. 20041.

Mysto the Great, 25 min/color. Produced by American Film Institute, Distributor: Perspective Films, 369 West Erie Street, Chicago, IL 60610.

ELEVEN

MUSIC AND THE MANAGEMENT OF GRIEF REACTIONS

Ruth Bright

It is a recurrent problem for those in the helping professions that in order to function effectively, to "enjoy" being a good doctor, nurse, clergyman, lawyer or whatever, they must allow themselves to approach, and, to a degree, to share the distress of those they are attempting to help.
C. M. Parkes, 1972

LEARNING OBJECTIVES

- List four areas in which music therapy can be helpful to the elderly client.
- Describe the process of music therapy.
- Recognize and define obstructed grief and list three symptoms which may indicate an abnormal grief response.
- Explain the normal ambivalent feelings frequently associated with grief at the loss of a loved one.
- List seven guidelines for the use of music therapy with clients suffering from grief and/or anxiety.

Music therapy can be helpful to the elderly patient in four areas: (1) communication, (2) self-expression, (3) improving motivation for physiotherapy (and other therapies), and (4) providing a dimension of living seldom found in the hospital or the nursing home—sheer fun! This sense of enjoyment is essential to successful rehabilitation, because enjoyment can make the aged person want to continue living. Lack of desire to live makes treatment for the old person most difficult. It has been my experience that music therapy for the long-term patient helps to give to each a sense of individuality and also increases opportunities for decision making (Bright, 1972).

Music therapy is defined as the controlled use of music in the treatment, rehabilitation, education, and training of both children and adults who are suffering from physical, mental, and emotional disorders (Alvin, 1966).

Old age is characteristically a time of loss, which can include loss of competence in living because of increasing age and frailty; loss of independence through disability associated with stroke, amputation, etc.; and loss of spouse, peers, memorabilia, etc. (Burnside, 1970). The aging inevitably lose significant figures in their lives, and, finally, all must face the ultimate loss—that of life itself.

INHIBITED GRIEF

It is common to associate grief only with bereavement, but in fact one may grieve deeply over any significant loss; however, in loss situations experienced by the elderly, grief is often inhibited, which has adverse effects both emotionally and physically (Gramlich, 1968, Brandon, 1974). From the work and writings of such people as Lindemann, Kübler-Ross, and Parkes, we have in recent years become more aware of people's needs in times of grief and the risks which occur when feelings are bottled up (Lindemann, 1944; Kübler-Ross, 1970, 1974; Parkes, 1972). Yet people still have difficulty expressing their feelings. In some cultures, expressing and discussing death are still taboo; grieving persons may be encouraged to wear a smiling face to pretend that they are too strong to need tears and/or sighs. The comforter may truly believe

that tears are harmful or that to cry is to pity oneself, which may lead to discouragement. It may also be that the onlooker cannot face his or her own responses to loss and, therefore, tries to prevent the grieving person from showing emotion (Brandon, 1974). Some people fear that, if they give way to grief, they may experience a total loss of self-control and even insanity (Barnacle, 1949). (For a more complete survey of the literature and discussion of grief in the elderly, see Chapter 10.) Lindemann (1944) also described such fears of insanity.

Because of such widely practiced taboos, it is not uncommon to find people in hospitals and nursing homes suffering from obstructed grief for a short or long period of time and with a variety of effects. The effects may result in illnesses, and occasionally the patient is referred to a psychiatrist. The symptoms may seem unrelated to grief until a closer investigation shows that the illness has resulted from a long-obstructed grief. Helping the patient to ventilate the grief has extinguished the symptoms (Lieberman, 1978).

The following vignette describes not only bereavement overload, but also obstructed grief.

VIGNETTE 1

As music therapist I was asked by the nursing staff to see Mrs. F. because they felt that the patient was in an abnormal state of mind: she did not seem to realize that her husband was dead. The patient had suffered a stroke which affected her left side and been admitted to a nursing home in the country town where she lived. Unfortunately she was severely scalded during a bath there. A few days later her husband died from a heart attack. Soon after this she was flown by an aerial ambulance to Sydney for skin-grafts. When I saw her she was generally confused and disoriented in place and time—which, in view of the succession of serious events in her life, was not surprising. She was also incontinent.

My first session with her consisted only of playing a few pieces of music which I thought would probably be familiar to a person of her age, and also some comments to the patient about where she was, why she had come there, and, of course, what date and day of the week it was. The patient mumbled something about people "on the veranda in the cottage over there." There was no veranda or cottage to be seen.

The following week I spoke about her husband's death and suggested that anyone who had suffered such a disastrous sequence of events might have feelings of confusion. I asked whether she was still "seeing" her husband. I should add that this is the approach used by the psychiatrists at the hospital because many bereaved persons have quasi hallucinations of the deceased. Although a few persons are comforted by these hallucinations, many fear that they indicate mental illness and so do not tell anyone about them. Her face revealed mingled shock and relief. She had obviously been frightened by her hallucinations and kept them secret. I reassured her that seeing the dead person is quite normal and that it would pass off in the near future, but that it was all right to "see" someone who is dead in any case. Our interview ended with playing music.

The third week, the patient opened the conversation as soon as I arrived by saying eagerly, "Do you know, since that conversation last week, I haven't seen my husband once?" It was obvious that she felt great relief at this. She went on to ask me to play the Irving Berlin song "I'll Be Loving You, Always," a song which her husband had often sung to her. She started to cry and, in fact, continued to cry for some time. This was the first expression of grief she had shown. From that time on, she was able to show her grief and to speak of her feelings of confusion and bereftness. Her rehabilitation was not without problems, mostly caused by her perceptual losses; however, there were no further problems with disorientation or obstructed grief.

While Parkes (1972) has said that grief should be neither cut short nor accelerated by tugging at the heartstrings, it seems likely that this applies more to normal grief. Where grief has been, or is in grave danger of being, obstructed, this plucking at the heartstrings may bring relief and improvement of general health.

MUSIC HELPS EVOKE IMPORTANT FEELINGS

Because music tends to reach people at a physical or emotional level rather than an intellectual one, it can help to evoke feelings long repressed and even unsuspected. Kübler-Ross (1974) described the effects of music on a dying patient. The woman was thought to be beyond communication verbally. The musician-therapist's visit started the patient talking again, so that other members of staff were able once more to feel a rapport with her. Lieberman has described treatment of a delayed grief by using mementos of the deceased such as photographs to encourage grief work (Lieberman, 1978). In my own work I have observed that the response to music helps to create even stronger links than photographs with the deceased person and enables the patient to ventilate the obstructed grief. Thus, in the vignette presented earlier in this chapter, hearing the song her husband used to sing to her put Mrs. F. in touch with her feelings and allowed her to begin the healing process by expressing her grief.

Clearly such therapeutic interventions are not to be undertaken lightly: the emotions connected with grief are strong, and, as Bowlby pointed out, the way we react to a grief in adult life is affected by experiences of loss in earliest infancy (Bowlby, 1961). The bereft person feels anger and guilt as well as grief and sadness. We must be fully aware of these responses to grief to intervene successfully. Ideally, the music therapist should consult with the psychiatrist, or with social workers, nurses, counselor, or psychologist if a psychiatrist is not available.

AMBIVALENCE AND THE NEED FOR REASSURANCE

In almost every relationship (and some therapists would allow no exceptions), there is an element of ambivalence, some measure of love-hate. When one participant in that relationship dies, the survivor recalls those times when he or she wished the relationship ended, or even wished the partner dead, and feels guilt over such wishes. One observes this intensely with a child who has lost a parent, when there is often a strong sense of guilt because the child fears that his or her angry thoughts about the parent or bad behavior killed the parent. Even in relationships between adults there is frequently a parallel to these feelings.

In this matter, the tradition of speaking only well of the dead is not helpful. If the survivor feels a sense of relief at the death of a difficult partner, or remembers with guilt the occasions of wishing the partner "away," these guilty feelings will be exacerbated by having comforters dwell only on the good side of the deceased. It will, in fact, be more helpful to speak of the deceased as a real person, who "had difficult moments," thus giving to the survivor the opportunity of remembering the deceased in a more realistic fashion. Such realism in remembering the deceased will help the survivor to overcome or come to terms with guilt and anger about death. I have found that it is necessary to give a clear opening for the grieving survivor to express such feelings, so strong is the tradition of speaking no ill of the dead. This can be done easily by a comment such as, "I expect that, like all of us, he (or she) was sometimes difficult to live with!" but expressed in whatever mode of speech comes naturally in the circumstances. This remark, even when expressed in a casual tone of voice, gives an opening to those who are feeling guilty about aspects of the relationship with the deceased. They can then speak openly about these feelings and be given appropriate reassurance that such feelings are universal and not a matter for shame and remorse.

It is important to understand one's own feelings about grief; otherwise one's interventions may do harm rather than good. In encouraging people to show their grief, one sometimes meets the response already mentioned—that to grieve will lead to loss of self-control and insanity. It is necessary in such cases to reassure the patient that, when there has been enough grieving, the self-control will reassert itself—that the person will not cry forever.

One also meets the attitude, "I must not grumble—there are lots worse off than I am." In such instances the therapist needs to show empathy to help patients express their real feelings in the face of loss, disability, or impending death. The person needs to be encouraged to put all these feelings into words and to be reassured that it is not considered grumbling.

VIGNETTE 2

Mrs. T. was an elderly woman who watched her husband suffer a long illness and eventually die. The institution staff observed that he was not an easy man to work with. Mrs. T. had shown great devotion to him and was admitted into shared accommodation in order to participate in the task of caring for him. After his death, while Mrs. T. was a day-care patient at the same hospital, her mother died under distressing circumstances. She burned to death when an electric blanket short-circuited and caught fire as the result of the elderly woman's incontinence.[1] Shortly after her mother's death, Mrs. T. was at a music therapy session, and when one particular song was played, she started to cry. Private conversation with the music therapist after the session revealed that she felt guilty because she believed that she had grieved more over her mother's death than over her husband's. She was then encouraged to listen to music which she had enjoyed with her husband and to cry over these songs. The therapist also explained that in a grief reaction it is normal to have feelings of guilt and anger. They discussed the possibility that her husband's long illness had made it harder for her to grieve over his death, and that sudden death, like that of her mother, is harder to cope with than a long-expected bereavement (Levinson, 1972). The discussions were continued over a 2-week period, and the patient began to better understand her own feelings and experience less guilt.

The following vignette concerns a group of people not generally recognized as being at risk, those who are in the hospital when their spouse becomes ill and dies. Hospitalized people in this situation often feel intense guilt ("It's all my fault that he died—I should never have left

---

[1] Editor's note: In Australia, where this history took place, electric blankets are placed beneath the bottom sheet.

him'') or self-questioning ("If I had been there to care for him, would he have become ill?"). Similar reactions can sometimes be seen among young mothers in the hospital when a child becomes ill, who feel intense guilt at not being home to care for the child. In these circumstances guilt feelings seem illogical, since the patient did not choose to be in the hospital when the spouse or child became ill, and so that guilt may be unrecognized or denied by staff members. Hospitalized patients in this situation need help to ventilate, to put into words, their feelings of grief and guilt.

VIGNETTE 3

Mrs. M. was one of these at-risk individuals. She was in the hospital for rehabilitation, and she had been institutionalized for a long time following a subdural hematoma. While she was in the hospital, her husband died. It is rare for a staff to arrange to attend a funeral, but she did. However, although being able to attend the funeral assisted a satisfactory resolution of grief, Mrs. M. found it difficult to grieve, partly because of her own severe illness but more particularly because she found that the ward's communal atmosphere and environment was not conducive to the free expression of feelings.

She was encouraged to sit on the veranda alone. A family member was asked by the music therapist to bring in tape recordings of music that she had enjoyed with her husband. While listening to these tapes, she was able to express grief in privacy.

When working with people who have undergone, or are about to undergo, surgery, or who are suffering from a severe medical condition which is threatening to life or to life-style, one adopts a similar approach to that already described, playing music on request or offering music which seems likely to be appropriate. The patient who feels that the operation may not be successful and that, for instance, sight may not be restored or that an inoperable malignancy may be disclosed will often feel that the music, and the warmth of atmosphere which it brings, give him permission to speak of anxieties (anxieties which are closely akin to grief), to receive comfort and, if possible, reassurance. Similarly,

patients who have learned that the future is not hopeful to them, or who have undergone a mutilating procedure such as amputation or colostomy, will usually feel free to talk about their feelings in this situation.

VIGNETTE 4

One such woman, in her late seventies spoke quite abruptly at the end of the song which she had requested, saying in an apparently matter-of-fact tone of voice and without any explanation, "Of course I have to wear a bag now." It seemed probable that she was seeking reassurance and an opportunity for expressing her feelings, so I replied by saying, "I guess that takes a lot of getting used to. How do you feel about it yourself?" We went on to talk about adjustment to colostomy, the fact that a stoma therapist would be available to visit her at home, etc.; her fears about whether people would want to be near her and whether there would be odor from the bag were allayed. It was clear that all these matters had been discussed by the surgeon and nursing staff, at least in outline, but that the patient still needed additional support in her grief and anxiety about relationships with people, and in her emotional shock and fear resulting from the operation. Music provided the necessary atmosphere, and her willingness to speak in that atmosphere gave the therapist the opportunity of passing on this need to the social worker for further support.

SUMMARY AND GUIDELINES

These vignettes show how people have been helped in one way or another to express their grief and sadness with the use of music: music was played for them and followed with appropriate discussion and/or reassurance. Music serves as a facilitator or catalyst. The aged person is not only given permission to feel sad but encouraged to show it. How does one know what type of music to play to persons who need such a therapeutic approach? The patients themselves will tell you their needs, both emotional and musical, by the music they request. Their choice of songs, of renderings, is the integral component of therapeutic approach to grief work and facilitating the grieving process. There are implications for nurses who work with grieving patients or clients. I would suggest the following guidelines:

1. Work through your own feelings about grief to determine how well you have coped with loss situations in life.
2. Use a portable instrument so that you can work at the bedside if necessary; this is especially important if your work is to include acute medical or surgical areas.
3. Ask the client what musical selection he or she would like to hear.
4. Learn an extensive repertoire of music from the appropriate eras; when a song is so important to someone that he or she requests it, it is very daunting not to have that request fulfilled. Sometimes even the best musician is unable to play a particular request; one should apologize for this and try for a second choice.
5. Recorded music can be a help to expand one's repertoire, but it is in general too impersonal to form the backbone of a music therapy program.
6. From time to time one meets younger patients in geriatric units because of the nature of their illness; their musical needs will be different, and some may like to play instruments for themselves—guitars, drums, etc. But on the whole, the elderly prefer to listen or to sing with the accompaniment.
7. Allow plenty of time for discussion or just for quiet companionship. Holding the hand of a grieving patient may be just as important as conversation. One must also realize that the elderly patient who has been shocked by the news of impending surgery may even appear to forget what is happening and need repeated reassurance and explanation.

REFERENCES

Alvin, Juliette: *Music Therapy,* Humanities, New York, 1966.

Barnacle, C. H.: Grief reactions and their treatment, *Diseases of the Nervous System,* **10**:173–177, June 1949.

Bowlby, J.: Processes of mourning, *International Journal of Psychoanalysis,* **44**(4–5):317–340, 1961.

Brandon, S.: Grief, *Practitioner,* **212**(1272):867–875, June 1974.

Bright, Ruth: *Music in Geriatric Care,* Angus & Robertson, Sydney, Australia, 1972.

Burnside, Irene Mortenson: Loss: A constant theme in work with the aged, *Hospital and Community Psychiatry,* **12**(6):173–177, June 1970.

Gramlich, E.: Recognition and management of grief in elderly patients, *Geriatrics,* **23**:87–92, July 1968.

Kübler-Ross, E.: *On Death and Dying,* Tavistock, London, 1970.

————: *Questions and Answers on Death and Dying,* Macmillan, New York, 1974, p. 43.

Levinson, P.: On sudden death, *Psychiatry,* **35**:150–173, May 1972.

Lieberman, S.: Nineteen cases of morbid grief, *British Journal of Psychiatry,* **132**:159–163, February 1978.

Lindemann, E.: Symptomatology and management of acute grief, *American Journal of Psychiatry,* **101**(2):141–148, September 1944.

Parkes, C. M.: *Bereavement: Studies of Grief in Adult Life,* International Universities, New York, 1972.

TWELVE

SUICIDE IN THE AGED PERSON

Irene Mortenson Burnside

In their loneliness, in their lack of love and craving for it, the troubled are ever in danger of drifting to meaning's edge.
Huston Smith

LEARNING OBJECTIVES

- List two times of great risk in treatment of suicidal individuals.
- List six forces toward living for the aged.
- List 13 forces toward suicide in the aged.
- Define self-destructive behavior.
- Describe seven self-destructive behaviors.
- List steps for a nurse to follow to study self-destructive behavior.
- List four life-threatening maneuvers.
- Describe three possible reactions of staff members to a suicidal person.
- List guidelines from Payne for use in interventions.
- Discuss four aspects of presenting complaints.
- List important questions to ask in high-risk clients.

TABLE 12-1

DEATH RATES FOR SELECTED CAUSES OF DEATH BY AGE: UNITED STATES, 1968, 1976, AND 1977*

Cause of Death (Eighth Revision International Classification of Diseases, Adapted 1965)	Year	Total	Under 1 Year	1–4 Years	5–14 Years	15–24 Years	25–34 Years	35–44 Years	45–54 Years	55–64 Years	65–74 Years	75–84 Years	85 Years and Over
All causes	1977	878.1	1,485.6	68.8	34.6	117.1	136.2	247.5	620.7	1,434.9	3,055.6	7,181.9	14,725.9
	1976	889.6	1,595.0	69.9	34.7	113.3	136.2	254.1	634.8	1,475.6	3,127.6	7,331.6	15,486.9
	1968	967.9	2,265.7	89.6	43.0	123.7	157.2	319.8	751.3	1,704.4	3,724.0	8,293.5	19,582.7
Diseases of heart	1977	332.3	23.1	1.9	0.9	2.5	8.5	49.3	194.1	530.8	1,250.5	3,198.3	7,095.8
	1976	337.2	23.1	1.8	0.9	2.6	8.5	50.8	199.8	552.4	1,286.9	3,263.7	7,384.3
	1968	373.5	12.3	1.6	1.0	2.8	11.9	70.8	251.7	686.9	1,632.8	3,825.4	9,278.3
Malignant neoplasms, including neoplasms of lymphatic and hematopoietic tissues	1977	178.7	3.8	5.2	4.3	6.5	14.5	50.9	182.5	440.5	792.6	1,267.5	1,445.6
	1976	175.8	3.2	5.3	5.0	6.5	14.5	51.5	182.0	438.4	786.3	1,248.6	1,441.5
	1968	159.8	4.9	8.0	6.4	8.2	17.3	61.0	183.0	413.5	749.2	1,133.8	1,475.3
Cerebrovascular diseases	1977	84.1	5.3	0.8	0.5	1.2	3.1	10.3	28.7	79.5	259.9	970.7	2,425.2
	1976	87.9	4.4	0.7	0.5	1.2	3.4	11.5	31.4	85.8	280.1	1,014.0	2,586.8
	1968	106.0	5.3	0.9	0.7	1.7	4.9	16.5	44.6	121.7	409.5	1,317.6	3.605.9
Accidents:	1977	47.7	37.1	27.3	17.3	62.5	44.2	37.8	40.3	47.8	61.8	134.4	284.2
	1976	46.9	41.4	27.9	17.0	59.9	43.5	37.1	39.9	47.7	62.2	134.5	306.7
	1968	57.6	74.9	32.6	20.5	69.2	52.5	47.6	53.6	64.7	90.0	188.8	513.7
Motor vehicle accidents	1977	22.9	8.0	10.1	8.5	44.1	26.1	18.9	17.7	18.9	21.0	31.6	25.5
	1976	21.9	8.0	10.5	8.5	41.0	24.7	18.4	17.4	18.2	21.7	32.3	26.0
	1968	27.5	9.5	11.5	10.1	49.8	32.6	24.9	25.8	28.5	35.0	47.4	39.7
All other accidents	1977	24.8	29.1	17.2	8.7	18.4	18.2	18.9	22.6	28.9	40.8	102.7	258.7
	1976	25.0	33.4	17.4	8.4	18.9	18.8	18.7	22.5	29.5	40.4	102.2	280.7
	1968	30.1	65.4	21.1	10.5	19.5	19.9	22.7	27.8	36.2	55.0	141.5	474.0
Influenza and pneumonia	1977	23.7	53.2	3.1	0.9	1.3	2.0	4.4	9.6	21.9	58.5	236.2	731.2
	1976	28.8	64.8	3.9	1.0	1.5	2.4	5.4	11.6	26.3	70.1	289.3	959.2
	1968	36.9	234.9	9.9	1.8	2.8	4.4	9.3	19.9	41.9	106.0	330.7	1,167.8
Diabetes mellitus	1977	15.2	0.3	0.1	0.1	0.4	1.5	3.7	9.6	27.2	65.9	142.8	203.8
	1976	16.1	0.3	0.1	0.1	0.4	1.8	3.9	9.8	28.4	70.0	155.8	219.2
	1968	19.2	0.5	0.2	0.2	0.7	2.6	5.3	13.1	38.7	96.3	188.2	257.9
Cirrhosis of liver	1977	14.3	1.0	0.1	0.0	0.3	3.8	15.3	33.8	45.4	42.6	30.2	16.9
	1976	14.7	1.1	0.1	0.0	0.3	3.7	16.9	35.0	47.6	42.6	29.3	18.0
	1968	14.6	1.5	0.2	0.1	0.4	4.2	18.1	36.8	46.1	40.3	29.6	22.7
Arteriosclerosis	1977	13.3	.	.	0.0	0.0	0.0	0.2	1.1	5.3	25.4	146.0	659.2
	1976	13.7	0.0	0.0	.	0.0	0.0	0.2	0.9	5.2	25.8	152.5	714.3
	1968	16.8	0.0	0.0	0.0	0.0	0.0	0.2	1.2	6.8	40.7	220.7	1,121.7
Suicide	1977	13.3	...	...	0.5	13.6	17.7	16.8	18.9	19.4	20.1	21.5	17.3
	1976	12.5	...	...	0.4	11.7	15.9	16.3	19.2	20.0	19.5	20.8	18.9
	1968	10.7	...	...	0.3	7.1	12.0	16.1	19.7	21.5	19.0	21.3	22.1
Bronchitis, emphysema, and asthma	1977	10.3	2.2	0.4	0.2	0.3	0.4	1.3	5.1	20.4	54.4	94.3	91.7
	1976	11.4	2.3	0.5	0.2	0.2	0.5	1.3	6.0	23.0	60.7	101.4	108.5
	1968	16.6	5.2	0.9	0.3	0.5	1.0	2.9	10.9	40.8	94.4	139.1	154.5
Homicide	1977	9.2	5.6	2.7	1.2	12.7	16.5	14.5	9.8	7.4	5.2	4.9	4.7
	1976	9.1	5.6	2.5	1.1	12.4	16.5	14.3	10.0	7.3	5.3	5.3	4.9
	1968	7.4	4.8	1.5	0.7	10.1	15.3	12.9	9.1	6.3	4.4	3.4	3.7
Nephritis and nephrosis	1977	3.9	2.0	0.2	0.1	0.3	0.6	1.2	2.8	6.5	14.9	34.8	61.7
	1976	4.0	1.2	0.2	0.1	0.3	0.7	1.4	3.1	6.6	15.2	34.1	64.6
	1968	4.7	0.8	0.2	0.4	1.0	1.5	3.4	5.2	9.2	15.8	32.1	74.5
Septicemia	1977	3.3	34.4	0.6	0.1	0.2	0.3	0.8	1.9	4.5	9.5	25.3	49.4
	1976	3.0	35.6	0.6	0.1	0.2	0.4	0.8	1.8	4.0	8.6	22.8	41.6
	1968	1.5	23.8	0.7	0.1	0.2	0.3	0.5	0.9	2.0	4.2	8.4	17.0

* Refers only to resident deaths within the United States. Excludes fetal deaths. Rates per 100,000 population in specified group.

NOTE: Rates for 1968 are based on revised intercensal estimates of the population.

SOURCE: Department of Health, Education, and Welfare, Monthly Vital Statistics Report, Final Mortality Statistics, 1977, May 11, 1979, p. 23.

The suicide rate among the elderly in the United States should be cause for great concern by health workers. A great deal of attention is being paid to the prevalence of suicide among young people, especially college students. And a recent segment of the TV show "60 Minutes" investigated the rate of suicides among physicians, particularly the high incidence of suicide among psychiatrists. Current media reports, however, rarely discuss the incidence of suicide among the aged, just as, in general, less attention is paid to this phenomenon than to other forms of suicide.

STATISTICS

Statistical and research studies offer a clear indication of the scope of the problem of suicide among the elderly and a glimpse of some possible causes and high-risk situations. According to a recent U.S. Public Health Service study, white males over 80 have the highest suicide rate of any group (broken down by age, sex, and race). And that rate is between 2 and 10 times as high as the suicide rate for people of college age. Table 12-1 provides a clear indication of the high suicide rates among the elderly.

Edwin Schneidman and Norman Farberow (1957) have looked at suicide notes as one of the clues to suicide and at the distribution of suicide note writers according to age groups (Table 12-2).

Barraclough (1971) reviewed suicide among the elderly in a study of 30 people over the age of 65 who killed themselves. Eighty-seven percent

of his subjects were mentally ill. Many suicides occurred after an illness of less than 1 year's duration, and 83 percent of his subjects had consulted with a doctor within 3 months prior to their suicide. A significant number had lived alone for less than 1 year and were living alone because of the death of their spouses or for a lack of caretakers.

Other researchers have attributed a general predisposition to commit suicide to the loss of parents, the lack of parental care, and/or other deprivations in childhood (Tabachnick, 1957). This lack of parental care for depressed individuals is called *underbonding* (Parker, 1978). See Chapter 10 of this book for a discussion of underbonding.

The suicide wish of an elderly person is, according to J. Haggerty (1973), "usually the culmination of inner and outer problems," and it may indicate a need to change the person's social milieu.

DANGEROUS TIMES

The two times of greatest risk in the treatment of the suicidal patient are the dangerous period when arrangements for treatment are being made and the time during the stage of recovery when the person seems to be much improved. When recovering patients leave the hospital and its support systems, their former loneliness, grief, and isolation frequently return. The risk remains high during the first 6 months to a year following discharge (Payne, 1975). I have observed staff members feel completely crushed when, after discharging a patient who seemed much improved, they learned that the individual committed suicide at home.

Payne has argued that "the most important element in keeping a suicidal patient alive is the wish of a responsible person that he remain alive, expressed in the person's vigilance, and conveyed to the patient by means of the psychotherapeutic relationship" (Payne, 1975). Payne's conclusion is quite relevant to nurses, who are often in a position to maintain a close relationship with an elderly client. Nurses should also be aware of the point made by Jerome Motto (1965), a psychiatrist, that most

TABLE 12-2
Distribution of Male and Female Suicide-Note Writers According to Age

Ages	Male	Female	Number
20–39	99	38	137
40–59	215	52	267
60+	175	40	215
Total	489	130	619

SOURCE: Schneidman and Farberow, 1957.

completed suicides which take place after hospitalization occur among individuals with whom caretakers could not maintain the therapeutic relationship and follow-up.

LIFE AND DEATH FACTORS

The doctoral work of Marv Miller, which focuses on suicidal elderly males, is the most complete material available at present on suicide among the elderly (Miller, 1977, 1978a, and 1978b). Miller has composed a balance scale of life-promoting and death-encouraging factors which encompasses the conclusions of many of the researchers I have discussed and which graphically illustrates some of the forces which caretakers should watch for when considering the possibility that an aged client might commit suicide. (See Figure 12-1.)

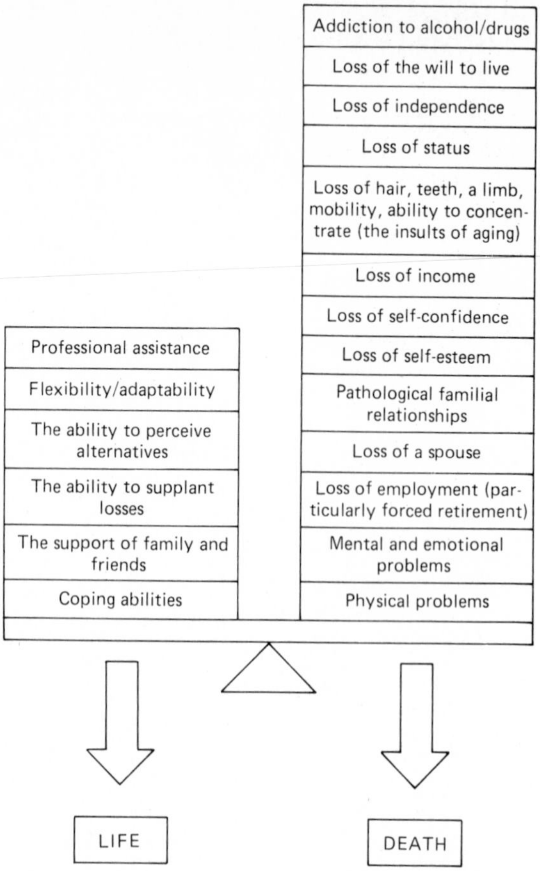

FACTS AND FABLES

Many misconceptions about suicide in general also affect people's understanding of suicide among the aged. Table 12-3, compiled by the National Institute of Mental Health, lists some of the most common mistaken beliefs about suicide and the corresponding facts which caretakers should keep in mind.

DIRECT SELF-DESTRUCTIVE BEHAVIOR

Self-injurious behavior has been observed to occur frequently among the aged who reside in nursing homes (Kastenbaum and Mishara, 1971; Mishara et al., 1973). Professionals tend to expect such behavior in a mental hospital or on a psychiatric ward, but they are frequently surprised to see it in a long-term care facility. But one should keep in mind that many patients in state hospitals have been transferred to nursing homes and that many mental patients from Veterans' Hospitals are ultimately placed in nursing homes. Nor do all suicide attempts by elderly patients necessarily result from the kind of history of mental illness that would have caused

FIGURE 12-1 Life-versus-death forces in the context of geriatric suicide. (*Courtesy of Marv Miller, Ph.D., Consultant in Suicidology, San Diego, Calif.*)

them to be classified as mental patients prior to the attempt.

Direct self-destructive behavior is the obvious overt attempt at self-destruction which could include any of the following: (1) overdoses of medications, (2) gunshot wound, (3) hanging, (4) slashing wrists or neck with a knife, razor blade, or piece of broken glass, (5) placing a plastic bag over the head, (6) putting the head in a sink of water to attempt drowning, or (7) jumping from a building.

A director of nurses has written the following description of one typical case.

Suicide is fairly acceptable among the Issei (first generation Japanese). One week ago Mr. H. took a pocketknife and lacerated his

TABLE 12-3
SOME FACTS ABOUT SUICIDE

Fable	Fact
People who talk about suicide do not commit suicide.	Of any 10 people who kill themselves, 8 have given definite warnings of their suicidal intentions. Suicide threats and attempts *must* be taken seriously.
Suicide happens without warning.	Studies reveal that the suicidal person gives many clues and warnings regarding suicidal intentions. Alertness to these cries for help may prevent suicidal behavior.
Suicidal people are fully intent on dying.	Most suicidal people are undecided about living or dying, and they "gamble with death," leaving it to others to save them. Almost no one commits suicide without letting others know how he or she is feeling. Often this "cry for help" is given in "code." These distress signals can be used to save lives.
Once people are suicidal, they are suicidal forever.	Happily, individuals who wish to kill themselves are "suicidal" only for a limited period of time. If they are saved from self-destruction, they can go on to lead useful lives.
Improvement following a suicidal crisis means that the suicidal risk is over.	Most suicides occur within about three months following the beginning of "improvement," when the individual has the energy to put morbid thoughts and feelings into effect. Relatives and physicians should be especially vigilant during this period.
Suicide strikes more often among the rich—or, conversely, it occurs more frequently among the poor.	Suicide is neither the rich person's disease nor the poor person's curse. Suicide is very "democratic" and is represented proportionately among all levels of society.
Suicide is inherited or "runs in a family."	Suicide does *not* run in families. It is an individual matter and can be prevented.
All suicidal individuals are mentally ill, and suicide always is the act of a psychotic person.	Studies of hundreds of genuine suicide notes indicate that the suicidal person, although extremely unhappy, is not necessarily mentally ill. His or her overpowering unhappiness may result from a temporary emotional upset, a long and painful illness, or a complete loss of hope. It is circular reasoning to say that "suicide is an insane act," and therefore all suicidal people are psychotic.

SOURCE: *Some Facts about Suicide,* National Institute of Mental Health, Bethesda, Md., n.d.

left temple. (We did not know he had the knife.) He managed a deep enough cut to get a good, sloppy blood flow and a black eye from it. About five days later he died of a cardiovascular accident. He was 95 years old with osteoporosis. He had arteriosclerotic heart disease without edema, which was fairly well controlled by medication and diet. He would spit his medications into the urinal because he said he did not wish to get well. He was severely depressed because of pain. His nearest relatives were nephews who did as well as possible to care for him, but not adequately enough to make him feel needed and loved. He lamented about his deteriorating physical condition, which made it impossible to care for himself. He never articulated his feelings, but they were pried out of him by Japanese-speaking personnel. (Mummah, 1974)

The more violent means of self-destruction are not nearly as common as the indirect self-destructive means which occur in nursing homes. Indirect self-destruction has been called "benign suicide" (Finch, 1974), and Butler and Lewis (1973) write about "subintentional suicide." Indirect attempts at self-destruction are often so subtle that they sometimes are not really viewed as suicide attempts by the staff members. Refusing medication can be easily written off and charted as the patient's being stubborn and cantankerous. Taking medications incorrectly can be seen as confusion rather than suicidal. Ignoring or delaying treatment can be viewed as part of the forgetfulness of the aged, and taking unusual physical risks can be easily charted as carelessness. The intent behind the behavior is not often studied or considered. Continued association with patients often seems to dull our sharpness when it comes to observation of new, different, or changed behavior. We more easily accept behavior that we see on a day-to-day basis, and so we have to be continually alert for a behavior that is even slightly different from usual. Ancillary workers should be encouraged and rewarded for reporting changes in behavior in elderly clients, since they often are the ones closest to the older person (Burnside, 1973). It seems sensible for nurses to begin to design continuing education programs on "benign suicide" and methods of alleviating the miseries that cause such behavior in the elderly.

Patterson, Abrahams, and Baker (1974) have observed that "alcoholism, heavy smoking, neglect of health care, and psychological stress can be just as lethal as suicide." In a survey of 445 people over the age of 65 in a lower-middle-class town in the Boston area, they discovered the following types of self-injurious behavior: (1) lack of concern about overweight, 25 percent; (2) untreated vision problems, 15 percent; (3) no visit to a physician for over 2 years, 14 percent; (4) untreated hearing problems, 13 percent; (5) smoking 20 or more cigarettes daily, 11 percent; (6) neglect of illnesses, 9 percent; (7) neglect of diet for obesity, 8 percent; (8) inadequate medical emergency plan, 5 percent; and (9) underweight, 4 percent. These findings should alert nurses in health clinics to watch for and assess such behavior among their elderly clients. The high incidence of untreated hearing and vision problems should be areas of real concern to caretakers.

Mishara et al. (1973) have listed steps to follow which might be useful in the study of self-destructive behavior. These are (1) observation, (2) reflection, (3) intervention, (4) assessment, and (5) follow-up.

One must be careful in making a judgment, because some behavior that may seem abnormal may be due to organic problems and not for self-destructive purposes. The researchers Kastenbaum and Mishara (1971) observed the following behavior during a 1-week period on a chronic geriatric ward. The remarks enclosed in brackets are mine.

1. Injury due to the inability to walk adequately, falling down.
2. Bumping into objects such as the wall.
3. Climbing out of wheelchairs and falling.
4. Scratching self.
5. Undressing self.
6. Injury due to careless use of cigarettes. [This is a real concern and worry for caretakers in any facility. The widespread publicity about the fires in nursing homes has intensified the concerns about smoking.]
7. Scalding hands by turning on hot water. [Hot water tanks must be adjusted to a lower heat.]
8. Eating foreign objects. [I have seen elderly mental patients rip up bed sheets and eat the strips, take the feathers out of their pillows and eat them, strip geranium plants of their leaves. One begins to appreciate the ability of the gastrointestinal tract to handle some unusual assignments considering the list of objects ingested.]
9. Choking due to eating too fast. [Deaths do occur both from feeding too fast and from the elderly person eating too fast.]
10. Fighting, pushing, etc.
11. Tripping over one another and being injured.
12. Striking the wall or window.
13. Injury due to hostility evoked by stealing another's cigarettes.

LIFE-THREATENING MANEUVERS

The life-threatening maneuvers are categorized by Kastenbaum and Mishara (1971).

1. Refuses medications. [This could include oral medication, intravenous medication, and intramuscular medications.]

2. Fails to follow the orders of the physicians. [Smoking is a common problem with the circulatory condition, Buerger's disease. One also observes chain smokers who have severe emphysema or lung cancer. Staff members may become angry about the patient disobeying the doctor's orders and may issue punitive orders which often only seem to make the patient even more resistant to the treatment plan. Chronic brain disease secondary to alcoholism is common. Alcoholism is another problem that is frequently seen in the long-term care settings, and staff members may treat the elderly alcoholic unkindly. I have noticed this to be particularly true of bitter staff members who have had alcoholic persons in their own family.]

3. Refuses to eat or accept food. One very subtle way is to take it but to ingest or to retain very little. [It always amazed me that patients who ate very poorly during mealtime in the institution ate voraciously at group meetings when served out-of-the-ordinary sweets and treats. One psychotic old man used to gulp down the milk shake I brought him during our time together. The following vignette describes a depressed elderly man who refused food and an exasperated staff who tried to make him eat.]

4. Situates self in hazardous environment—by drafty window.

VIGNETTE 1

The refusal of Mr. A. to eat shows how complicated and frustrating these life-threatening maneuvers can be, but it also shows that a humane and creative staff can always hope for a solution. Mr. A. was an 83-year-old divorced, white male who had been in a veterans' hospital, and was subsequently discharged to an "L" facility (light mental, long-term care) after treatment for bilateral lower-lobe pneumonia and pleural effusion. He also had these diagnoses: (1) cardiovascular accident, (2) chronic organic brain syndrome (CBS), (3) abdominal aneurysm, (4) a history of duodenal ulcer, and (5) psoriasis. His only significant other was a landlady who phoned occasionally to inquire about him. The physician wrote on his chart: "Patient has been afebrile and clinically much improved *except for extreme depression and consequent anorexia.* Patient lost 15 pounds during hospitalization because of not eating. Patient needs much encouragement before he will eat. . . . He gradually improved and now is able to be up and about, but does not want to do anything for himself. Needs to have an area near the bathroom, otherwise becomes incontinent. Patient can verbalize but not in context. Cannot follow simple instructions. Needs to be left alone, as he can do more for himself without encouragement. Increased confusion without evidence of fever, cough, melena, hematemesis or trauma prior to admission. . . ."

The patient refused to eat, no matter how much the staff coaxed and cajoled him. In December 1973, he weighed 109 pounds. Finally, more in desperation than because of rationale, the staff began to take his meals to him and set them down beside him without any fuss. They also quietly left wine, eggnog, and snacks for him. He stayed in bed for 2 to 3 weeks and then gradually began to eat. On April 23, 1974, he had gained 29 pounds and, though still somewhat confused, was less depressed. He got out of bed, became more active, and physically looked better. The staff was not sure what had happened. It could be argued that their behavior was "an invitation to die" (Jourard, 1970). On the other hand, I prefer to believe that he had been given the decisions to make for himself and this may have been the turning point for him. He could decide when to eat, what to eat, how much, and he could also decide when he was ready to get up. *Perhaps we underestimate the importance of the decision-making process for the aged, and most especially the institutionalized aged.*

TREATMENT OF POTENTIALLY SUICIDAL PERSONS

One way to begin treatment of suicidal persons is to work with the nurse or with the staff. Suicidal patients have a tendency to bring out the worst in us, the caretakers. Several reactions are often observed: anger, despair, depression, fear, and guilt.

ANGER

Anger directed at the suicidal patient is often seen expressed especially toward the younger patient. The treatment staff in effect is going "to show him so he won't try it again." In one emergency ward I recall a resident physician using the largest-size tube available as a lavage in a patient because she had taken an overdose of aspirin. Anger seems to be based on the feeling that the patient is "copping out." Another reason for the staff's anger and hostility may be the thought that the patient has not appreciated all the good medical care and treatment and thus reacts by attempting suicide. In fact, it is not uncommon for the patient to sense that he or she *has* had good treatment, and instead of committing suicide in a hospital unit waits for a pass or until discharged from the hospital. Moriwaki (1974) reported that she studied suicidal behavior for psychological autopsies and that elderly patients hanged themselves on the grounds away from their ward or had gone home on pass to complete the act.

DESPAIR AND DEPRESSION

Feelings of despair and depression often arise in patients as well as in members of the staff. One cannot help thinking of one's own old age and ask, "Is this what is ahead for me?" The plight of the aged sometimes drives one to despair as one begins to solve problems with them. The need to acknowledge one's feelings and to maintain objectivity in the care of such patients is frequently easier written about in a textbook than it is done in reality!

FEAR

The initial fright when one finds a person who has committed suicide can be traumatic. A night nurse once described to me finding a body hanging from a tree outside a window. On every shift she described at length how she still often saw the body hanging in the tree. Another nurse, who found a patient in the lobby in a pool of blood from slashing his wrists, discussed the impact on other residents and the staff members. For new staff members, such emergencies on a ward jar them considerably. Change-of-shift reports can serve several purposes other than relaying information about patients. The report can serve as a catharsis, a true sharing of one's own personal feelings. In a relaxed, informal atmosphere, even the most inarticulate employee often verbalizes some rather intense feelings. In-service education and change-of-shift reports both can be utilized to help staff deal more effectively with feelings based on suicide.

GUILT

It is not uncommon for caretakers to feel guilty when a patient has attempted suicide. One wonders where one missed the boat, what could have been done to prevent the patient's suicide attempt. It is important for staff members to be able to discuss the attempt and find interested listeners.

VIGNETTE 2
An elderly man in a long-term care facility went to the front lobby and slashed his wrists. The bloody scene and the suddenness of the incident unnerved the personnel. The staff quickly cleaned the bloody lobby and pretended nothing had happened. Several persons were able to discuss their guilt feelings in a class they attended much later.

Guilt feelings can provide a valuable lesson for caretakers, because members of the patient's family often have many of the same feelings. Thus the caretaker's own guilt feelings can serve as a reminder that family members, particularly the patient's spouse, need help and support during the crisis caused by a suicide attempt.

INTERVENTION

McLeod (1978, p. 14) states,

Patients often express surprise when the therapist asks about suicidal feelings or ideas. It is wise to approach this subject gently, asking how the patient feels about the future or whether the patient ever felt that life was not worth living, and lead into the subject from there; the question is important but often alarms patients and on occasion encourages them to be evasive when answering. Most successful suicides have sought medical advice in the month preceding their death, which suggests that the doctor has not asked the proper questions, or that if he has, the answers have either been unheard or misunderstood.

Drye et al. (1973) have described one approach to the suicidal person. After expressing thoughts of suicide, a client is asked to make this statement to the therapist: "No matter what happens, I will not kill myself, accidentally or on purpose, at any time." If the client cannot confidently make the statement, the client is judged to be a serious risk. The authors report no fatalities with 600 individuals with the "no-suicide decisions" over a 5-year period.

The following guidelines are suggested for intervention (Payne, 1975):

1. Elicit direct information from the client.
2. Actively solicit client's cooperation.
3. The client can estimate his or her own emotional position if given a method to work with.
4. Strengthen the therapeutic relationship.
5. Look for alcohol abuse and psychosis, for if confusion or decreased cognition is present, the judgment is unreliable and one cannot consider the statement valid.

Assessment and management of the potentially suicidal depressive person is diagrammed in Figure 12-2. The treatment of potentially suicidal persons should consider the following:

1. A protective environment should be provided for the aged suicidal person.
2. If there is a psychotic depression, especially one due to a strict superego and hostility turned inward, use firmness but not too much firmness (Weiss, 1968). The following is a case of too much firmness which did not accomplish the therapeutic results intended.

Mr. K., a man in his late sixties, was admitted to an acute psychiatric hospital with a psy-

chotic depression. The treatment plan, intended to make the former engineer lose his temper, stated he was to pick up the papers in the yard and do menial tasks. The worst task was scrubbing the floor of the occupational therapy room with a toothbrush. The man saw it as punishment, complied obediently, and withdrew even more. One night during the recreation period, the 4:00 P.M. to midnight nurse asked him to dance. Because her feet were bothering her, she took off her shoes. With great surprise he said, "You mean you trust me enough to dance with me without your shoes on?" Often a very small gesture can bolster a depressed person.

3. The passive, dependent older person with depression due to losses may be suffering from a "bereavement overload" (as Kastenbaum well phrased multiple deaths) and responds favorably to empathy, understanding, and kindness. Staff members are too often afraid of spoiling a person who is dependent and grieving.
4. The development of interest in hobbies requires a concerted effort on the part of the staff, but it may take away the meaninglessness of life that so many oldsters complain about.
5. Electroshock therapy (EST) is often used, but some patients may be terrified of it. They are afraid of losing consciousness and hate the amnesia that follows the therapy; e.g., they cannot remember where their rooms are. A careful explanation about the treatment and its results may relieve a patient's anxiety.
6. Group therapy is not always successful. (A pair of psychiatric students once selected a group entirely of suicidal patients and found that the experience was too much for them to handle.)
7. Antidepressive drugs may be helpful, but the correct dosage is necessary and may have to be adjusted for an aged person.
8. Careful physical examination is always in order to rule out physical problems. Kastenbaum and Mishara (1971) suggest the importance of four factors in the elderly: (a) Encourage continuity of care; do not shift personnel on these people. (b) Discourage relocation; do all you can to prevent "translocation shock." (c) Foster interpersonal mutuality. Do not place an elderly person in the role of a powerless human being. (d) Reinforce comfort-giving behaviors. No matter how self-destructive someone may be today,

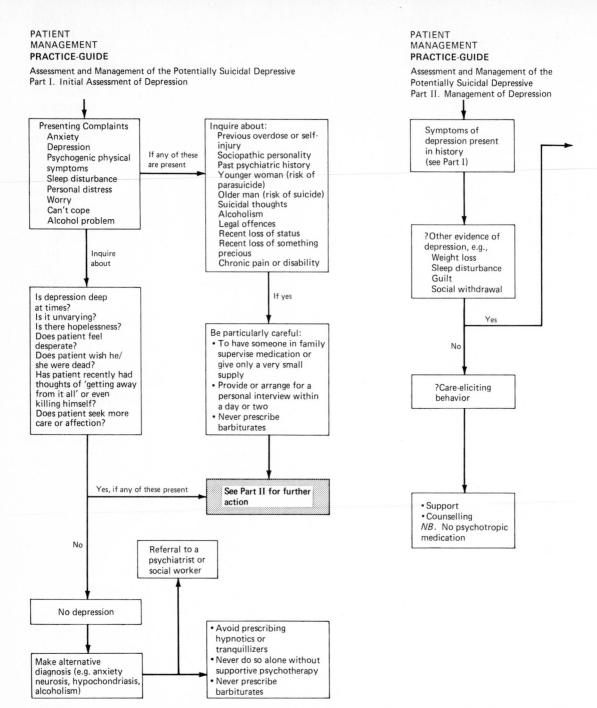

PATIENT
MANAGEMENT
PRACTICE-GUIDE

Assessment and Management of the Potentially Suicidal Depressive
Part I. Initial Assessment of Depression

PATIENT
MANAGEMENT
PRACTICE-GUIDE

Assessment and Management of the
Potentially Suicidal Depressive
Part II. Management of Depression

Presenting Complaints
  Anxiety
  Depression
  Psychogenic physical
  symptoms
  Sleep disturbance
  Personal distress
  Worry
  Can't cope
  Alcohol problem

If any of these
are present

Inquire about:
  Previous overdose or self-
  injury
  Sociopathic personality
  Past psychiatric history
  Younger woman (risk of
  parasuicide)
  Older man (risk of suicide)
  Suicidal thoughts
  Alcoholism
  Legal offences
  Recent loss of status
  Recent loss of something
  precious
  Chronic pain or disability

Inquire
about

Is depression deep
at times?
Is it unvarying?
Is there hopelessness?
Does patient feel
desperate?
Does patient wish he/
she were dead?
Has patient recently had
thoughts of 'getting away
from it all' or even
killing himself?
Does patient seek more
care or affection?

If yes

Be particularly careful:
• To have someone in family
  supervise medication or
  give only a very small
  supply
• Provide or arrange for a
  personal interview within
  a day or two
• Never prescribe
  barbiturates

Yes, if any of these present

See Part II for further
action

No

Referral to a
psychiatrist or
social worker

No depression

• Avoid prescribing
  hypnotics or
  tranquillizers
• Never do so alone without
  supportive psychotherapy
• Never prescribe
  barbiturates

Make alternative
diagnosis (e.g. anxiety
neurosis, hypochondriasis,
alcoholism)

Symptoms of
depression present
in history
(see Part I)

?Other evidence of
depression, e.g.,
  Weight loss
  Sleep disturbance
  Guilt
  Social withdrawal

Yes

No

?Care-eliciting
behavior

• Support
• Counselling
NB. No psychotropic
medication

FIGURE 12-2   Assessment and management of the potentially suicidal depressive. [*Patient Management, 2(7):43–45, July 1978, ADIS Press Australasia Pty Ltd., Sydney, Australia.*]

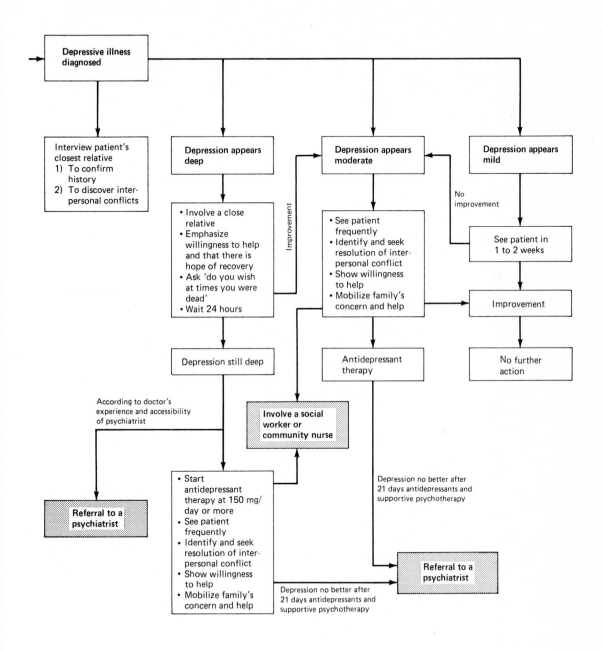

Depressive illness diagnosed

Interview patient's closest relative
1) To confirm history
2) To discover interpersonal conflicts

Depression appears deep

Depression appears moderate

Depression appears mild

- Involve a close relative
- Emphasize willingness to help and that there is hope of recovery
- Ask 'do you wish at times you were dead'
- Wait 24 hours

Improvement

- See patient frequently
- Identify and seek resolution of interpersonal conflict
- Show willingness to help
- Mobilize family's concern and help

No improvement

See patient in 1 to 2 weeks

Improvement

Depression still deep

Antidepressant therapy

No further action

According to doctor's experience and accessibility of psychiatrist

Involve a social worker or community nurse

Referral to a psychiatrist

- Start antidepressant therapy at 150 mg/day or more
- See patient frequently
- Identify and seek resolution of interpersonal conflict
- Show willingness to help
- Mobilize family's concern and help

Depression no better after 21 days antidepressants and supportive psychotherapy

Referral to a psychiatrist

Depression no better after 21 days antidepressants and supportive psychotherapy tomorrow that person may be deeply grateful that these feelings were respected but not obeyed.

Treatment should be meaningful and based on the psychodynamics of the depression of the older person. This means careful assessment of the many losses, and especially recent losses; changes in health which cause pain or change in body image; and recent anniversary dates of loss of loved ones. The patient should be continually assessed as to suicidal risk, and behavior should be noted daily. Butler and Lewis (1973) emphasize that the depression-based suicide may be prevented through treatment. The reader is referred to an in-depth discussion of suicide assessment (Hatton, et al., 1977).

VIGNETTE 3

A woman in her seventies was being seen by a nursing student working toward a master's degree. The woman and student had developed a close relationship over the school term.

The student felt that the woman was depressed and withdrawing and was concerned about her. She became especially concerned when she visited one day and discovered that the woman had gone through her apartment and placed all the pictures face down.

The concerned student alerted the aged woman's physician and the public health nurse/supervisor, who did not show much concern about the clue the student described. Since the client had threatened suicide in the past, this action was felt to be "just another threat" and was not to be taken seriously. The student was left feeling she had overreacted.

When the woman died, the student felt she had taken an overdose of pills, but there was no note and no definite proof that she had a lethal number of pills. No postmortem was done, and it was said that she died in her sleep.

In many cases the cause of death is murky, and families may be reluctant to grant permission for autopsies, particularly when they are in the throes of denial. The effect of suicidal deaths on the survivors can be great, as shown in Vignette 4.

Payne offers these suggestions in working with the depressed, potentially suicidal, individual:

1. Treat the underlying depression.
2. Keep the client alive until the treatment begins to take effect.
3. Ameliorate the psychosocial problems which have increased the client's despair.

A review of the literature would suggest these guidelines for intervention:

1. Improve the general health including minor ailments.
2. Plan for retirement so there is no cessation of self-esteem support.
3. Recognize the high-risk clients.
4. Organize cross-referrals to all agencies.
5. Talk about death.
6. Seek community help.
7. Educate the relatives.
8. Recognize the importance of aftercare.
9. Watch for "bereavement overload" (Kastenbaum, 1969).

VIGNETTE 4

A man in his mid-eighties had been greatly saddened by the loss of vision after his retirement. He could no longer drive or fish or go camping, and he missed all three forms of leisure. His wife had to assume the driving and more and more of the responsibilities around the home.

He had been on reserpine for some time, and his depression apparently was well masked, especially from his wife, physician, and close friends who visited.

His wife thought he had given away all his guns and did not know that he had kept one revolver and placed it under his mattress. (They slept in separate bedrooms because one of them had a snoring problem which disturbed the other.)

One night he placed the gun in his mouth and killed himself. His wife discovered him the next day when she went in to call him for breakfast. She never did really recover from the shock of that scene and rather quickly gave away things, sold the house, and moved to a distant part of the country. She subsequently had a stroke. Because of her severe problem in speaking, a distant relative took power of attorney, and soon she was in a nursing home where she died. In a pathetic, shakily written letter to a friend she described how she had lost complete control of her life after the stroke. "They think I do not know what they are doing, but I have not lost my mind. They are selling my things and do not ask me about my business affairs" (Anonymous, 1969).

As professionals we need to be aware of the message being sent by the self-destructive behavior observed. Lipsitt (1969) wrote, "The anguish arising from emotional starvation is profound and lingering and it ultimately leads to despair, preoccupation with bodily function, reliance upon others, physical and mental deterioration, hospitalization, and even death." And Kastenbaum and Mishara (1971, p. 81) wrote, "Organic illness or no, treated or no, the patient seems to require sensitive support if he is to remain interested in surviving." I see sensitive support as an important nursing role in care of depressed aged.

"The most significant aspect to the study of the phenomenon of suicide in the aging population is the sensitive indicator to the source of despair with which it provides us" (Payne, 1975, p. 310). Unfortunately, we often fail to heed the despair manifested by old people.

The poet Housman describes thoughts of suicide in words which reflect very movingly the isolation felt by an older person surrounded by people insensitive to his despair.

> Good creatures, do you love your lives
> And have you ears for sense?
> Here is a knife like other knives,
> That cost me 18 pence.
> I need but stick it in my heart
> And down will come the sky
> And earth's foundation will depart
> And all you folk will die.
>
> A. E. Housman

REFERENCES

Barraclough, B. M.: Suicide in the elderly, in D. W. Kay and A. Walk (eds.), *Recent Developments in Psychogeriatrics,* Headly Brothers, Ashford, Kent, England, 1971, pp. 89–97.

Burnside, Irene Mortenson: Multiple losses in the aged, *Gerontologist,* **13**(2):157–162, Summer 1973.

Butler, Robert N., and Myrna I. Lewis: *Aging and Mental Health,* Mosby, St. Louis, 1973.

Drye, R. C., R. L. Goulding, and M. E. Goulding: No-suicide decisions: Patient monitoring of suicidal risk, *American Journal of Psychiatry,* **130**(2):174, 1973.

Finch, Caleb: Physiology of aging, implications for nursing, lecture for class, Andrus Gerontology Center, University of Southern California, Jan. 7, 1974.

Haggerty, J.: Suicidal behavior in a 70-year-old man: A case report, *Journal of Geriatric Psychiatry,* **6**(1):43–51, Fall 1973.

Hatton, Corrine Loing, Sharon McBride Valente, and Alice Rink: *Suicide Assessment and Intervention,* Appleton-Century-Crofts, New York, 1977.

Housman, A. E.: "I Counsel You Beware," *More Poems,* Barclays Bank, Poole, Dorset, England, 1936.

Jourard, Sidney M.: An invitation to die, *American Journal of Nursing,* **70**(2):269–275, February 1970.

Kastenbaum, Robert: Death and bereavement in later life, in A. H. Kutscher (ed.), *Death and Bereavement,* Charles C Thomas, Springfield, Ill., pp. 28–54, 1969.

———, and Brian L. Mishara: Premature death and self-injurious behavior in old age, *Geriatrics,* **26**(7):70–81, July 1971.

Lipsitt, D. R.: A medico-psychological approach to dependency in the aged, in Richard A. Kalish (ed.), *The Dependencies of Old People,* Ann Arbor Institute, University of Michigan, Ann Arbor, 1969.

McLeod, W. R.: Making the most of the interview: Psychological and psychiatric aspects, *Patient Management,* **2**(7):9–16, July 1978.

Miller, Marv: *Suicide after Sixty,* Springer, New York, 1979.

———: *Suicide among the Elderly: The Final Alternative,* 1977, in press.

———: Suicide after suicide, *Aging,* (289–290):28–31, November/December 1978a.

———: Toward a profile of the older white male suicide, *Gerontologist,* **18**(1):80–82, February 1978b.

Mishara, Brian, et al.: Self-injurious behavior in the elderly, *Gerontologist,* **13**(3):311–317, Autumn 1973.

Moriwaki, Sharon: Personal communication, 1974.

Motto, Jerome: Suicide attempts: A longitudinal view, *Archives General Psychiatry,* **13**(6):516–520, 1965.

Mummah, Hazel: Personal communication, 1974.

Parker, Gordon: *The Bonds of Depression,* Angus & Robertson, Sydney, Australia, 1978.

Patterson, Robert, D., Ruby Abrahams, and Frank Baker: Preventing self-destructive behavior, *Geriatrics,* **30**(7):115–131, November 1974.

Payne, Edmund C.: Depression and suicide, in John G. Howells (ed.), *Modern Perspectives in the Psychiatry of Old Age,* Brunner/Mazel, New York, 1975, pp. 290–312.

Schneidman, Edwin, and Norman Farberow (eds.): *Clues to Suicide,* McGraw-Hill, New York, 1957.

Tabachnick, N.: Observations in attempted suicide, in E. S. Schneidman, N. L. Farberow (eds.), *Clues to Suicide,* McGraw-Hill, New York, 1957.

Weiss, J. M. A.: Suicide in the aged, in H. C. P. Resnick (ed.), *Suicidal Behaviors,* Little, Brown, Boston, 1968.

OTHER RESOURCES

Suicide: Causes and Prevention, 32 min/16 mm/color. Two-part filmstrip (also available in cassettes). Part I provides a historical and cultural overview of suicide and explores some of its possible causes. Part II explores various ways to help prevent suicide. Distributor: Human Relations Media, 175 Tompkins Avenue, Pleasantville, NY 10570.

THIRTEEN

PARANOID BEHAVIOR IN THE ELDERLY

Irene Mortenson Burnside

Trust, the sense of being supported by the scheme of things, the feeling that one receives from life at least as much as one gives.
Huston Smith

LEARNING OBJECTIVES

- Define paranoia.
- Define paraphrenia.
- Describe the relationship of perceptual losses and paranoia.
- List three techniques to reduce anxiety in aged persons with paranoid reactions.
- Describe behavior of the aged paranoid individual who also has a brain syndrome.
- Describe two behaviors of an alcoholic paranoid aged person.
- List interventions for caretakers when delusions concern the fidelity of the spouse.
- List interviewing techniques with the suspicious, guarded aged client.
- List two common delusions which may occur in the aged paranoid.

PARANOIA IN THE ELDERLY

Busse and Pfeiffer (1973) state that, though older people may manifest any of the mental illnesses seen in younger adults, the majority of psychiatric disturbances in the elderly fall into a fairly small cluster of psychiatric syndromes, including affective disorders, paranoid reactions, hypochondriacal states, situational disturbances, organic brain syndromes, and alcoholism. Of these syndromes, paranoia is among the more common and troubling. Paranoia is a mental disorder which is characterized by delusions of persecution, or illusions of grandeur, or a combination of both (Miller and Keane, 1972).

Geropsychiatrists Busse and Pfeiffer (1973, pp. 126–127) note,

> While younger paranoid patients often blame powerful but somewhat remote and esoteric forces for their misfortunes, old people often blame persons either geographically or emotionally close to themselves. Thus paranoid ideas in old age often center on neighbors or passersby, on the mailman or milkman, or on members of the aged person's own household; for instance, neighbors are accused of laughing or talking about the old person, of maligning his or her character.

Some psychiatrists consider paranoid states in old people to be the other side of the coin of depression—the person's abnormal mood is turned against others, rather than against one's self (Caird and Judge, 1977). Women are affected more frequently than men, but paranoid states are common in both sexes in late life (Butler and Lewis, 1977).

DIAGNOSED PROBLEMS

Paranoid syndromes account for about one-tenth of the admissions to mental hospitals of persons over the age of 60. They can also be associated with a senile character-change, an acute confusional state, depressive illness, arteriosclerotic dementia, or a chronic illness called *paraphrenia*, which will be discussed later in this chapter (Anderson, 1971). Although the data on cases of paranoia in the aged population are not clear, one community sample showed that 17 percent of the subjects exhibited suspiciousness (Lowenthal, 1964).

Many of these elderly paranoid individuals are unmarried women, and one-third of them are affected by disorders of vision or, more commonly, hearing. They have often exhibited paranoid tendencies throughout their life, but in later life they also develop delusions. Short-lived paranoid reactions can be observed in the states of exhaustion of persons who are kept awake by pain or by dyspneic problems (Anderson, 1971).

Davidson (1964) states that paranoid symptoms can be seen after severe infection and are probably as common as the depressive symptoms associated with influenza, hepatitis, use of steroids, and vitamin deficiencies as in pellagra and pernicious anemia. The treatment is based on the treatment of the organic disease. One must remember, however, that the paranoid symptoms may not end when the physical illness has been cured (Anderson, 1971).

Paranoid syndromes can be difficult to diagnose. Diagnosis is easy when the patient has obvious delusions or discusses persecution by others. However, if the delusions are more restricted and are discovered only after prolonged interrogation about physical symptoms and daily routine, then diagnosis of paranoia can be difficult. But Caird and Judge (1977) believe that the diagnosis of such cases is frequently not of major importance. The primary need for detection of mild cases lies in the uproar that paranoid behavior can cause; it is frequently more of a problem to neighbors and family than to the client. Paranoia responds reasonably well to phenothiazine therapy, however, which can be a good reason for detecting any paranoid state.

MEDICALLY TREATABLE

It is important to remember that paranoid patients are medically treatable but there is a lower degree of success with them if they are not given the medications which are known to help them. And although there is currently much furor and concern about overmedicating individuals, good sense does indicate that in cases where there is a tremendous need for medication which is therapeutically effective, it should be used.

Drugs of choice include chlorpromazine (Thorazine), thioridazine (Mellaril), and haloperidol (Haldol). Generally the aged person will have to take these drugs for long periods of time for lasting results (Busse and Pfeiffer, 1973).

There is evidence that the drug tripluoperazine has been helpful in the management of elderly clients who suffer from paraphrenia and have systematized persecutory delusions. Post recorded favorable results in 72 subjects who were over the age of 60 and had paranoid psychosis. The treatment must be undertaken in a hospital because the dosage can be up to 30 mg daily and may continue for months (Post, 1962; A. N. Exton-Smith and A. C. M. Windsor, 1971).

Neadly (1977) has reported on a difficult and complicated nursing care study of paranoid depression. A 62-year-old man had the following problems: delusions, incontinence, diabetes, cataracts, depression, a suicide attempt, and myocardial infarction. The patient's aggressivity abated after he had "settled in" following his admission to the hospital.

PARAPHRENIA

Paraphrenia is late-onset schizophrenia in the form of a persecutory state. Eisdorfer (1977, p. 120) once remarked that "at one time I didn't believe there was such a thing as paraphrenia; I thought it was something the British made up to confuse American psychiatrists; I was wrong."

The paranoid delusions in paraphrenia are often about a neighbor. One man who lived in a low-cost housing unit felt that the people who lived above him had designed an intricate plot to kill him. The strange noises he heard and described as part of the plot were actually rather strange gurgling noises in the water pipes.

These conditions most often occur in people who have been loners and have led withdrawn lives, often isolated spinsters. They tend to "have well-preserved if eccentric person-

alities and often maintain their independence surprisingly well" (Hodkinson, 1975, p. 84). One nurse has described such an eccentric nonagenarian spinster who was in both group and one-to-one interactions with a nurse. Her delusions and paranoid behavior took her to a locked unit (Burnside, 1978).

LIFE-STYLE

It is helpful to assess the life-styles of clients because some people do have a life-long pattern of suspiciousness, guardedness, and aloofness. Charatan (1978) states that "while the premorbid personality may have contributed to the development of the paranoid defense, the old person is, in fact, weak and relatively dependent, often experiencing the environment as more hostile than helpful. He therefore is more likely to feel persecuted and victimized."

Weinberg (1970) has pointed out that the tendency of paranoid people to lose things may often account for their thinking that items are being stolen from them. One elderly woman I knew carefully hid her silverware so that it would not be stolen, then promptly forgot where she had hidden it and accused the neighbors of stealing it.

Paranoid states can be of short duration and tend to occur under such adverse conditions as imprisonment, deafness, isolation, disfigurement, infections, drunkenness, involution, or blindness. Incoming stimuli are misinterpreted, and there can be isolation from human contact. (See Chapter 34 for a full discussion of sensory deprivation and blindness.)

The personality features of paranoid people do have a particular maladaptiveness in old age. But often much is happening in their lives which does reinforce the feeling that the problems are all "out there." Added to that, hearing and other sensory losses may increase the inability to handle threatening forces and compound the isolation of aged persons with paranoid tendencies (Butler and Lewis, 1977).

Aged, paranoid individuals can appear more helpless than they really are. Sometimes they use their age, disease, or perceptual losses as a defense so that, for example, they may hear only what they want to hear. Others may react with rigidity, despair, or depression, which can make them maladapted and apparently helpless (Butler and Lewis, 1977).

PARANOID REACTION AND ORGANIC BRAIN SYNDROME

Paranoid reactions are commonly associated with organic brain syndrome. These paranoid phenomena, which are secondary to cerebral decompensation, are lacking in sophistication and systematization, says Verwoerdt. The person manages to improvise on the spot, and the story will change and be inconsistent. As the physical condition improves, the paranoid delusion or the hallucination tends to clear up as well (Verwoerdt, 1976).

The paranoid type of senile dementia is observed in quarrelsome and demanding behavior. There may be chronic complaints about maltreatment.

ALCOHOLISM AND PARANOID STATE

The paranoid state in chronic alcoholics (usually in men) is manifested by extreme jealousy and frequent delusions regarding the fidelity of the spouse. Nurses often must handle such individuals.

DELUSIONS OF INFIDELITY

I recall one old man who thought his wife rendezvoused often in the basement with her lover. It was difficult to convince him she was unable to descend or climb the flight of stairs.

At the onset of senile dementia, abnormal behavior can occur and includes a rather common delusion—the delusion of infidelity. Such delusions are the most common form of deviant sexual behavior associated with senile dementia and are usually seen in aged men. Grauer (1978) says that they are often related to a decline in sexual performance and occur more often in men who have had a tendency to overvalue their sexual potency.

When these delusions occur in women, they may be provoked by misinterpreting the partner's sexual deterioration as rejection and then projecting that into a belief that the husband (or the lover) is having sexual affairs with other women. Such delusions can create obvious severe marital and family upsets and may block the person's chances for sexual readjustment. They may also build up to a crisis situation in which children or neighbors have to intervene. Such delusions of infidelity, however, do not usually lead to deviant sexual activity (Grauer, 1978).

The caretaker should explain and interpret the dynamics of the delusions to the client's spouse and also to the family. When it is possible, the couple should be encouraged to resume sexual relations or closeness. If the delusions are fixed, antipsychotic or phenothiazine therapy is sometimes helpful. But such drugs must be used cautiously because they might interfere with sexual potency, and if diminished potency is already playing a role in the delusion of the aged person, their use may only exacerbate the problem and be contraindicated. If depression is a part of the diagnosis, then antidepressive medication may be combined with the phenothiazines (Grauer, 1978).

REFUSAL TO EAT

Another common problem of aged delusional people is a refusal to eat because they fear that the food is poisoned. Such individuals require excellent nursing interventions to prevent dehydration or malnutrition, and it takes real skill to encourage them to eat. The nurse will have to learn what seems to work best for each individual (Burnside, 1971). I have personally found that sharing food or beverage with the aged person helps. Also much time needs to be spent with staff members and family to find out what is helpful. And sometimes nothing helps, as in the case of Gramp (Jury and Jury, 1976).

NURSING CARE OF PARANOIA

The immediate goal in treatment of paranoia is to reduce the anxiety which leads to the formation of paranoid ideas. Busse and Pfeiffer (1969) suggest three related but differing techniques (all may be used): (1) psychotherapeutic intervention, (2) reduction of threat from external environment, and (3) tranquilizers.

Nurses can sometimes be effective in helping to reduce the anxiety of paranoid clients by their presence, especially if clients are very fearful. They can also help bolster sagging self-esteem; this often takes real skill in communication. Assigning student nurses in one-to-one relationships can produce beneficial changes in elderly mentally ill. This technique can also have an effect on staff members; it frequently makes the students selected become more interested in the care of the aged. They may even emulate the behavior of a therapeutic student. However, the one-to-one relationship can be difficult, since the patients' delusions may be constantly expressed, and at times the nurses may feel that little therapy is occurring.

It is important to do whatever one can to break down the isolation of the paranoid patient or client, but such individuals usually put everyone off by their bristly, offensive manners and consistent abrasiveness, or their far-out stories about the FBI tapping wires, etc.

ENVIRONMENTAL MANIPULATION

Environmental manipulation may be necessary; providing a stable environment that is not too complicated may be the nurse's responsibility.

Attention to sensory deficits is imperative. Visual deficits and hearing losses must be attended to by checking for adequate lighting and whatever else needs correcting to improve sensory performance for the aged. See Chapters 33 and 34 for pragmatic suggestions. Abarca (1980) has described interventions needed with an elderly lonely hallucinating individual.

INTERVIEWING PARANOID CLIENTS

Interviewing the paranoid client at any age is difficult, but it becomes increasingly difficult when the old person is not only suspicious, guarded, mistrusting, and/or delusional but has

hearing problems, vision problems, or problems with personal safety.

Many elderly persons hide their delusional system, and the nurse may require some time to discover its intricacies (Burnside, 1978). My first realization of delusions in one client occurred when she thought my pendant was a tape machine recording our conversation.

McLeod (1978, p. 10) reminds us of another point to remember in interviewing. "An authoritarian interviewer is likely to evoke a hostile response. One needs no skill to generate more anger in the angry, or fear in those who are afraid; the anxious can be made more so, and feelings of worthlessness and hopelessness in the depressed patients can be aggravated." The therapist's skill lies in the ability to diminish, resolve, or otherwise handle such feelings.

Hostile responses come rather quickly and easily for the mistrusting paranoid individual and can sometimes throw the new interviewer off guard or at least increase the timidity of the interviewer. The patient's caustic, sarcastic demeanor can be difficult to work with, and so can the crazy talking of some patients suffering from chronic brain syndrome who have an overlay of paranoia.

USE OF TAPE RECORDERS

It is well for instructors to caution students rather vigorously about refraining from the use of any type of tape recorders with paranoid individuals because the aged person may feel it is part of a plan or the FBI is spying and that you will use the tape against them in some harmful way. The building of trust is extremely important, and the use of a tape recorder might prevent the student from even beginning to build a comfortable relationship with the client. Also, patients who are confused or have been institutionalized for a long time may not comprehend what a tape recorder is.

HOSTILITY

When hostile behavior does appear in the aged paranoid client, the nurse needs to remain objective and recognize that the hostility is part and parcel of the underlying disorder. One clinical tool to learn is to observe in such a detached manner that one does not react to the hostility in a highly personal manner. Attempting to understand the underlying problem of which the hostility is symptomatic is better than reacting with counterhostility, avoidance, or obviously cringing with hurt. Criticism, sarcasm, and haughty ways can be manifested as well as outbursts of anger or hostile behavior.

HONESTY

The nurse must be honest at all times with the paranoid person; these persons want closeness, but it must come gradually and slowly. These people have had "years of 'training' at recognizing phony talk. Irony and humor—referring to the universities of the human condition are valuable" (Butler and Lewis, 1977).

The interviewer should be on the alert for the theme of aloneness. The semantics of the client's conversation may be a clue if no discrete circumscribed delusion is elicited. The following interview illustrates the way a covert theme may be discovered through the language of a client.

VIGNETTE 1

During the class on psychosocial care of the elderly, I was interviewing a man over 60 years of age in Hawaii. While I could pick up that he was guarded and suspicious, his social grace, politeness, and grooming fooled me for awhile. He described his travels all over the world with the merchant marine, and then he talked about wanting to go to the North Pole and discussed Byrd. His interest in the coldness, being alone at the end of the earth, came through to us all. I ultimately ended the interview feeling I had been on an ice floe with him.

These are some signs to watch for which may indicate isolation and/or paranoia: (1) the theme of being a loner; (2) guarded behavior—e.g., asking the interviewer, "Why do you need to hear that?"; (3) unwillingness to share or reveal; (4) tangential replies; (5) putting the interviewer down; and (6) lack of eye contact. In regard to the latter, however, be sure you are aware of any existing eye problems when you work on eye contact. One paranoid lady in her eighties in one of my groups avoided eye contact, and it was some time before she sadly told me how self-conscious she was about her crossed eye and so kept her eyes downward.

PARANOID INDIVIDUALS IN THE COMMUNITY

Paranoids who develop late in life do not lose their speech patterns and sometimes function quite well. Most of the problems are created by the ones who imagine plots, abuses, and conspiracies and who demand protection from the police or assistance from the fire department. I vividly recall the exasperation of the nurses in a long-term care facility for the mentally ill aged who had to cope with one such individual. The woman often got a dime during the daytime; then at about 3 A.M. she would go to the pay phone on the ward and call the police or fire department. Policemen once appeared at the door because "they had gotten a phone call saying that they had better get down there quick as she was being held prisoner and they were beating everyone up."

Such individuals can be a significant problem even when they live in the community, as the following vignette will show.

This example is taken from the paper of a student nurse who formed a therapeutic relationship with Mrs. C., a 77-year-old widow who was living, and causing problems, in the community. The student nurse, in her work with Mrs. C., was quite successful in achieving some of the major nursing goals in work with paranoid people. She not only broke through the client's isolation herself, but she also helped the client increase her contact with others and helped to reduce the woman's anxiety.

VIGNETTE 2

Mrs. C. lived alone in a public, federally subsidized housing complex. She was alert, in good physical condition, and, although *her sight and hearing were beginning to go,*[1]

---

[1] I have italicized important sentences which reflect the dynamics of paranoid thinking and/or behavior (IB).

she managed to maintain good conversational skills and mobility. She had never learned to drive because "it makes her too nervous," which limited her travels somewhat. Her general appearance was one of a very prim and proper English lady with every hair on her head in place and her clothing very clean, neat, and without a wrinkle.

She greeted the student cheerfully at the door and quickly reminded her that she "was right on time" and "my, aren't you a beautiful young woman." Such comments initially took the student by surprise, and at first she was not sure whether they were a good or a bad sign. *Mrs. C. seemed to be suspicious of younger people in general.* Within a matter of minutes, however, she began to talk about the *"tape talk" that she was hearing late at night and in the early hours of the morning. She recounted voices saying,* "I'll see you, dear," "Hello there," and "It's not nice to be poor," to mention a few of the phrases.

She was very serious in describing what she believed to be an attempt on the part of a certain "colored" lady *to make it look like she was going crazy.* The tape talk apparently had been following her for 18 months, and she had moved twice in an effort to be "rid of them." She even slept over at a friend's house for several nights to get away, but the *tapes* and the *knocks* followed her there. She seemed very tired and reported not having been able to get a good night's sleep in months.

Seeing two or more of the younger residents talking together immediately made Mrs. C. nervous because *she believed they were talking about her.*

The student initially intervened in this woman's situation by simply allowing her to talk about the suspicions, fears, and general confusion about what was really happening to her. Just knowing that someone was taking the time to listen to her seemed very important to her. *She had called the police and fire departments three different times.* They told her that they could not do anything without a warrant, but they did come out to check her place for unusual wiring, electronic "bugs," etc. However, they did not have time to sit and listen to her story. She repeatedly bemoaned the fact that "they just don't care here in America. They wouldn't treat me that way in England."

Mrs. C. did make some attempts to adapt, however. For example, she began to leave the television on in the evenings to cover up the voices late at night. She even bought some earplugs which did not work. She no longer uses them.

She did agree to see the staff psychiatrist in order to obtain a prescription for medication for sleep. An appointment was made for the following week. The student agreed to meet with her again following her appointment with the psychiatrist. Medication was prescribed for "the voices" as well as to help her sleep.

The psychiatrist who prescribed the medication was due to retire within the next 6 months. The student nurse expected him to be sensitive to her needs and to general recommendations that she required only nighttime medication for sleep. However, he gave her high dosages of a drug, which resulted in a severe medication reaction and which caused even more fear and anxiety (Walters, 1974).

LONERS RELATE TO BIRDS OR PETS

In several parts of the world I have noticed that old women relate to pets. It is not uncommon to see such loners in city parks, usually away from the groups and crowds, feeding animals or birds. If one tries to share the feeding with them, they can become quite nasty. I learned this rather quickly while traveling abroad.

VIGNETTE 3

I was crossing a lovely city park in Sydney, Australia, one day about 6 A.M. to catch a bus. As I sauntered along I came upon a tiny old woman feeding many, many pigeons. They were on her shoulder, on her arm, trying to get to a large bag of corn. When I came close to her, she watched me carefully, and then apparently became very afraid and rushed at me with her shopping bag held over her head, screaming at me, "You have your nerve coming down here all dressed up and snooping on me!" (I was in jeans and boots and hardly "dressed up," but that is how she perceived my garb.) She yelled at me for not buying bird food and feeding them as she did, and that she bet I would not get up at three in the morning to come down and feed those birds. I was too surprised to respond, and she did not allow time for a reply. She had reacted with alacrity and vehemence when I moved in close to her and her birds; it was her territory and she came at me with such aggressivity I was caught completely off guard.

MOVING IN CLOSE

It is usually important not to move into a paranoid person's territory too quickly and not to be overly warm or friendly, because this can lead to a quick rejection. In several instances, though, I have been able to move in closely and touch or hold a quite paranoid old lady. This has been especially true of the paranoid individuals who also had chronic brain syndrome. It is particularly important to consider touch with those elderly who have vision or hearing losses and are without family or friends.

VIGNETTE 4

I interviewed Mrs. A., a woman in her seventies, who had once been a pharmacist. I wanted her to join a group for a demonstration to student nurses. I had been warned by staff nurses that she was paranoid in her behavior and not to move too quickly with her. Mrs. A. and I talked for awhile and she seemed uncomfortable— fiddling with her buttons on her sweater and making nervous hand motions. When I noticed that her anxiety had abated somewhat, I asked her to join in the group. She immediately came back with "Why would you want to talk to me?" Her low self-esteem and her awareness of where she had ultimately been placed in late life came

through clearly. Her haughty manners and paranoid ways had tended to put me off, but she did let me move closer and closer to her, which gave me the idea of trying to embrace her. When she said, "I am not worth the head of a pin," I slowly moved close and put my arms around her shoulder (she was much smaller than I, so I could be braver than if she had been a gargantuan woman). She remained very still in my arms and let me gently pat her back and say that I did not think that about her and respected her because she knew about drugs.

I also found that another very paranoid woman who was in her nineties would let me hold her for a few moments and never tried to disengage herself from my hold (Burnside, 1978).

It takes careful assessment to know when to stay where one is and when to move closer. This applies to psychological stance as well as to physical position.

STATEMENTS FROM THE LITERATURE REGARDING PARANOID BEHAVIOR IN THE ELDERLY

1. Paranoid syndromes account for one-tenth of admissions to mental hospitals (Anderson, 1971).
2. Paranoid syndromes present diagnostic problems (Anderson, 1971).
3. Paranoid states tend to occur under adverse conditions, e.g., imprisonment, drunkenness, involution, blindness (Butler and Lewis, 1977).
4. Paranoid symptoms may be seen following severe infections in the elderly (Anderson, 1971).
5. Paranoid individuals are often affected by disorders of vision or, more commonly, of hearing (Anderson, 1971; Butler and Lewis, 1977).
6. Paranoid reactions may occur in either acute (reversible) or chronic (irreversible) syndromes (Busse and Pfeiffer, 1973).

7. Depression may also be part of a diagnosis along with paranoid behavior (Grauer, 1978).
8. Delusions may alter over the years (Neadly, 1977).
9. Women are more frequently afflicted with paranoid states than men (Butler and Lewis, 1973).
10. Spinsters are often victims of paranoid behavior (Anderson, 1971).
11. Paranoid ideas in old age often are centered on neighbors or persons close by (Busse and Pfeiffer, 1973).
12. Alcoholic paranoid states are often characterized by extreme jealousy and delusions regarding the faithfulness of the spouse (Grauer, 1978).
13. Paranoid patients are medically treatable (Busse and Pfeiffer, 1969; Exton-Smith and Windsor, 1971).
14. The immediate goal in treatment of paranoia is to reduce the anxiety (Busse and Pfeiffer, 1969).
15. Honesty is absolutely crucial in working with paranoid individuals (Butler and Lewis, 1977).
16. It is important to listen for the semantics as indicator of tone of the interview and mood of the interviewee.

SUMMARY

Paranoia may occur across the life-span, but it occurs frequently in late life and is seen more in women than in men. While youthful persons who are paranoid blame esoteric forces, old people tend to attack and blame people nearby, either psychologically or geographically.

Projection, anger, hostility, depression, alcoholism all may be a part of and complicate the clinical picture. The skill of the interviewer depends on being scrupulously honest, showing self-confidence in interviews, not moving in too rapidly, and attending to sensory losses and to environmental and other special problems.

These special problems can be (1) isolation, (2) delusions of infidelity, (3) delusions regarding food. Students will need strong preceptorship support when handling these individuals, especially the aggressive ones or those who are constantly sharing wild, grandiose delusions or verbally attacking the student.

The elderly paranoid patient comes to mind in a poem entitled "Across the Broken Pavement."

What is across the broken pavement, the ribbon of cement?
A hope, vanished of the night, borne into the day on the feet of one who doubts and refuses, sulks and pines
A crazy cruel existence of one's own work and one that shouldn't be.
May whatever is almighty save me from my hell, for I can trust no other.

Rosemary Brant

REFERENCES

Abarca, Maria C.: One-to-one relationship therapy: A case study, in Irene M. Burnside (ed.), *Psychosocial Nursing Care of the Aged,* 2d ed., McGraw-Hill, New York, 1980.

Anderson, W. Ferguson: *Practical Management of the Elderly,* 2d ed., Blackwell, Oxford, England, 1971.

Burnside, Irene Mortenson: Eulogy for Ms. Hogue, *American Journal of Nursing,* **78**(4):625–626, April 1978.

————: Gerontion: A case study, *Perspectives in Psychiatric Care,* **9**(3):103–109, May-June 1971.

Busse, Ewald W., and Eric Pfeiffer (eds.): *Behavior and Adaptation in Late Life,* Little, Brown, Boston, 1969, pp. 188, 196–199.

———— and ———— (eds.): *Mental Illness in Later Life,* American Psychiatric Association, Washington, 1973.

Butler, Robert N., and Myrna I. Lewis: *Aging and Mental Health: Positive Psychosocial Approaches,* Mosby, St. Louis, 1977.

Caird, F. I., and T. G. Judge: *Assessment of the Elderly Patient,* Pitman Medical, Kent, England, 1977.

Charatan, Frederick B.: The psychopathology of old age, *Journal of the National Association of Private Psychiatric Hospitals,* **10**(1):28–35, Fall 1978.

Davidson, R.: Paranoid symptoms in organic disease, *Gerontologica Clinica,* **6**:13–21, 1964.

————: Discussion, in A. N. Exton-Smith and J. Grimley Evans (eds.), *Care of the Elderly,* Grune & Stratton, New York, 1977.

Eisdorfer, Carl: *Care of the Elderly,* A. N. Exton-Smith and J. Grimley Evans (eds.), Grune & Stratton, New York, 1977.

Exton-Smith, A. N., and A. C. M. Windsor: Principles of drug treatment in the aged, in Isadore Rossman (ed.), *Clinical Geriatrics,* Lippincott, Philadelphia, 1971.

Grauer, H.: Deviant sexual behavior associated with senility, *Medical Aspects of Human Sexuality,* **12**(4):127–129, April 1978.

Hodkinson, H. M.: *An Outline of Geriatrics,* Academic, London, 1975.

Jury, Mark, and Dan Jury: *Gramp,* Grossman, New York, 1976.

Lowenthal, Marjorie: *Lives in Distress,* Basic Books, New York, 1964.

McLeod, W. R.: Making the most of the interview: Psychological and psychiatric aspects, *Patient Management,* **2**(7):9–16, July 1978.

Miller, Benjamin, and Claire Brackman Keane: *Encyclopedia and Dictionary of Medicine and Nursing,* Saunders, Philadelphia, 1972.

Neadly, A. W.: Paranoid depression: Nursing care study, *Nursing Times,* **73**(41):1590–1592, Oct. 13, 1977.

Post, F.: Impact of modern drug treatment on old age: Schizophrenia, in A. N. Exton-Smith and E. Woodford-Williams (eds.), *Proceedings of the Third Meeting of the European Clinical Section of the International Association of Gerontology,* Karger, Basel, 1962.

Smith, Huston: *Condemned to Meaning,* Harper & Row, New York, 1965, p. 47.

Verwoerdt, Adrian: *Clinical Geropsychiatry,* Williams & Wilkins, Baltimore, 1976.

Walters, Mary Margaret: Unpublished paper for course, Psychosocial aspects of aging, Arizona State University, Tempe, Ariz., May 1974.

Weinberg, Jack: Lecture, Summer Institute, Andrus Gerontology Center, University of Southern California, Los Angeles, July 20, 1970.

OTHER RESOURCES

The Disturbed Nursing Home Patient, film produced by Hugh James Lurie, University of Washington, Seattle, Wash. Funded by an NIMH-PS grant to the Bureau of Mental Health, DSHS, Olympia, Wash.

FOUR

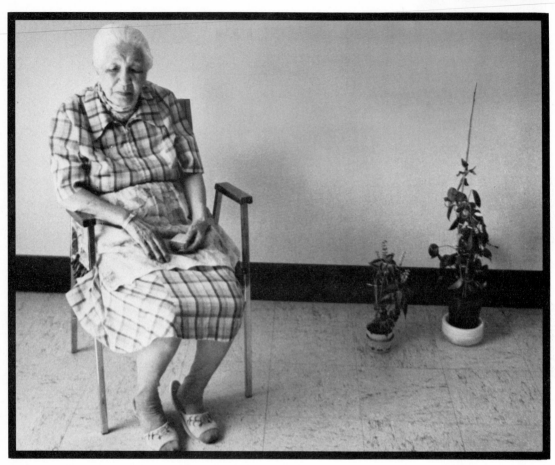

Anthony J. Skirlick, Jr.

ORGANIC BRAIN SYNDROME: THEORY AND THERAPY

I found her sitting in the lounge, in the spot we had shared so many times before. She wore a blue-and-green-plaid housedress, and as she sat there, her fingers traced the pattern over and over again. Once in a while her hand wandered to a small raveled spot, and a soft finger twisted itself through the loose thread. Her eyes met mine as I sat down.

"Hello," I said. "How are you?"

"Oh, pretty good," she replied. "And you?"

"Just fine," I answered. She hadn't visited with anyone for many days, and she seemed to enjoy my company.

"It's a lovely day," I said. "Cool but sunny."

"Is it? Where did all the leaves go?"

"Away," I replied. "It's fall now, and everything is getting ready for winter."

"I used to be so busy in the fall," she said, "but I haven't done anything at home yet."

"My garden was great this year. The strawberries were really nice," I replied.

Her eyes were so blue, so clear. Her face so pleasant. Her hair, always so well-groomed, fell in soft waves, pure white and soft as a thistledown.

I spoke again. "Let's go have some coffee. I brought some cookies Karen baked"

"Do you have a daughter?" she questioned.

"Yes, Karen is my daughter. She is 12 now."

"She bakes lovely cookies. You must always encourage her, even if they don't turn out just right. Otherwise she will lose interest in baking."

I crumbled a cookie. "Our boy is 16 now."

"What is his name?" she asked.

"Mark, and he's such a tall boy. Almost six foot four inches tall now."

"My, that is big," she agreed. "I knew somebody called Mark, I think, but he was a little fellow."

And so we sat, talking of small things, common things. Once she mentioned "him." I didn't have to ask his name. I knew him well. He had been dead for many years.

Slowly the sun dipped behind the trees. It was time for dinner. Lights blinked on here and there. The nurse stood waiting at the door.

"I must be going," I said. "I have a long drive ahead of me."

"Do you live very far away?"

I answered slowly. "Almost 300 miles south of here."

She walked with me to the front door. "This has been nice," she said, "but I don't even know your name."

The words choked me. "It's Loraine. . . ." I could say no more.

Then, for just one second, blinding recognition flashed across her face. Then shame. Then sorrow. Then nothing.

Softly she whispered, "Yes, my Loraine, and you are so pretty."

I turned and ran—the compliment clutched to my heart to ease its pain. I carried the words even more closely than I used to carry the cookies she handed out years ago, to ease my childhood hurt.

Dear Lord, thank you for letting Mother call me pretty.

Loraine Bridge
"Crumbs for my Heart"
The Lutheran Standard, 1977, by permission of Augsburg Publishing House, Minneapolis.

FOURTEEN

ORGANIC BRAIN SYNDROME

Irene Mortenson Burnside

Injury to the cerebral cortex means injury also to the ego functions, . . . the cerebral functions are highly valued by man, and any diminution in their efficacy causes apprehension and concern. . . . An organism uncertain of its spatial-temporal-social relations (disturbances of the comprehension of the environment) as brain-damaged cases are, is much more vulnerable to suffering than the normal person.
H. W. Brosin, 1952

LEARNING OBJECTIVES

- Define organic brain syndrome, acute and chronic brain syndrome, benign and malignant senescence, presenile dementia, senile dementia, Alzheimer's disease.
- List diseases that present as dementia in later life.
- Contrast acute and chronic brain syndromes.
- List reasons for mistaking depression for chronic brain syndrome.
- List the pentad of characteristics of chronic brain syndrome.
- Summarize causes of acute brain syndrome.
- Describe the brain changes in Alzheimer's disease.
- Describe a catastrophic reaction.
- Describe 10 nursing interventions for the cognitively impaired person.
- Describe four treatment modalities used in nursing care of the regressing aged individual.

This chapter is about the condition of organic brain syndrome (OBS) in the older person. The chapter is divided into three sections: the first gives definitions used, discusses acute and chronic brain syndromes, and describes diagnostic issues. The second explains presenile dementia but focuses only on one of the diseases, Alzheimer's disease. The third is concerned with nursing care of the person suffering from cognitive impairment.

DEFINITIONS AND ORGANIC BRAIN SYNDROMES

Because the terms used to describe the degrees of cognitive impairment are so varied, it is important to establish definitions immediately. The meaning of *dementia* is difficult to fix (Wells, 1977). The current usage of *dementia* comes from *demence,* a Latin word used by Pinel when he was attempting to develop a rather simple taxonomy of the clinical syndromes he was finding in his practice in France (Rush, 1962). *Dementia* can have two meanings. Used as a descriptive term, it means that certain changes have taken place in a person as, for example, during the growth of a brain tumor which causes changes in the functioning and the behavior of the individual. Used in this way, the word could apply to a wide range of conditions. Used in the diagnostic sense, it refers to a specific category of diseases. The latter is the usage of *dementia* in this chapter; for example, referring to diseases which are organic brain syndromes.

Presenile dementias occur in late middle age; those which occur after 60 to 65 are called *senile dementias.* The presenile dementias include (1) Alzheimer's disease (the only one to be discussed in this chapter), (2) Pick's disease, (3) Huntington's chorea, (4) Jakob-Creutzfeldt's disease, (5) normal pressure hydrocephalus, and (6) neurosyphilis. Diseases are also designated as vascular or nonvascular in origin.

ACUTE AND CHRONIC BRAIN SYNDROMES

A commonly used term is *organic brain syndrome* (OBS), and subsumed under this are *acute brain syndrome* (ABS) and *chronic brain syndrome* (CBS). ABS and CBS are differentiated by the fact that ABS is reversible, CBS is not. ABS is usually rather sudden in onset. A correct diagnosis must be established so that aggressive treatment can be planned. Chronic brain syndrome can be mistaken for depression, since the behavior of the very depressed can mimic behavior of the person with chronic brain syndrome. It can be difficult to measure capacity and dysfunction in the elderly—partly because of severe sensory losses and also because of the tendency to vacillate from day to day, or even within a 24-hour period. Try, say, examining the confused person upon awakening him at 2 A.M. (I know of one confused woman in a nursing home who did so! She sneaked a stethoscope out of the examining room and, pretending to be the doctor, went around at night awakening individuals to "check their heart!") We need to consider how our actions and treatment increase or compound confusional states.

Organic brain syndrome is caused by or associated with impaired tissue function leading to behavior disturbances and dysfunction. The following symptoms are observed: impaired memory, orientation, intellectual function, judgment, and shallow affect (*Diagnostic and Statistical Manual of Mental Disorders,* 1968). Peth (1973) uses the helpful mnemonic JAMCO for the pentad of characteristics of CBS: *j*udgment, *a*ffect, *m*emory, *c*onfusion, *o*rientation.

MAGNITUDE OF THE PROBLEM

Gurland et al. (1979) state that dementia is found in about half of the severely dependent elderly in or out of institutions. "It has been estimated that 5 percent of persons 65 and older and 20 percent of those 85 and older manifest such problems seriously enough to require assistance" (Eisdorfer, 1979a). Kay (1977) of the United Kingdom clearly indicates that there is a significant increase in the symptoms of dementing illness beyond the age of 65. The frequency of occurrence of these symptoms almost doubles with every 5 years of life past 65 through the ages of 85 to 90. See Table 14-1 for the number of hospitalized mental patients in the United States with diagnosis of OBS.

"Severe" dementia may be present in 1.0 to 9.1 percent of the aged population; "mild"

TABLE 14-1

NUMBER OF RESIDENT PATIENTS IN STATE AND COUNTY MENTAL HOSPITALS BY SEX AND AGE FOR SELECTED DIAGNOSES, UNITED STATES, 1969–1975: ORGANIC BRAIN SYNDROMES ASSOCIATED WITH CEREBRAL ARTERIOSCLEROSIS AND SENILE AND PRESENILE BRAIN DISEASE

	Total	Under 15	15–24	25–34	35–44	45–54	55–64	65–74	Over 75
Both sexes:									
1969	45,477	1	10	44	180	711	4,326	13,721	26,484
1970	41,241	*	14	72	216	764	4,344	12,643	23,188
1971	36,038	6	26	63	182	673	3,919	11,126	20,043
1972	31,203	*	22	72	158	596	3,491	9,734	17,130
1973	26,173	2	17	41	139	421	2,717	7,988	14,848
1974	19,340	*	3	27	111	313	2,033	6,019	10,834
1975	18,254	1	4	30	55	285	1,871	5,613	10,395
Males:									
1969	18,207	*	6	22	74	354	2,157	6,026	9,568
1970	16,485	*	8	39	113	359	2,107	5,602	8,257
1971	14,168	5	13	32	86	325	1,877	4,924	6,906
1972	12,135	*	11	37	65	269	1,654	4,348	5,751
1973	10,417	2	13	17	61	191	1,288	3,648	5,197
1974	8,375	*	2	16	54	147	1,042	3,043	4,071
1975	7,123	*	*	20	31	130	863	2,540	3,539
Females:									
1969	27,270	1	4	22	106	357	2,169	7,695	16,916
1970	24,756	*	6	33	103	405	2,237	7,041	14,931
1971	21,870	1	13	31	96	348	2,042	6,202	13,137
1972	19,068	*	11	35	93	327	1,837	5,386	11,379
1973	15,756	*	4	24	78	230	1,429	4,340	9,651
1974	10,965	*	1	11	57	166	991	2,976	6,763
1975	11,131	1	4	10	24	155	1,008	3,073	6,856

* Quantity zero.

SOURCE: *Mental Health Statistical Note,* no. 146, Department of Health, Education, and Welfare (Dept. NIMH), DHEW Publication no. (ADM) 78-158, March 1978, p. 10.

dementia may be present in 2.6 to 15.4 percent (Wang, 1977, p. 15). Dementing syndromes, whether vascular or nonvascular in origin, account for a large percentage of nursing home and extended care placements. The memory loss, confusion, and disorientation (and sometimes wandering syndromes) tend to confound every aspect of medical and nursing care. An increasing amount of every health care dollar in the future will be devoted to the extended care of persons who are suffering from one of the dementing processes. In spite of this, there has been no systematic survey of the common daily care techniques which could maximize the quality of life for these individuals. Pending major breakthroughs in cellular and subcellular physiopathology, most health care systems need to markedly alter the efficiency and effectiveness of their therapeutic efforts directed toward this special and vulnerable population (Storrie, 1978). Yet discussion of therapeutic efforts is seriously lacking in current literature.

Slaby and Wyatt (1974, p. 24) remind us that "the level of sophistication needed to document cognitive impairment in a patient with dementia depends upon the stage of the illness when he is examined. Late in the course of the illness, a corner grocer can readily provide the diagnosis, but early recognition often takes remarkable skill."

Gerontological nurse practitioners (GNP) will need to be alert to the early signs of cognitive impairment in the physical and psychological examinations of their clients.

MOST PROMINENT EARLY SIGN: WANG

Wang (1972) points out that *the most prominent early manifestation of organic brain syndrome is recent memory loss, and further that the main problem of the early stage is not the memory deficit itself; rather, the problem is the individual's emotional reaction to the memory loss and the difficulties which result.* Wang feels that these reactions are determined by prior personality patterns. The caretaker or examiner should be alert to usual defense mechanisms used previously by the client when under duress or when threatened.

Well-adjusted aged individuals can accept difficulties in a realistic fashion, and many do find innovative ways to compensate for memory loss. Other individuals, who have been insecure, unstable, rigid, compulsive, or dependent, may reveal high anxiety and/or be depressed when they become aware of even a slight memory loss. (See Chapter 5 for elaboration of anxiety in

the aged and Chapter 10 for a discussion of depression.)

It is well established that the life expectancy is significantly less when the condition of organic brain syndrome begins early in life; however, little is known about the prognosis of persons who remain in the community because they are out of reach of the health care workers. Wang (1972) feels that the shortening of life in elderly persons who have organic brain syndrome could be related less to the disease than to therapeutic nihilism. Some persons develop dementia but then clearly stabilize, and the degree of cognitive defect remains stable for a time (Pfeiffer, 1978).

The attitude of the health care professionals influences the care they give (or do not give), and often they exude a hopeless what's-the-use attitude. Families are quite sensitive to staff apathy and negativism.

"SENILITY"

The word *senility* will not be used in this chapter since it is a pejorative description and *not a diagnosis.* Unfortunately, it is still frequently seen as a diagnosis, it is still included in our medical and nursing dictionaries, and it is still listed in indexes. It is also commonly used in the media—in both newspapers and journal articles,

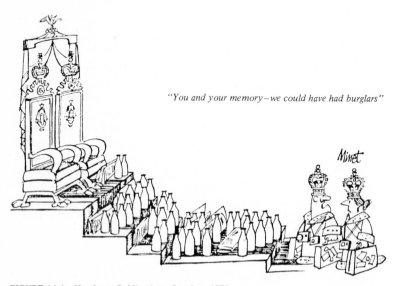

"You and your memory—we could have had burglars"

FIGURE 14-1   *Headway Publications, London, 1978.*

especially in titles. Nurses, it is hoped, will ban the word from their vocabularies entirely! *Senility* is pejorative, vague, and far too general. Symptoms or a syndrome are not specifically known when the word *senility* is used. I recall two of my former neighbors fighting; the expletive one used for the other was "you are senile." (See Table 14-2 for a list of fables about mental impairment in the elderly.)

An important role for nurses in the management of patients with organic or chronic brain syndrome was noted in the twenty-fifth anniversary issue of *Nursing Research.* The need for skilled nursing care should be given attention by nursing investigators and others in the health and helping professions (Gunter and

TABLE 14-2
FABLES ABOUT MENTAL IMPAIRMENT IN THE AGED

Changes in mental capability and behavior, such as confusion, forgetfulness, and depression, are just part of getting old.

Old people who are forgetful, confused, and disoriented are dangerous to themselves and to their families.

Organic mental disorders ("senile" dementia or Alzheimer-like disorders) are caused by insufficient blood supply to the brain.

The symptoms of chronic organic mental disorder are quite obvious and disruptive. Once they appear they cannot be reversed.

Old people who are uncooperative, unsocial, and argumentative display "senile" behavior and pose difficult management problems.

Inability to concentrate, apathy, impaired attention span, and memory loss in an old person are signs of "senility."

Old people are rigid; they do not respond well to new situations, and their ability to learn is limited.

We should not expect old people to engage in work or activity that requires more than a simple mental or physical effort.

Old people need 8 hours of sleep.

Old people react to drugs just as younger adults do, and they rarely have problems with overmedication.

SOURCE: Sidney Cohen, *Mental Impairment in the Aged,* scientific exhibit, Gerontological Society, Dallas, Tex., 1978.

Miller, 1977). The nursing profession has not thus far shown much interest in the study and/or improvement of care of this fragile group of elderly persons.

The reader is referred to two excellent (but technical) overviews on organic brain syndrome (Seltzer and Sherwin, 1978; Wells, 1978). Seltzer and Sherwin state that the division of brain disease into more specific diagnoses is crucial to better understand these diseases. Wells' article (1978) focuses primarily on the dementias, because Alzheimer's disease now is the fourth or fifth most common cause of death in the United States (Katzman, 1976). He points out that even barely perceptible organic brain disease may impair a person's capabilities in the areas of learning, work, and interpersonal relationships. Another fine article, by Libow (1973), is also recommended (see Table 14-3). See Tables 14-4 and 14-5 regarding institutionalized demented persons.

MODES OF BEHAVIOR: GOLDSTEIN

One of the outstanding theorists and clinicians was a neurologist, Goldstein, who worked with brain-damaged soldiers. He compiled a list of various modes of behavior associated with brain syndromes (Goldstein, 1969, p. 774). He discovered that the patient will fail if obliged to do the following:

1. To assume a definite mental act, for example, a simple subtraction problem
2. To give an account to himself or herself for acts and thoughts
3. To shift reflectively from one aspect of a situation to another
4. To keep in mind various aspects of a task or of any presentation simultaneously
5. To grasp the essential of a given whole, that is, break it up into pieces, isolate them, and synthesize them
6. To abstract common properties reflectively
7. To grasp concepts and symbols and to understand them
8. To evoke previous experiences (for example, images) voluntarily
9. To detach the ego from the outer world or from inner experiences

TABLE 14-3
CAUSES OF ACUTE AND "REVERSIBLE" MENTAL CHANGES IN THE ELDERLY

I. Medications
  A. Errors in self-administration
  B. Chlorpropamide (Diabinese) causes inappropriate ADH secretion leading to water intoxication
  C. L-dopa, indomethacin, steroids can induce psychoses
  D. Diuretics lead to subtle dehydration and electrolyte imbalance
  E. All drugs with a primary CNS-desired action, e.g., phenothiazines, barbiturates, tricyclic antidepressants, diphenylhydantoin

II. Metabolic imbalance
  A. Hypercalcemia secondary to
    1. Carcinoma of lung, breast, and other tissues
    2. Primary hyperparathyroidism
    3. Multiple myeloma
    4. Paget's disease coupled with immobilization
    5. Thiazide administration
  B. Hyperglycemia
    1. Easily recognized
      a. Ketoacidosis
    2. Less easily recognized
      a. Lactic acidosis, look for the "anion gap"
      b. Nonacidotic hyperosmolarity syndrome; blood sugar above 600 mg per 100 ml; serum bicarbonate normal; no urinary ketones
  C. Hypoglycemia secondary to insulin or sulfonylureas; not with phenformin (DBI) when used alone
  D. Hypothyroidism; "subacute" onset; low PBI, serum thyroxine (T_4), T_3 resin uptake and 24-hour ^{131}I uptake by thyroid gland; high SGOT, LDH, and CPK
  E. Hyperthyroidism; may be present in the elderly as depression and/or apathy; termed *apathetic hyperthyroidism*
  F. Hypernatremia; a hyperosmolarity syndrome secondary to
    1. Inadequate fluid intake in very ill or disoriented patients
    2. Cerebral concussion
    3. Iatrogenic factors; administration of hypertonic saline by intravenous or intraperitoneal route or tube feeding of high-protein mixtures
    4. Excessive sweating without increased water intake
  G. Hyponatremia; a hypo-osmolarity syndrome secondary to
    1. Increased antidiuretic hormone secretion; bronchogenic carcinoma; cerebrovascular accident; skull fracture; postoperative period; other
  H. Azotemia
    1. Worsening of a chronic mild nephritis by a urinary tract infection
    2. Medication-induced dehydration or hypokalemic nephropathy
    3. "Obstructive" uropathy
      a. Benign prostatic hypertrophy
      b. Neurogenic
        (1) Diabetes mellitus
        (2) Anticholinergics
        (3) Antihypertensives: reserpine, ganglionic blockers, hydralazine
        (4) Adrenergics: ephedrine, dextroamphetamine
        (5) Antihistamines
        (6) Isoniazid
    4. Potent diuretics causing acute bladder overload
      a. Furosemide (Lasix)
      b. Ethacrynic acid (Edecrin)
    5. Urate precipitation in treatment of lymphoma or leukemia
    6. Calcium precipitation in hypercalcemia syndromes

III. Depression or acute emotional stress; usually related to "losses"

IV. Nutrition. More than 10% of the elderly have simultaneous deficiencies of at least three of four important vitamins: thiamine, riboflavin, ascorbic acid, and vitamin A. Deficiencies may play a role in CNS dysfunction and may be due to inadequate intake, or secondary to chronic illness. Pernicious anemia, too, may have CNS manifestations.

V. Tumors
  A. Intracranial
    1. Gliomas 50–60% of all CNS tumors, mostly malignant
    2. Metastatic, 20–50%; lung, breast, others
  B. Remote effects of distant cancers
    1. Lymphoma, lung; both effects are rare

VI. Hepatic
  A. Cirrhosis, onset between ages 40 and 70 years
  B. Hepatitis; not uncommon in the elderly

VII. Cardiac
  A. Decreased cardiac output secondary to arrhythmia, congestive heart failure, or pulmonary emboli
  B. Acute myocardial infarction; 13% of patients have confusion as the major symptom

VIII. Vascular
  A. Transient ischemic attacks and cerebrovascular accidents
  B. Subdural hematoma; 20% of all intracranial masses in the elderly

IX. Any febrile condition

X. Pulmonary: Chronic lung disease (emphysema) with hypoxia and/or hypercapnia

SOURCE: Reprinted with permission of Leslie S. Libow, Psuedo-senility: Acute and reversible organic brain syndromes, *Journal of the American Geriatric Society*, 21:112–120, March 1973.

TABLE 14-4
AVERAGE AGES OF 81 PATIENTS WITH DEMENTIA

	Primary	Arterio-sclerotic	Parkin-sonism	Brain Tumor
Males	74	72	71	45
Females	77	70	71	63

SOURCE: A. J. Rosin, The physical and behavioral complex of dementia, *Gerontology,* 32(1):37–46, 1977, p. 39.

CATASTROPHIC REACTION

Goldstein (1942) also coined the frequently used term "catastrophic reaction," which is the heightened anxiety occurring during interviewing or questioning when the brain-damaged person cannot answer or perform. Nurses must be cognizant of such a reaction as they push the cognitively impaired for responses or performances.

Goldstein (1969, p. 792) noted, "Perseveration occurs particularly when the patient is forced to fulfill tasks with which he is unable to cope," for example, an arithmetic task as a part of a mental examination. (*Perseveration* is the constant repetition of a word or phrase.) Perseveration can be a most irritating behavior for nurses to cope with during an 8-hour shift. Staff

TABLE 14-5
CAUSES OF ADMISSION OF 81 PATIENTS WITH DEMENTIA

	Primary	Arterio-sclerotic	Parkin-sonism
Mental deterioration	17	1	1
Mobility problem	6	18	8
Wandering	5	1	
Nursing care	2	10	
Medical illness	3		
Fracture	5	1	

SOURCE: A. J. Rosin, The physical and behavioral complex of dementia, *Gerontology,* 32(1):37–46, 1977, p. 39.

must have frequent respites during care of such individuals. Once, when I worked the evening shift in a nursing home, a patient's endless repetition of "kitty, kitty, kitty, kitty" nearly drove all of us mad. It is fortunate that there was not a cat population to respond to such plaintive beckonings. The important lesson of this story, however, is that staff members who work with the demented feel normal, human frustrations and irritations, and that they need much support from peers (Poggi, 1978).

BENIGN AND MALIGNANT SENESCENCE: KRAL

"Benign" senescent forgetfulness is characterized by inability of the person to recall fairly unimportant data and parts of experiences. That is, a date or place may be forgotten, but not the experience.

The "malignant" type of senescent forgetfulness is characterized by the inability to recall events of the recent past, and not only unimportant data and/or parts of the experience, but the experience as such. Subjects suffering from organic brain syndrome with malignant senescent forgetfulness have a significantly higher death rate and a significantly shorter survival time than subjects with preserved memory function of the benign type (Kral, 1970).

Kral (1973) also states that old persons who have suffered emotional deprivation in childhood were represented to a significantly greater extent in the group which showed signs of organic brain syndrome. They showed difficulties in adjustment and had financial and other stresses in later life. Women in this particular group had also experienced more postpartum psychotic episodes than women who had not experienced childhood deprivations. Miller (1977), a psychologist, has written a thorough book on dementia; he criticizes Kral's work because "the predominantly clinical data used by Kral do not convincingly demonstrate that he is dealing with two distinct types of memory disorders rather than merely describing the milder and more advanced forms of the same process" (p. 45).

Dr. Alvin Goldfarb (1969) studied factors which influence survival of elderly institutionalized subjects. He found four characteristics to be associated with the highest mortality in the first year: (1) chronic brain syndrome of severe degree (which had been psychiatrically determined), (2) high rate of errors in the brief mental status questionnaire (MSQ), (3) diminished capacity for self-care and mobility, and (4) incontinence. (See Chapter 36 for an in-depth discussion of continence.)

STUDY OF A NURSING HOME: GUBRIUM

Gubrium (1975, pp. 22 and 23), in a study of a nursing home, reports his observations of common behavior of staff members interacting with residents. They are important observations:

Accounts offered by clientele who are considered by the staff to be completely senile are not honored, no matter how rationally presented. An allegedly disoriented patient who says he wants to "see someone in charge because I've got a complaint about what I have to pay here" is humored, . . . and coaxed back to his room. . . . Being disoriented officially means that his talk is believed to have no connection with his actions and to provide no clues to the causes of this behavior. The talk of such people is ignored by floor staff. . . . To ignore a disoriented person's talk as a way of managing him is the same as to ignore it altogether. The staff member provides the appearance taken into account while directing interaction toward a different end.

Staff members tend to focus on the "bed and body routines," as Gubrium neatly expresses their attitude. His report further emphasizes what was said earlier about nihilistic attitudes of personnel.

LONELINESS OF DEMENTIA

Not much has been written about the marked loneliness common in cases of dementia, yet that is one of the most noticeable characteristics to impress a person beginning to work with the mentally impaired elderly. Although many elderly people insist on having their privacy, very often that privacy and the related lack of stimu-

lation promote the cycle of withdrawal and loneliness. Work has been done by Bowers (1967) and by Ernst et al. (1978) to prevent such loneliness. In a study done in Australia, Bowers (1967) noted that the achievements of efforts to relieve alienation and withdrawal are lost if they are not sustained, and very often the boosting effect of increased stimulation simply cannot be sustained. When that happens, staff members are often very disappointed. Staff members who work with the mentally impaired elderly must have inordinate amounts of patience and compassion, since in cases of dementia the patient's basic personality functions of "drive" or "self-motivation" appear to be gone. Since much of the energy, motivation, and persistence must come from staff members, selection of the staff is very important. One should also remember that family members also experience loneliness when a loved one regresses (Hunt, 1979).

SUICIDE AND DEMENTIA

Sendbuehler and Goldstein (1977) state that even though the rate for suicide in the elderly is high, the rate for attempted suicide (unsuccessful) is low. Those who do attempt suicide in the elderly age group have more physical disorders, more psychoses, and more psychopathology. Fifty percent of the elderly attempters of suicide have organic brain syndrome. Sendbuehler and Goldstein point out that "what might be expected to be a high risk suicide population, OBS apparently interferes with the success of suicide attempts by impairing coordination, planning, determination, and awareness of reality" (p. 245).

DIAGNOSTIC ISSUES

The person with apparent dementia will need to be hospitalized for a complete physical examination and laboratory workup. The following tests should be done:

1. Chest and skull x-rays
2. Electroencephalogram
3. Electrocardiogram
4. Urinalysis
5. SMA 12
6. T3 and T4
7. Complete blood count

8. VDRL
9. Serum creatinine
10. Electrolytes
11. Serum B_{12}
12. Serum folate

Vision and hearing also must be carefully evaluated.

The presenting complaint may be depression, and further investigation will reveal that the depression may be a reaction to the client's awareness of the decreasing mental capacity (Cameron et al., 1977). The prognosis can be good in the treatment of a depression. Discontinue as many drugs as possible; monitor the person's intake of medications. Stop all the drugs which are not needed for life support (Cameron et al., 1977).

Drugs to check include: antiparkinsonian drugs, hypnotics, tranquilizers, analgesics, digoxin, hypotensives, diuretics, Valium, and Librium (Godber, 1979b). If you do begin withdrawal of drugs and the person is an outpatient, see the patient at least twice weekly (Cameron et al., 1977). Improvement in drug-induced dementias can occur in 48 to 72 hours, and at least within 2 weeks. If poor nutrition is suspected, do a nutritional assessment. (See Chapter 23 of this volume.)

ONSET OF SYMPTOMS

A sudden onset of symptoms should be considered as due to physical illness, drug toxicity, or a mental state (Godber, 1979a). A sudden deterioration may also occur in a dementia which is secondary to cerebrovascular disease, and acute decline is often followed by improvement (Godber, 1979a). The control of urine is usually lost well before that of feces (Cameron, 1977). (See Figure 14-1.)

PLAN OF MANAGEMENT[1]

For the Aged Individual Living with Others

1. Treatment of the physical disturbance is important.

---

[1] Adapted from Godber, 1979b.

2. Problems will arise if medications are not reviewed regularly.
3. Systematic and regular surveillance and assessment of the elderly at risk is an important target for the health team.
4. With the family and social services, plan the support the person is going to require as the disabilities increase.
5. Give every encouragement to the families caring for the disabled person.
6. Try to prevent the relatives from feeling overwhelmed by feeding in extra supports as the load gets heavier. Also make sure that the load is in some way intermittent. Use respite care in a hospital, preferably at regular intervals; the periods of hospitalization should be increased as the load gets heavier. For example, start a relief program by admitting the patient for 2 weeks in every 8 weeks and increase in the mild cases. Three or four such spells are a realistic goal.
7. Day-care centers are acceptable and stimulating to the individual. The centers must have flexible hours, however, if the care givers have to work.
8. Ensure that when a crisis occurs, help will be quick in getting there, so that extra nursing care can be assigned or medical attention can be increased.

For the Aged Individual Living Alone

1. The aim is to compensate for the disabilities by manipulating the environment.
2. Keep the client in as much harmony with the current setting as is possible (the normalization theory; see article by Burnside and Moehrlin, 1980).
3. Do not overload the neighbor who is caring for the person.
4. It is crucial not to have the client's disabilities (whether they are acute or chronic) overload and overwhelm those who are giving the care.
5. Dementia in most individuals is usually characterized by a loss of skills (memory, housekeeping, hygiene, dressing, continence, etc.) rather than by a florid behavior disturbance. The nurse needs to constantly assess what skills are being lost and how much.

Issues with the Family during Diagnosis[2]

1. Make a diagnosis from an adequate history and use someone who knows the client well, but do get the symptoms as experienced by the client.
2. Informants will dwell on aspects of behavior that are distressing to them, for example, restlessness, aggression, sleep disturbances, and incontinence. The examiner must probe for such things as unhappiness, loss of appetite, loss of interest.
3. Be wary; the relative or neighbor questioned may have diagnosed the case, found the cause, and selected the solutions!
4. Also realize that the client's disability may be covered up by a caring spouse, or, in the case of depression, the long-standing illness will be oversimplified and blamed on a grief reaction.
5. The client may be a scapegoat for larger family problems. The increasing difficulty with the patient may indicate that the family's intolerance is waning, not that the patient's condition is changing.
6. Remember that a resentful family may be reluctant to recognize improvements in the client's condition. If the family continues to reject the client, the negative behavior may continue.
7. Keep the questions directed to the client simple and brief to avoid embarrassment to the individual.

A poignant description of one family's coping with dementia was written especially for *Nursing and the Aged* (Pfeiffer, 1979):

VIGNETTE 1

We called my mother last week on her seventieth birthday.

"Hello, Mother?" I asked.

"Hello, Mother?" she repeated mechanically, without comprehension.

"Happy birthday!" Then all of us huddled around the receiver and sang the birthday song. But before it was over, we heard a click and knew she'd hung up, her attention

---

[2] Adapted from Godber, 1979b.

span unequal to our greetings. My father, on an extension, tried to call her back to the phone, and in the distance we heard her long shrill scream, a primitive substitute for lost vocabulary.

Heaven knows when her illness began. One doctor linked it to a childhood virus. Another blamed it on prolonged dehydration, accidentally induced a decade earlier by a combination of prescribed medications. But most doctors shrug at the cause.

The symptoms were subtle and were discounted at first. Five years ago, when my mother was 65, we began to notice some changes. She had always been active and trim (and looked at least 10 years younger than her age). Now she was putting on weight, sleeping much more, and seemed to be withdrawing from social contacts.

I flew to visit them about this time, when they were still living in Florida. My father showed me a bathroom cabinet jammed with toothpaste. "She keeps buying the same things over and over," he said. "Last week I got a delivery of bath towels from Sears—the exact same towels she ordered the week before. I had to take them back. It's the same story in the kitchen."

Even after we recognized the problem, we failed to identify it. Because she looked so young and healthy, we blamed it on adjustment to a new retirement condominium. But in time other symptoms appeared. She would lose her way on once-familiar terrain. One scary night she wandered on the freeways for several hours before she found her way back home. And once the police had to escort her.

Soon after these incidents, my parents moved to Sun City, and my mother applied for an Arizona driver's license. That, finally, was the moment of truth. Even after studying, she missed 23 of 25 routine questions. That week they consulted a neurologist. Extensive tests indicated advanced arteriosclerosis of the brain. X-rays showed quarter-inch blood vessels narrowed to threadlike conduits and much of the brain already atrophied for lack of oxygen.

The prognosis was depressing. There was no way to halt or reverse the disease; it could only be slowed down with some trial-and-error prescriptions to dilate the blood vessels. "In two years," the doctor told my father in confidence, "your wife will be virtually helpless."

His prediction proved tragically accurate. Gradually her short-term memory disintegrated until she could no longer perform ordinary household tasks. Soon she began having bathroom "accidents," and now she no longer has any control over bladder or bowels. Her vocabulary shrank to only a few stock responses, and she began to substitute those long, ear-shattering shrieks for words. Her compulsive hyperactive pacing throughout their two-bedroom duplex has actually worn threadbare paths in their new wall-to-wall carpeting. "The doctor gave us some tranquilizers, but I hate to use them," my father says. "When I give her the pills, she just sits around like a vegetable."

The rest of my mother's circulatory system is apparently undamaged, and her health is otherwise excellent. "She could live well into her nineties," the neurologist says, and my father sighs. Eight years her senior, he worries what will become of her when he can no longer care for her.

Although he accepts it with dignity, that care has already become a monumental burden. Their social life was the first to feel the impact of her illness. Even old friends found it difficult to relate to my mother's erratic behavior, and former pastimes like bridge or bowling became impossible. In the beginning, my father would take her along to Sun City's numerous activities, but she grew increasingly restless. She would often wander away from the recreation centers. Or, forced to stay in one place, she would cause confusion and embarrassment with her screams.

About 2 years ago, my father began to hire part-time help to baby-sit with my mother a few times each week to free him for golf and handicrafts. Now he has a woman come in 4 hours each weekday on a regular basis. But this kind of help is difficult to come by and even harder to keep. Few "companions" are willing—or able—to cope with the logistics of changing and shower-

ing (to combat recurring diaper rashes) someone physically strong enough to resist. And only one or two of the women he employed have tried to respond to her emotional needs. Luckily, my father has a better-than-average retirement nest egg to draw upon. But home care is expensive.

So is institutional care. Yet ultimately, he knows, he will have to resort to it. He gave it a try, in fact, 6 months ago and placed my mother in a small custodial facility. There were only six patients and the care seemed personal. But after 2 weeks he brought her back home. "She seemed too happy to see me each day. And she wasn't eating enough. I couldn't leave her there," he said over the phone. "Maybe when she no longer knows me or is totally unaware of her surroundings, that will be the answer."

"And I suppose it was lonely for you to come back to an empty house," I said gently. The silence at his end of the line told me he was crying.

"For as long as I can," he finally replied, "I'll take care of her."

PRESENILE DEMENTIA: ALZHEIMER'S DISEASE[3]

As stated earlier, the condition termed *presenile dementia* begins early in life, sometimes as early as the forties; the most common form that nurses need to know about is Alzheimer's disease. It was selected as a major focus of this chapter because it is the form of presenile dementia nurses will see often and only five articles exist in current nursing literature (Frost, 1973; Hayter, 1974; Pinel, 1975; Burnside, 1979; Bartol, 1979). Katzman (1976) estimates that Alzheimer's disease may rank as the fourth or fifth most common cause of death; however, the U.S. Vital Statistics do not even list Alzheimer's dis-

[3] I am deeply grateful to Michael Storrie, M.D., and Mari Ann Bartol, R.N., M.S., who shared their interest and empathy and their work in the care of men with Alzheimer's disease. Mari Ann Bartol helped with the "Literature Search," in which many of the findings are discussed later in this chapter.

ease, senile dementia, or "senility" in the 263 causes of death. Its prevalence and its poignant problems are good reasons for nurses to study it.

Lay persons sometimes refer to "old-timers' disease" when they mean Alzheimer's (Storrie, 1978). The name originated in Tubingen, Germany, in 1906 when Alois Alzheimer (1864–1915), a neuropathologist, presented the clinical findings of his study of a woman with the disease. The woman was 51 years old; her symptoms began with memory loss, disorientation, then depression, hallucinations, and profound dementia. She died 4½ years after the onset of the disease. In postmortem examination, her brain was atrophied, and distortions in the cortical neurofibrils were found and later named *Alzheimer's tangles*. In 1910, an Italian clinician demonstrated four cases of the disease.

The disease is rare before the fortieth year; the usual onset is between 50 and 60. About half the cases occur after the sixtieth year. (See Table 14-6.) The disease affects women more frequently than men. One study showed that 20 percent of women and 8 percent of men in geriatric hospitals have Alzheimer's disease (Hughes, 1970). Gøtestam (1980) reports a ratio of three women to two men. Another study reports three women to one man (Wilstenholm and O'Connor, 1970). The life-span after onset of full-blown Alzheimer's disease is only 4 years (Shelanski, 1975). See Table 14-4 for the average age of patients with dementia.

Gooddy (1969) pointed out that one of the sad conditions of presenile dementia is that the disease occurs in women and men when they are most powerful in human affairs. If unrecognized and untreated, it can have deleterious consequences not only for the patient but for society as a whole. The pathos such illness creates in a family can be seen in the photographs in *Gramp* (Jury and Jury, 1976).

PATHOLOGICAL CHANGES

Alzheimer's disease reveals three important characteristic pathological changes: (1) neurofibril tangles, (2) plaques, and (3) atrophy of the brain. The reader should complement the study of this chapter by reading an excellent article,

"Alzheimer's Disease" by W. Hughes (1970), a psychiatrist. For nursing literature read the five articles mentioned earlier.

PROGNOSIS POOR

Prognosis in the disease is poor. The patients have to be watched carefully as often a slight infection can cause death. The symptoms of the disease are described in a nursing article (Burnside, 1979). See Table 14-5 for causes of admission of 81 patients with dementia. Poor personal hygiene can be an early clue; memory loss is another. Sufferers seem emotionally unresponsive or, as Goldstein (1969) has observed, unable to experience joy; they never appear to enjoy anything as far as can be seen by their facial expressions and lack of animation. Rosin (1977) studied patients with Alzheimer's disease and noted that five were brought in for examination because of aimless wandering. (See Table 14-5.) Cameron (1941) studied the confused wandering patient and used the term *senile nocturnal delirium*. He also reported in that study that the same disorganized and confused behavior could occur during the daytime hours if the patient was placed in a darkened room. There may also be behavioral changes when persons with chronic brain syndrome are awakened. CBS subjects studied manifested behavioral disturbances on awakening from rapid eye movement (REM) sleep; nocturnal delirium and wandering may result from the inability of an impaired cerebrum to distinguish dreams from reality or the persistence of this REM phenomenon in the waking state (Feinberg, Koresico, and Heller, 1967).

However, while it may seem that the individual has no insight, Storrie (1978) observed that the men he studied often had remarkable insight into the doom of their condition. He also described some clever problem-solving in attempts to get out of the locked ward. Storrie's favorite story is about the retired army officer working on a jigsaw puzzle. Storrie observed the man, who was in his eighties, assembling a 500-piece jigsaw puzzle with ease. When the pieces of the puzzle did not fit, he simply took a small scissors and cut the pieces until they did fit! Stor-

TABLE 14-6
ALZHEIMER'S BRAIN SYNDROME IS A REALITY . . . AND A MYSTERY

Realities

- Alzheimer's is a disease of brain failure named for its discoverer.
- Many adults of normal intelligence may become afflicted with Alzheimer's disease which causes changes in their thinking and behavior from accustomed patterns to bizarre and disoriented confusion.
- People with Alzheimer's disease may act confused, paranoid, drunk, tired, or depressed, depending on personality variations. Sometimes they appear quite normal.
- Long known incorrectly as "senility" and as inevitable in life's later years, Alzheimer's is now thought to be a specific disease, not simply normal aging. It can occur at any adult age.
- The breakdown of the "computer" in the brain of a person with Alzheimer's disease is caused by accelerated loss of brain cells. Every person is born with a surplus of brain cells, and, as time goes by, cells normally drop out while cognitive functioning remains normal. Because brain cells do not rebuild or reproduce themselves, a dropout is gone forever. Persons with Alzheimer's disease have lost so many cells so quickly that their functioning is no longer normal.
- Memory loss is the basic disability and is the cause of many behavior and personality changes. From an occasional absentmindedness, the signs worsen to a complete loss of all remembered and learned procedures, facts, and functions.
- Many everyday activities depend on memory patterns, and so daily life eventually becomes chaotic and confusing when the client cannot remember how to put on a jacket, tune the TV, or brush the teeth.
- Controls over emotions, ethics, and values are lost. Personality changes and behavioral deviations may involve disregard for habitual manners and morals, sudden senseless mood swings from laughter to tears, or a turnabout from love to hate.
- Controls over physical functions are decreased. Walking becomes an unsteady shuffle. Posture sags. Appetite decreases. Hallucinations of sight and sound occur. Bowel and bladder control is lost. Disorientation in space and time turns day into night and home into a strange place.
- The person with Alzheimer's disease becomes increasingly difficult for normal persons to relate to, to understand, and to care for. Those who do care and support their afflicted loved ones find it a most devastating, frustrating, sorrowful experience. Most families feel totally isolated, not knowing that many people are enmeshed in a similar difficulty.
- Relatives and friends of persons with Alzheimer's disease have banded together in a group known as Alzheimer Support, Information, Service Team (ASIST). Their aims are to offer helpful support to all afflicted families, to offer accurate information to the general public, to encourage establishment of long-term care facilities, and to help solve some of the mysteries of the Alzheimer syndrome.

Mysteries

- What causes this disease? Research has not yet found the answer.
- How can it be cured? No cure is possible until the cause is known.
- Can it be prevented? No prevention can be devised until the cause is known.
- Can a certain diagnosis be made? Difficulties in diagnosis are a result of the similarity of Alzheimer symptoms to those of hypoglycemia, depression, arteriosclerosis, alcoholism, and other dysfunctions. Neurologists using brain-scan equipment (EEG) offer the best available diagnosis, but final certainty depends on an autopsy.
- What is the treatment? For the disease, no treatment is known. (For side effects such as insomnia and depression, help is available.) Supportive management and caring are the only options.
- Who cares for people with Alzheimer's disease? No specific care facility exists, except for one research ward. (Inadequate nursing home care or care at home with the family are the only alternatives.)
- Where are the solutions to these mysteries? ASIST asks you to join the quest for answers.

SOURCE: State of Washington, Department of Social and Health Services, Division of Mental Health, DHS 22-110 12/78.

TABLE 14-7

VARIANTS OF THE CLINICAL SYNDROME OF ORGANIC BRAIN DISEASE: GUIDELINES FOR PROGNOSIS OF DEMENTIA IN A NURSING HOME POPULATION*

Description of Cause of Dementia	Potential for Recovery†	Time
Acute multiple cerebral infarct disease (MID) with dementia (nondominant hemisphere)	Good; grade 4–0	Minutes to 90–100 days (multiple, unilateral, non-dominant infarct dementia has better prognosis than bilateral hemisphere dementia)
MID (dominant hemisphere) with aphasia and dementia	Fair to poor; grade 4–2	1 year or more to reach optimum recovery
MID, bilateral hemisphere with dementia	Permanent increments of dementia with some resolution of OBS; intermittent fluctuations due to intercurrent physical and psychogenic causes	Short-term improvement of dementia (30–90 days) when nondominant hemisphere involved; slower recovery when dominant hemisphere involved
Affective depressive disorders and pseudo-OBS	Good; grade 3–0.	Several weeks to several months
Exacerbation of clinical and sub-clinical dementia by depressant drugs	Good with drug withdrawal; grade 4 to preexisting level of dementia, provided permanent cortical damage not sustained	Several days to 60 days
Preexisting or subclinical dementia exacerbated by cardio-vascular decompensation, infection, etc.	Good with appropriate treatment; grade 4–0, or to preexisting level of cerebral function	30–90 days following subsidence of acute somatic stress
Dementia due to primary neuronal degeneration (Alzheimer's disease, senile psychosis) and/or diffuse nonfocal cerebral arteriosclerosis	Uniformly poor, although fluctuations occur with intercurrent depressions, MID, and cardio-vascular or infectious diseases	Indeterminate
Dementia due to traumatic brain damage	Probable improvement grade 4–3 or 2, depending on quantitative cortical cell and neuronal damage and preexisting substrate of neuron degeneration	Several weeks to 18 months
Nutritional deficiency (chronic alcoholism)	With alcohol withdrawal probable improvement to grade 3 or 4 to grade 1, depending on level of preexisting neuronal degeneration	1 year

* Parameters of brain functions evaluated: (1) orientation, (2) memory, (3) judgment, (4) comprehension, and (5) lability and shallowness of affect.

† Criteria of severity: grade 0, no organic brain deficits; grade 1, minimal deficits; grade 2, mild deficits; grade 3, moderate deficits; grade 4, severe deficits.

NOTE: Cases of primary infections of the brain and CNS (lues, encephalomyelitis), metabolic disorders (thyroid dysfunction, insulin shock, diabetic acidosis) were too few to evaluate.

SOURCE: Michael B. Miller, M.D., F.A.C.P., Medical Director, White Plains Center for Nursing Care, White Plains, N.Y. Presented at Gerontological Society Meeting, Louisville, Ky., Oct. 27, 1975.

rie uses it as an example of crystallized intelligence. (See Chapter 4 for a definition and description of intelligence.)

THE DISINTEGRATING OF INTEGRATION

Hughes (1970) quotes Sims who called Alzheimer's disease "the forgotten entity," and Hughes stated,

> For its economic importance alone it certainly deserves more attention. From an academic approach we know of no other disease which provides such interesting material for the analysis of human behavior. In the individual case we are witnessing the disintegration of integration. The dysphasia presents us with new ideas of concepts. The amnesia sets us thinking about our basic knowledge of knowledge and understanding of understanding.

It is the "disintegration of integration" which should be such a challenge to providing nursing care of the individual.

Zarit (1979) has been studying brain-damaged individuals for several years. He advises families of these persons not to be overprotective. The physician or care provider should support family members who are caring for the affected individuals by (1) providing information about the irreversibility of the memory loss, (2) trying to maintain them in independent activities, and (3) not taking over responsibilities until necessary. Godber (1979b) advises that we do not overwhelm the family. Crises arise from three behaviors which commonly occur in the demented: incontinence, disturbed sleep, and excessive wandering (Hunt, 1979). The family will need added support when these behaviors begin.

COMMUNICATION DIFFICULTIES

An excellent guide, *Communication Disorders of the Aged*, is recommended as supplementary reading (Schow et al., 1978). These authors state that there are few experiments in language functioning and dementia and that a "poverty of words" and "lack of language initiative" are common in dementia clients. The vignette above vividly describes such behavior in communication.

It has been pointed out by Ball (1977, p. 20) in Canada that the rate of study of this important disease will be directly related to the funding available for research in this area. He also emphasized that Alzheimer's is "a *disease* and not an inevitable result of 'normal aging.' " Let us hope that funds will be available and that there will be interested nurses to research some of the problems of these clients.

> Were the condition [dementia] rare, we might take comfort in devoting our efforts to other pressing problems. Unfortunately dementia is common and becoming more so. The pain and suffering it causes patients and their families are great, as are the frustration and discouragement. . . . The proper care of the demented patient requires uncommon time, effort, and devotion and makes uncommon demands upon the family and community resources. There is no question that these unfortunate individuals do not now generally receive the best care possible, even allowing that the best care possible falls short of our goals. (Wells, 1977, p. 273)

TABLE 14-8
FEATURES SUGGESTING DEMENTIA DUE TO CEREBROVASCULAR DISEASE

- Abrupt onset
- Stepwise deterioration
- Fluctuating course
- History or presence of hypertension
- History of "strokes"
- Focal neurological symptoms
- Focal neurological signs

SOURCE: Charles E. Wells, *Dementia*, 2d ed., Davis, Philadelphia, 1977, pp. 264.

NURSING CARE OF THE COGNITIVELY IMPAIRED OLDER PERSON

Do not imagine, because I am silent,
that I am not present,
and alive,
to all that is going on.

Mrs. Rooney in *Krapp's*
Last Tape
Samuel Beckett

Nurses often make one of two mistakes with the cognitively impaired. They either (1) set goals too high and expect too much or (2) anticipate too little. Sometimes, as implied in the quotation above, nothing is expected from the cognitively impaired individual. Often nurses have to cope with their own integral dilemmas and feelings of helplessness regarding intervention with cognitively impaired persons. Their philosophy of care is put to some severe tests.

The dilemmas faced by student nurses caring for demented individuals have been poignantly described by one student nurse writing about an 85-year-old client.

. . . I found myself getting more confused, upset and uncertain as to what to say. . . . How does one know how much hard reality to . . . [present to] this fragile, lonely, elderly lady? Does one tell her that her statements are incorrect and that she is in a hospital and doesn't have any belongings and that she can't write letters to dead people? How much can a person stand? How to deal effectively with this type of patient is not found in any textbook but, I guess, has to be learned by experience. . . . I wanted to help her but felt completely helpless. (Moses, 1970)

Her feelings of confusion point out another difficulty of work with the mentally impaired elderly which I have noticed—confusion seems to breed confusion. I have observed staff members of a locked ward who misplaced their keys or locked themselves out of the ward so often that they became concerned about their own mental acuity. I also have observed a number of blunders at a conference on senile dementia—the substitution of the names of prominent speakers, for example, or conversations over coffee prefaced with "Perhaps I am getting senile, but. . . ." Does work with demented individuals make us aware of our own vulnerability and fallibility? Instructors might well warn their students to expect to feel increasingly addled and confused when working with confused clients and also warn them that a sense of humor and perspective is essential when involved in incidents like the following one.

VIGNETTE 2

I was seated in a physician's office in a hospital reading and I was wearing street clothes. The door was open. A man with Alzheimer's disease sauntered in, mumbling. I could not understand his words, and he began talking to the object behind me—a physician's lab coat hanging on a coat rack. He picked up one sleeve, kept shaking it vigorously, and kept talking to the coat. Finally, he walked over to me, at the desk, looked me straight in the eye and said very distinctly, "She's not much help, is she?" And with that walked out. I studied the coat rack and, closing my eyes a bit, looked at the lab coat. I discovered that, if I saw the world with some distortion or illusions, I might also have seen the lab coat as a very thin, unresponsive female nurse!

LITERATURE SEARCH

Scattered articles can be found about care of the regressed elderly. Nursing literature, as stated earlier, is pitifully scant, possibly for several reasons:

1. Nurses who care for the demented persons are too exhausted to write.
2. These nurses are not motivated to write or publish.
3. Caretakers say, "Well, everyone knows this" (a common comment).
4. Students still do not receive enough encouragement to publish excellent papers or studies.

Mari Ann Bartol and I reviewed 65 articles or chapters on the care of the cognitively impaired older person. Articles were from the United Kingdom, United States, and Australia, from 1968 on and a few were from Canada. The authors were from psychiatry, psychology, nursing, and other related disciplines in the health field. Treatment modalities recommended were reality orientation, individual therapy, group therapy, behavior modification, family therapy, and music therapy. The following portion of the chapter is an extrapolation of important components of care delineated by the literature. (Because of lack of space, not all the reviewed articles are included in the reference list.)

ASSESSMENT AND DIAGNOSIS

Assessment and diagnosis are crucial because of the limited treatment often given to dementia clients. Depression mimics dementia, and often depressed individuals do not receive sufficiently aggressive intervention. Epstein (1976) says that depressed individuals with chronic brain syndrome will respond to treatment for depression. Other authors agree.

The clinical picture of chronic brain syndrome is greatly influenced by the patient's basic personality structure (MacKinnon and Michels, 1971). There is no disturbance of consciousness in the person with chronic brain syndrome in contrast to the one with acute brain syndrome (see Table 14-8).

"Psychosocial factors in the patient's life exert a direct influence on the form and prognosis of the chronic brain syndrome." Certain remote memories in the individual with chronic brain syndrome are retained as a result of being constantly reinforced through repetition (MacKinnon and Michels, 1971, p. 343). But the memory problems of the individual with CBS remind one of a child's definition of memory. "My memory is the thing I forget with."

However, Zarit (1979) states that memory loss can be a subjective symptom rather than an objective one. He states that complaints about poor memory often seem to be related to stereotypes about the aging process and to the presence of a depressive state, rather than to chronic brain syndrome. It is important to reassure the elderly that some forgetfulness is not a sure sign of "senility"; improving the morale in depressed older persons may be effective in reducing exaggerated memory concerns.

A point to remember is that the person's name is the last thing to be forgotten. Scarbrough discusses this more fully in Chapter 15. The story reported by a pharmacist about a confused lady he visited is not the most typical. He said, "Hello, my name is Ron Kayne," and she quickly and tartly came back with, "I don't care what the hell your name is, what's my name?" (Kayne, 1976).

Eisdorfer (1979b) also advises caretakers to push for precision when doing a mental assessment; you must get down to the date, the last president, etc., when you are doing a mental status questionnaire (MSQ). (See Table 14-9 for an example of an MSQ.)

Look for these and similar problems when a dementing process is suspected:

1. Drugs are not taken correctly.
2. The once-balanced checkbook is no longer balanced. (It is well to remember that some people have never had a balanced checking account in their lifetime!)
3. Any changes in personal appearance, e.g., buttons are buttoned wrong, zippers are not zipped, clothes are on backwards or in many layers, or the client has begun using other people's clothing.
4. Food is spilled frequently.
5. Sleep patterns are altered.
6. Social graces and manners wane.
7. Wandering behavior. (This can occur by car, on foot, or in wheelchair, and the individual is not aware of being lost.)

The face-hand test is used by some clinicians and can be found in Table 14-10. Pfeiffer (1975) developed a short, portable, mental status questionnaire that was tested at Duke University, and it is also widely used.

COMPENSATORY MECHANISMS IN ORGANIC BRAIN SYNDROME

1. *Circumstantiality.* Client uses descriptive phrases as substitutes for names or words he or she is unable to recall.

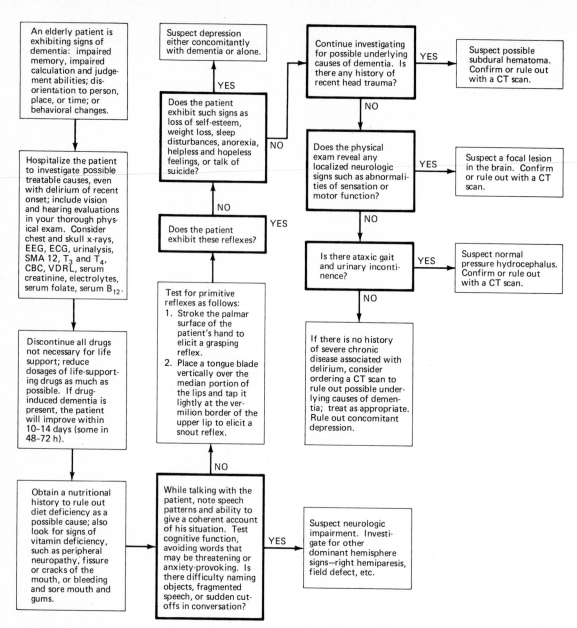

An elderly patient is exhibiting signs of dementia: impaired memory, impaired calculation and judgement abilities; disorientation to person, place, or time; or behavioral changes.

Hospitalize the patient to investigate possible treatable causes, even with delirium of recent onset; include vision and hearing evaluations in your thorough physical exam. Consider chest and skull x-rays, EEG, ECG, urinalysis, SMA 12, T_3 and T_4, CBC, VDRL, serum creatinine, electrolytes, serum folate, serum B_{12}.

Discontinue all drugs not necessary for life support; reduce dosages of life-supporting drugs as much as possible. If drug-induced dementia is present, the patient will improve within 10–14 days (some in 48–72 h).

Obtain a nutritional history to rule out diet deficiency as a possible cause; also look for signs of vitamin deficiency, such as peripheral neuropathy, fissure or cracks of the mouth, or bleeding and sore mouth and gums.

Suspect depression either concomitantly with dementia or alone.

YES

Does the patient exhibit such signs as loss of self-esteem, weight loss, sleep disturbances, anorexia, helpless and hopeless feelings, or talk of suicide?

NO

Does the patient exhibit these reflexes?

YES

NO

Test for primitive reflexes as follows:
1. Stroke the palmar surface of the patient's hand to elicit a grasping reflex.
2. Place a tongue blade vertically over the median portion of the lips and tap it lightly at the vermilion border of the upper lip to elicit a snout reflex.

NO

While talking with the patient, note speech patterns and ability to give a coherent account of his situation. Test cognitive function, avoiding words that may be threatening or anxiety-provoking. Is there difficulty naming objects, fragmented speech, or sudden cut-offs in conversation?

YES

Suspect neurologic impairment. Investigate for other dominant hemisphere signs—right hemiparesis, field defect, etc.

Continue investigating for possible underlying causes of dementia. Is there any history of recent head trauma?

YES

Suspect possible subdural hematoma. Confirm or rule out with a CT scan.

NO

Does the physical exam reveal any localized neurologic signs such as abnormalities of sensation or motor function?

YES

Suspect a focal lesion in the brain. Confirm or rule out with a CT scan.

NO

Is there ataxic gait and urinary incontinence?

YES

Suspect normal pressure hydrocephalus. Confirm or rule out with a CT scan.

NO

If there is no history of severe chronic disease associated with delirium, consider ordering a CT scan to rule out possible underlying causes of dementia; treat as appropriate. Rule out concomitant depression.

FIGURE 14-2 Evaluating the patient with apparent dementia (decision points in heavy outline). (*Patient Care, Nov. 30, 1977, pp. 101–102. Copyright 1977 by Miller and Fink Corporation. Reprinted by permission of FlowChart Service, Box 1245, Darien, CT 06820.*)

TABLE 14-9

MENTAL HEALTH STATUS QUESTIONNAIRE, RATINGS, AND GUIDELINES TO AID THE EXAMINER IN OBTAINING THE MOST ACCURATE RESULTS POSSIBLE FROM IT

Guidelines

1. Patients often say that the question is silly or that they do not want to answer, usually indicating that they do not immediately know the answer. Rephrase the question and *urge* the patient to answer. With urging, patients often do know the answer; they simply need more time to respond.
2. Tell the patient when an incorrect response is given and again urge them to try again.
3. When asking time-related questions, be sure that the patient has access to this information. Homebound and institutionalized patients often do not have access to calendars that they can read, and their daily activities do not vary enough to help them orientate themselves to time.

Mental Status Questionnaire

1. Where are we now?	Place
2. Where is this place located?	Place
3. What are today's date and day of month?	Time
4. What month is it?	Time
5. What year is it?	Time
6. How old are you?	Memory—recent or remote
7. What is your birthday?	Memory—recent or remote
8. What year were you born?	Memory—recent or remote
9. Who is president of the United States?	General information—memory
10. Who was president before him?	General information—memory

Ratings of Mental Status Questionnaire

No. of errors:	Presumed mental status:
0–2	Chronic brain syndrome, absent or mild
3–5	Chronic brain syndrome, mild to moderate
6–8	Chronic brain syndrome, moderate to severe
9–10	Chronic brain syndrome, severe
Nontestable	Chronic brain syndrome, severe

SOURCE: Modified from R. L. Kahn et al., Brief objective measure for the determination of mental status in the aged, *American Journal of Psychiatry,* 117:326, 1960. Copyright 1960, the American Psychiatric Association. Reprinted by permission.

2. *Confabulation.* Client fills memory gap with other materials. The nurse should remember that these have psychological significance, much like dreams or fantasies.
3. *Denial.*
4. *Complaints* of excessive fatigue, strain, or overwork, possibly indicating an increased effort by the client to cope with intellectual tasks.

Disorientation of time, place, and person may occur and first be noticed in the change from sleep and waking. This may be especially true in a strange environment. Later on the disorientation periods tend to grow longer. Such episodes will occur during the day and are often set off by a stressful situation.

The nurse should (1) watch for depression, irritability, angry outbursts, apathy, flat affect, labile moods, or perseveration; (2) observe for increasingly rigid attitudes which help to compensate for impairment; (3) observe for increased withdrawal from social activities, which

TABLE 14-10
FACE-HAND TEST

Instructions

The client sits facing the examiner, feet flat on the floor, hands resting on the knees. The client is touched or brushed simultaneously on one cheek and the dorsum of one hand, usually in a specified order. The face-hand test is done first with the client's eyes closed, then the series is repeated with the eyes open. Eighty percent of individuals who make errors with the eyes closed will show no improvement with the eyes open. In trials 1 through 4 the client becomes accustomed to the procedure. In trials 5 and 6 the examiner informs the client where he or she touches and reinforces a correct response by saying something such as, "That's right, both cheeks."

Common Order of Stimulation in Face-Hand Test

1. Right cheek—left hand	Initial trials. Response evaluated in context of further trials.
2. Left cheek—right hand	
3. Right cheek—right hand	
4. Left cheek—left hand	
5. Right cheek—left cheek	Teaching trials. Almost always correctly reported. Examiner informs, or reinforces response that there were two touches.
6. Right hand—left hand	
7. Right cheek—left hand	Incorrect response and stimulation not reported, felt but displaced, projected, or located in space are presumptive of brain damage.
8. Left cheek—right hand	
9. Right cheek—right hand	
10. Left cheek—left hand	

Results

A client who learns to correctly report where he or she is touched after the fifth and sixth trials is presumed free of brain damage. Only steps 7 through 10 (which is a repeat of 1 through 4) are considered presumptive of brain damage. The test results are highly correlated with the degree of brain syndrome as measured by the mental status questionnaire and by psychiatric evaluation. However, alert, well-educated people may score well even when some brain damage is present. If there is a discrepancy between the results of the MSQ and the face-hand test, it is possible that the cognitive functioning can be improved to the level of the better test performance.

In an acute brain syndrome all signs are not necessarily present at the same time. In chronic brain syndrome, while there may be variability in the degree of disorientation, memory, and intellectual function, all these are always simultaneously present.

SOURCE: As modified from R. L. Kahn et al., Brief objective measures for the determination of mental status in the aged, *American Journal of Psychiatry,* 117:326, 1960. Copyright 1960, the American Psychiatric Association. Reprinted by permission.

may also occur in depressed states; (4) observe for development of rituals in early life which also help to conceal the loss of abilities; and (5) be aware that adaptation will tend to follow earlier ways the individual adapted (as mentioned earlier by Wang).

Paranoid attitudes are quite common, and such behavior is difficult for staff members to handle. Often they take personally the remark or hostility. The nurse should be alert for these three behaviors: (1) irritability, (2) querulousness, and sometimes (3) preoccupation (Busse and Pfeiffer, 1973). One should be aware that

sensory losses may be compensated for with suspiciousness and/or paranoid thinking. Scrupulous attention to sensory losses is the hallmark of gerontological nursing care!

One does not often consider retaliatory manifestations as a part of a depressive episode rather than the result of an organic brain disease. Safirstein (1972) includes four case studies in his article to indicate that confusion, disorientation, and clouding of the sensorium could also be a form of retaliation used by the aged individual.

Regarding therapeutic management, Busse

and Pfeiffer (1973) say that, unfortunately, it is not possible to present a single treatment plan that will have general application to all older persons with organic brain syndrome. The procedure of choice involves carefully weighing all "the many interacting qualitative and quantitative variables." A comprehensive treatment plan will take into account (1) pathophysiologic status of the brain, (2) other diseases or physical disabilities, (3) treatment facilities available, (4) the family social environment, and (5) socioeconomic status.

Treatment techniques can be roughly divided into:

1. Ergotherapy: Work
2. Kinesitherapy: Movement and exercise
3. Ludotherapy: Play and games
4. Psychotherapy: Individual and group
5. Social therapy: Interpersonal and social skills

A depressed person may complain of memory loss, but, when tested, the memory will be intact. The very severely depressed person has the information but is too apathetic to give it to the examiner. Clients with organic brain syndrome try to cover up. They will say, "I forget right now," or "Ask my son about it." Or they will supply an answer employing one of the compensatory mechanisms mentioned earlier. I once climbed a hill near the ocean on the coast of Australia with a 76-year-old woman. She had severe memory loss. I pointed to the bay beyond and asked her what it was called. She calmly replied, "The ocean" but could not give me the name. And then as a retaliatory response when I asked her midway up the steep climb if she would like to rest, she said, "Why yes, dear, if you are tired." Touché.

It is important not to put clients on the spot too often and to help them save face. The pressure from interviewing may trigger the "catastrophic reaction" described earlier in this chapter. The examiner must be sensitive about provoking anxiety in aged clients who are struggling to make sense out of the situation. And we must remember that they truly are trying to interpret and explain—often according to their own previous experiences. Hence, it is important that we learn as much as possible about

who that individual was and about her or his life-style.

It is also important for nurses to check for vision problems in an interview. The patient's mental problems may seem greater than they are; it has been established that there is a relationship between "senile" behavior and vision loss. Researchers studied MSQs (see Table 14-9) and vision and found 20/70 to 20/100 vision in 35 percent of the sample. The people with visual deficiences did less well on the MSQ (Snyder, Pyrek, and Smith, 1976). The problems of behavior are related to the loss in vision and should be suspected as one possible cause of "senile" behavior.

On the basis of Cameron's findings (1941), nurses should not place regressed patients into a dark room during the daytime hours. If, for example, you must place drops in the eyes and place the patient in a dark room, then constantly orient and reassure the individual.

WANDERING BEHAVIOR

Management of wandering behavior is difficult in the care of the cognitively impaired. The following suggestions are taken from the literature. Protective environment is needed for the wanderers and room to move about (Cornbleth, 1977). Nocturnal wandering may be indicative of cardiac decompensation; a physical examination is, therefore, indicated (Anderson, 1971). Day care will help even when the wandering is nocturnal (Whitehead, 1974). Treatment of wanderers must have a double focus and be aimed at treating the symptoms and the underlying pathology (Whitehead, 1974). Use restraints discretely with a wanderer. Is it necessary to use a Posey belt or tie the individual to a chair? Be alert for the crisis signals telling us that the client has become lost in a familiar neighborhood (Cameron et al., 1977).

THERAPIST'S BEHAVIOR WITH COGNITIVELY IMPAIRED PERSONS

1. Reality tests.
2. Uses touch.
3. Uses patient's correct name.

4. Is verbally active—is dominant.
5. Assists in life review.
6. Encourages decision-making.
7. Supports denial if it is therapeutic.
8. Individualizes the care and recognizes uniqueness of each client.
9. Uses humor.
10. Avoids confrontation.
11. Teases lightly.
12. Approaches slowly.
13. Does not argue.
14. Does not take client's behavior personally.
15. Does not alter long-standing personality patterns.
16. Uses short contacts, frequent contacts, or both.
17. Meets client's needs; does not deny problems.
18. Leader is the unifying force in the group.
19. Reduces client's need to employ functions which have been lost; aims at maximal utilization of residual functions.
20. Identifies feelings and helps clients express them.
21. Assesses physical liabilities thoroughly.
22. Assesses psychological liabilities thoroughly.
23. Capable of symbolic giving.
24. Assesses preserved functions thoroughly; gains knowledge of premorbid personality characteristics.
25. Talks *with* patient (not *about* him or her).
26. Gains attention.
27. Uses affection.
28. Uses praise.
29. Enhances self-expression.
30. Increases hope.
31. Never pushes.
32. Never gives orders.
33. Has extra keen powers of observation.
34. Encourages use of client's former habits (Davidson, 1978).
35. Keeps open all options of discharge (Hunt, 1977).
36. Eliminates (or reduces) unexpected situations (Davidson, 1978).
37. Is aware of tone of voice and approach, knowing client will respond and react to them (Hunt, 1977).
38. Uses good-byes effectively.
39. Does not take problems home.

QUALITIES OF THE LEADER/THERAPIST OF THE COGNITIVELY IMPAIRED PERSON

1. Accepting
2. Respects the individual
3. Consistent
4. Interested
5. Warm
6. Kind
7. Sincere
8. Empathetic
9. Courteous
10. Patient
11. Reassuring
12. Nonjudgmental
13. Matter-of-fact
14. Does not nag
15. Is not punitive
16. Works physically close to the client
17. Is open
18. Is able to show high degree of caring (Trockman, 1978)
19. Is honest
20. Always uses humane approach
21. Is good-natured (Trockman, 1978)
22. Is calm (Trockman, 1978)
23. Can use cajolery and be persuasive (Linden, 1953)
24. Is able to tolerate frightful behavior

ASPECTS OF COMMUNICATION WITH DEMENTED CLIENTS

- Orient a new client to the unit (Hunt, 1977).
- Use nonverbal techniques whenever necessary (Morris and Rhodes, 1972).
- Open conversation with orienting information (Trockman, 1978).
- Use simple messages expressed in sentences (Morris and Rhodes, 1972).
- Find out the name the client prefers; use it consistently (Trockman, 1978).
- Speak as one adult to another.
- Talk as though the client understands.
- Move in close to the individual during communication (Trockman, 1978).
- Use repetitive verbal instructions.
- Use conversational shifts, e.g., acknowledge how individual feels, then shift to the familiar

(Trockman, 1978): "I know you must be depressed—to be divorced at 84 as you have been must be hard to accept."
- Keep your pace slow.
- Use face-to-face contact when communicating (Trockman, 1978).
- Gain attention.
- Speak slowly.
- If one sensory modality is not being used, increase the others (Trockman, 1978).
- Allow ample time for tasks.
- Try using paper and pencil if the client cannot speak (Trockman, 1978).
- Carefully explain all procedures to the client before beginning (Trockman, 1978). Show the client any instruments or materials to be used.
- When giving medications do not say, "It's to make you feel better." It may not (Hunt, 1977).
- Do not support disorientation (Morris and Rhodes, 1972).
- For aphasic individuals, ask questions which can be answered with a yes or no (Dodd, 1978).
- Reinforce realistic hopes or optimism (Trockman, 1978).
- Do not encourage expressions of anxiety (Trockman, 1978).
- Use open-ended questions (Trockman, 1978).
- Complete one step before beginning the next one.
- Secure an interpreter if necessary (Trockman, 1978).
- Encourage registration, recording, and recall of surroundings.
- Give much feedback.
- The client who asks questions is usually ready to hear the answers (Trockman, 1978).
- Use environment the same as or similar to the one the client is familiar with.
- Pick out meaningful comments in the conversation.
- Do not elaborate and do not refute delusional thinking (Trockman, 1978).
- Encourage communication and expression.
- If client drifts out of contact, repeat the orienting information (Trockman, 1978).
- Use writing pad to communicate if patient can read and cannot hear.
- Interpret environment in simplest possible terms (Trockman, 1978).
- Use black felt-tip pen for easily legible written messages.

- Allow sufficient time for responses (Davidson, 1978).
- Focus on topics most familiar to the client.
- Support the individual's self-esteem by internal reorientation, a reference point like hobbies, work, etc. (Trockman, 1978).
- Remember that good-byes and closure are important.

When interviewing or teaching a severely demented person, be sure (1) not to give more than one element (object) of visual input simultaneously (Flekkøy, 1976) and to remember that the patient may lack understanding of the task expected; (2) to be aware that relevant information may be remembered for a longer period than irrelevant; (3) to break tasks and learning into small, brief steps; (4) to give only one instruction at a time. Also remember to report, record, and chart using behavioral descriptions (Dodd, 1978).

MEMORY DEVELOPMENT

The following list of guidelines for memory development was adapted from *Memory and Memory Development* (Carroll, 1978).

1. Cues must be perceived and processed. (See also Chapter 33.)
2. Sufficient cues should be provided to aid memory and orientation (e.g., props to indicate change of seasons).
3. Cues should be consistent. (For example, when familiar landmarks are removed, they should be rapidly replaced. See the delightful story in Chapter 16 of this book.)
4. Cues should encourage recognition instead of recall—i.e., recognize information rather than recalling it. For example, furniture is set up which will indicate to them that there will be a group meeting.
5. Limit demands—give choices.
6. Cues should be issued to aid remote memory, e.g., discussion of familiar experiences.
7. Cues must convey accurate information, especially reality orientation boards.
8. Multiple cues are important (Pastalan calls this "redundant cueing"). Clocks, calendars everywhere must be of a type easy to read

(see Figure 33-10 for an example of a readable, seeable clock).

9. Use optimal conditions for learning (see Chapter 6).
10. Schedules are learned through practice.
11. Older people should not be overaroused in learning, i.e., no pressure to perform. Avoid "catastrophic reactions."
12. Meaningful material tends to be remembered.
13. Relevant material is more motivating.
14. Unique experiences are remembered well.
15. People remember better what they know they are expected to remember.

It is well to remember that when older people forget, "denial of reality is not an automatic assumption. . . . Possible explanations may include inaccurate or insufficient cues, a simple forgetting of the facts, communication problems, and true denial of reality" (Carroll, 1978, p. 13). To this I would add that the illusions so frequent in the elderly may be the result of vision problems.

INCREASE THE SELF-ESTEEM OF THE CLIENT

The following are some factors that may influence the client's self-esteem:

- Client wears own clothing.
- Makeup is available for women (clothing is marked, and clothes are fitted).
- Clients do not wear nightclothes during daytime hours.
- Men are shaved and shampooed, have wallets if possible.
- Women's hair is coiffed; they can carry their purses.
- Women's hair is removed from upper lip, chin.
- Clients wear dentures if they require them.
- Clients set their own pace.
- Clients have monthly allowance to spend (especially if check-writing privileges are taken away).

Recommended Nursing Behaviors

- Use praise whenever possible.
- Use affection.
- Let clients make decisions when possible, but offer only two choices.

- Help client maintain a self-image of strength.
- Be careful in removing pets from individuals.
- Do not restrain (Bayne, 1978; Bartol, 1979).
- Increase the usage of the telephone if possible.
- Leave the denial intact when it is not a serious risk.
- Encourage clients to begin a notebook called "This Is My Life" to increase the reminiscing and to increase self-esteem (Hellebrandt, 1978).
- Use memory joggers—frequent notes, messages on calendars, etc.—to reduce forgetfulness.
- Design a "shrine." Hirschfeld (1975), in an excellent paper which focuses on nursing care of cognitively impaired older adults, describes the importance of keeping "concrete symbols of one's self, of 'who am I?' to give continuity of sense of self." She describes a 52-year-old woman suffering from Alzheimer's disease who had made a shrine with all the tangible achievements of her past. This type of shrine helps a person "to be through having been" as Erikson (1959) once wrote.

ACTIVITIES AND SENSORY STIMULATION

The following activities are some of the methods that may be used to increase social interaction and reduce isolation and sensory deprivation (Burnside, 1978):

1. Orientation to the ward
2. Clocks that strike or chime the hour
3. Calendars, large and strategically placed
4. Music
5. Knitting
6. Growing, picking, and arranging flowers
7. Walks
8. Reading
9. Quizzes
10. Classes in applying cosmetics
11. Writing classes
12. Games
13. Drawing classes
14. Daily newspapers, discussions (and also publishing newsletters)
15. Sewing
16. Painting
17. Puzzles

18. Religious activities
19. Outings
20. Elevated heated sandbox with objects, e.g. marbles, stones shells, etc., hidden in the sand
21. Shopping trips
22. Social hours (e.g., serve tea, coffee, or wine)
23. Structured schedule for each day
24. Favorite and/or familiar objects close by
25. Groups: reality orientation, remotivation, reminiscing, art, poetry, exercise, dance, and social

GROUP APPROACHES FROM THE LITERATURE

One of the very first reports about group therapy with "senile" psychotics was the pioneering work of Dr. A. Silver in Montreal in 1950. Helpful points for nurse therapists extrapolated from Silver's work include:

1. Keep group close together in small room.
2. Refreshments improve rapport, interest, and participation.
3. The therapist has to be active and ingenious because of short attention spans and amnesia.
4. There is a carry-over value in having the patients come to the meetings in their Sunday best.
5. Families feel less distressed when the relative is in a group.

A group leader should also be thoroughly familiar with Dr. Maurice Linden's classic research on aged women (Linden, 1953; Burnside, 1978).

Ernst et al. (1977) reported that a group of six elderly persons who received biweekly sensory stimulation and group therapy for 3 months showed improvement on posttesting. One is reminded of Eisdorfer's frequent remark, "Because no one is doing much in treatment, everything tried seems to work" (Eisdorfer, 1979b). See Chapter 17 of this book for a nursing perspective on one group approach with demented elderly members.

Fischer and Fischer (1977) conducted art therapy with twelve 63- to 89-year-old residents of a nursing home who all had brain damage. The group met 2 hours weekly for 20 weeks.

They found no correlation between the degree of brain damage of the group member and the originality of the art work done. The leaders felt that the testing itself had an unexpected beneficial effect on some of the members.

MANIPULATE THE ENVIRONMENT

1. Night-lights are a must.
2. Provide strict surveillance, increased staff, and/or locked area for identified wanderers.
3. Use bright colors in decorating.
4. Use a variety of textures.
5. Color-code doors of special areas.
6. Provide work programs, if possible.
7. Keep consistent staff working with the individuals.
8. Provide redundant cueing, i.e., multiple cues.
9. Provide a safe environment (see "Prevention Strategies" below).
10. Environment must not be too boring but must not be overstimulating.
11. Environment must not threaten individual, e.g., there must be no use of dishonest approaches or cruel teasing.
12. Provide clocks and calendars (Morris and Rhodes, 1972; Dodd, 1978; Trockman, 1978; Burnside, 1970).
13. Special efforts must be made to provide a milieu that reduces sundowner's syndrome.

Every effort should be made to keep the patient oriented because the condition

is characterized by: disorientation, clouding of the sensorium, confusion, perplexity, stupor, visual hallucinations, fear, agitation, misidentification of objects and people, misperceptions leading to illusory phenomena and paranoid ideation which usually relates to fear of bodily harm. These conditions should not be treated with chlordiazepoxide, diazepam, barbiturates, or chloral hydrate. They may worsen the condition. Use low doses of thioridazine (25 to 50 mg), thiothixene (1 to 5 mg), or haloperidol (1 to 5 mg) at bedtime. (Steinhart, 1978)

PREVENTION STRATEGIES

1. Prevent translocation shock; staff members should learn client's routine at home and follow it. As much as possible, do not transfer staff members, and encourage the relatives to visit.
2. Prevent malnutrition.
3. Prevent dehydration; if in doubt about the fluid intake, push fluids (Morris and Rhodes, 1972).
4. Prevent choking.
5. Prevent infections.
6. Prevent decubiti.
7. Prevent physical disease (Davidson, 1978).
8. Prevent restlessness, agitation (watch for triggering signs or prevent hypoglycemia) or observe for pain.
9. Prevent injury to self or others (Bayne, 1978).
10. Prevent sundowner's syndrome.
11. Prevent falls (monitor antihypertensive agents, provide nonskid floors and rugs; keep objects out of way, observe stair usage).
12. Prevent acute stress which causes confusional states.
13. Prevent injury or suicide by checking for firearms at home (or when admitting new residents).
14. Prevent accidents by checking gas heat, outlets, etc., in the home.
15. Prevent immobility.
16. Prevent burnout of family; plan respite care (Powter, 1976).
17. Prevent burnout of staff. Rotate staff occasionally. Provide separate areas for coffee breaks, lunches, recreational activity for staff. Remember to convey praise, strokes, rewards, and also empathy for their work. Use in-service education incentives.

Bach et al. (1976) state that

The main therapeutic instruments for managing dementia in either a nursing home or a geriatric unit are the nurses and aides. They must be educated about the characteristics of the demented patient and understand that these patients often have lost their self-motivating capacity and are so-cially withdrawn and isolated. Regressive features (. . . rocking, spitting, and hoarding, incontinence, and sleep reversal) are common. Many patients are so amnesic that they wander into other patient's rooms and cause difficulties. At mealtime, gluttony and primitive habits can lead to choking. Other patients need coaxing to eat or help in feeding. . . .

AREAS OMITTED IN THE LITERATURE

Bartol (1977) suggested areas that are not well covered in the literature. They include (1) care for nails (long, uncared-for nails can scratch and also can cause infections); (2) nutritional care and fluid intake (the need for high protein and for observing the eating patterns and how food is handled); (3) bulimia and the stealing of food from others; (4) skin care; (5) infection and protection; (6) incontinence and how to handle this problem with the resident, with relatives, and with the staff. Other areas include: psychological interventions in the paranoid, depressive, manic or agitated states; the furnishing of the environment, or the actual setting up of a ward for these individuals; "catastrophic reactions" (not mentioned in the literature surveyed); detailed instructions about reducing translocation shock (not covered). There was almost nothing about preventing fires, the fire hazards with smokers, and the need for smoking rules. There was nothing about sexuality or masturbation—only that care providers should be affectionate. Professional writers occasionally misused the term *reality therapy* when they meant either *reality orientation* or *reality testing*. There are no studies (other than the one by Cameron) about nighttime behaviors. Yet nurses, more than members of any other discipline, see sundowner's syndrome. Nursing will, we hope, assume increasing responsibilities for care of the cognitively impaired individuals. So much of what happens to these persons ultimately rests on nursing care—quite literally their life depends on the quality of the nursing care that they receive. In the words of Miller (1977, p. 55), which should have a sobering impact on nurse readers, "For those demented patients who require admission to hospital, the quality of life depends almost entirely on the type of nursing care they receive."

RESEARCH AREAS

Research areas nurses might consider include:

1. The incidence and prevalence of organic brain syndromes in their own case loads—whether in the community, in schoolwork, or in an institution.
2. The effectiveness of the specific modalities: reality orientation, remotivation, reminiscing, music therapy, exercise classes.
3. The ameliorative and rehabilitative services nursing can offer in institutions and in the community.
4. The most cost-effective and economical ways to deliver services to the demented.
5. Programs, facilities, and personnel needed to provide services.
6. The family dynamics in families with a demented family member.
7. Trajectories of persons who have dementia.
8. The impact the gerontological nurse practitioner can have in the assessment and management of such individuals.
9. Ethnic and cultural differences seen in the individuals with organic brain syndromes.
10. Crises that tip the psychological equilibrium (either for the aged client or the supporting person).
11. Methods of motivating and/or training health professionals and/or new types of personnel to work with the demented.
12. The effectiveness of nurse-managed wards with these individuals.
13. The support systems needed to maintain regressing aged persons in their own homes.
14. The burnout of personnel.

SUMMARY

Dementia is perhaps the most frightening of diseases for persons in the middle or later years. Only now is there beginning to be a surge of interest in the condition of dementia. We nurses will have to continue to work on our own thera-

peutic nihilism. How sad that we as professionals have to read in a journal, "Use a humane approach." We do need to remind ourselves that we can be "the main therapeutic instruments" in many of the cases of dementia. Or we may be supporting those aged who are in the caring role and who say, "For as long as I can, I'll take care of her."

REFERENCES

Anderson, W. Ferguson: *Practical Management of the Elderly,* 2d ed., Blackwell Scientific Publications, Oxford, 1971.

Bach, Julius, et al.: Preventive medicine in a long-term care institution, *Geriatrics,* **31**(2):99–108, February 1976.

Ball, M. J.: Quantitative histology in Alzheimer's disease, *Research in Dementia,* **3**(1):17–20, February 1977.

Bartol, Mari Ann: Dialogue with dementia: Nonverbal communication in patients with Alzheimer's disease, *Journal of Gerontological Nursing,* **5**:(4):21–31, July–August 1979.

——: Personal Communication, 1977.

Bayne, J. R. D.: Management of confusion in elderly persons, *California Medical Journal,* **118**:139–141, Jan. 21, 1978.

Bowers, Herbert M.: Sensory stimulation and the treatment of senile dementia, *Medical Journal of Australia,* **1**(22):1113–1119, June 1967.

Brosin, H. W.: Contributions of psychoanalysis to the study of organic cerebral disorders, in F. Alexander and H. Ross (eds.), *Dynamic Psychiatry,* University of Chicago, 1952.

Burnside, Irene Mortenson: Alzheimer's disease: An overview, *Journal of Gerontological Nursing,* **5**(4):14–20, July–August 1979.

——: Clocks and calendars, *American Journal of Nursing,* **70**(1):117–119, January 1970.

——: *Working with the Elderly: Group Process and Techniques,* Duxbury, No. Scituate, Mass., 1978.

—— and Barbara Moehrlin: Health care of the confused elderly living at home, *Nursing Clinics of North America,* Saunders, Philadelphia, 1980.

Busse, Ewald, and Eric Pfeiffer: *Mental Illness in Later Life,* American Psychiatric Association, Washington, 1973.

Cameron, D. E.: Studies in senile nocturnal delirium, *Psychiatric Quarterly,* **15**(1):47–53, January 1941.

Cameron, Ian, et al.: Assessing and managing dementia, *Patient Care,* **11**(18):90–116, Nov. 30, 1977.

Carroll, Kathy: *Memory and Memory Development,*

Ebenezer Center for Aging and Human Development, Minneapolis, 1978.

Cornbleth, Terry: Effect of a protected hospital ward area and wandering and non-wandering geriatric patients, *Journal of Gerontology,* **35**(5):573–577, September 1977.

Davidson, Robert: The problem of senile dementia, *Nursing Times,* **74**(22):932–933, June 1, 1978.

Diagnostic and Statistical Manual of Mental Disorders, 2d ed., American Psychiatric Association, Washington, 1968.

Dodd, Marylin J.: Assessing mental status, *American Journal of Nursing,* **78**(9):1501–1503, September 1978.

Eisdorfer, Carl: Aging and mental health: An introduction, *Generations,* **3**(4):5, Spring 1979a.

————: Keynote address, workshop, Focus on mental health and aging, Salt Lake City, January 1979b.

Epstein, Leon J.: Depression in the elderly, *Journal of Gerontology,* **31**(3):278–282, May–June 1976.

Erikson, E. H.: *Identity and the Life Cycle,* Psychological Issues, **1**(1):166, monograph no. 1, International Universities, New York, 1959.

Ernst, Philip, et al.: Isolation and the symptoms of chronic brain syndrome, *The Gerontologist,* **18**(5):468–474, September–October 1978.

———— et al.: Treatment of the aged mentally ill: Further unmasking of the effects of a diagnosis of chronic brain syndrome, *Journal of the American Geriatrics Society,* **25**(10):466–469, October 1977.

Feinberg, I., R. Koresico, and N. Heller: EEG sleep patterns as a function of normal and pathological aging in men, *Journal of Psychiatric Research,* **5**(2):107–144, June 1967.

Fischer, Trudy, and Roland Fischer: Nonverbal dialogue with the brain-damaged elderly, *Confinia Psychiatry,* **20**(1):61–78, January 1977.

Flekkøy, Kjell: Visual agnosia and cognitive defects in a case of Alzheimer's disease, *Biological Psychiatry,* **11**(3):333–334, March 1976.

Frost, Monica: Pre-senile dementia, *Nursing Mirror,* **137**(17):34, Oct. 26, 1973.

Godber, Colin: Demented—or just a scapegoat? *Nursing Mirror,* **143**:29–30, July 19, 1979a.

————: Don't overwhelm the family! *Nursing Mirror,* **143**:30–32, July 26, 1979b.

Goldfarb, A. I.: Predicting mortality in the institutionalized aged, *Archives General Psychiatry,* **21**:172–176, 1969.

Goldstein, Kurt: *Aftereffects of Brain Injuries in War and Their Evaluation and Treatment,* Grune & Stratton, New York, pp. 71–73, 77–78, 93, 1942.

————: Functional disturbances in brain damage, in S. Ariet (ed.), *American Handbook of Psychiatry,* vol. 1, Basic Books, New York, 1969, pp. 770–793.

Gooddy, W.: Introduction to the problems of dementia, *Proceedings of the Australian Association of Neurologists,* **6**:9–11, 1969.

Gøtestam, K. Gunnar: Behavioral and dynamic psychotherapy with the elderly, in James E. Birren and Bruce Sloan (eds.), *Handbook on Mental Health and Aging,* Prentice-Hall, Englewood Cliffs, N.J., 1980.

Gubrium, Jaber F.: *Living and Dying at Murray Manor,* St. Martin's, New York, 1975.

Gunter, Laurie M., and Jean C. Miller: Toward a nursing gerontology, *Nursing Research* **26**(3):208–221, May/June 1977.

Gurland, B. J., et al.: *Depression and Dementia in the New York City Elderly,* proceedings of a research utilization workshop, Community Council of Greater New York, April 6, 1979.

Hayter, Jean: Patients who have Alzheimer's disease, *American Journal of Nursing,* **74**(8):1460–1463, August 1974.

Hellebrandt, Frances A.: Comment: The senile dement in our midst, *The Gerontologist,* **18**(1):67–72, January–February 1978.

Hirschfeld, Miriam: Nursing care of the cognitively impaired, in Carl Eisdorfer and Robert O. Friedel (eds.), *Cognitive and Emotional Disturbances in the Elderly,* Year Book, Chicago, 1977.

Hughes, W.: Alzheimer's disease, *Gerontologia Clinica* (Basel), **12**:129–148, 1970.

Hunt, Penny: The caring family needs support, *Nursing Mirror,* **145**:24–25, August 1979.

————: Confusion in the elderly, *Nursing Times,* **73**:1928–1929, Dec. 8, 1977.

Jury, Mark, and Dan Jury: *Gramp,* Grossman, New York, 1976.

Katzman, Robert: The prevalence and malignancy of Alzheimer's disease, *Archives of Neurology,* **33**(4):217–218, April 1976.

Kay, D. W. K.: The epidemiology of brain deficit in the aged: Problems in patient identification, in Carl Eisdorfer and Robert O. Friedel (eds.), *The Cognitively and Emotionally Impaired Elderly,* Year Book, Chicago, 1977.

Kayne, Ronald: Personal communication, 1976.

Kral, V. A.: Clinical contributions towards an understanding of memory function, *Diseases of the Nervous System,* **31**(1):23–29, January 1970.

————: *Managing the Disturbed Elderly in Family Practice,* McNeil Laboratories, Inc., Fort Washington, Pa., 1973.

Libow, Leslie S.: Pseudo-senility: Acute and reversible organic brain syndromes, *Journal of the American Geriatrics Society,* **21**(3):112–120, March 1973.

Linden, Maurice E.: Group psychotherapy with institutionalized senile women: Study in gerontologic human relations, *International Journal of Group Psychotherapy,* **3**:130–170, 1953.

MacKinnon, Roger A., and Robert Michels: The organic brain syndrome patient, *The Psychiatric Interview in Clinical Practice*, Saunders, Philadelphia, 1971.

Miller, Edgar: *Abnormal Aging: The Psychology of Senile and Presenile Dementia*, Wiley, London, 1977.

Morris, Magdalena, and Martha Rhodes: Guidelines for the care of confused patients, *American Journal of Nursing*, **72**(10):1630–1633, October 1972.

Moses, Dorothy V.: Reality orientation in the aging person, in Carolyn E. Carlson (ed.), *Behavioral Concepts and Nursing Intervention*, J. B. Lippincott Company, Philadelphia, 1970, p. 171.

Pastalan, Leon: Keynote address, Conference on Sensory Losses, Geriatric Research Institute, Dallas, Texas, December 1974.

Peth, Peter: Personal communication, 1973.

Pfeiffer, Eric: A short portable mental status questionnaire for the assessment of organic brain deficit in elderly patients, *Journal of the American Geriatrics Society*, **23**(10):433–441, October 1975.

———: Treatment of senile dementia, in Kalidas Nandy (ed.), *Senile Dementia: A Biomedical Approach*, Elsevier/North-Holland, New York, 1978, pp. 171–182.

Pfeiffer, Pat Scheuerman: Personal communication, 1979.

Pinel, Carl: Alzheimer's disease, *Nursing Times*, **71**(3):105–106, Jan. 16, 1975.

Poggi, Raymond: Personal communication, October 1978.

Powter, Sue: Senile dementia, *Nursing Mirror*, **143**, Nov. 30, 1976.

Roberts, Ida: Planning care at home, *Nursing Times*, **74**:154–156, Jan. 26, 1978.

Rosin, Arnold J.: The physical and behavioral complex of dementia, *Journal of Gerontology*, **32**(1):37–46, January–February 1977.

Rush, B.: *Medical Inquiries and Observations: Diseases of the Mind* (facsimile of Philadelphia edition), Hafner, New York, 1962.

Safirstein, Samuel L.: Psychotherapy for geriatric patients, *New York State Journal of Medicine*, **72**(2):2743–2748, Nov. 15, 1972.

Schow, Ronald M., et al.: *Communication Disorders of the Aged*, University Park, Baltimore, 1978.

Seltzer, Benjamin, and Ira Sherwin: Organic brain syndromes: An empirical study and critical review, *American Journal of Psychiatry*, **135**(1):13–20, January 1978.

Sendbuehler, J. M., and S. Goldstein: Attempted-suicide among the aged, *Journal of the American Geriatrics Society*, **25**(6):245–248, June 1977.

Shelanski, Michael: The aging brain: Alzheimer's disease and senile dementia, *Epidemiology of Aging*, Department of HEW, DHEW Publication No. (NIH) 77-711, 1975, p. 6.

Silver, A.: Group psychotherapy with senile psychotic patients, *Geriatrics*, **5**(3):147–150, May–June 1950.

Slaby, Andrew Edmund, and Richard Jed Wyatt: *Dementia in the Presenium*, Charles C Thomas, Springfield, Ill., 1974.

Snyder, Lorraine Hiatt, Janine Pyrek, and K. C. Smith: Vision and mental function, *The Gerontologist*, **16**(4):491–495, Winter 1976.

Steinhart, Melvin J.: Drugs for the elderly psychiatric patient, *Consultant*, **18**(6):137–139, June 1978.

Storrie, Michael: Personal communication, 1978.

Trockman, Gordon: Caring for the confused or delirious patient, *American Journal of Nursing*, **78**(10):1495–1499, October 1978.

Wang, H. S.: Organic brain syndrome in the elderly: A re-evaluation of concepts, *Postgraduate Medicine*, **2**:237–244, February 1972.

———: Dementia in old age, *Dementia*, Charles E. Wells (ed.), Davis, Philadelphia, 1977.

Wells, Charles E.: Chronic brain disease: An overview, *American Journal of Psychiatry*, **135**(1):1–12, January 1978.

———: *Dementia*, 2d ed., Davis, Philadelphia, 1977.

Whitehead, J. A.: *Psychiatric Disorders in Old Age*, Springer, New York, 1974.

Wilstenholm, G. E. W., and Maeve O'Connor: *Alzheimer's Disease and Related Conditions*, Ciba Foundation Symposium, London, 1969, J. and A. Churchill, London, 1970, p. 260.

Zarit, Steven H.: Helping an aging patient to cope with memory problems, *Geriatrics*, **34**(4):82–90, April 1979.

OTHER RESOURCES

Booklets

Diagnostic Forms for the Elderly Patient: A Checklist for Organic Brain Syndrome, 48 pp., Roerig (Pfizer) Pharmaceuticals, New York, NY 10017, January 1978 (has tearsheets).

Goldfarb, Alvin I.: *Managing the Disturbed Elderly Patient in Family Practice*, 9 pp., McNeil Laboratories, Inc., Camp Hill Road, Fort Washington, PA 19034, July 13, 1973.

Graham, Thomas F.: *Mental Status Manual*, 21 pp., Sandoz Pharmaceuticals, East Hanover, N.J., May 5, 1969.

Kral, V. A.: *Managing the Disturbed Elderly Patient in Family Practice*, 5 pp., McNeil Laboratories, Inc., Fort Washington, PA 19034, March 8, 1973.

Management of Confusion in the Elderly, tape and booklet, 18 pp., and self-assessment examination,

Fred B. Charatan, Roerig (Pfizer) Pharmaceuticals, New York, NY 10017, January 1979.

Organic Brain Syndrome I, Organic Brain Syndrome II (brochure and quiz booklet): Carl Eisdorfer and Leon Epstein. Distributor: Sandoz Pharmaceuticals, East Hanover, N.J.

Films

Aging and Organic Brain Syndrome (with booklet), Alvin J. Goldfarb and Shervert Frazier, McNeil Laboratories, Camp Hill Road, Fort Washington, PA 19034.

The Confused Person: Approaches to Reality Orientation, Concept Media, Costa Mesa, Calif.

Gramp: A Man Ages and Dies, 16 min/b&w. Based on the book, *Gramp,* by Dan Jury and Mark Jury. Distributor: Mass Media Ministries, 2116 North Charles Street, Baltimore, MD 21218.

Learning Module

Reality Orientation for the Confused Elderly Person, Virgil Parsons. Assessment, planning, intervention, evaluation, and independent learning module, San Jose State University, School of Nursing, San Jose, Calif., 1976.

FIFTEEN

INTERVENTION IN CONFUSED STATES IN THE ELDERLY

Dorothy R. Scarbrough

Mental breakdown, confusion, and disorientation can and do occur at any age. However, if an individual is both old and mentally disabled, he is in double jeopardy.

James C. Folsom, Barbara L. Boies, Kenneth Pommerenck, 1978

LEARNING OBJECTIVES

- Give descriptive definitions of confusion, disorientation, and memory loss, and compare each using behavioral terms.
- Describe at least three nursing interventions for those who are confused, without specific regard to age or cause.
- Describe 24-hour reality orientation.
- Explain at least four environmental changes which will improve the orientation of an individual.
- Identify the appropriate responses for interaction when a person has nocturnal confusion.
- Identify at least three approaches a nurse can use to teach family members about coping with confusion.

The health professions should place emphasis on ability rather than disability, prevention rather than curing. The incidence of confusional states could be lowered if proper emphasis were placed on early detection and better assessments of the older client. A patient with intellectual impairment deserves a comprehensive physical and psychosocial examination just as a patient with any other complaint does. There is great need to improve both our attitudes and expectations so that we can promote sound therapeutic interventions after an accurate diagnosis is made.

SCOPE OF THE PROBLEM

It is estimated that at least 3 million Americans over age 65 have some form of dementia which results in a confusional state, and two-thirds of these people live in the community (Besdine, 1978). (See Vignette 1 in Chapter 14 for a discussion of an elderly person being maintained in the community.) The problem is serious and costly both in dollars and in human energy, and confusional states cause a major loss of human potential—now and in the future.

DEFINITION OF TERMS

To use therapeutic approaches effectively in the management of confusional states and disorientation, terms need to be better understood. It is little wonder that a confused individual is often ignored and untreated, when an operational definition of the term *confusion* is rarely included in the literature. Many different terms are used to describe the confusional state; this creates problems for those who work in the health professions.

A dictionary definition of confusion is "turmoil or uncertainty or mind disorder." *Disorientation,* a term used synonymously with *confusion,* is stated to be "a state of confusion; to cause to lose bearings or a sense of identity or location" (Webster, 1977, p. 238). How can one best describe mental confusion? First, it is not a diagnosis! The phrase does not define a disease entity—just as "aging" is not an illness

(Brocklehurst and Hanley, 1976, p. 59). Mental confusion is a symptom of a disorder of cerebral function. Cerebral dysfunction may be brief or prolonged, mild or profound. There is rarely one single causative factor, especially in older persons.

The Merck Manual (1977, p. 1392) refers to delirium and confusional states as periods in which patients are disoriented for place or time, are mixed up in their interpretation of sensory stimuli, may have hallucinations, particularly visual, have a short attention span, and are often drowsy or agitated. Kerstein and Isenberg (1974) describe confusion as characterized by thinking with less than accustomed clarity and coherence, inadequate perception, and forgetfulness, resulting in a state of bewilderment.

Memory loss is commonly associated with a confused person's behavior. Memory loss per se is not a disease nor a diagnosis, and we must remember that it occurs in young, middle-aged, and old people. For purposes of this chapter, *memory loss* will be considered a *symptom* when the patient or the family complains about it; it will be a *sign* of illness when the physician records it. (It can also be a part of a syndrome found in a particular illness, such as Alzheimer's disease. See Chapter 14 for a further discussion of Alzheimer's disease.)

Confusion and *disorientation* as they are defined and used in much of the literature often refer to the same or similar behavior. Memory loss, confusion, and disorientation are all used to describe behavior related to various mental conditions. Memory includes the ability to register, store, and retrieve information. Memory loss is evident when this ability is impaired. *The most significant factor is the degree of intellectual impairment, regardless of what it is called.*

CAUSATIVE FACTORS

The causative factors must be considered along with the confusional state or disorientation. The symptomatic confusional states often indicate temporary disruptions of cerebral function caused by physical illnesses; such states are not easily or sharply defined except in behavioral terms. Nurses should constantly be alert to detect the causative factors of confusion in an older person. Wolanin and Holloway (1980) have studied nursing interventions for elderly clients in confusional states and have spelled out in detail the steps to take. Space does not permit the outlining of steps, but the reader is referred to their work (1980, in press).

ORGANIC BRAIN SYNDROME

Organic brain syndrome (OBS) has traditionally been a diagnostic term associated with confusion, disorientation, and memory loss. In Besdine's (1978) recent report, the following categorization for the syndrome was made by several experts in the field of geriatrics.

Acute organic brain syndrome develops abruptly, generally has been present for hours or a few days, may not progress, and has an easily identifiable time of onset. Delirium is a major feature, with restlessness and diminished attention span. Decrease in amount and quality of sleep with day-night reversal is common.

Chronic organic brain syndrome develops slowly, generally has been present for several months when detected, is progressive, and has an uncertain time of onset. It can be detected by mental status tests reflecting intellectual losses.

Dual organic brain syndrome is the development of an acute organic brain syndrome in a patient with preexisting chronic organic brain syndrome. Although not a commonly used psychiatric or neurological term, the dual syndrome is common in old age.

Each category has reversible and irreversible causes. The nurse should remember that each syndrome describes a number of characteristic behavioral manifestations and features which must be individually evaluated to plan appropriate nursing interventions. Often a precise identification of chronic, acute, or dual syndrome cannot be made unless very comprehensive diagnostic screening is done. The most common misconception is that the causes of chronic organic brain syndrome are definitely irreversible, which is clearly and emphatically false according to Besdine (1978). Drug intoxication, metabolic conditions, infections, and anemia are only a few of the causes that are reversible when

identified promptly and treated properly. It is well to remember that old people have a tendency to underreport diseases, and symptoms that may be considered within normal range for a younger person could be a classic disease entity in an elderly client.

At any age when intellectual dysfunction or dementia is allowed to progress, *orientation* becomes increasingly disturbed. *Time orientation usually fails first.*[1] Then it becomes more difficult to recall directions and one's place of residence. For example, an elderly woman who is having a problem remembering the time may also begin to think that she is in a home of long ago. Following the time and place disorientation, the individual may begin to misidentify people in the present situation—such as calling the dietitian by a daughter's name. In addition, past acquaintances can become less and less familiar until, finally, no one is familiar.

Drummond et al. (1978) point out that no matter what the cause, a person's first symptoms of confusion may accompany a physical illness, or a person may gradually become absentminded, forget common facts, or wander aimlessly. *In mental decline, the first thing to be forgotten is the awareness of time, then place and recognition (in that order).* Next, the ability to count disappears, and as the mental impairment becomes worse, the person forgets his or her own name.

RECENT AND REMOTE MEMORY

For clinical purposes, the nurse should know that memory is divided into three types: immediate, recent, and remote. Dementia can affect all or any of these, but one should not be too hasty in attributing all apparent memory loss to some cerebral dysfunction. For an old person, the yardsticks of existence, familiar people, places, and things disappear as the years pass. Often the aged individual lives in a world which

---

[1] A wife of a patient with Alzheimer's disease once described with pathos the first indications she had of his disease. During breakfast one day her husband repeatedly asked her what time it was. She got a clock to show him and then realized he could not tell time (*IB*).

is increasingly unfamiliar and has little or no control over current events. Also, if an acute illness requires hospitalization, the patient is removed from familiar surroundings. Consequently, the patient may suffer from immediate memory loss which is not part of the symptomatology of the acute illness. Observations over a period of time may also show evidence of recent memory impairment. For the patient, forgetting details of the illness or where he or she is can cause great distress. When the aged person has no recall that the illness exists and even denies its existence, then the memory deficit is greater. During memory gaps some individuals cope with such devices as confabulation (making up answers) and fantasy. These coping devices need to be evaluated in relation to the cause of confusion and not accepted as simple "forgetfulness" (Verwoerdt, 1976, p. 43). *Remote* memory refers to early experiences and is often seen during reminiscing. Even a very confused person will often, for example, recall the name of a dog owned while a child.

In addition to disorientation and memory loss, various functional or organic states can affect a person's concentration, calculation, judgment, learning ability, and affect. When the causative factor for any of these is generally thought to be "old age," "senility," or similar labels, there is a need for education. Family and patient education are excellent beginning points. A nurse must constantly assess the therapeutic responses of the patient and work with other health professionals to obtain the greatest possible benefits for the client. The causes of confusion are multiple and are often difficult to recognize, and the nurse needs to be constantly aware of the nonorganic factors which cause confusional states.

THERAPEUTIC APPROACHES IN MANAGEMENT OF THE CLIENT

The nurse can make major contributions to the management of confusional states because of having frequent contacts and expertise in communication skills. The nurse needs to be skilled in using and teaching various isolation-reducing therapies, such as reality orientation (RO), re-

socialization, reminiscence, sensory stimulation methods, and medicopharmacological therapies, all of which can maintain or restore equilibrium. *It is essential that the person exhibiting confused behavior, regardless of the cause, have therapeutic interventions constantly available within the total support system surrounding the patient* (Scarbrough, 1974). Folsom et al. (1978) stress that an effective rehabilitation program is only as good as the knowledge and practice of those conducting the program; too often the therapies seem to be held separate from the rest of the treatments and are given only for isolated periods of time.

TWENTY-FOUR-HOUR REALITY ORIENTATION

Twenty-four-hour reality orientation (RO) is a therapeutic measure which, when used consistently, can provide the patient with a means of adapting to the surroundings. It involves both people and the environment. According to Drummond et al. (1978) 24-hour reality orientation provides a means of structuring the environment throughout the 24 hours so that the staff can intervene appropriately and consistently with each confused person. The interactions are planned to prevent confusion or to assist an aged person to regain awareness of identity and the concrete, existing realities in the surrounding environment. Nurses are the ones who work with patients on a 24-hour basis; therefore, all shifts need to be taught the importance of 24-hour RO.

Environment The environment is an essential part of the RO process and should include these items: (1) directional signs, (2) clocks, (3) up-to-date calendars, and (4) RO boards. Contrasting colors in the environment are also essential, as is the presence of some of the patient's personal possessions. Clues such as directional signs should be located in conspicuous places and should be large enough to compensate for the sensory deficits which often occur in later life.

The entire staff should promote contact with reality by means of personal interaction including the involvement of visitors, volunteers, and family. These people need to understand the reasons behind the orientation process and the approaches useful in time, place, and person orientation. The nurse is a key person in providing the education necessary to ensure their active participation. Too often, the task of educating and counseling family, volunteers, and others is ignored and results in "wasted human potential." The family must be recognized as an integral part of the team working to reinforce oriented behavior. Knowing the concepts and process of RO can enable everyone in contact with a patient to provide preventive maintenance for those with minimal memory loss (Drummond et al., 1978).

Classroom RO, a supplement to 24-hour RO, is a structured, intensive small-group activity for the very confused. It provides an opportunity for staff to concentrate on time, place, and person orientation with those who have a short attention span or who need extra stimulation (Drummond et al., 1979).

Changes in Milieu Other simple but effective alterations are needed in the environment to prevent decompensation in the person who has only a marginal reserve (Verwoerdt, 1976, p. 193). Some suggestions are:

1. Keep the environment as constant as possible, avoiding transfers to other areas and unnecessary staff changes.
2. Speak to the patient with a voice of expectancy, explaining actions and mentioning one's name and function at regular intervals.
3. Structure the hours and days of the week so there is a noticeable difference in the patient's routine.
4. Provide opportunities for specific group experiences, such as RO class, exercise groups, remotivation groups, and others, beginning at the patient's level of comprehension.

These relatively minor considerations can be enough to help those with minimal confusion cope with day-to-day stresses in their environment. They offer mental and physical stimulation which promotes self-worth, social participation, and overall personality integration and tends to lessen the degree of isolation (Ernst et al., 1978).

OTHER BEHAVIORS WHICH MUST BE MANAGED

Behaviors which occur in confusional states can range from noisy, distracting actions to quiet withdrawal. In temporal-spatial relationships, the confused persons may wander aimlessly, enter other people's space, or feel "lost or mixed up." They may wander because of a desire to establish themselves in their own environment. Other general behavioral manifestations of confusion include the inability to concentrate, forgetting staff or family names, diminished emotional responsiveness, and occasionally confabulation, rambling, or incoherent speech (Verwoerdt, 1976, p. 43). At times these individuals are emotionally unstable; they may cry for no apparent reason, act impulsively, lose their temper, and even threaten other people.

These behaviors are often poorly tolerated by staff and are unacceptable in any social environment. Family members seek explanations. They wonder why a confused relative shows a lack of common sense by giving money away or buying useless things. Both family and staff react negatively to hoarding of useless items. They cannot understand why confused people hoard things that are readily available (Wolff, 1970, p. 89).

THERAPEUTIC GOAL

The therapeutic goal most helpful in nursing interventions is to provide support while searching for insight into the behavior. Focus must be on counteracting the confusion and the accompanying feeling of helplessness, which can be done by constant basic, matter-of-fact informing and educating. The repetitious reminders must be offered in a nonthreatening, noncritical way. The entire treatment staff must be accepting, understanding, supporting, and reassuring to the confused person. It must be remembered that confused people, regardless of the specific problem behavior, are complex individuals who are attempting to respond to the environment they perceive within the limits of their ability (Drummond et al., 1979, p. 4).

GROUP SESSIONS

In group sessions, there are coping behaviors which require intervention because the behavior is harmful to others, disruptive for the group experience, or reinforcing to the confusional state. Drummond et al. (1979) divide these behaviors into three categories: (1) distracting remarks and behaviors, (2) hostile-aggressive remarks and/or behaviors, (3) uninvolved remarks and behaviors. These authors include a list of the possible causes for the behaviors and some suggested responses, and they make the point that much problem behavior can be attributed to the fact that staff is working with confused, disoriented, regressed people.

Most acceptable behavior in an RO group can be related to the categories above; negative behaviors can also be provoked by the staff. For example, a group leader's action may show a lack of personal interest or press an individual for a rapid response, or the required work may be at a level which is too basic for the individual's cognitive ability. A nonthreatening but involved group atmosphere can best be achieved when the group leader is well informed about confusion, sensitive to individual needs, and demonstrates a positive attitude about the particular therapeutic intervention being used.

THE PROBLEMS OF NOCTURNAL CONFUSION

Patients who are not confused at other times may become so at night, and this nocturnal confusion is more prevalent in acute conditions. This sleepless state is sometimes referred to as *sundowner's syndrome*. According to Verwoerdt (1976, p. 192), nocturnal confusion is common in organic brain syndrome and is frequently a major complaint of both family and staff personnel.

Confusion after dark may be caused by difficulty in adjusting to darkness because of loss of sight and hearing. Noises and shapes grow monstrously out of proportion. The curtains become ghosts and images of people out of the past. Siderails become prison bars. An environmental change such as a relocation within a facility can require a major readjustment to the environment. A rapidly paced clinical setting creates anxiety and tension, which can result in insomnia and heightened confusion.

Kerstein and Isenberg (1974) verified that darkness, not fatigue, was the major contributor to nighttime disorientation. Patients who become confused at night should be frequently oriented to their rooms so that they can see and locate familiar things around them. If siderails must be used, orientation should be positive by explaining that the rails will keep them from falling and will protect them. These people need a night-light, a call button within reach, and an understanding, caring staff available when they do use the call signal (Conahan, 1976).

Nocturnal confusion is a major concern, and the solution does not always lend itself to the "traditional" rules of an institution. The nurse must seek every means to individualize the plan of care and avoid the disruptive atmosphere created by nocturnal confusion. To avoid the feeling of insecurity and isolation at night, the nurse may move the confused person's bed near the nurses' station or into the hall. The nurse's close presence and conversation, which offers basic orienting information, and the use of touch will do more for the patient than drugs or restraints. *Restraints will rarely end the disturbing behavior and can create more fear and discomfort for the patient.*

These behaviors and possible solutions emphasize the need for a greater understanding of each individual, contact with reality, the here and now, and a consistency of approach to help resolve the problem (Scarbrough, 1974).

SPECIAL NEEDS

SENSORY LOSSES

Sensory losses are directly related to confusion in many instances. These aged people will become confused simply because of an inaccurate perception of the environment around them. To compensate for these losses, both 24-hour RO and classroom RO emphasize identifying reality through the use of all senses. Staff can promote extrasensory stimulation by using touch and by identifying foods, smells, and objects in the environment (Drummond et al., 1978, p. 573). The important point is that nursing staff working with the confused should recognize their sensory deficits and compensate for these special needs as a part of the total rehabilitation program (see Chapters 33 and 34).

COMMUNICATION DISORDERS

People with communicative disorders are often considered confused and treated accordingly, especially if they are also old. Research studies of the relation of language functioning among patients with dementia and confusion are fragmentary (Schow, 1978, p. 273). After a stroke, a person may have a language problem which is interpreted to be intellectual impairment and memory loss. The person may comprehend what is said but need special assistance in expressing thoughts. This skill can be secured for the patient by getting a thorough assessment by a speech pathologist. It is best for the patient to have such an assessment before corrective exercises are begun. If memory impairment does exist, rehabilitative measures can be beneficial provided the following communication tips are used.

When patients with memory impairments speak in a rambling, poorly integrated way, they may be tactfully returned to the present by a direct question or reminder. If the disabled person is very disoriented, it may be most appropriate to end the conversation and resume at another time. Prodding or treating the person like a child should be avoided. Because intellectual processing is impaired, however, presenting the information slowly with short, simple statements will make it easier to comprehend. Allow adequate response time and repeat the sentence as necessary. Sometimes, the confused person may need to have the attention aroused. Touching the person or prefacing remarks by calling his or her name are simple but effective approaches. The key to therapeutic intervention with patients who are communicatively impaired is determining whether confusion exists. One never assumes that confusion is present.

Many health professionals do not like to work with old people. The multiplicity, duplicity, and the chronicity of the aged person's condition can become very frustrating. Problems seem overwhelming. The aged themselves often have such low expectation about progress that remaining ill and "sick" can be a self-fulfilling prophecy. *Confusion may simply be an effective coping device rather than the result of organic dysfunction.*

STABLE DISEASE

In truth there is a prevalence of chronic disease as one ages and little is known about preventing the onset of these slow killers, especially in late life. Health professionals need to utilize the new, descriptive term, a *stable disease* state, to describe chronic disease. A stable disease is one which is controlled to the extent that the person can be maintained at a level of functional ability most of the time (Byl and Clever, 1977). When confusion does occur in patients with such chronic illnesses, the cause may be more difficult to determine. Reality orientation and other approaches must be used to help keep the confusion at a minimal state for these individuals.

FAMILY SUPPORT: HELPING THE FAMILY UNDERSTAND

The family must be recognized as an integral part of the team working to reinforce oriented behavior. They need assistance in setting realistic expectations and in determining ways they can be helpful. When taught the concepts of the therapies, they have tools which help them communicate. They can also provide suggestions for helping a confused person become better oriented to the surroundings. Some individuals with minimal confusion may become preoccupied with reminiscing, and families often consider this a sign of deterioration. In counseling relatives of aged persons, it is important to explain the function of reminiscing and suggest how to react to it. They can be taught to allow times for reminiscence, to encourage the elderly person to verbalize facts and feelings from the past. If the person begins to confuse the past with the present, family members should assist with keeping the facts reasonably accurate and related to the past.

NURSES ARE A KEY LINK

Nurses provide a key link in family support since they are present 24 hours a day and 7 days a week. Staff must be encouraged to take time during family visits to teach family members the process of RO and reminiscence therapy. Family support and involvement will help provide the consistency needed to prevent confusion or deal with it therapeutically when it occurs.

A confusional state may be temporary and clear up adequately so the person can return home. Visits from a homemaker or nurse could assist with the adaptations needed and lend support to both the patient and family. Minor environmental alterations can sometimes be made to help overcome the problems which occur. Visual perception can be improved simply by using more powerful light bulbs and a night-light. Likewise, large, readable aids can be installed in the home to facilitate the overall orientation. Persons can be taught to mark off the calendar daily. A person can read timely events in the news and discuss these with the family regularly. Red hands on hot water faucets will make it easier to recall which can cause scalding and remind them that there is a difference.

Orientation is also affected by prosthetics such as glasses, dentures, and hearing aids. These need regular checks so that they are clean and in good working order. These simple considerations concerning living at home may avoid prolonged institutionalization and create a better-oriented person.

MAINTAINING QUALITY OF LIFE

Is it therapeutic to plan interventions for confused persons? Is it necessary to determine goals for the confused, disoriented client? There are health professionals who maintain that the confused are happy and better off in a confused state when their reality is harsh. Over a lifespan, individuals will age in different ways at different rates. If confusion does occur, it is our goal to be therapeutic. If we base our goal on the value of human life per se, our goal must be to help the confused person reach and maintain the maximum potential for functioning *Armstrong (1978) reminds us that with a constantly deteriorating client, specific goals will have to be adjusted downward—something that the therapeutic-minded person is reluctant to do.* Health care providers would rather "cure," but often the reality is that we can only "care."

Interventions such as touch and verbal communication are of critical importance to maximize personal awareness (see Chapter 35 for a discussion of therapeutic touch). Repeated explanations, questions, and simple cues to self-care will make the disoriented less vulnerable. An environment which arouses, stimulates, and provides options and choices will help promote orientation. Staff members should not feel a sense of failure when these skills do not work and the person remains confused. Cohen (1978) pleads for greater clinical understanding of the causes, diagnosis, course, and treatment of organic brain syndrome through research. In the meantime, quality of life may be the basic goal of therapeutic maintenance—medical and psychosocial.

Finally, although some of these confused persons may have multiple handicaps, there are those who are in fairly good health. They may have a lengthy period of time to live in spite of their confused state, with only a steady deterioration of functioning expected in all areas. Surely nursing care should be oriented toward helping the client to live as fully as possible during this time, rather than simply to "make him comfortable" until death (Armstrong, 1978). Folsom et al. (1978) speak of the use and abuse of rehabilitation therapies in their recent article, and they point out that the successful application of any intervention relies on the *people* using the tool. The entire health care team needs to take actions which promote the quality of life for confused individuals.

REFERENCES

Armstrong, Priscilla W.: More thoughts on senility, *The Gerontologist,* **18**(3):315–316, June 1978.
Besdine, Richard W.: *Treatable Dementia in the El-*

derly, Department of Health, Education and Welfare, National Institutes of Health, National Institute on Aging, Bethesda, Md., May 1978, p. 1–19, in press.

Brocklehurst, J. G., and T. Hanley: *Geriatric Medicine for Students,* Churchill Livingstone, New York, 1976, p. 59.

Byl, Nancy W., and Linda H. Clever: Stable chronic disease: A behavioral model, *Journal of the American Geriatric Society,* **25**(9):408–414, September 1977.

Cohen, Gene D.: Comment: Organic brain syndrome, reality orientation for critics of clinical interventions, *The Gerontologist,* **18**(3):313–314, June 1978.

Conahan, Judith M.: *Helping Your Elderly Patients, a Guide for Nursing Assistants,* Tiresias, New York City, 1976, p. 35.

Drummond, Linda, Lorraine Kirchhoff, and Dorothy Scarbrough: *Leading Reality Orientation Classes: Basic and Advanced,* Intercraft Associates, Arlington Heights, Ill., 1979, p. 4.

————, ————, **and** ————: A practical guide to reality orientation: A treatment approach for confusion and disorientation, *The Gerontologist,* **18**(6):568–573, December 1978.

Ernst, Philip, et al.: Isolation and the symptoms of chronic brain syndrome, *Gerontologist,* **18**(5):468–474, November 1978.

Folsom, James C., Barbara L. Boies, and Kenneth Pommerenck: Life adjustment techniques for use with the dysfunctional elderly, *Aged Care & Services Review,* **1**(4):1–12, 1978.

Kerstein, Morris, and Sarah Isenberg: Dealing with the confused elderly patient, *Hospital and Community Psychiatry,* **24**(3):160–161, March 1974.

Merck Manual of Diagnosis and Therapy: Robert Berkow (ed.), Merck & Co., Inc., Rahway, N.J., 1977 p. 1392.

Scarbrough, Dorothy R.: Reality orientation: A new approach to an old problem, *Nursing,* *74,* **(11)**:12–13, November 1974.

Schow, Ronald L., et al.: *Communication Disorders of the Aged: A Guide for Health Professionals,* University Park, Baltimore, 1978, p. 273.

Verwoerdt, Adrian: *Clinical Geropsychiatry,* Williams & Wilkins, Baltimore, 1976, p. 43, 192, 193.

Webster's New Collegiate Dictionary: Merriam, Springfield, Mass., 1977, p. 238.

Wolanin, Mary Opal, and Janet C. Holloway: *Confusion in the Elderly,* Mosby, St. Louis, in press.

———— **and** ————: Relocation confusion: intervention for prevention, in I. Burnside (ed.), *Psychosocial Nursing Care of the Aged,* McGraw-Hill, New York, 1980.

Wolff, Kurt: *The Emotional Rehabilitation of the Geriatric Patient,* Charles C Thomas, Springfield, Ill., 1970, p. 89.

OTHER RESOURCES

MANUALS

Professional Services Division: *Policy and Procedures Manual: Reality Orientation,* Hillhaven, Inc., Tacoma, Wash., 1978.

This Way to Reality, training kit containing five sets of slides with accompanying audiocassettes. Available from National Audiovisual Center (NAC), General Services Administration, Order Section, Washington, DC 20409.

FILMS

Return to Reality, 16 mm/color/35 min, introduces concept of RO. National Audiovisual Center (NAC), General Services Administration, Order Section, Washington, DC 20409.

December Spring: 24-Hour Reality Orientation, 16 mm/b&w/29 min, illustrates application of 24-hour RO. National Audiovisual Center (NAC), General Services Administration, Order Section, Washington, DC 20409.

A Time To Learn: Reality Orientation in the Nursing Home, 16 mm/color/28 min, demonstrates the "how to" in implementing RO. National Audiovisual Center (NAC), General Services Administration, Order Section, Washington, DC 20409.

Peege, 16 mm/color/28 min, shows dynamics of family relationships. Phoenix Films, 743 Alexander Rd., Princeton, NJ 08540.

AUDIOCASSETTE

Drummond, Linda, Lorraine Kirchhoff, and Dorothy R. Scarbrough: *Leading Reality Orientation Classes: Basic and Advanced,* booklet and audiocassette which provides information on organizing and conducting RO classes, 1979. Available from Intercraft Associates, Box 613, Arlington Heights, IL 60006.

MISCELLANEOUS

Ernst, Marvin, and Herbert Shore: *Sensitizing People to the Processes of Aging: The In-Service Educator's Guide,* University Center for Community Services, Box 5344, NT Station, Denton, TX 76203.

24-Hour Reality Orientation at Home, brochure from Community Services Program, VA Medical Center, Tuscaloosa, Ala.

I Happen to Be Older, training packet on reality orientation. Available from Intercraft Associates, Box 613, Arlington Heights, IL 60006.

SIXTEEN

DEVELOPING A WORKING RELATIONSHIP WITH A CONFUSED CLIENT

Janet E. Porter
Theodore J. Rasmussen
Irene Mortenson
Burnside

Grief can take care of itself; but to get the full value of a joy you must have somebody to divide it with.
Mark Twain, 1861

LEARNING OBJECTIVES

- Define a working relationship.
- Explain the necessity for multisensory input.
- Describe at least three staff behaviors which are useful in getting the client's attention.
- Give two examples each of verbal and nonverbal techniques.
- List five behavioral areas (staff) that are important in developing a working relationship.

- Given any one of the above five behavioral areas, describe two related staff behaviors.
- Describe interventions with the withdrawn apathetic client.

THE WORKING RELATIONSHIP

A working relationship with confused clients provides an opportunity for clients to participate in a cooperative venture to the limits of their abilities. They are helped to feel that they are part of what is happening. To the extent that they understand what others expect of them and what they can expect from others, their care will be easier to provide. They will be less resistive to necessary care and will be less inclined to be demanding at inappropriate or inconvenient times.

Of special importance is the fact that the care giver offers one of the most significant elements in a healthy life—a meaningful relationship in which dignity and mutual respect can grow. As the care giver relates to the confused client at the present functioning level of the client, the client is offered someone with whom to share feelings of frustration, grief, and joy. We cannot afford to provide less than this as we strive toward quality of life for all.

DEFINITION

Relationship, as described by Kramer and Kramer (1976, p. 35), "is all that goes on between and among people—their feelings, thoughts, and actions—including not only things we are aware of but also what we are not aware of." Content and process, verbal and nonverbal behaviors, are all important aspects of a relationship. A working relationship between the confused client and care giver includes all messages, verbal and nonverbal, the nurse or

Many thanks to Milton Northway, B.S., B.A., O.T.R., whose observations and suggestions have contributed to this chapter.

care giver is forwarding to the client. Interestingly, there is some clinical indication that the individual suffering from senile dementia may "read" body language messages more spontaneously and accurately than verbal messages (Storrie, 1978). The care giver, in turn, must be prepared to observe the confused client carefully for responses, some of which may be subtle or inappropriate but nonetheless relevant to the felt concern of the client.

A working relationship between the confused client and the care giver is described as a mutual sharing of information, both verbal and nonverbal, which takes place anytime the care giver is with the client. The major responsibility for establishing and maintaining the working relationship is upon the care giver or staff member. In a working relationship it is evident that the care giver is working *with* the client rather than *on* him and that the care giver is responding to the confused client as to an adult rather than as to a child.

The client is repeatedly informed as to what is happening and what is expected of him. He is repeatedly invited to respond and to participate. The client may or may not respond directly to what the care giver is saying, but the lack of evidence of response is not automatically assumed to indicate lack of awareness or disinterest on the client's part. Almost every health professional who has worked in a long-term care facility has at least one story of the confused, incontinent, helpless client thought to be "out of it" who surprised the staff member by making a statement which revealed the client's awareness of the situation and insight into the staff member's frustration in trying to provide care.

A working relationship means that the care giver responds to the confused client with dignity and uses words appropriate to the chronological age of the client. The unconscious trap of infantilizing the confused client may partially allay anxiety and anger of the care giver who must often feed, bathe, and clean the client as one would an infant. To avoid this trap, care givers must be alert to their own feelings in such situations and deal with them in a manner that is constructive to themselves and their clients. To continue to talk to elderly confused clients as if they were children may be to condemn them to helplessness indefinitely.

A working relationship must be developed and maintained concurrently with regular care routines. Interaction takes place during bathing and dressing, at mealtimes, when medications are given, when clients are escorted from place to place and moved in the bedroom, ward, or floor, when care givers and routines are changed, and at numerous other occasions. *Development of a working relationship does not require more staff, more money, more equipment, or more supplies!* It does not require a separate room and special time each day for one-to-one interaction. All these, of course, can enrich and improve client care, but they are not at issue in the present discussion of a working relationship.

The following sections on sensory input and getting the client's attention are concerned with communication between the confused client and the care giver. Adequate communication is essential to a working relationship. Communication may be hampered by sensory deficits.

SENSORY LOSSES AND SENSORY INPUT

Many elderly clients display sensory losses or dysfunction. Limitations in seeing and hearing are frequently encountered. There may be loss or diminution of smell, taste, and touch. Kinesthetic losses may contribute to unstable gait, or difficulty in performing various movements, a situation which is disconcerting to the client and adds to his confusion. The care giver must check whether the client has any sensory loss and which senses appear to be functional. The care giver who is communicating with a blind client must give more detailed verbal information and more messages via touch. The deaf client will look for body language and will require more written information (usually in large dark letters on light paper). Clients who are both blind and deaf will require careful attention as to what they seem to understand and through what senses they appear to obtain that information. In the meantime the care giver must rely on touching the blind or deaf client as the primary means of "speaking."

Generally, the staff member will find it useful to develop the habit of expressing informa-

tion, a request, or a feeling via more than one sensory mode. Speech is most commonly used. Key words or important information may be written or posted as well, perhaps with copies put in strategic places. Many requests can be expressed via body language, e.g., "Come with me" (finger or arm gesture), "I'm leaving you now" (wave good-bye). Touch can convey a number of meanings including anger, concern, sympathy, goodwill, encouragement, a pull saying "Come with me," and a firm pressure saying, "Stay here." See Chapter 35 for a discussion on touching the aged client.

Since sensory losses are frequent, it is recommended that the staff person caring for any elderly client routinely watch for previously unrecognized losses and seek proper diagnosis and treatment. In a recent study of 295 elderly residents a relationship between vision and mental status was indicated (Snyder et al., 1976). The study raises the question of whether an older client with unrecognized vision needs might be labeled as confused because of acting dazed and slow. Wells (1976) points out that early diagnosis of sensory losses and appropriate therapy for the elderly may forestall or avoid possible related withdrawal, apathy, and symptoms of confusion. See Chapter 14 on organic brain syndrome and Chapters 33 and 34 on the senses for elaboration of these points.

It should be noted that while the label *confused* might incorrectly be applied to the elderly client who is suffering from the limitations of unrecognized sensory loss, there are other elderly clients whose senses are intact but who are not responding to input. They may have been living in a sensory-deprived environment or an environment without meaning where they learned to expect little stimulation. These clients often display symptoms of confusion. Sensory stimulation programs have been shown to be useful in such cases (Sandel, 1978; Ernst et al., 1977).

In developing a working relationship with the confused client with complex sensory losses, it may be useful for the care giver to seek information from available resource persons, a psychiatrist, or a neurologist. Some difficulties, such as hemianopsia, may be difficult to diagnose but, once identified, are fairly easy "to work around." (Hemianopsia is blindness for a part of the field of vision in one or both eyes.) Central nervous system deficits may complicate sensory input and response, adding to confusion. Shore (1976) has designed a training program for understanding sensory losses in aging.

The care giver must communicate with the confused client in spite of sensory loss as the working relationship develops. This may require "speaking" to the client without use of written or spoken word, or it may require multisensory input. It is important to gain the client's attention.

GETTING CLIENTS' ATTENTION

The first step in communicating with confused clients is to get their attention, a task which is often made more difficult by a short or fleeting attention span. If clients tend to wander or move about frequently, they may resist attempts to restrain them in one place. Occasionally a confused client seems unable to separate significant input (the care giver's voice) from other sounds in the environment (television, vacuum cleaner, dishwasher, etc.,) and, therefore, does not respond.

The following suggestions for staff behavior have been found useful in gaining the attention of the confused client:

• Wear clothing of bright colors (reds, oranges, yellows). This will increase the chance that the client will notice you.
• Call the client by name frequently from a position within arm's distance as you try to gain his or her attention.
• Touch the client on the hand, arm, or shoulder. Try gently jiggling the confused person's forearm or hand (Northway, 1977).
• Watch for the instant the client looks into your face. At that moment smile broadly, call the client's name, and try to hold his or her gaze while you say a few words. If you have difficulty getting eye contact, try gently wiggling your fingers about 12 inches from the client's face until the client looks at your fingers, then, keeping your fingers moving, raise them slowly to your eyes. Raise your fingers slowly enough that the client is able to track their

movement upward with his or her eyes. When your fingers are close alongside your eyes the client will be looking at your face. At that moment call the client by name and smile broadly.

You may need to repeat this procedure many times. Eventually the confused elder will have learned to look at you directly when you are close and call him or her by name. With daily practice during which a few simple words are exchanged, the span of attention will increase. Regular practice with the same routine is important.

The following section is concerned with additional verbal and nonverbal (body language) techniques and behaviors that can help the care giver develop a working relationship.

USEFUL VERBAL AND NONVERBAL TECHNIQUES

The way in which one communicates with the confused client is as important as the message to be conveyed. The client may have physical or psychological problems which interfere with the ability to receive and comprehend information. Careful attention to the way one speaks and acts when communicating will enhance the possibility of success (Burnside, 1980a, 1980b; Blazer, 1978; Mead, 1977). When clients see you telling them nonverbally with your body language that you like and respect them, they will want to be cooperative. Many clients read nonverbal messages when they cannot speak or understand spoken words.

Suggestions for Effective Verbal and Vocal Techniques

• Get the client's attention (eye contact) first.
• Sit down beside the client if possible.
• Maintain eye contact while talking. Remember, however, that some cultures consider eye contact during conversation disrespectful or offensive, so check this for clients who may be from a different cultural background.
• Speak in a low, clear, slow voice, accentuating consonants. Speak loudly only when necessary. Try different pitches.

- Face the client so that he or she can see your face directly.
- Keep your hands away from your mouth. A male staff member who has a mustache should keep it away from his upper lip as many clients lip read to assist hearing.
- Use short sentences and repeat key words if necessary.
- Use simple, appropriate words. Remember that words are only tokens or symbols for the meaning we wish to convey, so do not quibble over the dictionary definition of words. Use words that are meaningful to you and your client.
- Give only one instruction at a time. Break down a large request into simple steps and ask for one step at a time.
- If the client uses a hearing aid, be sure it is turned on and has a functioning battery.
- When clients are speaking to you, show that you are listening by nodding your head and repeating key words they are saying. Ask them about anything that is not clear to you. Summarize out loud what you think they are telling you and ask whether you have it right.

Suggestions for Use of Body Language

- Keep your posture relaxed. Be aware of the different ways you could position your body to give someone the impression that you do not like that person, or that you are bored or repulsed. Facial expressions are especially important because people focus their eyes on the face most. Be aware of frowning or of setting your jaw. Note that a simple gesture can give a message; for example, if you light a cigarette while working with a client, he or she may conclude that you are nervous, impulsive, or bored.
- Move slowly and deliberately when around a client (within 4 feet). (See Figure 16-1.)
- Do not move hands or arms into your client's intimacy circle.
- Be sure you have made your presence known before you touch your client. Do not startle clients by approaching from the rear and suddenly touching them. (See Figure 16-1.)
- Use authoritarian postures only when you want to appear to be "the boss."
- If your clients are from cultures different from your own, learn the meanings of various nonverbal behaviors in those cultures.

- Avoid body positions and movements that could be interpreted in a negative way.
- Use touch with care and discrimination. Some clients need and like it, others do not. Touching can express affection, can calm, can interrupt, depending on the context.
- Reach out and offer your handshake but let the client touch your hand first. Many older people believe that a handshake is indicative of a person's character, so use a firm, positive grip (but not too tight!).
- Explain what you want with movements in addition to asking or telling the client to do something; for example, when asking the client to stand up or sit down, or to eat, drink, or walk with you.
- When talking with clients, have your eyes on the same level as theirs. Stoop or kneel if talking to a wheelchairbound client, especially if you are a big or tall person.
- Work at a steady, even pace.
- Keep your voice level, even, and calm.
- Have a regular routine.
- Always follow through with what you say. Avoid threats and promises.
- Find out the individual routine each client follows (or insists upon) and try to follow it each day.
- Try to keep your mood the same from one day to another.

It is human and normal to swing slowly up and down in moods over a period of a year. However, if your moods and resultant behavior swing drastically from day to day, practice self-awareness. It is almost impossible to hide a bad mood from a client. You may need to deal with your problems and settle them. You may be unintentionally bringing your personal problems into your work and making your clients go through your worry and emotional turmoil.

An understanding and accepting staff group will sometimes allow an upset staff member to back off from all client contact while having a bad day. If the bad days are frequent, however, the staff member should seek help, perhaps through a local mental health center or from the consulting psychologist in the work setting.

The following section deals with five particular areas that concern the confused client and useful staff behaviors relating to each of those areas.

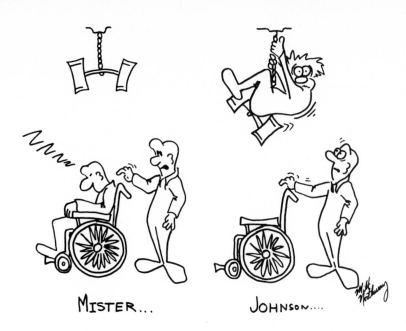

MISTER... JOHNSON.....

FIGURE 16-1 *Courtesy of Milt Northway.*

USEFUL STAFF BEHAVIORS

How the care giver handles the client's needs in each of the following areas will determine how the relationship develops or whether, indeed, any relationship is established:

1. Arranging the physical environment to meet clients' needs
2. Giving clients their own territory
3. Giving rewards for desired behavior
4. Giving necessary information to clients
5. Making opportunities for clients to express their independence

Staff behavior in these five areas indicates whether a custodial model of care is in operation or whether the client is allowed, encouraged, and assisted in a working relationship with a staff member caring for him.

ARRANGING THE PHYSICAL ENVIRONMENT TO MEET CLIENTS' NEEDS

It is an accepted fact that one's environment affects one's feelings and behavior. An attractive, functional work setting contributes to productivity. Interior designers and a vast array of home furnishings are available to personalize, organize, economize, and glamorize private homes. Because confused clients are usually limited to the same physical environment 24 hours a day, it is important that their living settings be arranged so as to help them overcome their problems, help them achieve their health potential, and be "at home." Harris et al. (1977) studied eight "homes for old people" selected to represent factors of size (large and small), design (institutional and family), and mental designation of residents (confused or rational). Verbal exchanges among residents were analyzed. The data suggested that several elements of architectural and spatial design could be modified between levels of client function.

The effects of different arrangements of furniture on the verbal expression of geriatric behavior were studied by Peterson et al. (1977). Their results suggest that rate of verbalization can be affected by arrangements of tables and chairs. They observed that there were advantages to modifying behavior by using physical stimuli because changes in the physical environment do not have to be costly and maintaining staff motivation is not a problem. Anderson (1970) studied the relationship of two different institutional environmental settings to frequency and nature of disturbed behavior in elderly demented clients. It was suggested that incidences of disturbed behavior could be reduced by having a simple ward plan with a minimum of doors, adequate day space to allow maximum movement for walking, clearly marked toilets, attractive decor, and reality orientation aids. This study also stressed that furniture should be arranged to foster talking and interaction. Mooney (1978) states that at present many of the psychological problems of old age seem to be a consequence of the demoralizing effects of our society where being old often means, among other unappealing options, living in an unattractive, barren, drab setting. Here are some suggestions for staff to follow as they seek to make the environment of the confused client helpful:

- Arrange furniture, especially chairs and tables, so that clients can easily see each other and talk to each other. Do not line up all the chairs in a row against the walls because that causes isolation of clients from one another.
- Keep the furniture in the same place as much as possible. Many clients orient themselves to certain chairs, pictures, etc. They will be "lost" for a few days if their "cue" is moved or missing. Two of the authors of this chapter were told the incident of an elderly confused man who had resided in a local nursing home for several years without problem. One evening the staff on duty was alarmed to hear screaming and yelling coming from the hall near the old man's room. They found that he had entered the room of the woman whose room was next door and had climbed into her bed. He appeared surprised to find her there, and she was outraged. The intruder was scolded, the mistake carefully pointed out, and his own room identified. For the next two evenings this problem repeated itself while the staff discussed possible interventions. Then the problem ended. The man began going directly to his own room without error. Careful investigation by staff revealed that when he went down the hall he proceeded as far as a red chair placed opposite the door to his room. At the chair he stopped. Then without looking at the number or name on the door, he immediately opened it and went on to bed. Several days previously the chair had been moved in order to clean the carpet. It had accidentally been placed opposite the door of the room of the offended woman!

- Make signs for the clients in extra large print. They should be in a color that is in a sharp contrast to the background. Put clients' names on their bedroom doors. Label the toilet and the dining room. Find a calendar with large numbers.
- Put reality orientation aids at strategic places. These aids include clocks, calendars, information boards, names of staff on duty, daily menu, pictures of familiar objects. Staff name tags should be large if confused clients are expected to read them. Be alert to sensory and perceptual losses, however, remembering that not all confused clients will be able to use all orientation aids. A Dutch study of clock-reading by 50 psychogeriatric nursing home clients (Cahn and Diesfeldt, 1977) showed that most had difficulty of some sort telling time from the clock face.
- Make doors, doorknobs, and light switches stand out by use of paint, colored paper, or cardboard.
- Include different kinds of textures and bright colors. This is important in selecting furniture, walls, pillows, blankets, rugs, wall decorations, etc., so that clients receive varied sensory input by touching and looking (Northway, 1977).
- Give extra sensory input to bedridden clients. Use backrubs, help them touch things of different textures and temperatures, play music, and vary the lighting.
- Keep a rocking chair handy for use by hostile clients. This rocking movement can provide a calming, soothing effect.
- Arrange for sensory input of touch by having group activities in which patients touch each other or objects. Such activities include holding hands in a circle to say hello or good-bye after an event, tossing a ball to one another, rolling a ball back and forth in a sheet.
- Notice the various sounds in the environment—eliminate unnecessary noises. Frequent sources of unnecessary noise are telephone, loudspeaker, electric floor buffer, dishwasher, vacuum cleaner, yelling and talking of patients, staff, and visitors. Many clients cannot "filter out" sounds that are not relevant to their needs, as most adults do without think-

ing. You will, therefore, be competing with all these extraneous sounds when you try to get the client's attention.

GIVING CLIENTS THEIR OWN TERRITORY

The importance of personal space and possessions in the lives of clients is receiving increasing attention, and appropriately so (Stillman, 1978; Trierweiler, 1978; Sherman and Newman, 1977–1978).

Those who have space and possessions of their own feel more secure and safe. They experience less need to hit out and feel happier and more important. Each of us needs some private space (or territory) where we can escape the attention of our fellows and relax and replenish our energies. Then we can ready ourselves for the stresses of renewed interaction with other people. The most important territory we own is our own body. Other important territory includes personal possessions and space. The closer the space is to our body, the more personal and intimate it becomes. (See Figure 16-2.)

Suggestions for ways the care giver can help confused clients feel that they have a place, both physically and psychologically, are these:

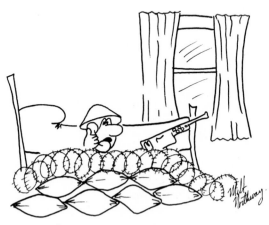

YES SON, I FINALLY SECURED MY OWN TERRITORY...

FIGURE 16-2 *Courtesy of Milt Northway.*

- Keep clients' clothes and personal belongings safe from others and in a place where they can be used by their owners.
- Ask permission of clients before you move them or their possessions, when this is practical. If there is no choice, then do not ask, but do explain.
- Remind families who bring pictures and personal mementos to place them where clients can see and handle them.
- Encourage long-term clients to decorate their side of the room in a way they like. (But observe fire-code regulations.)
- When talking about a client with another staff member, do so in a place where the client cannot see or hear you. Do not talk about clients in their presence or within their hearing (as if they were not there). Show respect for a client's physical presence by either including him or her in the conversation as an equal or waiting to have your talk with other staff in private. Do not talk about a client in front of other clients.
- Work close (within $1\frac{1}{2}$ feet of the client's body) with confused clients. This will help give them a feeling of trust and safety.

GIVING REWARDS FOR DESIRED BEHAVIOR

People usually do what makes them feel good and is rewarding. Use rewards to strengthen desired behavior. Rewards that a staff person can give a client include (1) words, (2) eye contact, (3) smiling, (4) touching, and (5) spending a few extra minutes with the client.

More suggestions for staff behavior are:

- When a client cooperates with you, say, "Good," "Good for you," "I appreciate your helping," "Great," or something else that communicates that you are pleased. Occasions when you can give such praise are mealtime, bath, toilet, getting up in the morning, going to bed at night, combing hair, shaving, brushing teeth, dressing, or any other time you are together.
- Smile at the client when he or she is cooperating.
- Look directly at the client you are complimenting.

- Give the cooperating client an affectionate pat on shoulder, hand, or arm if this seems appropriate.
- Compliment the client in the same manner and tone as you would a coworker or friend: as an adult with respect, not in a high-pitched voice as you would a child.
- Give rewards for desired behavior as often as you can. Remember that if you give clients attention (eye contact, touch, calling by name, being with them) when they are doing something you do *not* like, you may actually be fortifying the undesirable behavior. The old saying is that when one is starving for attention, it seems better to get the attention of punishment than no attention at all. It is unfortunate when a client must yell or hit out in order to get attention (rewards) from the staff.

VIGNETTE

A description of how rewards were used to change the behavior of an 80-year-old woman who displayed chronic "screaming" behavior is given by Baltes and Lascomb (1975). A resident of a nursing home for about 3 years, she had started calling out the name Mary about $1\frac{1}{2}$ years previously when she fractured her hip. At the time of the study she remained in her drab room all the time and did not walk, although there appeared to be no reason for this limitation. By carefully rewarding behaviors other than screaming (i.e., holding eyes open, answering questions, trying to touch) and by carefully not rewarding screaming behavior, the investigators were able to reduce the amount of screaming to almost none. Rewards used were (1) praise, (2) smile, (3) touch, (4) verbal contact, (5) recorded music, and (6) cereal, raisins, and ice cream.

When a confused client displays problem behavior, it is essential that the care giver examine what is done by staff in response to such behavior. Possibly the staff is in fact rewarding the client for the display of problem behavior by increased response at those times. Is the client receiving sufficient rewards for desired behavior or is the desired behavior ignored?

GIVING NECESSARY INFORMATION TO CLIENTS

Clients who have little difficulty asking questions tend to get answers to their questions. Clients who are confused and unable to express questions verbally do not get necessary information unless their care givers make a point of getting their attention and telling them in a way that optimizes their chances of understanding. Clients need information about their environment in order to act appropriately and not become unnecessarily anxious. Knowing the reasons behind changes in routines, medication, ward, personnel, etc., or being told ahead of time that a change will take place will reduce their anxiety.

Suggestions about giving necessary information:

- When new clients arrive in your area, tell them what they need to know about daily routine, activities, staff and patients, other client's behavior and possessions. They may not remember the details of what is said, but they are likely to remember your effort and attitude.
- Introduce new clients to staff and clients.
- If another client has "taken possession" of some special chair in the dayroom or place at the table and gets angry when that territory is used by someone else, the new client needs to know about this. (A staff member can keep a written list of orientation information to use with each new client.)
- Refer to reality orientation aids frequently (calendar, clock). Keep them up-to-date.
- Help a client find answers to questions if you cannot answer them. For example, a client may inquire about writing a will or contacting a distant relative. Do not just ignore the question. Tell the client whom to ask to get the information or where to look for it. If the client needs assistance, help him or her find the right source. Sometimes a confused client will try to ask a question but mix up the words. Try to get the gist of what is being said and reword or paraphase it. Then find an answer.
- Remind the client of regular events such as meal or bath a few minutes ahead of time and explain what is happening.

- Tell the client when a change in medication has been made and why.
- Tell the client why he or she is being moved to another room and when.
- Tell clients why the usual person is not caring for them. When a staff person leaves permanently, have some kind of traditional "goodbye" party with clients to help them understand the change.

It will probably be necessary to repeat the same information over and over. Remember that the confused client may be reading your tone of voice, facial expression, and body language, so it is important that these be consistent with what is said.

MAKING OPPORTUNITIES FOR CLIENTS TO EXPRESS THEIR INDEPENDENCE

As stated earlier, the confused client is often unable to identify or express needs and wishes effectively. The responsibility to see that these needs and wants are reasonably fulfilled is upon the care giver. Apart from food, clothing, and shelter, clients' needs may not be obvious; an example is the need for independence. The care giver must provide opportunities for confused clients to assert some independence within the limits of their capacity. (See Figure 16-3.)

- Give the client choices whenever possible. Questions can be part of morning care, e.g., "Do you want to wash your face alone or do you want some help?"; part of dressing, e.g., "Do you want to wear the red dress or the blue dress?"; part of hair care, e.g., "Do you want to have your hair parted on the side or in the middle?"; part of bathing, e.g., "Do you want a bath or shower?" "Do you want a man or woman to help you?" "Do you want your bath this morning or tomorrow morning?" and so on. Ask only questions for which either choice is satisfactory with you. And if the client does not really have a choice about something, do not ask; for example, when it is time to get up from a chair to go to bed, do not ask, "Do you want to go to bed now?" Say, "Time for bed!"

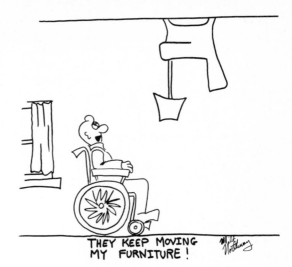

THEY KEEP MOVING MY FURNITURE!

FIGURE 16-3 *Courtesy of Milt Northway.*

- Help the client do as much self-care as possible (brush teeth, comb hair, dress, wash). Do this by giving encouragement and gathering materials together. Do the hard parts such as zipping up pants yourself. Help clients to help themselves. Do not make quick judgments about how much they can do. Give them a chance to show you.
- Know what each client can be expected to do. For example, say, "I am looking forward to seeing you do . . . ," or, "Try doing this today." *Encourage the more capable clients to assist the frailer clients if they show interest in doing*

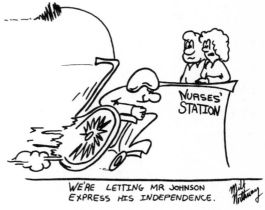

WE'RE LETTING MR JOHNSON EXPRESS HIS INDEPENDENCE.

FIGURE 16-4 *Courtesy of Milt Northway.*

so. Be sure to give honest praise when clients try to do a job. Praise their effort even if they cannot complete the job.

Helping clients to be as independent as possible is a goal that staff members must consistently work toward, and it usually requires that they become less directive and overprotective as a beginning step (Robinson and Owen, 1974). Feelings of helplessness and boredom which are often experienced by staff of long-term care facilities can be replaced by a healthier, more optimistic view when residents become more independent and involved in their own care (Rodstein, 1975) (see Figure 16-4).

SUMMARY

This chapter has presented basic concepts directed toward understanding care of the confused client, as well as a number of specific suggestions for staff behavior. Much of the information in this chapter will be familiar to some staff care givers. It sounds like plain old common sense which, however, is often more rare than common. A working relationship with a confused client must be developed as a special and valuable experience; it does require self-awareness, astute observation, tact, humility, persistence, and understanding.

REFERENCES

Anderson, J. F.: A study of disturbed behavior in patients with dementia in two hospital populations, *Gerontologia Clinica* (Basel), **12**(1):49–64, 1970.

Baltes, M. M., and S. L. Lascomb: Creating a healthy institutional environment for the elderly via behavior management: The nurse as a change agent, *International Journal of Nursing Studies*, **12**(1):5–12, March 1975.

Blazer, D.: Techniques for communicating with your elderly patient, *Geriatrics*, **33**(11):79–84, November 1978.

Burnside, Irene Mortenson: Interviewing the aged, in *Psychosocial Nursing Care of the Aged*, 2d ed., Irene Mortenson Burnside (ed.), McGraw-Hill, New York, 1980a.

———: Interviewing the confused aged person, in *Psychosocial Nursing Care of the Aged*, Irene Mor-tenson Burnside (ed.), McGraw-Hill, New York, 1980b.

Cahn, L. A., and H. F. A. Diesfeldt: To know what time it is (Dutch), *Nederlands Tijdschrift Gerontol.*, **8**(4):213–220, April 1977.

Ernst, P., et al.: Treatment of the aged mentally ill: Further unmasking of the effects of a diagnosis of chronic brain syndrome, *Journal of the American Geriatric Society*, **25**(10):466–469, October 1977.

Harris, H., et al.: Architectural design: The spatial location and interaction of old people, *Gerontology*, **23**(5):390–400, 1977.

Kramer, Charles H., and Jeannette R. Kramer: *Basic Principles of Long-Term Patient Care*, Charles C Thomas, Springfield, Ill., 1976, p. 35.

Mead, B. T.: How to relate to the elderly patient, *Geriatrics*, **30**(10):73–77, October 1977.

Mooney, C. M.: Psychologic problems of the aged, *Journal of the American Geriatrics Society*, **26**(6):268–273, June 1978.

Northway, M. A.: Personal communication, 1977.

Peterson, R. F., et al.: The effects of furniture arrangement on the behavior of geriatric patients, *Behavior Therapy*, **8**(3):464–467, June 1977.

Robinson, G. C., and J. Owen: No one told me to, *Nursing Outlook*, **22**(3):182–183, March 1974.

Rodstein, M.: Challenging residents to assume maximal responsibilities in homes for the aged, *Journal of the American Geriatrics Society*, **23**(7):317–321, July 1975.

Sandel, S. L.: Movement therapy with geriatric patients in a convalescent home, *Hospital and Community Psychiatry*, **29**(11):738–742, November 1978.

Sherman, E., and E. S. Newman: The meaning of cherished personal possessions for the elderly, *Journal of Aging and Human Development*, **8**(2):181–192, 1977–78.

Shore, H.: Designing a training program for understanding sensory losses in aging, *The Gerontologist*, **16**(2):157–165, February 1976.

Snyder, L. H., J. Pyrek, and K. C. Smith: Vision and mental function of the elderly, *The Gerontologist*, **16**(6):491–495, 1976.

Stillman, M.: Territoriality and personal space, *American Journal of Nursing*, **78**(10):1670–1672, October 1978.

Storrie, M.: Lecture at staff development program, Western State Hospital, Fort Steilacoom, Wash., May 1978.

Trierweiler, R.: Personal space and its effects on an elderly individual in a long-term care institution, *Journal of Gerontological Nursing*, **4**(5):21–23, September/October 1978.

Wells, Charles E. D.: Helping stave off a dimming of the five senses, *Medical Opinion*, **51**(2):20–35, February 1976.

SEVENTEEN

GROUP WORK WITH REGRESSED AGED PEOPLE

Irene Mortenson Burnside

Just because the message may never be received does not mean it is not worth sending.
Segaki (David Stockton, translator)

LEARNING OBJECTIVES

- Describe the theoretical requirements essential for conducting group therapy and the characteristics for effective leadership.
- Discuss the therapeutic use of touch in group work with the aged.
- Discuss pros and cons of props in group work.
- Define a contract.
- List at least four goals that would be therapeutic for a group of old people.
- Discuss two possible pitfalls of goal setting.
- Identify at least six problems that can present in group work with the elderly and give suggestions for intervention.

Although the literature contains little about group work with regressed aged persons, one cannot assume that working with these aged persons is not undertaken by nurses or other professionals. This chapter presents literature and focuses on one approach to group work as used by a nurse.

The problem of care of persons with chronic brain syndrome in institutions is one of great magnitude. It is not likely that the number of such individuals will decrease; in fact, with the steady increase in the aged population, nurses will have to find improved methods of caring for the regressed elderly. There is no accurate count of those who live in the community, and although many have varying degrees of organic brain syndrome, they have somehow managed to escape institutionalization. Public health nurses are acutely aware of such individuals, probably more so than other nurses. Group work with the person who is suffering from chronic brain syndrome is much different from group work with alert elderly (who may be disabled physically but still function well in a group), and an entire chapter is devoted to the organic brain syndromes in Chapter 14 of this book. Butler (1977, p. 97) stated that "a good target area for collaboration is senile dementia" and that "the National Institute on Aging (NIA) . . . is dedicated to improving the quality of life of the old in America through biomedical, social, and behavioral research."

OVERVIEW OF THE LITERATURE

There has been interest in group work since Silver (1950) wrote his article. Linden (1956) wrote the first comprehensive review of group psychotherapy with the elderly, and his report was the first to describe group psychotherapy with the "senile" elderly, which was an ongoing controlled program. Goldfarb's (1971) excellent review of the literature on group therapy with aged clients describes therapy by psychiatrists. There is also a survey of selected literature of group work conducted by people in different disciplines and in a variety of settings (Burnside, 1970).

THEORETICAL CONSIDERATIONS

Nurses have only recently begun to publish their experiences in group work with the elderly (Burnside, 1978c). Knowledge of group theory and dynamics is essential for nurses if they are to conduct group therapy with a degree of professional sophistication; it is also helpful if they themselves have had some type of group experience which was subject to evaluation. Group work with the aged is just as diverse as group work with any other group, and the group work conducted with regressed aged in the form of reality orientation is well documented (Taulbee, 1973). Leaders of such groups usually have an initial training period and also are supervised. Supervision should be available to anyone who is beginning group work with the aged. Nursing assistants, student nurses, and beginners from other disciplines should be screened for leadership ability. There are persons who cannot tolerate the many variables that exist in group work and prefer to function on a one-to-one basis with patients. The nurse who is skilled in nonverbal communication, psychodynamics, and interviewing should be the one to lead the way and demonstrate effective group leadership. Also it is sometimes good teaching strategy to demonstrate the ineffective methods. The importance of giving the rationale for the leader's choice of intervention is important with new group leaders. If written process recordings are assigned, rationales should be spelled out clearly by the student. Elsewhere I have described pragmatic approaches in group work with the elderly (Burnside, 1978b).

LEADER

The leader for group work with regressed aged must have the patience of Job, the perseverance of a nag, the stamina of an Olympic athlete, and an abundance of empathy. These traits are mandatory for effective leadership. While empathy is important in all work with the aged, it is crucial for the regressed aged, who receive only custodial care (and sometimes scarcely that in our present health-care system). Some of the aged have been treated as subhuman, something less than mortal beings. One cannot help but believe that some have also been mistreated, because innumerable times I have reached out to touch an aged person or to pat a cheek, only to have him or her draw back in fright, as though I were going to strike. Slowness of the motions of the leader helps prevent such fearful responses to the leader, and also speaking to them simultaneously as one touches or moves toward them is helpful.

TOUCH

The leader has to learn to use self. The spontaneity of the leader, the ability to care and be affectionate, the tolerance of silences, and the copious use of touch are all important in group work with the regressed. Touching these individuals and helping them reach out to touch one another is powerful therapy (Burnside, 1973b). Barnett (1972a and b) and McCorkle (1972) have contributed to the nursing literature on the subject of touch.

The use of touch with regressed aged persons cannot be overemphasized. Greenberg (1972) noted in her observations of psychiatrically ill patients that many of them were isolated from human touch, and she observed this to be the usual situation unless a form of routine nursing care was being given. Chapter 35 deals entirely with therapeutic touch. (See Figures 17-1 and 17-2.)

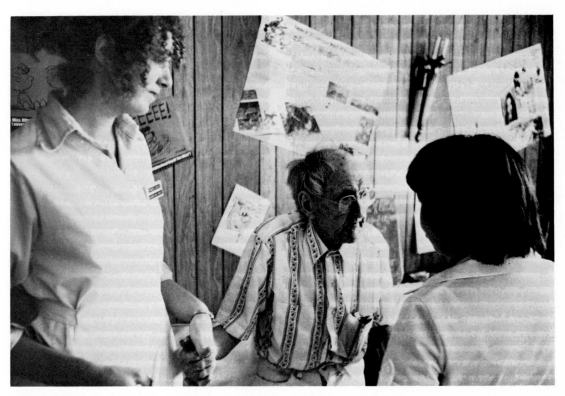

FIGURE 17-1 It is important for the leader to learn to use self, and the use of touch is especially important in group work with regressed elderly people. (*Courtesy of Anthony J. Skirlick, Jr.*)

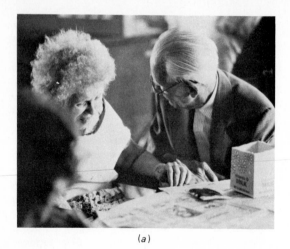 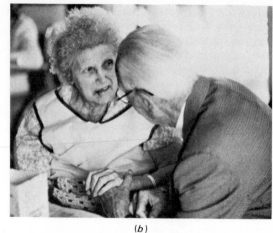

(a)   (b)

FIGURE 17-2 It is important that the group leader encourage friends and family to visit because they can help in reality orientation, they provide socialization, and they can supply the closeness and touch that are needed. (*Courtesy of Anthony J. Skirlick, Jr.*)

HELPFUL PROPS IN GROUP WORK WITH REGRESSED AGED PEOPLE

Some leaders have found that props are useful for several reasons. Props do provide some structure to the group, and structure helps to lower anxiety in both leader and the group members. Props are also important because they provide much needed stimuli in environments that may be quite sterile for the residents (Burnside, 1969b). Props offer variety and they launch subjects for discussion. Those which provide sensory stimulation in more than one sense are to be considered, for example, the aroma of a cigar, the taste of champagne (preferably pink champagne, as it can be seen better), cologne for the women, and shaving lotion for the men. Music and records are enjoyed, and invariably patients will begin to tap out the rhythm with their feet or clap their hands. Food and beverages, as previously stated, are important means to reach these persons. Jokes can often be enjoyed. Exercises in drawing can be surprisingly successful, but one has to be careful that there are not too many persons in the group who cannot use their hands. For instance stroke victims, those with parkinsonism, or arthritic

persons could not easily participate in such an exercise. There are, however, simple exercises that can be done by a person in a wheelchair which would be helpful.

Visual stimuli, pictures, photographs, slides may need to be carefully selected. I found that one group was not interested in slides I had taken of them. It could have been a visual problem; i.e., they could not see the slides very well. On the other hand it could have been that they did not wish to see themselves in their present state, or it may have been that they were anxious because for the first time I had changed the group's meeting place and moved participants to a dark room. In fact, the move so disoriented one of the less stable members that she kept trying to get out of the room and would walk into the wall on which the pictures were being shown.

LOCATION OF GROUPS

Group work with such frail aged persons is usually in long-term care institutions, but a leader could seek out a similar group in a psychiatric day-care center for the aged or perhaps other appropriate places. There are elderly confused persons living in old rundown hotels in the geriatric ghettos of our inner cities; perhaps there are old persons in prison, although no one has told me about them.

CONTRACT FORMATION

A contract is an agreement between the leader and a member concerning the group experience and needs to include a thorough explanation of the group's objectives (Burnside, 1978a). It is important for the group leader to meet each person individually and to evaluate the person's potential for group membership. Contract formation with the regressed aged is an arduous task in itself, because interviewing them can be so difficult (Burnside, 1980). Whether the leader is understood or not, an initial contact should be made and then an effort to negotiate a contract with the individual for group participation should be attempted. The staff gave me a list of people they thought might have some potential for group, and screened out the persons who were incontinent, too agitated to sit still, or too feeble to tolerate the stress of sitting among strangers. The new leader then should double-check the persons on the list. Sometimes staff members encouraged me to take a certain person into the group. When I have taken a patient into a group against my better judgment, I have almost always regretted it. On the other hand, I have had patients who wanted to be in the group—apparently from things they heard, or just from observing the festivity. One patient, who was not in the group, used to greet me, "Well, I see that you are having the party again."

GOALS

Whitaker and Lieberman (1964) wrote, "The purpose of the therapy group is to establish conditions under which each patient can change. Hopefully, each patient can achieve a less painful existence, learn new behavior, and learn to think of himself and others in new terms."

The most difficult aspect of goal setting for the regressed aged is to keep all the goals realistic enough to be fulfilling experiences for both the leader and the members. Student nurses may become depressed, discouraged, or both when they begin to work with the aged; therefore, every effort must be made to prevent the new group leader from feeling overwhelmed. Leaders should not complete their group experiences with a sense of failure. Once we realize that improving the quality of any aged person's life is a viable goal in itself, we will have made progress. Also, if the new leader can realize the challenge that exists in reaching regressed aged persons, the experience can take on added meaning, for the challenge with these regressed persons is just as great as is the challenge with regressed schizophrenics. Birren (1973) once described my group work with regressed aged as "ego-enhancing." That in itself could be a goal.

A very intellectual verbal leader bent on reaching preset goals would be detrimental as a group leader for regressed aged persons. The leader also should plan on a reasonable length of time in which to conduct the group and to allow group processes to evolve. The time needed to develop trust and to "catch on" to what the group is all about takes much longer for regressed elderly than it does with alert elderly. Usually, 10-week groups, run for research purposes, leave a lot to be desired. Plans should be made concerning continuation of the groups or other activities to replace the group meetings when the group leader terminates.

The goals originally lined up for one group were as follows: (1) to increase the various kinds of stimuli for these people to see if they would become more alert and responsive; (2) to consistently reality test; and (3) to use food as an adjunct to group therapy (Burnside, 1973b). In the past I had always found that food and beverages were important in group work with the aged in institutions. The people in this group were on five meals a day; therefore, at first we had only coffee. Later I changed the time of the meetings and introduced a variety of sweets and beverages.

PROBLEMS

There are many different problems in group work with the alert aged that one does not encounter with younger persons; namely, sensory deficits and diminished mobility. These problems are rampant in the regressed aged! *The leader must expect to deal immediately with diminished vision, hearing, and mobility.* There are other problem areas, and leaders have to cope with them in their own ways, trying various interventions to discover which ones work best for that particular group. Other problems could include relatives, staff behavior, visitors, and crises in the individual or in the milieu. One particular difficulty is the problem of assessing the anxiety of the aged person who is frail both mentally and physically.

Anxiety has been covered in detail in Chapter 5. Keen observation is required to assess the cues of anxiety in the aged person and most especially the anxiety of the wheelchair patient or the mute person.

The slowness of pace necessary for both the member and leader may require the leader to carefully consider his or her intentions. A group of aged regressed persons requires even more gentle handling and slower pace by the leader than a group of alert elderly. Working with such a frail group of elderly requires active participation by the leader.

Transportation problems are especially difficult if the staff does not help to get the patients to and from the meeting room. Many facilities are hard pressed for space, and in some institutions it is not always easy to find a large, quiet, warm, easily accessible room to use; yet these criteria for a meeting place are most important (Burnside, 1969a).

The leader also may have to tolerate staff negativism or disinterest or both. One is sometimes viewed by the staff as a rather sophisticated baby-sitter. Sometimes new leaders in a facility where the staff is not accustomed to group work (especially by nurses) face hostile beginnings. They may be looked on as being a threat by some of the staff members. Hostility may be manifested overtly or covertly by the staff. It is often necessary to prove one's self before the staff seems to take any interest in the project.

The leader will also receive information from the regular employees about the individuals in the groups selected, which may not correlate with his or her own observations. "He hallucinates all of the time," the leader may be told, but upon checking it out, find that the patient hallucinates more at night and when he is alone in his room. "She is out of it; she does not understand a thing." Yet, in a group meeting this woman might be a gracious hostess and help serve coffee and sweets or be the one to go and shut the door when it is noisy outside. Because generalization of patients' behavior by staff members is fairly common, the new leader must always think of the person as seen in the group, and not as described by staff. Reading charts before beginning a group can sometimes influence one in the wrong direction, as much charting is negative, repetitive, meaningless, or all these.

SUPERVISION IMPORTANT

Supervision is an important aspect of new situations and learning experiences, and guidance from a group leader is very helpful. Although each group develops its own distinct personality and each leader has a particular style, some guidelines can be helpful. Steffl (1978) wrote about her experiences in preparing students for group work under educated supervision.

SILENCES

The long silences which occur in such a group must be comfortable for all. Silences are usually comfortable for the members, for they are used to sitting all day long among people and being silent, but this is not so with the leader. Practice in handling silence is an essential component of expert leadership with the regressed aged. The poem "Baroque Pearls" describes such a silence (Burnside, 1973a):

Words come infrequently—if at all,
And often with effort so great
I wish I had opted for silence.
But they teach me that
Silence is its own communion.
One blind member talks to God.
Time has faded their eyes.
If they will look at me,
They remind me of yesterday's smooth lusterless
*   stones*
From my walk on the beach.

STUDY OF HUMAN BEHAVIOR

It is easy to consider any group work with the regressed aged as simply a remotivation or reality orientation group. Reality orientation and remotivation are components of it, to be sure, but it is more because it involves studying human behavior, responding to it, altering one's own behavior if necessary, and continually role modeling for the group and the staff members. If the behavior of the aged in the group does not change appreciably, the leader should not be discouraged, because changes in affect are not readily discernible. The slides taken during the 14 months of group work with one group demonstrated that quite vividly. Changes from depressed miens to some smiling faces, from apathy to greater interest and alertness, and in personal appearances as time went on were apparent. The staff should be warned that there will be no miracles and that at no time will the leader walk on water (perhaps this should be reconsidered, if there are incontinent patients in a group). Realistic expectations by staff and leaders are most important. If a preceptor is involved, there should be realistic expectations of student performances by the instructor. Instructors in gerontological nursing will have to do all they can to ensure "success" in student nursing experiences with the aged because we so desperately need them in the field of gerontology.

I have described my own personal struggle to solidify a style of group leadership with regressed aged people in institutions. In these groups, I have intervened in depression, paranoia, illusions, babbling, muteness, incoherence, disorientation, and delusions of semigrandeur. The physical frailties have been too numerous to enumerate, but I have also found the human qualities that are often ignored or not seen in regressed old people. In these groups I have found dignity, in spite of massive traumas and losses (and memory loss is a great trauma), faith, forebearance, gentleness, concern for one another, humor, responsiveness, willingness to try new things with me, spontaneity, trust, and sometimes, but not often, a glimmer of hope. Always I found appreciation and gratitude from the aged group members for what I brought to the group. As Mrs. S. always said when she got close enough to see me, "God love you, I know who you are, but I just can't remember your name. I am glad you came." In the 14 months I led the group she never knew my name, but she did know me as a leader and friend, which was more important.

Few of the persons in the groups described in this chapter were discharged from the facility. The greatest changes noted were in the affective states. To change the affective state of an elderly regressed person is a valid reason for a nurse to attempt group work with this frail neglected group of people.

REFERENCES

Barnett, Kathryn: A survey of the current utilization of touch by health team personnel with hospitalized patients, *International Journal of Nursing Studies,* **9**:195–209, 1972a.

————: A theoretical construct of the concept of touch as they relate to nursing, *Nursing Research,* **21**:102–110, March–April, 1972b.

Birren, James E.: Aging: issues and concepts, Andrus Gerontology Center conference, Sheraton-Universal Hotel, North Hollywood, Calif., January 1973.

Burnside, Irene M.: "Baroque Pearls," *American Journal of Nursing,* **73**:2061, December 1973a.

————: Contracts for group work, in Irene Mortenson Burnside (ed.), *Working with the Elderly: Group Process and Techniques,* Duxbury, North Scituate, Mass., 1978a.

————: Group work among the aged, *Nursing Outlook,* **17**:68–72, June 1969a.

————: Group work with the aged: Selected literature, *Gerontologist,* **1**:241–246, Fall 1970.

————: Group work with the mentally impaired elderly, in Irene Mortenson Burnside (ed.), *Working with the Elderly: Group Process and Techniques,* Duxbury, North Scituate, Mass., 1978b.

————: History and overview of group work with the elderly, in Irene Mortenson Burnside (ed.), *Working with the Elderly: Group Process and Techniques,* Duxbury, North Scituate, Mass., 1978c.

————: Interviewing the confused aged person, in Irene M. Burnside (ed.), *Psychosocial Nursing Care of the Aged,* McGraw-Hill, New York, 1980, pp. 19–33.

————: Sensory stimulation: An adjunct to group work with the disabled aged, *Mental Hygiene,* **54**:381–388, June 1969b.

————: Touching is talking, *American Journal of Nursing,* **73**:2060–2063, December 1973b.

Butler, Robert N.: Mission of the National Institute on

Aging, *Journal of American Geriatrics Society,* **XXV**(3):97–103, March 1977.

Goldfarb, Alvin I.: Group therapy with the old and aged, in Harold I. Kaplan (ed.), *Comprehensive Group Psychotherapy,* Williams & Wilkins, Baltimore, 1971.

Greenberg Barbara M.: Therapeutic effects of touch on alteration of psychotic behavior in institutionalized elderly patients, unpublished master's thesis, Duke University, Durham, N.C., 1972.

Linden, Maurice E.: Geriatrics, in S. R. Slauson (ed.), *The Fields of Group Psychotherapy,* International Universities, New York, 1956.

McCorkle, Ruth M.: The effects of touch on seriously ill patients, unpublished master's thesis, University of Iowa, Iowa City, 1972.

Silver, A.: Group psychotherapy with senile psychiatric patients, *Geriatrics,* **5**:147–150, 1950.

Steffl, Bernita M.: Perspectives on group work in professional curricula, in Irene Mortenson Burnside (ed.), *Working with the Elderly: Group Process and Techniques,* Duxbury, North Scituate, Mass., 1978.

Taulbee, Lucille: Reorientation means independence and dignity, *Modern Nursing Home,* pp. 50–51, September 1973.

Whitaker, Dorothy S., and Morton A. Lieberman: *Psychotherapy through Group Process,* Atherton, New York, 1964, p. 161.

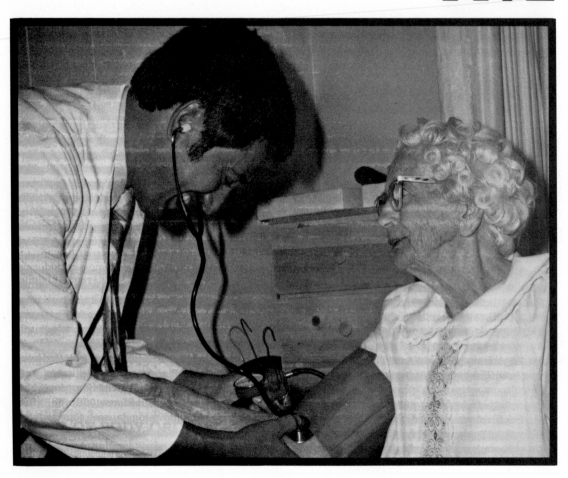

FIVE

Will Patton

SPECIAL CONCERNS OF THE AGED: THEORY AND THERAPY

For illness runs like a thread through every life; in
some it is a thin gossamer, barely discernible
filament; in others it is like a heavy line which, as it
grows with time, loops, bends, and strangles.

Alvin I. Goldfarb, M.D.

EIGHTEEN

CARDIO-PULMONARY ABNORMALITIES IN AGING

Sharon L. Roberts

Aging is a part of living. All living matter ages, and, as it ages, changes. . . . It begins with conception and ends only with death. Thus growth, development and maturation are just as much consequences of the occult processes of aging as are the atrophies and the degenerations of senility.
Edward Stieglitz

LEARNING OBJECTIVES

- Discuss the cardiac parameters used in assessing cardiac status of the aged individual.
- Discuss the pulmonary parameters used in assessing pulmonary status of the aged.
- Discuss bronchopulmonary movement, pulmonary function, and bronchoelimination as they change according to the aging process.
- List four major cardiac abnormalities associated with the aging process.
- Discuss four major cardiac abnormalities associated with the aging process.
- List three major pulmonary abnormalities associated with the aging process.
- Discuss three major pulmonary abnormalities associated with the aging process.
- Discuss each component of FANCAP as it specifically applies to the aged individual with cardiopulmonary disturbances.
- Construct a nursing care plan or assessment tool around the concept FANCAP.

As we nurses explore various nursing approaches to ensure the safety and well-being of the aged patient, we are, in fact, safeguarding our own future. The future of today's aged individual is threatened by the leading pathophysiological problem, namely, heart disease.

In discussing cardiopulmonary abnormalities of aging, I would like to focus on three general areas. First, the nurse needs to have a basic knowledge of the physiological changes involved in the aging heart and lungs. Attaining such knowledge requires a discussion of both cardiac and pulmonary parameters in the aging individual. The parameters provide the nurse with a physiological basis for nursing interventions. For example, if the nurse understands that the aged patient expends 70 percent of elastic work in moving the chest during breathing versus 40 percent expended by a younger individual, the nurse is better motivated to protect the patient from overexpenditure of valuable energy in other less significant ways. Second, since space does not permit a lengthy discussion of all cardiopulmonary abnormalities confronting the aged patient and the nurse, only major pathophysiological abnormalities will be discussed. And last, nursing and medical interventions will be discussed under the concept FANCAP, an acronym standing for *f*luids, *a*ctivity, *n*utrition, *c*ommunication, *a*eration, and *p*ain, originally developed by Professor June Abbey at the University of California, School of Nursing, San Francisco.

THE AGING CARDIOPULMONARY SYSTEM

Even though the health team cannot counteract the natural process of aging, life may be prolonged and disability reduced by improved nursing and medical care of the patient's cardiac and pulmonary dysfunction or disease. Improved care implies better understanding of the aging process and particular features pertaining to cardiac and pulmonary disease. One hopes that in the near future, death due to cardiopulmonary abnormalities and the high cost of such abnormalities will be reduced for the aged patient. Since the cardiac and pulmonary systems are closely interrelated, it is difficult to discuss one system without referring to the other. Even though heart disease is the leading cause of death in people over age 65, it can also lead to secondary pulmonary abnormalities. Likewise, pulmonary abnormalities subsequently can lead to cardiac abnormalities. For example, the individual's ability to exercise and maintain physical mobility depends on a normally functioning pulmonary system. Exercise in turn helps to sustain an adequately functioning cardiovascular system. Therefore, alteration in the individual's pulmonary system creates alteration in the cardiac system. Each major system has its own normal aging parameters. These parameters give the nurse insight into why certain physiological responses occur when the systems are placed under stress, whether the stress be internal or external.

CARDIAC PARAMETERS IN AGING

Harris (1971), in his discussion of cardiac parameters of aging, focuses on three major areas: (1) gross and microscopic structure of the heart, including heart size, endocardial changes, and valves; (2) physiological characteristics; and (3) the electrocardiogram. Each cardiac parameter leads into eventual discussion of major cardiac abnormalities confronting the aged individual.

Changes in the gross and microscopic structure of the heart develop as a result of hemodynamic stress and the aging process. It is interesting that hearts once enlarged from valvular heart disease, stress, or hypertension may shrink in old age. Such shrinkage may be the result of rest and reduced activity. It is also the result of cardiac atrophy due to prolonged illness, immobility, or malnutrition. The gross appearance of the heart changes with age. Harris (1971) states,

Fat appears at the entry of the pulmonary veins, the superior vena cava posteriorly, the base of the aorta, and extends from the left circumflex coronary artery upward over the left atrium to involve the region of the sinoatrial nodes and the intercaval band.

Endocardial changes also occur with aging. Such changes are the result of hemodynamic stress on the endocardium itself. Eventually, endocardial thickening and sclerosis develop. These appear as white patches and can be found in the endocardium, left atrium, right atrium, papillary muscles, and apical endocardium of the left ventricle (Harris, 1971).

The last change in the heart's structure deals with the valves. Like the endocardium, the valves are subjected to hemodynamic stress. In addition, the valves become more rigid and thickened owing to sclerosis and fibrosis (McMillan and Lev, 1964; Sell and Scully, 1965). The mitral valve is most severely affected. "In old age, there is marked thickening of the base of the aortic cusps. . . . These changes, due to aging, distort the mitral and aortic valves, render the valve closing less accurate and produce murmurs simulating acquired heart disease" (Harris, 1971). Any additional burden on the aged individual's heart valves, such as infection, pneumonia, and pulmonary hypertension, could lead to congestive heart failure. Therefore, the nurse must protect the aged patient from additional stress upon an already stressed cardiac or pulmonary system.

According to Harris (1961), the aging heart can function adequately in most older people as long as the coronary system is not damaged. Certain physiological alterations may occur with age, and these alterations have implications for nursing. The following are the most significant alterations:

1. The cardiac reserve diminishes and the heart reacts poorly to sudden stress (Harris, 1971).
2. The estimated left ventricular work declines at rest (Landowne, Brandfonbrener, and Shock, 1955).
3. The maximum blood flow through the coronary artery tree at the age of 60 is about 35 percent lower than in youth (Dock, 1941; 1956).
4. The aged myocardium shows a delay in the recovery of contractility and irritability. Despite its slow rate of recovery it functions well when there is an adequate period of rest between beats, but reacts poorly to tachycardia (Harris, 1971).
5. The heart is less sensitive to the effect of atropine and more sensitive to carotid sinus stimulation (Harris, 1971).
6. The aged heart has a decreased ability to utilize oxygen (Harris, 1971).

Additional physiological alterations have to do with blood pressure in the aged individual. Blood pressure measurement in the aging individual depends on loss of elasticity in walls of the larger arteries and the increased lability of vasopressor control. In extreme old age an individual's blood pressure may vary between 100 and 140 mmHg systolic and 70 and 90 mmHg diastolic (Harris, 1971).

The last cardiac parameter of aging to be discussed here deals with the electrocardiogram. Harris (1971) wrote,

In general, the normal electrocardiogram of the aged has no characteristics that distinguish it from that of younger persons. With aging, minor electrocardiographic changes may result from the cellular changes of age, neurogenic effects and minor fibrosis of the conduction system. The voltages of all waves may be diminished and there may be a slight prolongation of all intervals due to slowing of impulse conduction through the pacemaker, conduction system and the myocardium.

When changes do occur they may indicate myocardial damage, ischemia, or myocardial infarction. The changes may be a result of fibrosis or diminished coronary artery blood flow.

PULMONARY PARAMETERS IN AGING

Balchum (1971) discusses pulmonary parameters of the aging lungs. He divides these areas into three categories: first, changes in lung structure and function with age; gaseous exchange and pulmonary circulation; and homeostasis and ventilatory control.

Some of the more significant alterations in lung structure discussed by Balchum deal with elasticity and functioning, the control of ventilation, and capacity of the aged individual to exercise. The alterations have greater implications for the patient whose pulmonary system is compromised because of stress or illness. The aged lungs lose their elasticity. "The elasticity of the lungs is in part dependent upon the nature, properties, and arrangement of its connective tissue. This consists mainly of collagen (or fibrous protein) and elastin."

In terms of functional changes in the aging lung Balchum (1971) claims, "There is a decline in degree of osmotic swelling or absorption of water in collagen with aging." The pulmonary vasculature also changes with age. During the aging process there occurs a loss of elastic tissue in the blood vessels. Because the elastic fibers split, their extensibility decreases approximately 50 percent. Eventually what happens is intimal fibrosis of the pulmonary arteries and enlargement of both pulmonary arterioles and venules. Subsequently, progressive arteriosclerosis with aging occurs. According to Balchum (1971),

> Alterations in the properties and distribution of elastin result in a decrease in lung elasticity and a change in the volume pressure behavior of the lungs. . . . There is fairly general agreement that the elasticity or compliance of the chest wall decreases with age, the reduction being slightly greater than the increase in lung distensibility. This results in the total thoracic compliance being only slightly decreased in older individuals.

The nurse must realize that the aged patient may not have sufficient energy to maintain an adequate level of ventilation. In addition, since the patient's energy level may be compromised owing to other diseases, the nurse must actively seek to provide an environment conducive to energy conservation.

Balchum (1971) discusses the second pulmonary parameter in aging, i.e., gaseous exchange and pulmonary circulation. Pulmonary diffusing capacity between the air in the alveoli and the pulmonary capillary blood depends upon the surface area of capillaries exposed to ventilated alveoli. Cohn et al. (1954) and Chosy, Gee, and Rankin (1963) state that there is with age "a decrease in diffusing capacity with age which amounts to about 8 percent per decade." Furthermore, writes Balchum (1971), "the decrease in gas transfer may be due to a loss of lung capillaries with aging."

This pulmonary parameter is significant to the nurse caring for the aged patient with a pathological condition of the lungs, e.g., emphysema. The nurse, realizing that both normal aging and pulmonary pathological conditions reduce diffusion, must intervene to facilitate diffusion or to support its existence. The nurse may pay particular attention to the patient's blood gases, especially the pO_2 level. In addition to reduction in diffusion capacity, underventilation of the alveoli of the lower lung fields or bases occurs. Gravity is an important influence because that area of lung which is dependent is more poorly ventilated, in part owing to the weight of lung above it. However, it is better perfused because of the hydrostatic pressure of the weight of the volume of blood reaching from the dependent point to the right atrium. "With aging, lung elasticity decreases to a point where the smaller bronchioli are not held open by the now lessened force of lung recoil" (Balchum, 1971).

The last pulmonary parameter deals with homeostasis and ventilatory control. "Acid-base balance, pCO_2, and plasma and total blood volume do not significantly change with advancing years. However, even moderate stress may be less well handled in old age. . . . The bellows function decreases, ventilation capacity becomes less, the lungs lose part of their retractive force, and the chest wall becomes less compliant" (Balchum, 1971). Table 18-1 lists some of the physiological considerations of the pulmonary system during the aging process.

Both cardiac and pulmonary parameters clearly indicate how aging processes alter the function of each system. Stress, such as major illness specific to the cardiopulmonary system superimposed on reduced function, may seriously incapacitate the aged patient.

MAJOR CARDIOPULMONARY ABNORMALITIES

According to Bickerman (1952), Saxton has defined "a disease of old age in a species as one which increases in frequency and/or severity to the end of the life span; and depending on the organ or system affected and upon the degree of interference with function of a vital organ, may become a determining factor of that life span." One of the leading diseases causing death in the aged individual is heart disease; other major health problems of the aged are pulmonary cancer and emphysema.

TABLE 18-1

PHYSIOLOGICAL CONSIDERATIONS AS INFLUENCED BY AGING

Physiological Consideration	Aging Process
I. Bronchopulmonary movement	Reduction in movement due to increase in fibrous connective tissue and lymphoid elements; both factors leading to rigid and stiff bronchopulmonary tree
II. Pulmonary function A. Ventilatory function involving the exchange of air between lungs and environment	Reduced due to obstruction of pulmonary airway or restriction in pulmonary expansion and contraction
1. Lung volumes a. Vital capacity: the maximal volume of air expired after maximal inspiration	Decreases with age.
b. Residual air: the volume of air remaining in lungs following maximum expiration	Increase with age
c. Maximum breathing capacity: largest volume of air moving in and out of chest	Negative correlation with age
B. Respiratory gas exchange function which is concerned with distribution of air to functioning alveoli, and diffusion of gases across alveolocapillary membrane	Impairment due to underventilation of well-perfused alveoli or overventilation of portions of lung receiving little or no blood
1. Distributory and diffusion factors a. Index of intrapulmonary mixing: index of distribution of tidal air through alveolar spaces during quiet breathing	Factors altering intrapulmonary mixing: decreased elasticity; regional obstruction to air flow; decreased expansibility of certain areas
b. Respiratory gas exchange consisting of relationship between pulmonary ventilation and respiratory gases at rest and after exercise	Decreased respiratory rate; decrease in amount of expired CO_2; decrease in oxygen saturation
2. Elasticity and pressure-volume measurements	Impairment in pulmonary elasticity and decreased mobility of chest cage

III. Bronchoelimination
  A. Reflex activity
    1. Coughing
	Decreases due to diminished muscle tone and decreased sensitivity to stimuli

2. Ciliary mechanism	Effectiveness reduced due to drying and atrophy of epithelium

MAJOR CARDIAC ABNORMALITIES

Regardless of their causes, the two most important diseases that increase with age are (1) hypertension and aortic disease and (2) coronary artery disease with insufficiency or eventual myocardial infarction. Therefore the major cardiac abnormalities to be discussed are (1) hypertension; (2) coronary artery disease including myocardial infarction and congestive heart failure; (3) valvular disease; and (4) arrhythmias unique to the aged patient. It must be kept in mind that various factors contribute to heart disease. These factors include the aging process, disease or other precipitating factors such as infection, anemia, pneumonia, trauma, arrhythmias, surgery, emotional stress, fever, and diarrhea.

Hypertension Traditionally, hypertension has been defined as the elevation of arterial pressure above 150/90 mmHg. It seems that there is a continuum of increasing systolic, diastolic, and mean blood pressures which represents risk factors in the development of target organ damage. Therefore, hypertension is assessed to be a risk factor in the development of atherosclerotic disease of the brain, kidney, and heart.

According to Timiras (1972),

Many factors regulate blood pressure—blood viscosity and blood volume, cardiac output and elasticity of the arterial walls, peripheral resistance—and alterations in one or more of these parameters may induce a hypertensive condition. . . . Of particular interest in the genesis of hypertension, especially in the aged, are changes in peripheral resistance, which is normally regulated by circulatory adjustments effected, in turn, by neural and chemical mechanisms that change the caliber of the blood vessels, especially the arterioles, responsible for the maintenance of peripheral resistance.

Any changes in constriction of arterioles obviously result in alteration of arteriolar caliber and can then cause large changes in total peripheral resistance. In the aged individual, arteriosclerotic changes in the arteries and arterioles cause a decrease in the caliber of these vessels. Consequently arteriosclerosis signifies one of the principal causes of hypertension in the aged patient. Besides changes in the arteriolar caliber leading to hypertension in the aged, the abnormality may also be associated with other age-related changes. Furthermore according to Timiras (1972),

For instance, a diseased kidney, whether due to infection, circulatory disturbances, or congenital lesions, increases the production of pressor substances and thereby may lead to arteriolar vasoconstriction; or the hyperfunction of an endocrine organ inducing abnormally high blood levels of hormones . . . is also capable of raising blood pressure. Infections and circulatory disturbances of the kidney are frequent in old people.

Hypertensive arterial disease is one of the most urgent health problems of the aged individual. The abnormality is urgent in the sense that it impairs circulation to vital organs of the body. According to Harris (1971), "hypertension impairs circulation in the brain, heart and kidneys, increases cardiac work, precipitates congestive failure and aggravates arteriosclerosis. . . . Hypertension should be diagnosed only when a diastolic pressure over 95 mmHg and a systolic pressure over 170 mmHg are repeatedly found in the patient during several visits." The aged patient's blood pressure may fluctuate widely. It is when such elevation persists that arterial hypertension is diagnosed. In addition to hypertension being persistent, it may create other symptoms or consequences. The major symptoms or consequences of hypertensive disease arise from neurologic, cardiac, and renal injury.

Neurological symptoms of hypertension include impairment of memory, dull morning headache, and a slow coarse tremor. Nurses may instruct aged patients about an aspect of their care, only to discover that they cannot remember the instruction. During hypertensive periods, aged patients may have difficulty remembering which medications they took or when they last took them. Such lapses of memory can lead to serious problems. Tremors may frustrate patients and cause them to accidently drop objects. Consequently, nurses must alleviate patients' frustrations and protect them from unnecessary injury. Hypertension may even lead to disorientation or confusion. Such behavior may already be compounded by existing arteriosclerosis, resulting in cerebral insufficiency.

Prolonged hypertension in the aged can lead to hypertensive encephalopathy and is associated with some degree of cerebral edema. Two subproblems which may occur with arterial hypertension are worth mentioning. These problems or changes are cerebral apoplexy and injury to the eye. The aged patient may present symptoms of retinal hemorrhage, headaches, and epistaxis. Cerebral problems associated with hypertension can be due to hemorrhage, thrombosis, or embolism. The resulting effects are due to sudden ischemia to the brain, causing necrosis of the nervous tissue in the immediate vicinity and diffuse cerebral edema. The peripheral functional loss (paralysis, aphasia, sensory disturbance) due to destruction of nerve cells is permanent. The nurse needs to make frequent assessment of the individual's blood pressure and whether other symptoms directly caused by hypertension are present. Furthermore, these patients need constant reassurance and encouragement, since they live in fear of repeated hypertensive crises with their accompanying symptoms.

The second neurological subproblem associated with hypertension is injury to the aged patient's eyes. The symptoms may be compounded by visual changes that normally occur with aging. In any respect the patient experiences blurring of vision. Again the nurse must protect the patient from injury associated with poor vision.

The second consequence of hypertension involves cardiac injury. Hypertension eventually leads to impairment of nutrition and oxygenation of the myocardium. The aged patient's myocardium may not be able to keep pace with the increasing load of left ventricular work. The nurse discovers that the patient experiences dyspnea with less and less exertion. The aged patient may have difficulty moving from bed to commode or walking to the bathroom. Again rest periods may need to be provided so as not to overtax an already overcompensated heart. Therefore hypertension accelerates cardiac damage. Such cardiac damage takes the form of cardiac decompensation, angina pectoris, and coronary occlusion.

The last consequence of hypertension focuses on renal injury. Ischemia of renal tissue liberates a pressor substance. "The greater the renal anoxia, the greater the generation and/or the liberation of the pressor mediator and thus the greater the renal arteriolar constriction and the aggravation of the renal ischemia. This vicious circle undoubtedly constitutes a potent perpetuating force contributing to the persistent progression of the disorder" (Stieglitz, 1954). Hypertension as previously mentioned is not an isolated problem. Instead, it leads to other related problems; these were viewed as neurological, cardiac, and renal in nature.

Coronary Artery Disease Coronary atherosclerosis is a normal aspect of the aging process.

> The abnormality comes when the degree of coronary atherosclerosis is enough greater than the compensation afforded by an inadequate collateral circulation to cause symptoms or obvious signs; but happily it is also normal for a collateral circulation to develop rapidly enough to keep pace and so to bypass possible points of obstruction (White, 1952).

Atherosclerosis of the coronary arteries is the major cause of heart disease in the aged. It is important for the nurse to be aware of differences in symptoms presented by the aged patient versus those of the young adult or middle-aged patient. Each group of individuals may manifest different symptoms with the same problem. The symptoms in the aged may seem less severe because they deviate from the traditional angina. However, this does not negate their significance to either the patient or the nurse. Basically, symptoms of coronary atherosclerosis depend upon the amount of coronary artery disease and cerebral damage. According to Harris (1971),

> As in younger patients, angina pectoris may begin with substernal pressure, dyspnea or pain which radiates down the left arm and to the neck. In the extreme aged, reduced activity and greater collateral circulation decreased the incidence of angina pectoris. Coronary thrombosis should be suspected when angina pectoris persists or progresses. Acute coronary thrombosis is found in about 5 percent of patients in geriatric wards.

Pathy (1967) noted that another significant point of uniqueness is "an acute coronary occlusion in an older person presents with less pain but more dyspnea and congestive heart failure than in a younger person." Harris (1971) refers to the incidence of "silent" myocardial infarction in the aged. He believes that the decreased pain is due either to the patient's brain disease or to the extensive collateral circulation in the heart built up over the years.

Major abnormalities resulting from coronary artery disease include angina pectoris, myocardial infarction, and congestive heart failure. It is recognized that the latter abnormality can also occur as a result of hypertension or myocardial infarction, or both. The aged patient experiencing a myocardial infarction may present the traditional picture of precordial pain, accompanied by shock and a fall in blood pressure, and followed by fever and leukocytosis. The aged individual may not have sufficient myocardial reserve to survive an acute myocardial infarction. The nurse taking care of the aged patient with myocardial infarction must be aware of the poor prognostic signs manifested by the patient. Signs of a poor prognosis consist of severe shock, persistent dyspnea, severe cyanosis, persistent low blood pressure (90 mmHg or less systolic), acute left ventricular failure, rising fever, leukocytosis, arrhythmias, or congestive heart failure. The nurse must view these signs as not representing the normal picture of the myocardial infarction patient. Rather, the signs coupled with the individual's age produce a grave danger; therefore, the nurse must anticipate the potential problems in an effort to recognize and/or intervene to alleviate them. Myocardial infarction resulting in congestive heart failure may thrust the aged patient into frequent hospitalizations. It is not unusual to see the same patient hospitalized with congestive heart failure or pulmonary edema several times throughout the year.

Cardiac failure is a condition in which cardiac output is inadequate to meet the aged individual's metabolic demands. Cardiac failure involves risk factors associated with increased metabolic demands, increased preload, decreased compliance and contractility, and increased afterload. The causes of congestive heart failure in the aged patient can be grouped into two categories, as identified by Sharpe and Stieglitz (1954). The two groups consist of "(1) those giving rise to a lowering of effective output, resulting in low-output failure, and (2) those which tend greatly to increase peripheral blood flow, inducing high-output failure." Low-output failure includes such pathophysiological problems as valvular lesions, myocardial infarction, hypertension, and anoxemia due to anemia or to arteriosclerosis. Also contributing to low-output failure are diseases of the pulmonary circuit, such as pulmonary infarction and fibrosis, tumors, and arrhythmias with a rapid ventricular rate. On the other hand, Sharpe and Stieglitz say, "High-output failure may be due to fever, hyperthyroidism, excessive exertion or exercise, anemia, beriberi, pneumonia and emphysema, and arteriovenous shunt, including Paget's disease." Nurses may have greater influence in intervening to alleviate or minimize problems leading to high-output failure. They are in a position to detect early signs of fever, overexertion, and hypostatic pneumonia. All three of these problems, besides those previously cited, increase the workload beyond the capacity of the heart. The increased workload leads to high-output congestive failure. Knowing the physiological reasons leading to high-output failure, the nurse can intervene to prevent their occurrence by skillful care. How to intervene will be discussed under the heading "FANCAP: Nursing and Medical Care," in this chapter.

Valvular Disease   Bedford and Caird (1960) believe that much valvular heart disease in older people is due to rheumatic infection, syphilitic aortic insufficiency, and arteriosclerosis. Harris (1971) notes, "Valvular heart disease in the aged is less correctly diagnosed because most murmurs are attributed to arteriosclerosis, and other etiologies are overlooked." White (1952) states,

It is not rare to find either mitral or aortic valve disease in a person of 60 to 65 or even 70 years old which has been present ever since childhood; usually it is of less marked degree than the average, but nevertheless it may be clearly diagnosable. The commonest lesions so found are mitral stenosis of slight to moderate degree, aortic stenosis of slight to moderate degree and aortic or mitral regurgitation of slight or very slight degree.

It has been said that acute rheumatic fever and rheumatic heart disease constitute important facets of geriatric cardiology with a relatively high incidence of activity during the fifth to eighth decades of life (Rothschild, Kugel, and Gross, 1934; Adatto et al., 1965). The aged individual is affected differently by acute versus chronic rheumatic heart disease. Acute rheumatic fever in the aged can be recurrent. In addition, it is characterized by slight fever, moderate joint symptoms, and a low incidence of cardiac damage. On the other hand, chronic rheumatic heart disease follows a benign course; e.g., some aged individuals have had rheumatic heart disease for many years without symptoms. It is significant to note that, although rheumatic heart disease may be benign, the condition may become more critical as the individual develops hypertension or coronary artery disease. Harris (1971) says that according to Priest, "myocardial damage and valvular deformities from earlier attacks of rheumatic fever may remain dynamically insignificant until the addition of coronary or hypertensive cardiovascular disease in old age makes them serious."

The aged patient with rheumatic heart disease presents a different clinical picture than does the younger patient. The nurse should be familiar with both symptoms and problems unique to the aged rheumatic heart disease patient. Compensated rheumatic heart disease in the elderly shows clinically minimal cardiac lesions, dyspnea, and cyanosis because of emphysema, pulmonary arteriosclerosis, or anemic hypoxia (Kaufman and Poliakoff, 1950). In the aged the most common problems associated with rheumatic heart disease are congestive heart failure, pulmonary infarction, and pneumonia. The valves most often involved are the mitral and aortic. Aortic stenosis may be due to a combination of arteriosclerosis and rheumatic lesions or to arteriosclerosis alone. According to Kløvstad (1956), in uncomplicated mitral stenosis there may be no symptoms until death, and the disease is four times more frequent in older women than in men. The reason is a slower progression of coronary heart disease in women, also their greater longevity. When coronary artery disease, sclerosis, and calcification of rheumatic aortic lesions are added to an existing pathological condition of the heart, heart failure may develop. Such complications as coronary artery disease and advanced calcific aortic stenosis are two of the main causes of heart failure in old persons, and both increase in incidence and severity with age. These complications develop earlier and occur more frequently in men than in women. The aged patient with valvular disease due to rheumatic heart disease may have a relatively good prognosis. The factors supporting a good prognosis are the degree of physical mobility the patient enjoys and the presence of a normal heart rhythm. On the other hand, a poor prognosis is supported by the aged patient's inability to tolerate exercise and atrial fibrillation. The patient who is unable to tolerate exercise may enter the hospital experiencing severe dyspnea or congestive heart failure. It is not unusual to see the aged patient admitted to a cardiac care unit (CCU) with atrial fibrillation.

Arrhythmias The normal pulse rate is between 60 to 100 beats per minute. However, there are times when a sinus bradycardia of 30 beats per minute occurs in aged patients. The reduced rate may be found in aged patients on medication such as reserpine or digitalis, or with increased vagal tone, or with arteriosclerosis of the artery to the sinus node; or it may indicate heart block. Conversely, a heart rate of 90 beats per minute in an aged patient who normally maintains a rate of 50 per minute may constitute tachycardia.

According to Harris (1971),

The heart rhythm of most elderly patients with clinically normal hearts is sinus, but marked sinus arrhythmia due to arteriosclerosis of the artery to the sino-atrial node is frequently observed in the aged. Severe sinus bradycardia may be difficult to distinguish clinically from complete heart block. Both can cause vertigo, syncope of the Stokes-Adams type, runs of paroxysmal ventricular tachycardia, atrial flutter or fibrillation.

Sharpe and Stieglitz (1954) state,

Whereas cardiac arrhythmias in themselves may be either primary or functional, the most common cause of arrhythmia in older patients is myocardial damage. Conduction changes may be secondary to coronary vascular impairment with relative myocardial ischemia or may result from valvular incompetence with secondary involvement of the neurogenic mechanisms of cardiac function.

It was mentioned earlier that the aged patient's heart rate may decrease. As Carlson (1954) has pointed out,

The electrocardiogram shows lessened voltage and some slowing of conduction in old people. This probably indicates some impairment of the conductive system. On the other hand, there appears to be an increased sensitivity of the carotid sinus cardio-inhibitory reflex with the advancing years.

Conduction irregularities, such as premature contractions, tachycardia, atrial fibrillation, and heart block, increase in aged patients. These are the arrhythmias confronting the gerontological nurse. Premature contractions as they pertain to the aged patient are mainly atrial and ventricular in origin. Cardiac arrhythmias in old age are due to changes in the conduction system, e.g., muscle fibers losing their elasticity. Frequent atrial premature contractions can lead to paroxysmal or chronic atrial fibrillation. Ventricular extrasystoles are due to excessive use of tobacco, tea, coffee, and alcohol and to digestive disturbances. As Harris (1971) points out, "Unifocal ventricular extrasystoles are usually benign, but multifocal ventricular extrasystoles indicating myocardial damage or digitalis toxicity are bad prognostic signs foreshadowing a ventricular arrhythmia." The nurse, therefore, realizing that premature atrial contraction can indicate impending atrial fibrillation and that premature ventricular contractions can precede the more serious ventricular arrhythmias, must be on the alert to intervene.

Tachycardia in the aged patient can be of several types and can have various origins. The more significant types are paroxysmal atrial tachycardia and ventricular tachycardia. It is important to note that paroxysmal atrial tachycardia is not necessarily the result of heart disease. The nurse needs to realize that tachycardia may be a compensatory mechanism; for example, it may be due to hyperthyroidism, emotional disturbance, coronary artery disease, or congestive heart failure. In each instance, tachycardia is compensatory; when congestion is relieved, the heart rate becomes normal. Paroxysmal atrial tachycardia may then be advantageous for the aged patient. Prolonged tachycardia may have negative effects on the aged patient. It may lead to impairment of cerebral circulation, hypotension, and congestive heart failure. The latter problem may be due to increased workload on the patient's heart. The nurse, therefore, must be knowledgeable about the advantages and disadvantages of tachycardia on the aged patient. If tachycardia is permitted to continue, the nurse must be skillfully observant for signs and symptoms indicating cerebral perfusion impairment or congestive heart failure. Ventricular tachycardia is the most serious of all tachycardias. It is frequently associated with severe cardiac ischemia or infarction. The arrhythmia is serious in the sense that it is life threatening for any patient, regardless of his age.

The dominant arrhythmia of aging to be considered is atrial fibrillation. Atrial fibrillation is commonly associated with acute infection, surgical operations, cardiac ischemia, pulmonary embolism, thyrotoxicosis and heart failure, especially when due to rheumatic heart disease (Thompson, 1969). " 'Lone' atrial fibrillation is almost exclusively seen in the aged individual" (Harris, 1971). Aged patients may not realize that they are experiencing atrial fibrillation, because their heart rates are slow or otherwise described as atrial fibrillation with a slow ventricular response. Even though patients themselves may cope with the arrhythmia, the condition, atrial fibrillation, does carry with it some problems. The nurse must realize that atrial fibrillation interferes with the normal hemodynamics of the heart. The atrium dilates, and this can lead to intracranial clotting with the ultimate danger of embolism. It is not unusual for the nurse to see the geriatric patient suffer from cerebral embolism or microembolism in both mesenteric and renal arteries. Therefore, the nurse must observe for changes in color of urine, behavioral changes, or complaints of abdominal discomfort. The latter complaint may not be due to constipation, which is frequently associated with the aged; rather it may indicate the much more serious problem of infarcted bowel due to microembolism of the mesenteric artery.

The last conduction irregularity of the aged patient to be generally discussed is heart block. According to Lev (1964), heart block is usually attributed to arteriosclerosis, increased vagotonia, and changes in the cardiac skeleton. Harris (1971) believes,

> Digitalis and electrolyte imbalance should always be ruled out. Complete AV heart block is far more common in patients after 60. Older patients with heart block are most susceptible to cardiac standstill and Stokes-Adams attacks than are the younger adult. Syncope is often the presenting complaint in such patients.

Treatment associated with the major conduction irregularities will be discussed within the concept of FANCAP. Figure 18-1 summarizes major cardiac abnormalities affecting the aged patient.

MAJOR PULMONARY ABNORMALITIES

The pulmonary system involves several normal functions. These include ventilation, diffusion, distribution, and circulation. Ventilation is movement of air into and out of the alveoli. Diffusion is responsible for the exchange of gases across the alveolar-capillary membrane. The gases must be distributed evenly throughout the lungs. Lastly, circulation is responsible for disseminating oxygen-carrying hemoglobin throughout the lungs.

As Bickerman (1952) so aptly said, "The respiratory system in general and the lung in particular possesses an organ type physiologic time clock which governs the day to day inexorable alterations of senescence. Upon this base is engraved the countless insults of a hostile environment." It is difficult to know whether aging is primarily a genetic or environmental problem; however, we know that both play a vital role in the aging process. The lungs of the aged patient are more rigid. The rigid changes in the lungs coupled with reduction in muscle power create nursing-care problems. Since the aged patient suffers from a lessened ability to cough and breathe deeply, it becomes of particular concern when undergoing surgical correction for one or more cardiac abnormalities. The patient is prone to various respiratory complications. Besides res-

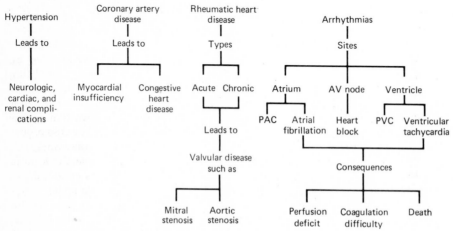

FIGURE 18-1 Major cardiac abnormalities affecting the aged patient.

piratory complications, the patient may enter the hospital with already existing pathophysiological pulmonary abnormalities. The primary pulmonary abnormalities to be discussed are lung cancer, bronchitis, and emphysema.

Lung Cancer Factors that lead to respiratory cancer are chronic damage to lung tissue resulting from scar formation, smoking, and environmental pollutants. There appears to be a relationship of scar tissue to lung cancer. Chronic damage to tissues, e.g., fibrosis, pneumonitis, and other causes of lung scarring, has been recognized as an important predisposing factor (Solovay and Solovay, 1965). The tumor may surround the scar and infiltrate the adjacent areas. Raeburn and Spencer (1957) suggest that as much as one-fourth the lung cancers are related to lung scars. The presenting symptoms are dyspnea and chronic cough. Other symptoms include a sense of heaviness and chest pain. At least three of the cited symptoms can be mistaken for impending cardiac abnormalities.

It is not surprising to learn that approximately 90 percent of individuals with lung cancer are also smokers. Research is still being done to determine the relationship of air pollution to lung cancer. Any relationship between the two is speculative; however, there is a relationship between heavy occupational exposures to dust containing radioactive materials, asbestos, chromates, and tar to an increased incidence of bronchogenic carcinoma.

Bronchitis Chronic bronchitis is the most common pulmonary abnormality of the aged. Christopherson and Broadbent (1934) do not believe that chronic bronchitis is a bacterial disease. They feel that it is due to continued irregularity of the vagus nerve and sympathetic nervous system. Along with bronchiectasis, emphysema, and asthma, it is considered to be a disturbance of the respiratory autonomic nervous system. The pathological findings of bronchitis are varied. For example, the mucous membrane may become atrophic or hypertropic; changes in the bronchial walls include fibrosis with occasional destruction of the muscle elements and extensive fibrotic replacement. With recurrent infection, all factors involved in raising sputum from the bronchial tree become impaired.

Clinically, the nurse sees symptoms of persistent cough and sputum production with or without dyspnea. Chronic bronchitis can be serious to the aged patient because it can result in airway obstruction severe enough to cause respiratory failure and death, even without emphysema. The pulmonary abnormality, chronic bronchitis, may be difficult to distinguish from emphysema. The physician may have difficulty determining whether emphysema is present in addition to chronic bronchitis. Probably the most frequent pulmonary abnormality seen by nurses in aged patients is emphysema. With the growing trend toward development of respiratory care units, more patients are seen with emphysema. In addition intensive care units are experiencing a rise in the number of aged patients with pulmonary emphysema.

Emphysema Emphysema increases progressively with age and reaches severity in the seventh decade. It is thought that the causes have a cumulative effect over a period of many years (Azcuy, Anderson, and Foraker, 1964). Increased residual volume and decreased vital capacity both are found in aged and emphysematous subjects, presumably because of alterations in lung elasticity. "The chief functional differences are usually a greater degree of flow resistance, more uneven ventilation of the lungs, and more diffusion impairment seen in emphysema, as compared to the changes seen with aging" (Balchum, 1971).

Kountz and Alexander (1934) have differentiated two forms of emphysema: (1) postural emphysema and (2) chronic hypertrophic or obstructive emphysema. The first form to be discussed is *postural emphysema*. Another name for postural emphysema is "senile" or "alveolar emphysema" and is often encountered in older patients. Some physiologists believe that practically all aging patients have some degree of emphysema. There are two views concerning the pathogenesis of postural emphysema. Kountz and Alexander (1934) believe this condition results from changes in the thoracic spine, especially in the intervertebral disks. The size of the thoracic cage is enlarged because of changes in the vertebrae and the lungs. As the lungs over-distend, there is thinning and atrophy of the alveolar septum with frequent rupture, usually at the free margins and periphery. Macklin and Macklin (1942) believe that "internal sclerotic" changes in the lung parenchyma are due to the increased fibrosis which limits normal movements of the tracheobronchial tree and includes the lung root. This fibrotic condition may be a part of the aging process. It could also be caused by numerous infections. The movement of the central portions of the lung is particularly hampered; only the periphery is able to expand along with the thoracic cage. The continuous stretching and overdistention of the peripheral alveoli cause a breakdown of the alveolar walls.

The second form of emphysema identified by Kountz and Alexander (1934) is *obstructive emphysema,* also called "chronic hypertrophic emphysema." There are two principal considerations involved in the pathogenesis of obstructive emphysema. The first is impairment in elasticity or retractility of the lung. The second is the existence of obstruction to the free flow of air in and out of the alveoli. Macklin and Macklin (1942) believe that intermittent or persistent spasm of the smooth muscle system will lead to narrowing of the air passages. The smooth muscle spasticity results from an inherited state of hypersensitivity or allergy. The disparity in force between the two phases of respiration causes air to be trapped within the lungs and not be completely evacuated during expiration. Overdistention of the lungs will eventually impair elastic recoil. Emphysema can be the result of single or repeated episodes of a pulmonary infection such as pneumonia. The nurse must keep in mind that any type of respiratory infection can produce obstruction. It becomes imperative that the nurse protect the patient from infection caused by hypostatic pneumonia, aspiration, or improper tracheal suctioning. Infection causes edema of the bronchial mucosa and infection superimposed on an already compromised pulmonary system could lead to severe complications for the aged patient. The nurse's goal becomes that of strengthening and maintaining the patient's pulmonary reserve. The nurse also realizes that a respiratory crisis increases the workload of the patient's heart. The patient who has had emphysema for a long period of time probably also has experienced cor

pulmonale. Thus both heart and lungs can become dangerously compromised with an infection.

The nurse's role is important in caring for the aged patient with cardiopulmonary abnormalities. It is through the nurse's creative intervention, knowledge of pathophysiology affecting the aged patient's cardiopulmonary system, and skillful implementation of medical therapy that the patient is restored to a level of wellness.

FANCAP: NURSING AND MEDICAL CARE

Nursing responsibilities are increasing in such dimension that today's nurses, no matter where they choose to work, are independent decision makers. Nurses are assuming responsibilities once belonging solely to physicians. The quality of care is improving to a high level. Today's nurses must understand patients' problems, needs, and treatments; but in addition, they must understand the human aspect of aged patients and focus on their total being. In nursing the aged patient with cardiopulmonary abnormalities, the nurse should attempt to support both psychosocial and physiological systems. Aged patients need to know that nurses view them as worthy and significant persons. Such emotional input helps to restore injured self-concept and torn integrity. Physiologically, the nurse has an even greater responsibility: to maintain and strengthen the patient's faltering cardiopulmonary system. Nursing care should be directed toward achieving and maintaining adequate circulation and ventilation. In order to accomplish these goals, the nurse must have an organized way of assessing the patient and implementing care. FANCAP becomes that organizing tool, a tool developed by June Abbey while teaching student nurses.

FLUID

Interstitial Edema The aged patient with cardiac abnormalities in particular often may have to endure interstitial edema. Interstitial edema can lead to such pulmonary complications as pulmonary edema. Since the patient already has diminished peripheral perfusion, peripheral edema eventually may lead to skin breakdown and ulcer formation. The nurse's goal is to decrease capillary venous pressure and pulmonary venous pressure. Mobilization of fluid in congestive heart failure is a potential hazard for the aged. Fluid associated with edema is not merely water, it also contains metabolic debris which is toxic. Too rapid mobilization of extensive edema may lead to profound intoxication and add further injury to an already seriously injured myocardium. The nurse can promote a decrease in capillary and pulmonary venous pressure by allowing the patient to sit up with the feet on a chair for support. This intervention promotes pooling of fluid in the abdominal cavity and extremities. Of course, the nurse realizes that interstitial edema resulting from pedal dependency can cause skin breakdown. The aged patient with sacral edema will need a change in position frequently to prevent additional skin breakdown due to pressure and poor tissue integrity.

Skin and back care are very important for the aged patient. The skin is assessed for pressure points and/or reddened areas. Skin care does not imply frequent bathing of the aged patient; on the contrary, frequent baths may be injurious to the patient, for they cause the skin to become rough, irritated, and prone to excoriation. Back care is of particular significance. Most aged patients with cardiopulmonary abnormalities find a degree of comfort by lying on their backs. Back care provides an opportunity for moving patients, stimulating them, and inducing subtle postural drainage from their lungs. Powder is not recommended for the patient who has a pulmonary condition or tracheostomy. The use of powder introduces the risk of inhaling an irritant. Beside providing effective skin and back care, the nurse must also provide care in returning an edematous patient to bed. As mentioned earlier, prolonged sitting in the upright position with legs dependent leads to peripheral edema. Therefore, the nurse must take particular care not to elevate an aged patient's extremities too quickly. Avoiding elevation of extremities avoids the possibility of right-sided congestive heart failure due to a rapid return of fluid to the heart.

Fluids that move into serous cavities, where infringement on respiration and/or cardiac function may occur, are best removed by thoracentesis. As Sharpe and Stieglitz (1954) remind us, "Caution against too rapid removal of intrathoracic fluid is important." The nurse should assess the patient for evidence of pain, dyspnea, or color changes during the procedure. Mechanical removal of fluid has two advantages over mobilization of fluids through diuresis. First, diuresis requires the heart to move all the fluid via the circulation to the kidneys. Second, diuresis may cause systemic intoxication subsequent to the movement of fluid from cavities to the bloodstream (Sharpe and Stieglitz, 1954). The aged patient with cardiopulmonary problems is subject to interstitial edema. The nurse's goal is to recognize its existence; to assess potential hazards from the problem itself and its treatment; and to provide care that serves to lessen its intensity or protect the system it most involves.

Intake Intake, as it applies to the fluid component of FANCAP, involves fluid intake both orally and parenterally, medications, and environmental intake. Type and amount of intravenous fluid depends upon the hydration level of the patient. The hydration status of the patient is assessed by comparing the relationship between total intake and output, by looking at skin turgor and mucous membranes, by comparing changes in daily weight, and by watching changes in vital signs, particularly arterial pressure and body temperature.

Fluid intake is very important to the aged patient. An inadequate consumption of water is common among hypertensive patients in general, and among the aged in particular. Water is probably the best, and certainly the safest, diuretic. In instances of cardiac impairment, water should be taken in small quantities at frequent intervals. With prolonged fluid restriction and diuretics, the aged patient can become seriously dehydrated. The dehydrated patient's skin will be warm and dry. In addition, body temperature may be elevated because heat can no longer be eliminated through evaporation of perspiration. Thirst is not always a reliable indicator of the need for fluid. Dryness of the pharyngeal membrane causes thirst, and dryness may be due to mouth breathing rather than from lack of fluids. A nurse may also assess the patient's hydration by checking the hematocrit, which is elevated in hemoconcentration; the urine specific gravity, which is increased if the urine is concentrated; and the blood pressure, which falls when the blood volume is markedly decreased (Secor, 1969).

Intravenous solutions may be infused simply to keep the veins open in the event of cardiopulmonary complications. In addition, they may be used to provide medication to lower blood pressure or reduce pulmonary impairment. The nurse must keep in mind that intravenous fluids should be administered slowly to eliminate danger of hypervolemia with congestive heart failure. Glucose solution should be terminated gradually. Too rapid infusion of glucose solution can lead to minor hyperinsulinism. The type of intravenous solution depends on the patient's unique problem. There is a trend with myocardial infarction patients to use what is referred to as *polarizing solutions.* A polarizing solution consists of 10% D_5W with 10 units of regular insulin and 20 to 30 meq potassium chloride (KCl). The solution has two basic functions. First, a 10% solution acts as a diuretic; second, insulin changes the permeability of the cell to foster the movement of potassium from extracellular fluid to intracellular fluid. With infarction resulting in tissue injury, potassium is liberated from the cardiac cell. Such movement increases toxic effects of digitalis and fosters creation of dangerous arrhythmias. The nurse's responsibility is to administer the proper amount, in the proper period of time, without overhydrating or underhydrating the patient.

The aged patient's condition may necessitate limited oral fluids. The amount of fluids received over a 24-hour period may be divided between parenteral and oral intake. The nurse must, therefore, carefully arrange the patient's oral intake to take place during meals and administration of medication. Because the patient may resent the need for curtailment of fluids, the nurse must carefully explain reasons behind the restriction. Fluids offered the patient should be taken into consideration. If a Foley catheter is inserted in the patient's bladder, the nurse may choose cranberry juice for the patient. Cranberry juice maintains an acid pH of urine in the blad-

der and thus prevents urinary calculi. Other juices to be offered, if possible, are orange and grape juice, both of which elevate the patient's potassium level. The aged patient may experience thirst. Thirst and dryness of mucous membranes are caused by several factors; they can be due to fluid restrictions, mouth breathing, or use of oxygen. Regardless of the reason, the nurse intervenes by offering the patient a cool cloth to suck on or by encouraging frequent oral hygiene.

The administration of medication is another significant aspect of fluid intake. A lengthy discussion of pertinent medications is not possible. Specific medications will be referred to and only those applicable to the aged patient in particular will be discussed. In addition to the type of medication prescribed, the route of administration is significant to the aged patient. Orally administered medications are absorbed more slowly and sometimes less completely. Urinary elimination is often retarded and diminished. Therefore, drugs are more likely to accumulate, especially if circulatory impairment is added to the effects of renal functional depreciation. Figure 18-2 indicates which drugs are of particular significance to the aged patient with cardiopulmonary abnormalities.

Drugs Primarily Affecting Cardiac System The goal in treating hypertension is gradually to reduce the pressure to the individual's optimal range. The intervention will help to control, if not prevent, the long-term cardiovascular consequences of uncontrolled hypertension. Such reduction avoids the hazards of hypotension. The nurse in monitoring the patient's blood pressure, degree of hypertension, and progress of treatment must remember that hypertension itself is a compensatory mechanism. The alteration of a compensatory mechanism may prove hazardous. According to Stieglitz (1954),

> Sclerotic arterioles cannot relax; too radical and too rapid reduction of pressure proximal to the arteriolar sluice gates dangerously impedes the circulation to the distal tissue cells. There is an optimum range for each individual, the lower limit determined by the physiologic necessity for compensatory

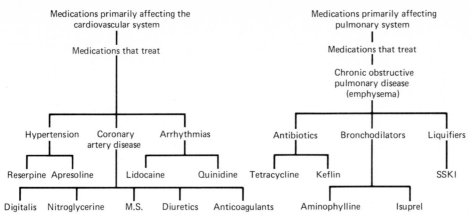

FIGURE 18-2 Medications of particular significance for the aged patient with cardiopulmonary abnormalities.

elevation of pressure, the upper limit by the margin of safety. As the disease progresses, these limits tend to draw together and the situation becomes increasingly precarious.

Since the desired outcome is gradually to reduce the aged patient's blood pressure, the nurse needs to accurately assess the patient's response to interventions and must skillfully assess the patient for signs of hypotension. These include such signs as dizziness, drowsiness, restlessness, or a rising level of blood urea nitrogen. The latter sign may indicate deterioration of renal function because of lower blood pressure. For diastolic hypertension with cerebral manifestations or congestive heart failure, greater salt restriction, reserpine, and diuretics are the treatment of choice. One of the problems with reserpine is that it may deplete the catecholamine content of the myocardium. Therefore, if the nurse observes sinus bradycardia, arrhythmias, or congestive heart failure, the physician should be notified and the drug stopped. If the patient should be more sensitive to effects of drugs than most others, potential side effects of antihypertensive drugs need to be weighed against their desired effects.

The elderly person's increased sensitivity to the effects of drugs on vascular, gastrointestinal, autonomic nervous systems, and the sphincter should be considered in the choice of medication. Ganglionic blocking agents, particularly those affecting the parasympathetic chain may produce urinary retention (usually in the elderly male with prostatic enlargement), constipation, diarrhea, and other distressing symptoms (Harris, 1971).

Digitalis is another important drug in treating cardiac abnormalities. It must be remembered that digitalis may not work in the elderly person with a badly damaged myocardium. In addition, the greater sensitivity of the aged cardiac patient to digitalis requires that smaller amounts be given. For the aged, digitalis is indicated in tachycardia or congestive heart failure if present. The nurse must assess the patient's response to digitalis. Any side effects, such as sinus bradycardia leading to congestive heart failure, arrhythmias, diarrhea, nausea, or visual changes, should indicate that digitalis be discontinued.

It is not unusual for the aged cardiac patient to experience angina. The drug most frequently utilized to relieve angina in the aged is nitroglycerin. Long-acting nitrates, which may not be as clinically effective as nitroglycerin, may be used in the aged patient with symptomatic coronary artery disease. A point of consideration is the relationship between long-acting nitrates and intraocular pressure. Since the long-acting nitrates tend to raise intraocular pressure, they should be avoided in the aged person with glaucoma. In addition, nitrates can also raise intracranial pressure, resulting in headaches or blood pressure changes or both. The nurse assumes the responsibility of recording how frequently the patient experiences angina necessitating nitroglycerin and the degree of relief attained. Depending upon the cognition level of the patient, the nurse may or may not leave a supply of nitroglycerin tablets at the bedside. The patient's alertness and ability to assume responsibility would need to be assessed carefully.

Diuretic mobilization and subsequent removal of fluid should be initiated early. The diuretic utilized depends on sensitivity of the patient, degree of edema, or acuteness of the patient's condition. There are various diuretics, ranging from the more potent furosemide (Lasix) or ethacrynic acid (Edecrin) to the mercurials. All the mercurial diuretics (e.g., Thiomerin) are toxic to the renal parenchyma and must be administered discriminately. The mercurial diuretics act upon the renal tubules by affecting the enzymatic processes concerned with transport and absorption of electrolytes. The nurse should keep in mind that diuretics may have serious side effects for the aged patient. For example, diuretics may aggravate dehydration; deplete important electrolytes such as sodium, potassium, and calcium; and elevate both blood sugar and uric acid levels. To avoid hazards of hypokalemia, the nurse should offer the patient orange juice or fresh bananas. The latter may lead to constipation in the aged patient. Therefore if fluid intake is possible, juices high in potassium content should be encouraged. Whenever possible hypokalemia is to be avoided in the cardiac patient on digitalis. The hypokalemic patient on digitalis is more vulnerable to digitalis toxicity and the problems that ensue.

Pain may be relieved with various types of analgesics or narcotics. Possibly, the most effective pain medication used in the treatment of acute myocardial infarction and congestive heart failure is morphine sulfate. Morphine may be utilized to alleviate the fear and restlessness associated with congestive heart failure. Dramatic improvements occur when morphine is given to the aged patient with pulmonary edema. The nurse must keep in mind that morphine produces an antidiuretic action and also a depressing effect on respirations. Interestingly, morphine may alleviate Cheyne-Stokes respirations sometimes associated with congestive

heart failure and tends to reduce the hyperpneic aspect of Cheyne-Stokes breathing, thus permitting the patient to sleep. The amount of morphine to be given must be taken into consideration. While morphine sulfate has its merits for the aged patient, it may also have its problems. Some aged patients may be sensitive to morphine and develop respiratory depression, hypotension, or urinary retention. As the intensity of pain subsides, meperidine (Demerol) may be substituted. The latter drug may suffice to reduce pain and constipating effects of morphine. Sedatives are not effective in reducing pain, for they lead to confusion in the aged patient with arteriosclerosis.

Anticoagulants, such as heparin or coumadin, are of little value in the average aged patient with acute coronary occlusion. According to Harris (1971),

Many old patients already have a reduced prothrombin time due to poor nutrition and liver damage or suffer from hematuria and melena which contraindicate anticoagulation therapy. Anticoagulants are best saved for elderly patients with shock, refractory heart failure, thromboembolic phenomena, a previous coronary thrombosis, or prolonged confinement to bed.

If anticoagulants are utilized, the nurse observes for any indications of side effects such as hematuria, bleeding gums, or bruises.

Lidocaine, Pronestyl, and quinidine sulfate are useful in the treatment of arrhythmias. Quinidine is useful if premature ventricular contractions or paroxysms of ventricular tachycardia occur in the absence of shock. Ventricular tachycardia is of concern to the nurse and patient because it can lead to ventricular fibrillation. Since quinidine is slow-acting, lidocaine may be safer in an attempt to prevent additional episodes of ventricular irritability.

Drugs Primarily Affecting Pulmonary System One major threat to the aged patient with pulmonary abnormalities is infection. Infection leads to unnecessary work for the pulmonary and cardiac system. Tetracycline and cephalothin (Keflin) are antibiotics employed in the treatment of such infections. Because many aged patients with emphysema have a persistent low-grade pulmonary infection, an acute exacerbation may not manifest itself beyond the symptoms of increased shortness of breath, changes in sputum, and increased cough. The nurses' goal is to protect patients from infection to which they are particularly vulnerable.

Bronchodilators relieve edema, swelling, and spasms associated with a chronic obstructive pulmonary disease such as emphysema. Aminophylline can be administered intravenously or rectally and isoproterenol (Isuprel) administered in the patient's nebulizer. Particular attention must be given to the patient receiving Isuprel, because it can lead to cardiac arrhythmias. Excessive use of nebulized bronchodilators should be avoided because the drug can produce the opposite effect. The mucosa becomes increasingly congested after the drug wears off.

Saturated solution of potassium iodide (SSKI) is used to thin secretions so that they can be better expectorated. Severe coughing may be very tiring to the already exhausted pulmonary patient. Such coughing may require administration of cough depressants. The nurse must assess the patient's cough in relation to its productiveness and in addition should assess the tenaciousness of expectorated secretions. If the nurse finds that secretions are excessive but cannot be removed through suctioning or coughing, a tracheostomy may be necessary.

Lastly, adrenal corticosteroids may be used in the treatment of emphysema. Prednisone is effective in relieving bronchial spasms; steroids help to reduce secretions and improve ventilation. Even though the therapy has its positive effects, it can be hazardous to the aged patient, who may not pay attention to signs indicating adverse reactions. The patient's primary concern is to relieve bronchial spasms and respiratory distress. Therefore, the patient may attribute rectal bleeding to hemorrhoids or the sharp pain in the stomach to indigestion. Both symptoms may indicate the larger problem of peptic or duodenal ulcer. The nurse must teach the patient the potential side effects of steroid therapy and the need for antacids. Together the nurse and patient should find the antacids that are best for the patient. Because some antacids cause either diarrhea or constipation, the antacids need to be alternated.

The last aspect of intake is environmental intake. Aged patients are taken from a familiar environment and placed in the unfamiliar world of a busy hospital. The environment may be frightening because it contains all the environmental props that remind them of their illness. These props consist of IPPB machine, IV apparatus, oxygen tubing, cardioscope, and restriction of visitors. Rightfully so, patients are concerned about their future biological status. Death may seem very close to patients who have severe respiratory insufficiency. As a result of such fear and anxiety, the patients' intake may be greatly reduced. They may fail to hear explanations regarding their progress and care and, therefore, may unintentionally disobey orders. Nurses need to accurately assess the origin of the patients' behavior. Confusion or defiance may be due to changes in blood gases, electrolyte imbalance, cerebral perfusion deficit, hypoxia, or hypotension. Once these possibilities have been eliminated, nurses can provide aged patients with support and encouragement. They need assurance that their biological integrity is stabilized.

Output   Output, as it relates to cardiopulmonary abnormalities, takes several forms. It involves fluid output, such as emesis, urine, and specific gravity; vital signs, including pulse, respiratory rate, temperature, arterial blood pressure, venous pressure, and weight; and information derived from laboratory studies.

Fluid or Volume Output   The aged patient with a cardiac abnormality, such as myocardial infarction or congestive heart failure, may experience nausea and vomiting. The amount and content of emesis should be recorded. Frequent emesis together with diuresis can contribute to the patient's dehydration and electrolyte imbalance. Vomiting may also increase the workload of the patient's heart, leading to the possible extension of myocardial infarction. The nurse also realizes that vomiting may be a side effect of one of the patient's drugs. If the latter is the origin of emesis, the nurse should report observations to the patient's physician. Vomiting may present problems unique to the aged patient with pulmonary abnormalities. Vomiting is produced by a sudden spasm of the diaphragm which momentarily halts respirations. Persistent vomiting or retching necessitates procedures for immediate relief because the breathing becomes irregular and rapid and aspirations can occur. Pulmonary patients may swallow their sputum, thus increasing their tendency to vomit. Nurses must assess the origin of patients' emesis, support them during the episode, and administer treatment to reduce its recurrence.

Urinary output is an important indicator of adequate or inadequate circulatory function. Besides assessing the amount of urinary output, the nurse also assesses the color, odor, and specific gravity. A reduction in urinary output may indicate renal problems associated with a perfusion deficit. Reduced urinary output together with concentrated urine can indicate dehydration. The nurse may need to assess the relationship between the patient's total volume intake and output including emesis, urine, or incidental, and may independently assess the specific gravity of the urine. Specific gravity provides information regarding the patient's level of hydration and ability of the kidney to remove wastes. A decreased output of urine may have specific implications for the aged male patient. He may have a concurrent prostatic disorder which leads to urine retention because of inability to completely empty his bladder. It may become necessary to insert a Foley catheter. The nurse must take great care in protecting the patient from unnecessary urinary tract infection due to improper catheter care.

The underhydrated patient may suffer from constipation. Constipation may be of particular importance to the aged patient with acute myocardial infarction. Straining may cause undue vagal stimulation leading to a slowing heart rate. The respiratory patient may be unable to strain at defecation because of weakness or fear that straining might cause dyspnea and coughing. Anal dilatation, as from the passage of feces, produces respiratory stimulation which could cause frightening breathlessness. Consequently, the nurse should assess the patient's bowel habits and assist in responding to the need to defecate. Both cardiac and pulmonary patients may suppress the need to defecate for fear of undesirable outcome. The patient's call light should be close at hand to signal for a nurse's assistance.

Vital Signs The patient's pulse provides information regarding cardiac and circulatory integrity and internal changes associated with pulmonary irregularities. An increase in pulse rate may indicate hypoxia, a need to be suctioned, presence of infection, impending cardiac failure due to pulmonary capillary hypertension (cor pulmonale), and shock from reduced cardiac output or blood loss. In addition, an increased heart rate may indicate airway obstruction. Therefore, the nurse must assess other parameters, such as blood pressure, urine output, neck vein distention, and respiratory rate. Once these parameters are assessed, the nurse is better able to formulate a nursing diagnosis and implement a plan of action.

The patient's respirations are another significant aspect of the output system. In assessing the patient's respiration, the nurse pays particular attention to the rate, rhythm, regularity, and color. According to Secor (1969),

Detection of subtle irregularities in the breathing pattern provides advance warning of impending trouble, which can be controlled by immediate intervention such as suction, oxygen administration, or ventilation assistance. . . . Rate, rhythm, depth, chest movements, evidence of discomfort or effort during either of the two phases of breathing, and sounds associated with the cycle are criteria for evaluating respirations.

Temperature is an important patient parameter. Elevation of the aged patient's temperature can be an early sign of infection. This becomes a serious complication for patients who have cardiopulmonary abnormalities. An increase in the patient's temperature leads to an increase in metabolism, increased need for oxygen, increase in workload of the heart, and a greater demand for pulmonary ventilation. On the other hand a decrease in temperature causes a decrease in rate of oxygen consumption and a decrease in CO_2 production. In this respect ventilatory needs are lessened. Perspiration is useful in lowering body temperature, because body heat is diverted to the skin. Evaporation takes place when the patient sweats. The aged patient who is dehydrated may not be able to sweat. Consequently the temperature usually becomes elevated. In taking the patient's temperature, the nurse must assess which route elicits the most accurate reading. For example, the patient with severe dyspnea may not be able to retain an oral thermometer. Because mouth breathing gives an inaccurate reading, a rectal thermometer is better. Some believe that rectal temperatures should not be taken on the patient with a myocardial infarction because the anal stimulation causes a vagal effect. Concern exists over whether the vagal effect can lead to such arrhythmias as sinus bradycardia or premature ventricular contractions. If not otherwise indicated, the nurse must decide which route would be most appropriate.

Arterial blood pressure is a reflection of left ventricular contraction, blood volume, blood viscosity, and elasticity of artery walls. Rigid artery walls or a reduction in their size lead to hypertension. Other factors which contribute to an increase in arterial pressure are stress, anxiety, and worry, which increase cardiac output and arteriolar constriction. The nurse must also realize that chronic hypoxia from impaired ventilation causes a rise in arterial blood pressure, which in turn causes hypervolemia resulting in an increased cardiac output. Factors of significance to the aged person, leading to decreased arterial pressure, are congestive heart failure with a reduced cardiac output, reduced blood volume, and vasodilatation. The nurse must assess what is normal arterial blood pressure for each patient and evaluate potential hazards if deviations from normal should develop.

Venous pressure is a reflection of how well the right ventricle is able to empty, thus reducing or increasing pressure in the right atrium. It represents a dynamic relationship between cardiac output, blood volume, and venous tone. A rise in central venous pressure is due to right-sided heart failure. Other factors leading to an increase are pleural effusion, emphysema, and extensive pneumonia. If direct measurement of central venous pressure is not possible, the nurse can assess for neck vein distention.

The patient's weight is a good indicator of the effectiveness of diuretic therapy. To ensure accurate measurement of weight, the patient should be weighed on the same scale and at the same time each day. In addition, any gowns, dressings, or sheets on the patient at the time of weight measurement should be weighed separately and subtracted from the total weight. Weight then becomes a good index of fluid retention or loss, tissue catabolism, and renal function.

Laboratory Studies The pertinent laboratory studies regarding the aged patient with cardiopulmonary abnormalities include (1) arterial blood gases, (2) serum electrolytes, (3) serum enzymes, (4) complete blood count (CBC) and prothrombin time. Arterial blood gases reflect ventilation efficiency, the ability of hemoglobin to carry oxygen and carbon dioxide, the rate of cellular metabolism, and the state of the buffer systems. The three significant aspects of arterial blood gases are pO_2, pCO_2, and pH. The pO_2 gives an indication of the amount of oxygen that has diffused through the alveoli into arterial blood. The pCO_2 measures carbon dioxide in the arterial blood. It reflects how well the lungs are able to ventilate.

Because the patient may be receiving diuretics, the serum electrolytes should be closely monitored. Secor (1969) identifies some of the problems associated with electrolyte irregularities.

Respiratory acidosis, a common disorder in chronic respiratory diseases, if not corrected or if inadequately compensated by the physiological buffering systems, can produce serious electrolyte irregularities, primarily of potassium. In an attempt to reduce acid factors of the blood, hydrogen ions move into the cells, forcing potassium ions out of the cells into the blood, from whence they are carried to the kidneys and excreted in the urine. The intracellular environment is particularly sensitive to slight potassium excesses or losses, and cells die if the potassium balance is not restored.

Being usually the first person to see the patient's electrolyte results, the nurse must know normal values to be able to recognize deviations and report them as necessary. The apathetic patient may actually be suffering from hyponatremia. The nurse must be able to correlate deviations with the patient's behavior.

Serum enzymes of interest are serum glutamic oxaloacetic transaminase (SGOT), lactic dehydrogenase (LDH), creatinine phosphokinase (CPK), and hydroxybutyrate dehydrogenase (HBD). Complete blood cell count consists of white blood cells (WBC) and red blood cells (RBC). The latter is significant because it represents the patient's hemoglobin and hematocrit level. Hemoglobin represents the amount of respiratory pigment protein available to combine with oxygen and carbon dioxide. A problem of the aged is anemia. In anemia the patient's hemoglobin is decreased, thus reducing the oxygen-carrying capacity. Hematocrit represents the relative volume of cells and plasma in blood.

ACTIVITY

Nursing care of the aged patient with cardiopulmonary abnormalities will be discussed in four ways. These include physical activity in general and cardiac, pulmonary, and mental activity.

Physical Rest is an important, though often ill-used, form of therapy for cardiac illness. When properly used, it may forestall the danger of refractory congestive failure. Prolonged absolute bed rest of the aged patient may result in negative nitrogen balance, osseous demineralization, urinary incontinence, constipation, and infection. If bed rest is overused, it may aggravate an increased venous return to an already overburdened heart. The patient's biologic problems must be assessed in comparison with complications derived from bed rest. The already weakened patient may become even weaker. Naturally, the patient with severe pulmonary problems will not have the energy to get out of bed. Likewise, the anemic patient may view ambulation to the commode, chair, or bathroom as being too exhausting.

Chair treatment for cardiac and pulmonary patients is gaining more recognition. Chair treatment has its advantages because it improves pulmonary ventilation and general circulation and decreases the possible risks of hypostatic pneumonia, thrombophlebitis, pulmonary embolism, and bed sores. It has been found that patients in severe congestive heart failure are more comfortable and improve more rapidly when allowed to sit in a chair. Orthopnea is reduced by permitting the patient to sit in a chair with his arms supported.

It must be kept in mind that before the nurse helps walk the patient, the stability of the cardiac rhythm and blood pressure must be assessed. Once these parameters are accurately assessed, the nurse is ready to help the patient to walk. Early ambulation of the aged patient offers physiological and psychological advantage. With prolonged bed rest the aged patient begins to feel hopeless about making progress. In this respect ambulation signifies improvement.

A degree of physical inactivity is necessary, but complete inactivity is injurious and impossible to achieve. The aged patient with hypertension may need to rest in bed. Stieglitz (1954) has pointed out,

> The fatigue of the spastic arteriolar medial musculature and of the myocardium are both lessened by arteriolar relaxation. The primary concern is with the average arteriolar tension rather than with transient elevations. Reduction of the diastolic pressure is the guide to the extent and the duration of vascular relaxation.

As the patient's arterial pressure returns to a more normal range, the nurse should encourage mobility and physical activity.

Cardiac Cardiac monitoring of the aged patient with acute coronary thrombosis is essential to detect early cardiac arrhythmias. It is also helpful when digitalis toxicity is suspected. The nurse uses the patient's cardioscope as a means of cardiac assessment but does not overreact to various alarms produced by the machine. Rather the nurse reacts to the clinical picture of the patient. Focusing on the equipment may create unnecessary anxiety within the patient. Arrhythmias of particular significance to the patient and nurse are Stokes-Adams syndrome or complete heart block.

It may be necessary to regulate the patient's cardiac activity by means of a pacemaker.

A pacemaker is the most effective way of restoring cardiac function. The arrhythmia associated with Stokes-Adams syndromes may occur during atrioventricular (AV) or sinoatrial (SA) block as well as sinus bradycardia. The pacemaker becomes a lifesaver for such aged patients. The patient may be too weak or ill for surgery; therefore, insertion of a transvenous catheter pacemaker is necessary. Care must be given to the site of pacemaker insertion to protect the patient against infection.

The patient with angina should be advised to curtail activities and to slow down the rate of performance, but encouraged to keep physically fit within the limits of his or her cardiac tolerance. According to Harris (1971),

> After a heart attack, the elderly patient should be encouraged to return to physical activity and social participation normally enjoyed by people of his age. . . . The senior cardiac has more to fear from sedation, social segregation and senility than from cardiac disease. . . . Although the heart of the senior cardiac may be enlarged, its rhythm irregular and its reserve diminished, it is ordinarily capable of providing sufficient cardiac output for his needs.

Therefore the aged patient must maintain a degree of physical activity to facilitate cardiac activity.

Pulmonary Pulmonary activity is assessed by means of chest x-ray, is altered by changes in position, and is assisted by use of a ventilator. A chest x-ray is helpful in obtaining direct visualization of the patient's chest. Assessment of the chest for infiltrates, such as fluid or secretions, can be made with an x-ray.

The position assumed by the patient affects breathing. Secor (1969) points out,

> When the individual is lying flat, there is less uniform gas distribution throughout the lungs than when he is upright. The sitting position causes the abdominal organs to sag away from the diaphragm, facilitating thoracic expansion. . . . When a normal person is supine, the total lung capacity is reduced by 300 ml. . . . Patients with emphysema have less difficulty breathing when they are in an upright position.

The sitting position permits gravity to move fluids to the dependent parts and prevents the pooling of blood in the pulmonary vascular structures. It does not matter whether patients are sitting up in bed, sitting in a chair, or standing; they should be encouraged to assume good posture. Patients who are more comfortable sitting in an armchair need to have their arms and head supported. If aged patients have difficulty exhaling, they have a tendency to lean forward in an attempt to compress the chest; however, such a position may cramp the chest, and thus their pulmonary inflation will be limited. Besides position changes to maintain adequate ventilation and circulation, the patient also needs sleep. This is especially true of the patient who tires easily, who works hard to breathe, and whose metabolism is affected by decreased oxygen. The nurse should attempt to position the patient comfortably, promote a quiet environment, and facilitate the sleep state.

The patient's pulmonary activity may be ineffective in supplying sufficient oxygen for metabolism and removing carbon dioxide produced by metabolism. In such instances the patient's faltering pulmonary system may need to be supported by a respirator. Intermittent positive pressure breathing (IPPB) machines serve to alter the quality of respirations by delivering a volume of air or oxygen under increased pressure to the airway at a set rate. With the IPPB machine, ventilation is either assisted or controlled. Controlled ventilation implies that the patient has no spontaneous respirations. Assisted ventilation occurs when the machine is triggered by the least inspiration from the patient. The nurse must be familiar with the type of ventilation, amount of pressure, and response of the patient.

Mental Mental or diversional activities are the best means of stimulation for both cardiac and pulmonary patients. The patient's mental activity and the need to learn, express, and relate should be considered. Any change in mental activity, such as confusion, restlessness, or irritability, should be cause for alarm. Changes that deviate from the patient's normal behavior may signify biologic problems which could include cerebral insufficiency, metabolic abnormalities, and electrolyte imbalance.

NUTRITION

One characteristic of aging is the fixation of habits. This is not the result of personality fixation. Instead, habits form and become fixed by repetition over a period of time. The longer the repetition is continued, the more rigid the fixation. Eating habits of the aged are affected by several factors. Appetite is not always a constant. Aged persons are frequently deficient in significant areas in their diet, i.e., minerals, such as calcium and iron, the vitamins, and proteins With rising food costs or reduced income, many elderly cannot afford variety in their diet. The hospitalized patient may have difficulty accepting changes in diet. In addition the nurse may unintentionally forget to offer patients their dentures before eating. Unless the food is soft, they may have difficulty "gumming" a steak. Anorexia may be a major nursing-care problem. Immobility, lack of interest or will to live, and drugs may depress the patient's appetite. Therefore, the nurse's goal is to provide an environment that encourages the patient to live.

In such an environment and with such care the patient is able to notice progress. Smaller servings of food can be offered and assistance given when necessary. A patient may be fearful of eating because of being interrupted by the need for a bedpan. The patient who associates diarrhea with eating may choose not to eat. Patients who have pulmonary abnormalities may eat poorly because they lack the strength or they fear eating will stimulate coughing, dyspnea, or other problems.

Anemia is frequently seen in hypertensive individuals. The existence of anemia increases the tissue injury seriously; it is not necessary that the reduction in hemoglobin content be great in order to be of considerable importance. The diet may need to consist of those foods with a high iron content. Nutritional deficiencies, whether due to lack of vitamins, glucose, or minerals or due to lack of oxygen because of anemia, may not be the most significant contributing factors in prolonging cardiac decompensation. Hypoproteinemia is frequently a con-

tributing cause of edema in the aged. Protein should not be unduly curtailed in aged patients, since protein restriction, especially prolonged restriction, depletes the body reserves and contributes to an exaggeration of any coexistent anemia. Protein is necessary for maintenance of tissue integrity. Therefore the daily requirements should be given as biologically appropriate to the patient's problem.

The aged cardiac patient may be placed on a low-salt diet. It is an accepted fact that an excess of sodium chloride contributes to development of edema; however, restrictions that are too rigid may be dangerous. A diet too restrictive of sodium chloride coupled with use of diuretics which cause increased sodium and chloride excretion can lead to hypochloremic alkalosis. The nurse must assess the patient's daily electrolyte panel. The diet, because it deviates from the patient's normal diet, may not be looked upon as palatable; therefore, whenever possible the patient should be permitted to make choices within the existing institutional restrictions. A dietitian can be of value to the aged patient and the nurse.

Another aspect of diet is important to the well-being of the aged cardiac or pulmonary patient, i.e., glucose. Of significance is the role of glucose combustion in the production of energy by the myocardium. Glucose is the chief source of cardiac energy. Aged patients do not tolerate even minor hypoglycemic levels. Interestingly, high blood sugar levels are necessary in aged patients. There is also a close relationship between glucose metabolism and blood potassium levels. There are three important factors that are required before effective combustion of glucose can occur. These factors are an adequate supply of oxygen, sufficient glucose, and enough insulin to catabolize the reaction. Consequently in acute cardiac decompensation, it is equally necessary to ensure an adequate level of glucose in the blood as it is to supply oxygen.

Nutritional status of the aged patient does not solely refer to the ability to ingest or digest. It also implies a need for spiritual nutrition. Spiritual needs of the aged patient are as significant as dietary needs. The patient may fear that death is imminent and, therefore, may seek the counsel of a minister, priest, or rabbi. Such a need must be fulfilled if we are to truly provide total or holistic nursing care. Religion may be a vital component in the aged individual's life and should be respected.

COMMUNICATION

Communication is a multifaceted concept. Within the larger concept FANCAP, communication involves facilitating biologic communication, through surgical or mechanical intervention, environmental communication, and human-to-human communication. In coronary artery disease, valvular disease, or conduction abnormalities, there exists a breakdown in circulatory communication between coronary blood flow and myocardium, valvular closing and cardiac output, and conduction pathway and cardiac regularity. Many cardiovascular diseases in the aged once thought to be hopeless are now corrected through surgery. Coronary artery blood flow is returned to the myocardium through surgical intervention of coronary artery bypass. The technique has been perfected by a number of hospitals so that risks are anticipated and quickly treated. Diseased valves creating congestive heart failure are replaced with artificial valves. As previously discussed under activity, conduction abnormalities of life-threatening significance can be corrected with use of a pacemaker. The breakdown of biologic communication with patient's pulmonary system is more difficult to correct. Respirators have helped sustain pulmonary function when patients could not spontaneously or independently sustain themselves. Lung transplants are still experimental and not realistic for the aged patient. Needless to say the aged patient might not cope with such major, radical surgical intervention.

Biologic communication directed externally can signify a change in the patient's condition. For example, sudden changes in behavior or sensorium may indicate impending biologic problems. These problems may include hypoxia, electrolyte imbalance, shock or metabolic disturbances. Likewise, changes in the aged patient's cardioscope pattern, blood gases, respiratory rate and rhythm, or arterial blood pressure indicate potential biologic threats. The nurse looks upon such changes as a means by which the patient's biologic system can communicate.

Environmental communication implies communication from equipment or treatment procedures to the patient, the environment in general, and diversional activities. The nurse observes that communication exists between the patient and the cardioscope, arterial line, IV apparatus, Foley catheter, respirator, nasogastric tube, or air mattress. There have been times when the patient and the respirator became separated, causing respiratory crisis. The patient who survives such an experience may be emotionally fearful of its recurrence. The patency of tubes must frequently be assessed to ensure proper flow of fluids or oxygen and communication.

Nurses create a protective environment. They protect patients from infections. Patients, because of their pathophysiologic problems, will have a lowered resistance to infection. The patient's environment should be free from wide fluctuations in temperature. A warm environment increases the patient's temperature (which earlier was said to increase metabolism), increases the need of oxygen, and increases workload of the heart. The aged patient with arteriosclerotic changes may not be able to respond biologically to the changes. A cold environment may induce vascular constriction. In either case, the environment should be comfortable for the individual. Diversional activities, such as television, radio, crafts, phone, or visitors, should be made available to the aged patient. Visitors may be temporarily restricted until the time the patient's biologic condition stabilizes.

The human-to-human communication that exists among patient, family, and nurse is most important. The aged patient looks to the nurse for support, understanding, and compassion. The nurse maintains the patient's sense of worth and dignity by personalizing care. The patient needs to feel more significant than the surrounding equipment. The nurse's presence helps with this feeling. Besides providing a personalized external environment, the nurse encourages internal personalization by allowing the patient to express fears. Stress may have a negative effect upon the patient's already compromised pulmonary system. Anxiety and fear alter the depth and rate of respiration, with the respirations becoming deeper and the heart rate and blood pressure increasing. These biologic responses get the patient in a state of readiness for physical activity. The aged patient's fears of being a cardiac or respiratory cripple need to be discussed by the physician with both the nurse and family members.

AERATION

Lungs and feelings both require aeration. Drugs and postural changes affecting aeration have already been discussed. Oxygen and humidification are important aspects of aeration. Anemia, cardiac problems, and pulmonary disease are the factors that interfere with oxygen transport. Oxygen therapy is indicated in the acute stage of left ventricular failure. In cases where failure may involve the right side, such as cor pulmonale, oxygen may be dangerous and cause death from carbon dioxide narcosis. To protect the patient the nurse should tape a sign on the oxygen unit specifying the maximum amount of oxygen to be given.

Oxygen administration may not be practical over a long period of time. It can be given by mask, nasal catheter, or nasal prongs. The actual amount of oxygen reaching the lungs is affected by the length and size of tubing used. Other factors influencing the amount of oxygen delivered are the nature of the aged patient's breathing, losses through the nose and mouth, and possible unreliability of flow meters. The two-pronged nasal cannula is the simplest means of delivering oxygen, but the tubing has a tendency to get in the patient's way or irritate the nostrils. Nasal catheter, another method of oxygen administration, is the most efficient way of providing oxygen and is less irritating to the patient. It does not interfere with eating or movement. If use of either the nasal cannula or catheter is not feasible, a face mask may be used. A face mask is less desirable for patients with congestive heart failure or severe pulmonary distress, because the mask often makes the patient feel claustrophobic. Regardless of the method utilized, oxygen has a tendency to dry the mucous membranes; therefore oral hygiene becomes an important nursing intervention. Humidification means provision of additional moisture to the inspired air. One goal in treating the pulmonary patient is to prevent dryness of the mucous membranes and their secretions.

Patients need an opportunity to air their feelings. (This is discussed earlier under "Communication.") Airing of feelings not only alleviates patients' fears, but also reduces the possibility of respiratory acidosis. As patients talk, they are removing carbon dioxide. It is worth mentioning that stress increases the secretion of mineralocorticoids with subsequent retention of sodium and water. Therefore, the nurses' goal is to identify and reduce the stress patients experience.

PAIN

The aged cardiac or pulmonary patient experiences two types of pain—physiological and psychological. Physiological pain is more definitive. It involves pain associated with an acute myocardial infarction or angina, headaches due to hypertension, and chest discomfort associated with pulmonary distress. Pain, regardless of its origin, can be exhausting to the patient. It takes energy needed for breathing or ambulating. Physiological pain associated with direct reflection of cardiac or pulmonary system is expected; however, abdominal pain is not to be expected. The nurse may suspect that the pain is due to constipation but must keep in mind that abdominal pain developing in the aged patient with an acute coronary thrombosis or with shock may indicate hemorrhagic infarction and necrosis of the intestines. All physiological pain experienced by the patient must be assessed. Pain associated with the pulmonary system may force the patient to splint the chest or avoid coughing. Therefore, the patient's chest must be supported while coughing or turning. Absence of pain where pain should be present is clinically significant. Decreasing sensitivity to pain associated with lethargy is a sign of brain hypoxia. If assessing the patient's problem, the nurse can change position and administer IPPB and oxygen if already ordered.

Psychological pain is equally as significant as physiological pain to the patient. Dyspnea, curtailment of activity, fatigue, and dependency are contributing factors to psychological pain. Besides the psychological pain associated with curtailment of activity or changes in life-style, financial loss due to hospitalization can also lead to psychological pain. Psychological pain may be more diffuse and less definitive, but it exists and should be alleviated.

In conclusion, the nurse working with aged patients experiencing pathophysiological abnormalities of the cardiopulmonary system needs to assess various significant cardiopulmonary parameters and pathological alterations in these parameters, and provide nursing care.

REFERENCES

Adatto, I. J., et al.: Rheumatic fever in the adult, *Journal of the American Medical Association*, **194**:1043, 1965.

Azcuy, A., A. E. Anderson, and A. G. Foraker: The morphological spectrum of aging and emphysematous lungs, *Radiology*, **83**:48, 1964.

Balchum, Oskar: The aging respiratory system, in *Working with Older People*, vol. 4, Department of Health, Education, and Welfare, 1971, pp. 115–118, 122.

Bedford, P. D., and F. I. Caird: *Valvular Disease of the Heart of Old Age*, Little, Brown, Boston, 1960.

Bickerman, Hylan A.: The respiratory system in the aged, in Albert Lansing (ed.), *Cowdry's Problems of Aging*, Williams & Wilkins, Baltimore, 1952, pp. 562, 592.

Carlson, Anton: *Geriatric Medicine*, Lippincott, Philadelphia, 1954, p. 70.

Chosy, L., J. B. L. Gee, and R. L. Rankin: The effects of smoking on the pulmonary diffusing capacity, *Clinical Research*, **11**:301, 1963.

Christopherson, J. B., and M. A. Broadbent: A new method of approach in certain respiratory disorders in elderly persons, *British Journal of Physical Medicine*, **9**:5, 1934.

Cohn, J. E., P. G. Carroll, B. W. Armstrong, R. A. Shepard, and R. L. Riley: Maximal diffusing capacity of the lung in normal subjects of different ages, *Journal of Applied Physiology*, **6**:588, 1954.

Dock, W.: Aging of the myocardium, *Bulletin of the New York Academy of Medicine*, **32**:173, 1956.

———: The capacity of the coronary bed in cardiac hypertrophy, *Journal of Experimental Medicine*, **74**:177, 1941.

Harris, Raymond: The heart in old age, in *Cardiology: An Encyclopedia of the Cardiovascular System*, vol. 5, pt. 23, McGraw-Hill, New York, 1961, chap. 3.

———: Special features of heart disease in the elderly patient, in *Working with Older People*, vol. 4, Department of Health, Education, and Welfare, 1971, pp. 82, 83, 86, 87, 89, 90–92, 94.

Kaufman, P., and H. Poliakoff: Studies on the aging heart: I. The pattern of rheumatic heart disease in old age (a clinical-pathological study), *Annals of Internal Medicine*, **32**:889, 1950.

Kløvstad, O.: Mitral stenosis in patients over the age of seventy, *Acta Medica Scandinavica*, **156** (Suppl. 319):99, 1956.

Kountz, W. B., and A. L. Alexander: Emphysema, *Medicine*, **13**:25, 1934.

Landowne, M., M. Brandfonbrener, and N. W. Shock: Relation of age to certain measures of the performance of the heart and circulation, *Circulation*, **12**:567, 1955.

Lev, M.: The normal anatomy of the conduction system in man and its pathology in A-V block, *Annals of the New York Academy of Science*, **111**:817, 1964.

Macklin, C. C., and M. T. Macklin: Respiratory system, in Albert Lansing (ed.), *Cowdry's Problems of Aging*, Williams & Wilkins, Baltimore, 1942, chap. 9.

McMillan, J., and H. Lev: The aging heart: II. The values, *Journal of Gerontology*, **19**:1, 1964.

Pathy, M. S.: Clinical presentation of myocardial infarction in the elderly, *British Heart Journal*, **29**:190, 1967.

Priest, W. S.: Anticipation and management of cardiac decompensation, *Geriatrics*, **12**:290, 1957.

Raeburn, C., and A. Spencer: Lung scar cancers, *British Journal of Tuberculosis and Diseases of the Chest*, **51**:237, 1957.

Rothschild, M. A., M. A. Kugel, and L. Gross: Incidence and significance of active infection in cases of rheumatic cardiovascular disease during the various age periods, *American Heart Journal*, **9**:586, 1934.

Secor, Jane: *Patient Care in Respiratory Problems*, Saunders, Philadelphia, 1969, pp. 72–74, 83.

Sell, S., and R. E. Scully: Aging changes in the aortic and mitral valves, *American Journal of Pathology*, **46**:345, 1965.

Sharpe, George, and Edward Stieglitz: Cardiac decompensation, in Edward Stieglitz (ed.), *Geriatric Medicine*, Lippincott, Philadelphia, 1954, pp. 372, 376, 378.

Solovay, J., and A. W. Solovay: Apical pulmonary tumors: Relation to apical scarring, *Diseases of the Chest*, **48**:20, 1965.

Stieglitz, Edward: Hypertensive arterial disease and hypotension, in Edward Stieglitz (ed.), *Geriatric Medicine*, Lippincott, Philadelphia, 1954, pp. 459, 460, 462, 465.

Thompson, M. K.: *Geriatrics and the Geriatric Practitioner Team*, Ballière, Tindall & Cassell, London, 1969, p. 79.

Timiras, P. S.: Diseases of aging, in P. S. Timiras (ed.), *Development Physiology and Aging*, Macmillan, New York, 1972, p. 474.

White, Paul D.: The heart and great vessels in old age, in Albert Lansing (ed.), *Cowdry's Problems of Aging*, Williams & Wilkins, Baltimore, 1952, pp. 279, 285.

NINETEEN

RENAL ABNORMALITIES IN AGING

Sharon L. Roberts

There are no greater forms of personal human tragedy than the disorders of urinary control and sexual performance. Too often, these losses are equated with and relegated to "the ravages of old age."
Jack Jaffe

LEARNING OBJECTIVES

- State the three general functions of the kidney.
- Compare functional and structural changes associated with aging.
- Contrast functional and structural changes associated with aging.
- Discuss problems associated with lower urinary tract disturbances.
- Identify five parenchymal or intrarenal disturbances confronting the aged individual.
- Discuss five parenchymal or intrarenal disturbances confronting the aged individual.
- List four postrenal disturbances confronting the aged individual.
- Discuss four postrenal disturbances confronting the aged individual.
- State the components of FANCAP.
- Discuss each component of FANCAP as it specifically applies to the aged individual with renal disturbances.
- Construct a nursing care plan or assessment tool around the concept of FANCAP.

Lately, attention has been given to renal disease and the problems it imposes. Renal disease, particularly renal failure, does not know age limits, skin color, economic status, or ethnic identity. Television programs have focused on the problems of renal failure victims. The public now can view hemodialysis units and watch films of patients as they are being connected to a hemodialysis machine. People tend to associate renal disease with hemodialysis and possibly renal transplant. Of course, these are the extremes of therapy and may be necessary after conservative approaches have been tried.

One must remember that chronic renal failure does not happen suddenly. Instead a chain of physiological events, such as renal disease, lower urinary tract infections, involutionary processes, extrarenal disease or injuries, and atrophy, occur over a period of time. Such physiological changes, if not corrected or altered, may lead to the final phase—uremia or renal failure—and necessitate drastic and costly lifesaving measures. The difficult task comes in deciding who shall benefit from modern technology and sophisticated surgical interventions. Unfortunately, one segment of our population, the aged, may be given low priority. It is understandable that renal transplant donors are not as plentiful as the recipients. Consequently, renal transplants are reserved for the younger patient. In addition, hemodialysis may require exchanges three times a week and be too expensive for the aged individual. Consequently, more conservative treatment approaches are utilized with the aged. Because all aged individuals with renal failure cannot benefit from hemodialysis or renal transplantation, the nurse has a tremendous responsibility to protect the patient from extrarenal problems that could in time lead to intrarenal abnormalities.

Fortunately, the aged individual may move through life never experiencing the threat of renal disease but experiencing only the normal physiological changes in the kidney associated with the aging process. According to Kahn and Snapper (1971),

The kidney in the elderly individual is affected by involutionary processes and atrophy, secondary to atherosclerosis and probable time-related phenomena independent of disease. Superimposed on these may be numerous other renal and extrarenal diseases.

Besides renal pathology, the aged individual may be confronted with psychosocial problems associated with incontinence and impotence; and since nurses care for the total individual, these problems become their concern. As Jaffe (1971) has said,

Total care of the elderly includes the maintenance of maximum activity, emotional security and physical comfort. Certainly, much can be offered by medical practitioners towards the relief of debilitating somatic and social distresses of the elderly presented by the commonplace disease of the lower urinary tract.

Renal abnormalities confronting the aged are varied in degree and complexity. First, physiological parameters of renal function will be discussed. Second, we will cover renal abnormalities pertaining to the aged patient. Renal abnormalities can be categorized according to their origins, such as prerenal, parenchymal, and postrenal. Last, significant nursing care will be discussed as it relates to the FANCAP concept.

PHYSIOLOGICAL CONSIDERATIONS

Kahn and Snapper (1971) have pointed out that approximately "one-third of patients 65 or older have normal glomerular and tubular function and more than two-thirds exhibit normal glomerular function." The aged patient's prognosis depends on the involuntary process itself or preexisting renal disease. Before presenting changes that occur in the aged kidney, it is important to discuss normal functions.

NORMAL PHYSIOLOGICAL RESPONSES

In general, the kidneys have excretory, secretory, and regulatory functions. The kidneys remove the end products of protein metabolism. In addition, the kidneys serve the vital homeostasis function of regulating extracellular fluid volume, electrolyte balance, and acid-base balance. The secretory function encompasses secretion of renin and erythropoietin. The former influences blood pressure while the latter influences the production of red blood cells.

Shock (1952) has identified specific functional activities:

> The functional activities of the kidney include the following: (a) the formation of an ultra filtrate of blood plasma, (b) the selective resorption of various substances from this ultra filtrate by enzymatic activity of cells comprising the epithelium of the tubule, (c) the selective excretion of substances from blood into the lumen of the tubule, and (d) the metabolic activity of the kidney in a formation of new compounds for excretion.

To accomplish their excretory function, the kidneys must be supplied with blood—1 L of blood per minute. One liter of blood per minute represents one-fifth of the total cardiac output.

> From the blood delivered to the kidney, a filtrate containing all the constituents of the blood plasma with the exception of the red cells and the plasma protein is formed. The rate of formation of this filtrate is dependent upon the amount of blood delivered to the filtering membrane and the pressure maintained by action of the heart. As this filtrate passes down the tubule certain of the substances present in it are reabsorbed, as for example, water, sugar, chloride, sodium, etc. Other substances may be actively secreted from the tubules and added to this filtrate which is subsequently excreted as urine. (Shock, 1952)

In summary, the kidney is an incredible organ because of its ability to maintain homeostasis. While doing so, it reacts to changes in plasma electrolyte levels and acid-base balance. The diseased kidneys can no longer perform their normal functions. Likewise aged kidney functions may be altered and subsequently less efficient.

THE KIDNEY

According to Shock (1952),

> With increasing age there is a gradual diminution in renal function as indicated by reduced rate of glomerular filtration, reduced effective plasma flow . . . the primary factor involved in the reduction in renal function is based on vascular changes. . . . The vascular bed remaining in the aged kidney is capable of responding to vasodilators as effectively as the vessels in young kidneys. In addition to the anatomical narrowing and loss of vessels, there is present in the aged kidney a persistent vasoconstriction which tends to reduce further the flow of blood through this organ.

Furthermore Oliver (1952) points out

> that the disturbance in renal function may be more the result of circulatory dysfunction than of renal structural change. The common cardiovascular disturbance of old age is the result of or is associated with or expressed by a hypertension . . . restrictions of blood flow through the renal arteries results in a continued elevation of general blood pressure.

The kidneys, as an organ, contain a tremendous amount of reserve in functional tissue. It is interesting to note that,

> As a biological problem ageing of the kidney derives interest more from its theoretical implications than from the practical aspect of ill effects produced by the senescent processes. The relatively small place that disturbances of renal eliminatory function occupy in the picture of old age is however not due to any lack of senile change in the kidney but rather to the fact that, like most glandular organs, it contains so large a reserve of functioning tissue as to be rarely exhausted to the point of appreciable dysfunction. (Oliver, 1952)

The aged kidneys undergo both structural and functional changes. Structural changes within the kidneys consist of both regressive processes and adaptive changes. Regressive processes take place in alteration in the renal arteries and subsequent modification in parenchyma resulting from vascular changes. Oliver (1952) discusses both regressive processes and adaptive changes and believes that the alterations in the renal arteries are part of processes occurring generally throughout the arterial system with the advance of years. The change in the terminal arterioles is of simple nature, consisting of a thickening and hyalinization of the vessel wall. The parenchymal modifications that follow the vascular change are the result of disturbances in the nutrition of the tissue and may be considered examples of ischemic atrophy. The distribution of these effects throughout the organ is determined by the distribution of the vascular change, so that a kidney not greatly reduced in size with a relatively smooth surface and scattered retracted scars is found. When the larger and middle arteries are irregularly affected, a general reduction of the size of the organ and a more diffuse granular scarring follow the involvement of smaller vessels and arteries. The glomerulus is affected either by collapse of its capillaries when the afferent arteriole is obliterated or by hyalinization which may extend into the tuft from the arterioles. Regardless of the process, the tuft is transformed into a fibrous nodule and may disappear. Examination of the aged human kidney has shown that in the seventh decade the number of glomeruli equals only two-thirds to one-half that of the early adult count. Arteriosclerotic changes bring about a reduction in the bulk of the nephrons. The interstitial connective tissue framework is condensed. Structural changes involve regressive processes and adaptive changes. The aging process brings about regressive changes in the narrowing of renal arteries. The narrowing is a result of arteriosclerosis associated with aging. The parenchyma and glomeruli are also affected because of vascular changes.

Besides structural changes, the aged kidneys also undergo functional changes associated with nephrosclerosis. Oliver (1952) states,

Structurally the kidney of the aged organ whose original parenchyma and vascular supply is reduced presents a varying and usually proportional degree of compensatory change in both of its constituent elements. In theory a functional balance might be expected. A complication, however, is found in the fact that though the parenchymal changes of atrophy and of hypertrophy may be considered a quantitative restitution in their functional effect, with the development of new vessels there has occurred a qualitative change in the sense that a different sort of blood supply has developed. The blood that formerly passed through the glomerular capillaries, and which there underwent certain modifications, is now being directed in ever increasing amount directly to the tubules.

The disturbance of vascular balance has its affects upon the function of the kidney. Oliver (1952) points out,

Due to its great reserve of tissue, the eliminatory capacity may be normal or any part of normal depending on the balance of parenchymal scarring and compensatory change that have occurred within the organ. In the majority of aged people depreciation of kidney function is not a major difficulty, for other systems, such as heart or brain, similarly involved by vascular change, fail more rapidly and more disastrously. It is perhaps true that those urinary disturbances that do occur are more the result of circulatory abnormality than of the change that senescence has produced in the kidney.

The primary circulatory dysfunction would be hypertension. Just as the aging process affects the kidneys themselves, so is the lower urinary tract affected.

Lower Urinary Tract In studying the renal system, one usually focuses primarily on the kidney itself to the exclusion of other anatomic and physiological components of the entire system. Attention is not always given to the process of urination. Urination is a function that is not as exciting as glomerular filtration, tubular secretion, or tubular reabsorption. The process of voiding or urinating is simply taken for granted until the process is altered through problems such as retention or incontinence. Furthermore, the role of the bladder as an organ comparable with the heart is taken for granted. Jaffe (1971) has stated,

> The voiding mechanism is a complex interaction of voluntary and involuntary processes. A delicate balance exists between the detrusor (bladder muscle) and the outlet. Changes from any cause which diminish efficiency of the motor component or increase resistance in the outflow tract result in incomplete emptying. A weak detrusor, as expected with loss of muscle tone in the aging processes, may turn a "normal" outlet towards an obstructed one.

Furthermore, Jaffe (1971) discusses how the bladder, like the heart muscle, obeys Starling's law.

> Gradual distention of the bladder produces a spasmodic contraction with compensation, until the point of the kicking off contraction is reached. Overdistention of the bladder, usually under chronic conditions, may produce complete decompensation with over stretched muscle fibers unable to reach a point of efficient coordination contraction. Often, relief of retention can allow for resetting of compensatory mechanisms. As in heart failure, judicious drug therapy can be used to increase bladder efficiency.

The lower urinary tract has particular significance for the aged. Urinary incontinence in the female aged patient can lead to understanding the factor causing genitourinary infection. Aged female patients who are on prolonged bed rest are plagued with the problem of urine collecting in their vagina. Like the female aged patient, the aged male patient also has unique problems associated with his lower urinary tract. His problem is associated with the process of urinating. The origin of disruption in the aged male's normal urinating process is his prostate gland. Prostatic enlargement, according to Jaffe, "is an unrelenting process initiating with puberty. . . . Some degree of prostatism (outlet symptoms) is present in three-fourths of the males 65 and over." Each unique problem associated with the lower urinary tract of the aged female and male will be discussed under "Renal Abnormalities in the Aged Individual." In order to understand abnormalities associated with the aged patient's renal system, the nurse must be familiar with both structural and functional changes associated with the kidneys and the functions related to lower urinary tract, i.e., urination.

It seems that, from discussion of basic physiological considerations of the kidney and lower urinary tract (see Figure 19-1), the determining factor for changes in the aged patient's renal function is primarily vascular alterations. Of course, this does not exclude those alterations in function created by renal diseases, resulting in

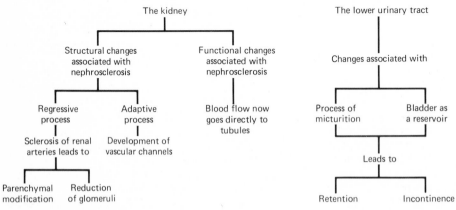

FIGURE 19-1   Physiological considerations in the aged renal system.

irreversible pathological conditions. There are several renal abnormalities that confront the aged patient, both female and male. Only those most frequently encountered by the elderly will be discussed.

RENAL ABNORMALITIES IN THE AGED INDIVIDUAL

Renal abnormalities can be categorized according to their causes. Therefore in order to present an organized and comprehensive discussion of major abnormalities confronting the aged individual, the following categories will be utilized: prerenal, parenchymal or intrarenal, and postrenal or extrarenal problems.

PRERENAL

A prerenal problem originates outside and prior to actually reaching the kidneys. The overall problem usually originates as a result of perfusion or renal blood flow deficit to the kidneys themselves. Other more specific problems nevertheless considered prerenal in origin are inadequate fluid intake; fluid loss due to vomiting or diarrhea; hemorrhage or traumatic shock; acute or chronic cardiac failure; septicemia due to gram-negative bacteria; and injudicious use of diuretics. Each is considered prerenal because of either a direct or indirect loss of volume normally circulating to the kidneys. It was stated earlier that the aging process brings about the progressive diminution in renal blood flow.

Prerenal failure is a consequence of diminished renal blood flow, usually resulting from decreased circulating blood volume. Take, for example, the aged patient who has congestive heart failure. The total blood volume may be normal for the individual; however, the heart as a pump is ineffective in its ability to deliver the required or normal blood volume. Therefore, with increasing cardiac failure, there is a decrease in the cardiac output. The left ventricle possibly receives the same amount of blood volume, but owing to hypertrophy or disease, does not eject the same volume of blood as it did when in a state of health. The nurse must keep in mind that a decrease in cardiac output leads to a decrease in renal blood flow. Thus the problem of prerenal failure due to blood volume deficit is created.

Frequently the aged individual who has a history of cardiac failure or pulmonary edema, or both, is placed on a regimen of limited fluids, restricted salt in the diet, and diuretics which may be mandatory in the critical phase of cardiac failure. However, as the patient's cardiac status stabilizes, the therapy may continue without modification. For example, a 70-year-old patient in congestive heart failure was placed in a coronary care unit (CCU). There his physicians treated him with diuretics, fluid restriction, and IPPB therapy. Subsequently, he was given Lasix 40 mg daily, and his fluid intake continued to be limited to 1200 mL per day. The latter amount included both oral and parenteral intake. After several days of therapy, the CCU nurse observed that the patient's urine output was scanty and concentrated and, furthermore, discovered that his hematocrit and blood urea nitrogen (BUN) levels were elevated. After the data were collected and presented to the physician, it was decided that the patient's clinical picture was due to hypovolemia. Therefore, all diuretics were stopped and the patient's fluid intake was gradually increased. In time, the patient's hematocrit, BUN, and urine output all returned to normal levels.

When reduced renal blood flow occurs as a result of cardiac failure; volume loss due to prolonged diuretic therapy, fluid restriction, diarrhea, or hemorrhage; or infection, such as septicemia, a chain of physiological events occur in an attempt to stabilize renal function. The body, in order to maintain its circulation and vascular integrity, secretes large amounts of the steroid hormone aldosterone and the vasopressor antidiuretic hormone (ADH). Aldosterone causes salt retention and thus water retention. The process would be ineffective if the body continued with diuresis. ADH produces water retention by increasing its reabsorption in the tubules. The overall effect is an increase or stabilizing of circulating volume until homeostasis is restored.

Prerenal failure must be treated quickly and safely. If not rapidly treated, prerenal failure will cause true parenchymal damage. Such is frequently the case in acute renal failure. In most cases of prerenal failure, restoration of blood pressure, blood volume, and cardiac output will quickly establish adequate to normal urine flow. The nurse must remember that the aged patient may not be able to physiologically compensate with too rapid a return of blood volume. Too rapid a return to normal may cause cardiac decompensation, further traumatizing already impaired renal functions. Those treating the aged must keep in mind that a large fluid load might be injurious, especially if the fluid cannot be excreted. Figure 19-2 summarizes prerenal abnormalities in aged patients.

One hopes that prerenal problems are transient. Once the cause is identified, it can be corrected before contributing to the more serious and potentially terminal problem associated with parenchymal damage.

PARENCHYMAL: INTRARENAL DISTURBANCES

Parenchymal or intrarenal problems affecting the aged patient primarily involve the kidneys themselves. The condition can be acute, as is the case in acute pyelonephritis or acute glomerulonephritis. Repeated infection or injury, however, can lead to a serious loss in renal function. Eventually, the problem can become less acute and more chronic. The ultimate chronic renal dysfunction is uremia or azotemia. The five major parenchymal problems confronting the aged individual are pyelonephritis, glomerulonephritis, renal calculi, renal failure, and uremia. Each abnormality will be comprehensively covered and medical and/or nursing interventions will be discussed under the concept FANCAP.

There are five intrarenal disturbances associated with the aging process or pathophysiological changes resulting from disease. These consist of the following: pyelonephritis, glomerulonephritis, renal calculi, renal failure, and uremia.

Pyelonephritis Guyton (1971) wrote,

Pyelonephritis is an infectious and inflammatory process that usually begins in the renal pelvis but extends progressively into the renal parenchyma. The infection can result from many different types of bacteria, including especially the colon bacillus and staphylococci. Invasion of the kidneys by these bacteria results in progressive destruction of renal tubules, glomeruli, and any other structures in the path of the invading organisms. Consequently, large portions of the functional renal tissue are lost.

Pyelonephritis usually affects the medulla before affecting the cortex. The medulla is responsible for the countercurrent mechanism that concentrates the urine. Therefore, rather than alteration in renal function, the ability to concentrate urine is impaired (Guyton, 1971). According to Kahn and Snapper (1971),

This entity is probably the most common renal disease in the aged male. The underlying cause is usually obstruction due to bladder neck pathology. Pyelonephritis is frequently responsible for acute failure in chronic renal disease, and if it can be treated, the failure may be at least temporarily reversed. . . . It is not even certain that for the disease to be progressive, active infection by micro-organisms must be continually present, especially in the later stages. Auto-immune mechanisms are now believed to play an important role.

Female aged patients are susceptible to pyelonephritis and other urinary tract infection.

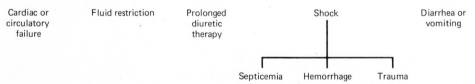

| Cardiac or circulatory failure | Fluid restriction | Prolonged diuretic therapy | | Shock | | Diarrhea or vomiting |

Septicemia   Hemorrhage   Trauma

FIGURE 19-2   Prerenal abnormalities resulting from a reduction in circulating blood volume.

The organisms present in the lower gastrointestinal tract enter the individual's urinary system via the urethra. The aged patient may manifest symptoms of pain over the area of the kidneys, and may have fever, chills, and gastrointestinal upset. The urine contains bacteria (bacteriuria) and often pus (pyuria). The overt symptoms of pyelonephritis disappear in a few days, with or without treatment, even though the urine still evidences infection.

The goal of therapy is to correct the causative factors which have led to the bacterial infection. It calls for the relief of obstruction, identification of bacteria, and improving of the aged individual's general health. Obstruction can develop outside the kidneys. Possible causes are urethral obstruction, bladder neck fibrosis, prostatic hypertrophy, prostatic carcinoma, interstitial cystitis with contraction of the bladder, bladder tumor, ureteral stricture, ureteral calculi, pelvic tumor, ureteropelvic obstruction, and tumor of renal pelvis (Kahn and Snapper, 1971). Pyelonephritis is a disease that can persist as a relatively asymptomatic infection which gradually destroys the kidney. The aged patient must be given adequate antibiotic therapy and be examined at intervals for quiescent disease.

Glomerulonephritis Acute glomerulonephritis is a problem that occurs frequently. In the aged individual glomerulonephritis is usually seen as a chronic disease or as an acute exacerbation of a chronic disease.

Acute glomerulonephritis is the result of an antigen-antibody reaction. The glomeruli become markedly inflamed. Many white blood cells collect in the inflamed glomeruli. . . . The inflammatory reactions cause total or partial blockage of large numbers of glomeruli, unblocked glomeruli develop greatly increased permeability of the glomerular membrane, and allow large amounts of protein to leak into the glomerular filtrate. . . . All degrees of glomerular dysfunction may happen in acute glomerulonephritis, including total renal shutdown. . . . Acute inflammation of the glomeruli usually subsides in ten days to two weeks. The nephrons may return to normal function. Sometimes, however, the inflammatory reactions are so severe that many or most of the glomeruli will be permanently destroyed. Furthermore acute glomerulonephritis frequently becomes chronic glomerulonephritis. Consequently more nephrons are destroyed and the result can be acute shutdown. (Guyton, 1971)

Therefore glomerulonephritis in the aged is looked upon as an extension of chronic disease. According to Kahn and Snapper (1971),

All recurrences of acute glomerulonephritis must be looked upon as acute exacerbations of a basically chronic disease. Both acute glomerulonephritis and exacerbations of chronic glomerulonephritis begin with non-specific symptoms which vary in each case—headache, fever, oliguria, nausea, vomiting and abdominal pain. The latter two may be so severe that an acute abdomen is simulated. The more specific signs include edema (usually periorbital), smoky or grossly bloody urine (latter is rare), hypertension and proteinuria.

It is worth reiterating that active glomerulonephritis in the aged patient is an exacerbation of a chronic process.

Renal Calculi Renal calculi are kidney stones which vary in size and shape. The intensity of pain and the symptoms also vary. Most patients complain of severe back pain. Kahn and Snapper (1971) have said, "The consideration of renal stones is particularly important in the aged because these calculi may be responsible for either acute or chronic renal syndromes, and if unrecognized, may lead to the loss of one or both kidneys." Kidney stones are caused by several mechanisms, among them increased urinary excretion of calcium, increased urinary excretion of uric acid, increased urinary excretion of cystine, and renal infection with formation of stones containing blood and pus. Kahn and Snapper describe the process by which kidney stones are formed.

Many of the constituents of calculi, particularly calcium, are present normally in the urine as supersaturated solutions and are maintained as such by protective colloids.

. . . If either the concentration or the pH changes, precipitation may result. At an alkaline pH, phosphates and carbonates are insoluble; acid pH will favor precipitation of uric acid and cystine.

The cystine and phosphate stones grow rapidly. As a result, they usually fill the cavity in which they have formed. In addition, their presence creates stasis which enhances continued growth because of three contributing factors: changes in concentration, deterioration of protective colloids, and infection (Kahn and Snapper 1971).

Other factors that contribute to the development of renal calculi are immobility and excessive elimination of uric acid. Immobility for a period of 2 weeks when due to paralysis or fracture can produce an increase in urinary calcium excretion. The normal amount of calcium excreted daily is 20 mg; however, prolonged immobilization may increase this amount to an excess of 500 mg per day. As a result of the dramatic increase, calcium stones form. Unfortunately, the aged patient who is particularly prone to fracture is also susceptible to stone formation because of the immobility. As Kahn and Snapper (1971) point out, "Excessive elimination of uric acid under a variety of conditions also presents favorable situations for formation of urinary tract stones. This would most commonly occur in gout and the myeloproliferation disorder." Renal calculi then can cause obstruction and if not removed can lead to the more serious renal abnormality—renal failure.

Renal Failure Renal failure signifies that the kidneys are unable to excrete the normal load of metabolites produced within the body. Acute renal failure has three phases: oliguric or anuric phase, diuretic phase, and convalescent phase. The oliguric (100 to 300 mL per day) and anuric (less than 100 mL per day) phases can last from a relatively short period of time to as long as several weeks. Depending on the amount of protein intake and degree of catabolism, the BUN level may rise 10 to 40 mg per day. Other significant laboratory findings reveal an elevated level of serum potassium, phosphate, and magnesium, but serum calcium, sodium, and chloride levels may be decreased. Serum potassium is the electrolyte that requires critical observation during the oliguric phase. The nurse must carefully observe the patient's potassium levels because hyperkalemia eventually leads to cessation of cardiac activity. In addition, the nurse should keep in mind that hyperkalemia is the result of catabolism due to potassium being liberated from destroyed cells, acidosis, and renal retention. The nurse will want to protect the patient from infection to prevent increased catabolism and subsequent hyperkalemia.

The second phase of acute renal failure is the diuretic phase. As the kidney begins to stabilize, urine output either gradually or abruptly increases. The sudden diuresis can lead to hyponatremia. Therefore, the nurse must observe the patient's serum sodium level and assess for signs or symptoms of hyponatremia.

Last, the kidneys, if not severely damaged, go through the phase of convalescence. It is during this time that the aged patient's kidneys may return to a normal state. If the stages of healing or phases beyond anuria do not take place, the patient then may experience the ultimate renal abnormality—uremia.

Uremia *Uremia* is the term applied to the clinical syndrome resulting from severe reduction in the excretory function of both kidneys. Its chief biochemical sign is an extreme degree of azotemia. The total clinical picture is a complex one, consisting of malnutrition, anemia, acidosis, water and electrolyte imbalance, hypertensive vascular disease, and circulatory insufficiency. Chronic uremia is most frequently the end result of the progressive destruction of renal parenchyma by a variety of diffuse bilateral renal disease. Extrarenal factors, such as circulatory failure, dehydration, and sodium depletion, or accelerated protein catabolism (as a fever or infection), frequently contribute to the pathogenesis of uremia. The clinical picture of uremia is variable. It is influenced by age, nutritional status of the individual, the nature of the underlying disease, and the rate of development of renal failure. Some aged patients do well despite advanced renal damage; others with similar damage may deteriorate rapidly.

The prognosis of the aged patient with uremia is determined by the nature of the underlying cause of renal failure. If uremia is caused by a reversible disease, such as obstruction, the prognosis is good. However, if renal failure is due to the loss of kidney parenchyma produced by progressive and irreversible diseases such as glomerulonephritis or pyelonephritis, uremia is bound to be a poor prognostic sign. Problems that alter the patient's parenchyma are varied in severity and complexity (see Figure 19-3). Acute infection, injury, or diseases can become chronic, causing irreversible damage to the nephrons, the ultimate outcome being renal failure or uremia.

In the aged individual, there is an increased potential of obstruction in the lower urinary tract coupled with an increased susceptibility to urogenital infection. These problems are categorized as postrenal or extrarenal in origin.

POSTRENAL

According to Jaffe (1971),

> The clinical features of lower urinary tract disease in the aged generally fall into two categories. The most dramatic and obvious types, typified by hematuria, fever, and acute retention, are undeniable. The relatively silent insidious ones, such as a change in voiding patterns, are easily overlooked. . . . Gradual but relentless progression is the rule in untreated lower urinary tract illness.

Postrenal problems consist of urethral stenosis or stricture, urinary tract infection, tumors, and urethral calculi. The patient may manifest the problem of incontinence. Other features of lower tract disease include those of the irritated outlet, such as urgency, frequency, nocturia and dysuria; urinary retention; and ill-defined pain referable to the low back, perineum, pelvis, groin, abdomen, or flank (Jaffe, 1971). The major postrenal or extrarenal problems confronting the aged are lower tract infection, urinary incontinence, acute urinary retention, prostatism, and impotence.

Lower Urinary Tract Infection One of the most common problems of the aged is lower urinary tract infection. Both males and females are susceptible to urinary tract infection. Problems unique to the male patient are urethritis, prostate enlargement, prostatitis, and atonic decompensated bladder. Female problems consist of prolapsed urethral mucosa, distal urethral stenosis, interstitial cystitis, and contracted bladder.

As Jaffe (1971) points out, "Both sexes can suffer from meatal stenosis, urethral stricture, urethral and bladder neoplasms, bladder neck contracture, diverticuli, calculi, reflux, ectopia, foreign body, neurogenic dysfunction, and the effects of prolonged recumbency."

Unfortunately the hospitalized aged patient may have an indwelling catheter. Such is the case for patients admitted to critical care units or those who are incontinent. Long-term catheterization leads to lower urinary tract infection. All too often the meatus around the catheter is not properly cleaned. Consequently, the area becomes a good medium for bacteria invasion and subsequent infection. In addition, chronic urethritis, bladder spasm, and bladder debris may also develop. The nurse must protect

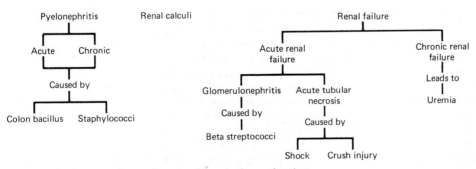

FIGURE 19-3 Summary of parenchymal problems in the aged patient.

the aged patient from further renal damage by preventing unnecessary infection. Urinary tract infection may be difficult to detect. The nurse must observe for changes in color or odor of the patient's urine and evidence of any precipitates. Furthermore the nurse listens for any complaints of bladder pain associated with a burning sensation or spasm. Any change in white blood cell count or in body temperature might indicate a lower urinary tract infection.

Urinary Incontinence Jaffe (1971) believes that the problem of urinary incontinence can consist of such pure and mixed components as neurogenic disease, urgency, stress, and overflow incontinence. Neurogenic incontinence can be subtle or dramatic in onset. Urination is a reflex act complicated by antagonistic action from sympathetic and parasympathetic nerve supply to both the bladder muscle and the outlet sphincter. Diseases that lead to neurogenic incontinence are tabes dorsalis, diabetic neuropathy, cerebral cortex lesions, and parkinsonism. The second component, urgency incontinence, depends on local mechanisms but may not be noted until the irritative focus develops secondary to supra- or extravesical disease. Contributing factors leading to urinary incontinence are diverticulitis, pelvic tumor, vaginitis, urinary tract infection, bladder tumor, or prostatic enlargement. The third component, stress incontinence, is dependent upon psychosocial pressures as well as bladder pressure. Aged patients may complain of incontinence when they cough, laugh, or sneeze. In the female stress incontinence may be due to uterine prolapse. Lastly, overflow incontinence is caused by obstructive lesions or incorrect drug therapy.

Regardless of its origin, urinary incontinence is both an inconvenience and an embarrassment. The aged patient takes pride in the ability to be independent. Illness can lead to dependency, and an inability to control the normal process of urination fosters feelings of childlike regression. The nurse's attitude can bolster the patient's sense of dignity. Sympathy for the patient's distressing problem is crucial; together they can discuss or plan for bladder training or control.

Acute Urinary Retention Acute urinary retention can be a serious problem to the aged; it can

even become life threatening. The nurse should assess the patient's urinary output every 8 hours. It is not unusual for a nurse to suddenly realize that the patient has not voided in 24 hours. In such cases the nurse must assess the patient for bladder distention, since urinary retention can progress to renal failure if not treated. Furthermore, if the condition is merely managed rather than treated, it can lead to cardiovascular and cerebrovascular impairment. Urinary retention in either males or females requires catheterization. If the retention is unlikely to recur or is only episodic, as in some patients with acute multiple sclerosis, a single catheterization may suffice, but chronic retention usually requires an indwelling Foley catheter. Occasionally, drugs may cause urinary retention. Again, the nurse must be aware of the patient's urinary output in terms of amount, color, odor, and precipitates.

Prostatism A problem confronting the aged male is prostatic hypertrophy. Early symptoms of the condition are hesitancy, decrease in force of urine, frequency, and nocturia. As the condition becomes more severe, obstructive symptoms are manifest. These include posturination dribbling, poor control, overflow incontinence, an irritated outlet, and sepsis. Any growth in the size of the prostate that leads to hematuria is more frequently benign than malignant. The degree of obstruction may vary. According to Jaffe (1971), "there may be little or no correlation between the size of the residual urine volume and the degree of obstruction. A chronically infected bladder may often have markedly decreased capacity."

If transurethral surgery is indicated, the patient and his wife need careful explanation regarding the possible outcome of the operation. The surgery itself does not cause impotence. Some men incorrectly believe that the surgical intervention will impair their sexual function or "demasculinize" them. The nurse can allay these fears through discussions with the patient and his family. While preoperatively teaching the patient, the nurse may seek knowledge regarding any changes in the patient's sexual performance. Most misunderstandings among the aged males stem from lack of scientific knowledge. Therefore, before actually beginning any teaching, the nurse should review with the patient the anatomy and physiology related to the genitourinary system. Even though impotence is not a result of transurethral surgery, it, nevertheless, is a problem among aged male patients.

Impotence Impotence is a complex problem that may be relative or complete and may involve any phase of the sexual act. Impotence may originate as a result of androgen deficiency, genitourinary disease, neurological disease, vascular insufficiency, poor nutritional status, or emotional disturbances. Emotional or situational difficulties may typify the problem of the younger male patient, not necessarily the aged male. If, however, impotence is the principal complaint of the aged patient, it is usually the result of an emotional disturbance. In such cases, androgen therapy is valueless and at times may even add to the psychic trauma. The aged male who has enjoyed sex and found it satisfactory should continue regardless of his chronological age. The sexual needs of patients are often overlooked when the patient is going through a biologic crisis. However, when biologic stability has been reached, his sexual activity should continue rather than terminate. See Chapter 25, "Normal Aging Changes in the Reproductive System," for a fuller discussion of this subject.

Postrenal problems (see Figure 19-4) are not as physiologically serious as parenchymal ones; however, both types have the potential of leading to renal insufficiency or failure. Emotionally, the problem may be just as serious. Patients who have based their lives on dignity, independence, and self-directedness suffer from the embarrassment of incontinence or impotence. For them, both problems are distressing and depressing; therefore the nurse must be sensitive to such feelings and alleviate them when possible.

FANCAP: NURSING CARE OF THE AGED

Treatment and nursing care of the aged patient with renal problems begins conservatively. A conservative approach involves diet management, medication therapy, and symptomatic management of uremic manifestations. The more radical treatment of the aged with renal abnormalities consists of peritoneal dialysis, hemodialysis, and renal transplantation. But realistically such radical treatment is usually reserved for the young.

FLUIDS

Fluid intake is balanced with fluid loss as the ability of the kidneys to maintain the delicate balance is impaired in renal failure. Therefore, a primary nursing goal is the accurate measurement of fluid loss so that correct fluid replacement can be administered. Fluid management involves the assessment of sensible and insensible losses.

Interstitial Edema Edema that occurs in uremia can be caused by sodium and water retention, congestive heart failure, or a decrease in serum protein. Hypoproteinemia results in interstitial edema. The proteins are the only dissolved substances of the plasma that do not diffuse readily into the interstitial fluid. When small

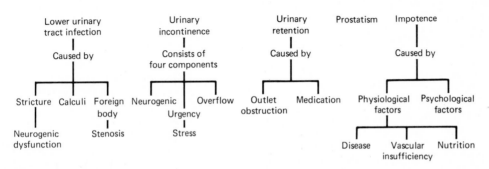

FIGURE 19-4 Major postrenal problems affecting the aged patient.

quantities of protein do diffuse into the interstitial fluid, these are soon removed from the interstitial spaces by way of the lymph vessels. Therefore, the dissolved proteins of the plasma and interstitial fluids are responsible for the osmotic pressure that develops at the capillary membrane. Hypoproteinemia, which occurs in the nephrotic syndrome and other conditions, results in a decrease in serum oncotic pressure and movement of fluid out of the capillaries and into body tissue.

The patient, whose kidneys are unable to excrete fluid, develops cerebral, pulmonary, and/or peripheral edema. The nurse should pay particular attention to the potential life-threatening problems created by pulmonary edema and assess changes in the patient's behavior, blood gases, chest sounds, respiratory rate, and color.

Interstitial edema creates problems associated with skin breakdown. Furthermore, the skin becomes a vehicle for insensible loss of fluid. The nurse should keep in mind that dry, flaking, itching skin often occurs in uremia which can be caused by disturbances in calcium and phosphorus balance. Also, the skin conditions may be due to an infection caused by the fungus *Candida albicans*. In terminal uremia, urea crystals precipitate out in the skin, forming "uremic frost." To remove the crystals from the skin, the patient should be bathed, but the nurse should remember that the crystals are soluble in water, and therefore, it is not necessary to use soap on skin that is already so dry. If soap is used, it should be a bland soap, i.e., one that does not contain perfume, the best examples being baby soaps and Ivory soap.

Besides bathing the patient's skin, the nurse should also assess reddened areas that might eventually lead to actual breakdown. Therefore, in the edematous states, the patient's position should be changed frequently. Areas of potential breakdown are those covering bony prominences where the tissue is thin. These include the sacrum, elbows, and ankles. Skin breakdown presents a problem because the broken area can become a site for infection. If the patient should have arteriosclerosis or vascular insufficiency, the broken skin may suffer from reduced blood flow and nutrients. Therefore the nurse, through care giving, becomes the patient's protective shield.

Intake Intake involves physiological intake of oral fluids, parenteral fluids or medications, and environmental intake. Because the kidneys may be unable to excrete fluid, oral intake may be restricted. The amount of oral restriction depends upon the degree of edema, as determined by the physical appearance of the patient and the amount of weight gain. The patient who has oliguria or anuria should not receive abundant fluid administration as a means of compensation. As Kahn and Snapper (1971) point out,

> Abundant fluid administration does not constitute the basis of therapy in all forms of acute renal failure. In parenchymatous renal failure, fluids must be restricted. This type of failure may be due either to prolonged renal ischemia as the result of uncorrected prerenal factors or to nephrotubular damage from heavy metals or drugs.

Intake is based on fluid loss the aged patient experiences. Oral intake may be limited to 1000 mL per day. The nurse must supervise the exact amount of fluid to be given each 8 hours. Fluids may be offered with medications and meals. In between, the patient should be provided with fluid substitutes, such as a wet cloth, chewing gum, or lemon swabs. The aged uremic patient's mouth is susceptible to ulceration, since the salivary flow is decreased and the possibility of infection is increased. If the patient's mouth is infected with *C. albicans,* as it frequently is, this can be treated with nystatin oral suspension 500 mg four times a day. The nurse should use judgment in deciding the types of fluids that should be offered to the patient; for example, orange juice and grape juice have higher levels of potassium than most juices. Also, the patient's potassium level must be assessed before offering these juices even though they may be a particular favorite. The patient may prefer water above all other juices because it is less irritating to a sore mouth. Ice cubes can be crushed and given to the patient, but the nurse should melt one ice cube to accurately determine the specific amount of fluid intake.

Parenteral intake may also be limited. There are instances in which the patient's total fluid intake may be 1200 to 1500 mL per day. This includes both oral and parenteral intake. Like oral intake, parenteral intake must be divided over a 24-hour period. The type of parenteral fluid depends on the needs of the aged patient. If the patient is hyperkalemic, 10% dextrose and water (D/W) with insulin may be given intravenously. Insulin causes glucose to go into the cell. As glucose moves inside the cell, it takes potassium with it and reduces the serum potassium. Throughout the past several years, parenteral hyperalimentation solutions have gained recognition as a therapeutic agent in treating patients with various debilitating problems such as renal failure. Hyperalimentation represents the infusion of large amounts of basic nutrients sufficient to achieve tissue synthesis and growth. The solution is mixed by using varying quantities of protein hydrolysate and hypertonic dextrose solutions. An example of a mixture is 750 mL of 5% fibrin hydrolysate in 5% D/W with 350 mL of 50% D/W. The resulting solution contains approximately 1000 calories and because it is very hypertonic, it is best infused through an indwelling catheter directed into a large vein, such as the superior vena cava (Metheny and Snively, 1974). The flow rate is constant over a 24-hour period and may not exceed 1 L if the patient is on restricted intake. Too rapid infusion may lead to osmotic diuresis. In turn, this can lead to dehydration and convulsion. While the patient receives hyperalimentation solution, the nurse assesses the patient's urine for glycosuria by checking the patient's fractional urine every 4 hours. Electrolytes will be included in the hyperalimentation solution. Depending on the patient's potassium level, potassium can be added to the solution. Potassium is needed for the transport of glucose and amino acids across the cell membrane. Magnesium, calcium, and phosphorus are given when needed. Normally hyperalimentation solution infuses by itself. This is because drugs may interact with the protein hydrolysate. Beside careful administration of the solution, the nurse assesses the infusion site for redness. The dressing covering the site is changed daily.

Medications are given with caution to the aged patient with renal problems. The damaged kidneys are unable to excrete drugs; therefore, they may build up in the patient. Medications of significance to the aged renal patient are antibiotics, antihypertensives, diuretics, digitalis, and antacids (see Figure 19-5). The nurse must assess the patient for potential side effects. Any drug which is metabolized and excreted by the kidneys must be given in decreased doses in uremia. Drugs that are metabolized to inactive substances by the liver and other means need not be given in decreased doses. Regardless of where the drug is metabolized, the nurse must observe for any toxic effects.

Hypertension develops in more than 80 percent of patients with chronic renal failure. The mechanism behind hypertension is not well understood. As Harrington and Brener (1973) point out,

Decreased blood flow to the kidney, caused, for example, by renal artery stenosis, stimulates the juxtaglomerular apparatus to release renin. Renin causes the liberation of angiotensinogen, angiotensin I, and angiotensin II. Angiotensin II stimulates the adrenal medulla to release aldosterone. Aldosterone causes sodium retention, which results in water retention and a rise in blood pressure, which should physiologically increase renal blood flow.

Hypertension is an important determinant of survival and can lead to further parenchymal damage, further sodium retention, and further hypertension. Rather than discuss the four specific antihypertensive drugs in detail, only

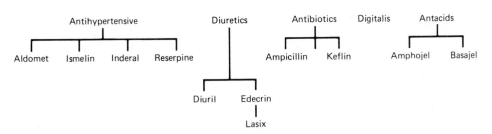

FIGURE 19-5 Medications of significance for the aged renal patient.

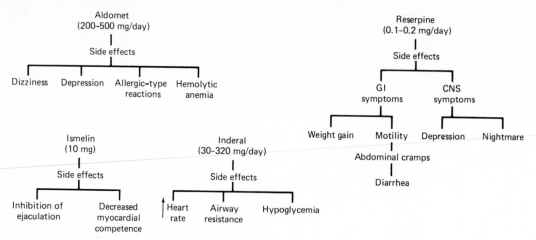

FIGURE 19-6 Common side effects of antihypertensive medications used in treating uremia.

their side effects will be discussed (see Figure 19-6).

It is interesting to note some of the side effects of drugs. Weight gain caused by reserpine further increases blood pressure. And the nurse is always observant for hypotension in any patient. The aged male patient receiving guanethidine (Ismelin) may become concerned when his sexual performance is reduced. Just as antihypertensive drugs lower the patient's blood pressure, so do diuretics. Patients with excessive salt and fluid retention may be helped by diuretics. The danger of toxicity from diuretics is reduced by giving intermittently rather than daily. Patients who require frequent diuretic therapy can be protected from toxicity by alternating drugs every few days.

As Figure 19-7 indicates, diuretics can have certain toxic effects. Therefore the nurse must observe for signs of electrolyte imbalance created by increased diuresis. Of particular significance is hypokalemia, since it can cause car-

diac arrhythmias and potentiate the toxicity of digitalis.

Antibiotics are used in the treatment of renal and urinary tract infection. The nurse must keep in mind that patients with chronic renal failure or uremia have a low resistance to infection. As has been mentioned earlier, lower urinary tract infection leads to renal failure. Antibiotics are necessary in treatment of infection; however, they should be used cautiously with severe renal damage. The kidneys are unable to excrete the drug; therefore, the levels may increase. Antibiotics like kanamycin, bacitracin, and neomycin are retained in high concentration in the kidneys. Furthermore, kanamycin and neomycin can lead to deafness. Streptomycin can have a mild nephrotoxic effect on the kidneys. Nitrofurantoin (Furadantin) which is sometimes used as a urinary antiseptic, can cause peripheral neuropathy. The antibiotics of choice are penicillin, ampicillin, and tetracycline. The nurse's primary goal is to prevent infection

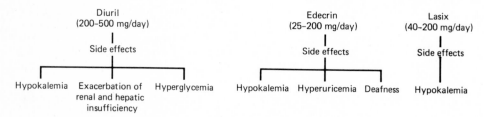

FIGURE 19-7 Common side effects of diuretics used in treating uremia.

so that antibiotics will not be necessary. When suctioning the patient's trachea, inserting or irrigating a catheter, or changing a dressing, the nurse must practice sterile techniques.

Digitalis is used in the treatment of congestive heart failure and pulmonary edema. Both problems can develop as a result of the kidneys' inability to excrete in volume. Digoxin can be potentially dangerous because of the patient's abnormal potassium level. A point for the nurse to remember is that a patient with hyperkalemia requires more digitalis for the same therapeutic effect than a patient with normal serum potassium. The nurse should note the patient's serum potassium level and report significant changes. In addition the nurse assesses the patient for signs of digitalis toxicity. The signs include arrhythmias, such as first-degree block, bigeminy, or premature ventricular contractions; nausea and vomiting; and disturbance of color vision.

Kayexalate, an ion exchange resin, is used for the treatment of hyperkalemia. It contains sodium in a compound that is not absorbed from the gastrointestinal tract. While in the gut, the sodium "exchanges" place with serum potassium, and the potassium becomes part of the nonabsorbable compound. The bound potassium is then excreted in the feces. The medication promotes osmotic diarrhea and thus ensures adequate gastrointestinal loss. Kayexalate is given orally or as a retention enema.

Antacids are given to patients for a variety of reasons. The antacids are specific for the aged patient with renal failure. In uremia, calcium level is decreased and phosphorus is increased. The nurse should give the patient aluminum hydroxide gel with meals to reduce absorption of the phosphorus in the ingested foods. The antacids used are Amphojel and Basaljel. Gels that contain magnesium in addition to aluminum are usually not used because of the danger of magnesium intoxication, e.g., Gelusil, Maalox, Mylanta, and milk of magnesia; therefore, the nurse should instruct the patient not to interchange antacids. Other patients interchange antacids because some cause constipation whereas others cause diarrhea. The aged patient with renal failure cannot be flexible in choice and can use only those antacids which bind phosphorus.

Testosterone is sometimes used in the treatment of patients with renal failure. Testosterone derivatives are so-called anabolic agents. They serve the purpose of reversing the catabolic processes that occur in the anuric phase. These may be given cautiously to the patient. Frequently the aged patient may receive the drug every other day or every third day. The nurse should assess the patient for toxic effects consisting of signs of hepatic toxicity and sodium retention.

The last aspect of intake is environmental intake. The nurse carefully monitors the amount of environmental intake and protects the patient from potential hazards in the environment. The aged renal patient is no exception. The most significant environmental hazard besides stress is infection. The nurse assesses the patient for signs of infection, which include malaise, fatigue, increased heart rate, high white blood cell count, and rapid respiration. The patient's resistance to infection may be greatly reduced, and when necessary, the patient should be isolated from other patients to ensure protection.

Output Output consists of sensible loss, such as urine, stool, and emesis; diagnostic procedures, including blood pressure, pulse, respiration, temperature, specific gravity, daily weight, and central venous pressure; and laboratory tests, such as serum electrolytes, BUN, creatinine, hemoglobin, hematocrit, uric acid, and WBC (white blood cells).

Sensible Loss Water losses, both sensible and insensible, are replaced with equal amounts of water in an attempt to maintain a state of balanced hydration. The urinary output of the aged patient can safely range from 25 to 500 mL per hour. The nurse should report hourly output below 25 mL or above 500 mL and an output of less than 500 mL for a 24-hour period. When assessing the patient's renal status, the nurse keeps in mind that urinary output is a much better guide than blood pressure in assessing the state of blood flow to the kidneys. The expected urinary output may vary with each patient and it is influenced by many factors. These factors are listed in Figure 19-8.

The nurse may observe two phases in the patient's urinary output. The first is oliguria, and it may be the first manifestation of acute renal

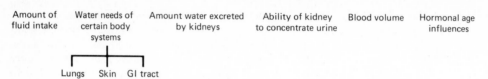

| Amount of
fluid intake | Water needs of
certain body
systems | Amount water excreted
by kidneys | Ability of kidney
to concentrate urine | Blood volume | Hormonal age
influences |

Lungs Skin GI tract

FIGURE 19-8 Factors influencing volume of urine output.

failure. A urinary output for 24 hours may be 50 to 150 mL. As mentioned previously the oliguric phase may last 1 day or several weeks. In the interim the nurse should observe for signs of excess volume, hyperkalemia, metabolic acidosis, and uremia. The second phase of diuresis begins when the patient has a urine volume of 1 L per day. This phase may not occur for 14 to 21 days. It is during the diuretic phase that the partially regenerated tubules are unable to concentrate urine and the glomerular filtrate is excreted unchanged. Therefore, the patient's condition does not necessarily improve during the initial days of the diuretic phase. The nurse may feel relieved when the patient's urinary output increases, but the crisis has not passed when such a phenomenona occurs. Laboratory tests such as BUN and creatinine may continue to remain elevated, thus reinforcing the fact that the kidneys are still unable to excrete waste products.

Besides assessing urine volume, the nurse also assesses the color and odor. The patient's urine may be bloody in the first few days of oliguria, becoming clear toward the end of this phase. If renal failure is due to hemolytic blood transfusion, then the urine assumes a dark red color. Deep amber urine may indicate dehydration. Straw-colored urine may indicate the kidney's inability to concentrate urine. Urine that is cloudy in appearance may indicate presence of pus or protein. A patient with nephrotic syndrome may be excreting large amounts of protein in urine. Naturally, urine should be somewhat odorless. The presence of precipitates in the urine, strong odor, or change in color should alert the nurse that a potential problem exists.

Other sensible losses consist of stool, emesis, and blood. Diarrhea and vomiting are troublesome symptoms of uremia. Intestinal hypermotility shortens the time for absorption of intestinal fluids and thus results in increased fluid loss in bowel movements. Liquid stools contain water and electrolytes derived from se-

cretions, ingested food and fluids, and extracellular fluid brought into the bowel to render ingested substances isotonic. The nurse should be alert for symptoms of volume depletion. Electrolytes lost through diarrhea and vomiting may further complicate the renal patient's clinical picture. The last form of sensible loss is blood. The aged uremic patient has a tendency to bleed. The bleeding is manifested by epistaxis, gastrointestinal bleeding, and easy bruising. The nurse should avoid any unnecessary trauma that might induce bleeding, for example, when inserting a nasogastric tube or performing nasotracheal suctioning. All losses derived from stool, emesis, or blood should be recorded and included in the total output.

DIAGNOSTIC PROCEDURES

Blood Pressure Variation in blood pressure is helpful in evaluating body fluid disturbances. Consequently, arterial blood pressure should be taken frequently in order to evaluate whether there is a real or potential water and electrolyte balance problem. The patient may be receiving antihypertensive drugs in an attempt to return blood pressure to normal. A too rapid decrease in blood pressure may be as harmful to the kidneys as elevated pressure. Lowering the blood pressure may cause a drop in glomerular filtration rate, decreased renal perfusion, and further renal damage. The nurse then must accurately measure the patient's blood pressure. According to Harrington and Brener (1973),

If the patient is receiving ganglionic blocking agents, the nurse measures the blood pressure when the patient is lying down, standing up, and after he has exercised, as these drugs cause exercise and postural hypotension. The nurse teaches the patient taking these drugs to stand up slowly in order to avoid dizziness and fainting. She checks that the patient is having normal bowel movements, as these drugs tend to cause diarrhea.

Pulse The aged patient's pulse should be evaluated in terms of rate, volume, and regularity. The nurse should be particularly observant of the patient receiving propranolol (Inderal). Since Inderal slows the patient's pulse rate, the drug should not be given if the pulse is below 50. The normal pulse rate is 70 to 80 beats per minute. A weak pulse may indicate volume deficit and electrolyte imbalance. A bounding pulse may indicate volume excess. The nurse should also assess the regularity of the patient's pulse. Because of changes in certain electrolytes, such as potassium or calcium, and drug therapy, such as digitalis, the patient may develop arrhythmias. Any irregularities should be communicated, and, if possible, a cardioscope connected to the aged patient.

Respirations Respirations become important in assessing changes of body pH. The nurse realizes that the lungs play a major role in regulating body pH by varying the amount of carbon dioxide retention. Just as with the pulse, the nurse assesses the patient's respirations for rate, depth, and regularity. Respirations change with metabolic acidosis and metabolic alkalosis. Figure 19-9 shows the respiratory change associated with each.

Temperature The aged patient's temperature is also assessed and is taken with pulse and respirations. The frequency is determined by absence or presence of fever. Fever causes an increase in metabolism and thus in formed metabolic wastes, which require fluid to make a solution for renal excretion; in this way, fluid loss is increased. Fever also causes hyperpnea, an increase in breathing resulting in extra water vapor loss via the lungs. Because fever increases

loss of body fluids, it is important that temperature elevations be reported and appropriate orders sought (Metheny and Snively, 1974). A decrease in "normal" temperature can indicate sodium depletion and/or fluid volume deficit. Likewise, an increase in temperature may indicate excess fluid loss or dehydration. In validating dehydration, the nurse should observe the patient's hematocrit level and assess skin turgor. Fever leads to diaphoresis and an increase in insensible loss of water.

Specific Gravity Specific gravity is another diagnostic procedure that provides the nurse with information regarding the kidneys' ability to concentrate urine. Specific gravity reflects osmolarity which is determined by the presence in the urine of substances of low molecular weight such as urea, potassium, sodium, and glucose. The aged patient with uremia has a decreased ability to concentrate urine. According to Harrington and Brener (1973),

> This decreased ability to concentrate occurs early in renal failure and is responsible for some of the early signs of renal impairment: nocturia, polyuria and polydypsia. As renal failure advances, there is a tendency for the urine to remain at about the same osmolarity as plasma (1.010); this is called isosthenuria.

A low specific gravity of 1.002 to 1.010 characterizes the oliguric phase. Other factors need to be assessed when a low specific gravity is discovered. It should be determined whether the patient is on a protein- or sodium-restricted diet and has received a diuretic. Each of these three factors is capable of producing a low specific gravity.

Daily body weights are necessary for determining the effectiveness of various therapeutic measures which alter fluid volume. Daily

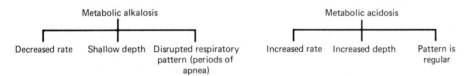

FIGURE 19-9 Character of respirations indicating metabolic alkalosis and acidosis.

weights of the aged patient are of value in obtaining an accurate measurement of intake and output. In addition, changes in the daily weight reflect changes in fluid volume. The patient who gains rather than loses weight may need an increase in diuretic therapy and a decrease in fluid intake. A body weight that reaches stability over a period of days should not necessarily foster the health team's sense of security. It must be remembered that fluids can pool in the body, creating volume deficit not indicated by weight changes. Therefore, the stabile-appearing daily weight may not accurately reflect the internal instability of shifting fluid volume. The nurse must remember that patients should be weighed daily at the same time, preferably in the morning before breakfast, on the same scale, and with the same clothing. This is particularly significant for the aged patient in renal failure whose daily weight is a measurement for volume replacement or removal.

Central Venous Pressure Another diagnostic procedure for determining volume status of the patient is central venous pressure. It provides momentary information regarding pressure in the right atrium of the heart. An increase beyond 4 to 10 cm can indicate problems such as hypervolemia, cardiac tamponade, and congestive heart failure. A decrease in venous pressure below zero level can indicate hypovolemia. Both problems, hypervolemia and hypovolemia, are of particular significance in establishing therapeutic guidelines for treating renal failure. Daily weight, central venous pressure, and intake-output become three diagnostic measures of significance in accurately determining the aged patient's fluid volume.

Laboratory Tests Laboratory tests of significance to the nurse are serum electrolytes such as potassium, sodium, and calcium; substances derived from protein metabolism including BUN, creatinine, and uric acid; hemoglobin and hematocrit; and WBC. Serum potassium is usually increased in uremia. Hyperkalemia can also be caused by several related factors, namely, increased dietary intake of potassium; protein breakdown, which releases intracellular potassium into the blood; acidosis; and hyponatremia. The nurse is alert to the patient's serum

potassium into the blood; acidosis; and hyponatremia. The nurse is alert to the patient's serum potassium levels in relation to the amount of protein intake either orally or parenterally. Furthermore, physiological events, such as tissue damage due to infection or increased temperature, all of which can increase potassium levels, should be observed. The nurse must also keep in mind the important interrelationship between sodium and potassium. The distal tubules of the nephrons secrete potassium, and a high level of sodium enhances this process. However, low sodium levels, possibly associated with dietary restriction or diuretic therapy, lead to an increase in potassium. When the patient's urinary output substantially decreases, the distal tubules do not secrete potassium.

Sodium levels of aged renal patients vary. They can be either increased or decreased in renal failure. In severe renal failure in which glomerular filtrate and urinary output are reduced, the kidney is unable to excrete sodium. A decreased sodium level can occur during the diuretic phase of renal disease. Hyponatremia can also occur through sensible loss due to vomiting or diarrhea and insensible loss due to sweating. Serum calcium is decreased in uremia; however, the calcium level is associated with an elevated phosphorus level. These two levels are interchangeable. The nurse must realize that an increase in one results in a decrease of the other. A decrease in calcium is significant because it can cause tetany. This is unusual in the uremic patient as acidosis created by the uremia protects the patient from tetany.

Substances derived from protein metabolism are urea, creatinine, and uric acid. Urea, the end product of nitrogen metabolism, is formed in the liver and excreted by the kidneys. BUN levels usually are elevated in uremia. The nurse should be aware that elevated BUN levels are not true diagnostic indicators of renal failure. It can be influenced by protein intake, rate of protein metabolism, and state of hydration. One isolated measurement of urea is not helpful in assessing the total picture of the aged renal failure patient. Serial studies are of greater benefit.

Creatinine is the end product of creatine metabolism. Serum creatinine levels increase in uremia. Because creatinine is related to muscle mass, it is less affected by extrarenal factors than BUN. Consequently it becomes a more reliable index of kidney function. Lastly, uric acid is the end product of purine metabolism. Purine is also a nitrogenous base. Serum uric acid is increased in uremia. Because uric acid can precipitate into body tissue, it causes joint pain associated with arthritis. The nurse should support painful joints when turning, positioning, or ambulating the aged patient.

Patients in renal failure have a tendency to be anemic and are susceptible to infection. The anemia is caused by lack of erythropoiesis, a process whereby red blood cells are produced by the bone marrow. The kidneys are normally responsible for secreting this substance. However, in renal failure the amount secreted is inadequate; consequently, the patient becomes anemic. Furthermore, azotemia seems to depress the bone marrow. Regardless of the origin, the patient's nurse must observe the patient's red blood count (RBC), including the hematocrit and hemoglobin. Because of the patient's lowered resistance to infection, the nurse must also be aware of changes in WBC.

ACTIVITY

The nurse must assess four major components of activity: (1) physical activity, (2) cardiopulmonary activity, (3) metabolic activity, and (4) mental activity.

Physical Activity Physical activity may need to be restricted in the early stages of renal disease and in the later uremic stages. A younger patient may be able to cope physiologically with immobility. However, the aged patient who must be immobilized is prone to develop specific problems. These problems consist of osteoporosis, thrombophlebitis, and more advanced arthritic changes. Immobilization should be terminated as soon as physiologically possible. The nurse should remember that the uremic patient who is anemic does not have energy to ambulate and fatigues easily, in all probability preferring immobility to mobility. The nurse should provide frequent rest periods so that when walking is necessary, it can take place. Furthermore, physical activity may be painful because of joint pain or gout associated with increased uric acid. The nurse prepares the pa-

tient for ambulation by gently exercising the joints and maintaining muscle tone. Mobility has other advantages besides preventing physiological complications, because it serves to encourage patients that their condition has stabilized or that they are getting well. Depressed patients become encouraged; their fear of dependence and loss of personal integrity or dignity is replaced with a feeling of independence and self-worth.

Cardiopulmonary Activity In assessment of the aged patient's cardiac status, a cardioscope may be necessary. This is especially true if the patient has congestive heart failure or arrhythmias associated with electrolyte imbalance, hypervolemia, or digitalis toxicity. The cardioscope is only a vehicle by which one aspect of the patient's cardiac status can be assessed. The nurse must continue to depend upon an ability to assess and appropriately intervene and must be aware of the patient's clinical picture, such as any change in behavior, vital signs, or color. All such changes can reflect changes in the patient's renal status.

The patient's pulmonary status may vary in accordance with changes in renal status. For example, as the patient moves toward metabolic acidosis associated with uremia, the pulmonary picture may indicate alkalosis. The nurse should then observe the patient's respirations for rate and depth, because rapid or deep respirations represent respiratory compensation. In other words, excess carbon dioxide is being exhaled by the lungs in an attempt to compensate for severe acidosis. Such rapid and deep breathing is called *Kussmaul's respiration*. The nurse who observes Kussmaul's respiration should not assume that the patient is anxious and attempt to slow the respiratory rate. Instead the nurse should assess the arterial blood gases, notify the physician, and further assess the patient.

Metabolic Activity Metabolic acidosis is associated with uremia. Like the patient with emphysema, the patient with renal problems can cope with acidosis. The uremic patient may have a serum bicarbonate level of 16 to 18 meq/L (normal 24 meq/L). If treatment is necessary, a conservative approach is initiated. This includes administration of sodium bicarbonate or sodium lactate. It may be difficult to return the bicarbonate level to within normal ranges. The process may also precipitate tetany in those patients with decreased calcium. Consequently calcium gluconate and sodium bicarbonate may need to be administered simultaneously. If the conservative approach fails to alter the acidosis or alleviate symptoms, a more drastic approach may be necessary. This would include peritoneal dialysis or hemodialysis. Peritoneal dialysis may be the treatment of choice because it does not involve general anesthesia. Either mode of treatment requires careful observation by the nurse.

Mental Activity The aged patient with renal abnormalities may experience psychological changes. These changes should not be looked upon as senility, rather, they are a reflection of renal status. The nurse may find that the patient is lethargic, less mentally acute, and unable to concentrate on a subject for more than a few seconds. Because of the possibility of confusion, the patient will need the nurse's protection even more. The tubes and wires that are inserted or attached must be secured to guard against unintentional or accidental removal. Furthermore, the confused patient may attempt to get out of bed and fall. In one instance the patient may be confused, then suddenly lucid. The nurse may assume a false sense of security during the patient's lucid moments. Until the metabolic status improves, the patient must be carefully observed and protected. In severe uremia, the patient even experiences periods of paranoia and hallucination, both of which can be frightening to the patient. The nurse's goal is to protect the patient from injury. In addition, the nurse should explain the patient's behavioral changes to the spouse and/or children. Should the once-quiet individual suddenly become combative, the nurse will realize that this behavior is a result of a pathologic condition.

NUTRITION

As Harrington and Brener (1973) point out, "Dietary regulation is extremely important in renal failure. Because the kidney cannot adequately balance the concentration of certain substances, the ingestion of these substances must be regulated. In the usual diet for patients with renal failure, protein, potassium, sodium and water are regulated." Depending upon the aged patient's specific renal abnormality, dietary protein may be either increased or decreased. For example, the patient with nephrotic syndrome experiences proteinuria. Patients may lose a tremendous amount of protein in their urine. The nurse must remember that protein is responsible for maintaining colloid osmotic pressure; loss creates volume shifts leading to ascites and edema. The patient with nephrotic syndrome will need a high-protein diet. On the other hand, aged patients with renal failure will usually be given a low-protein diet. In renal failure the end products of protein metabolism are excreted at a decreased rate. The nurse should take care to provide sufficient protein to meet the body's needs for maintaining and repairing body tissue. The minimum requirement is 10 to 20 g per day as compared with the normal requirement of 60 to 80 g per day. Furthermore, the diet must include calories to prevent the body's breakdown of protein for energy. The diet offered aged patients may not be to their liking, and their appetite is probably depressed; but all this is associated with immobility and uremia. Consequently, nurses will have a challenge in helping patients meet their daily requirements of protein and necessary caloric intake to prevent body breakdown of protein. Nurses must be sensitive to the amount and type of food intake by patients. If patients are unable to eat because of nausea or anorexia, it may be necessary to provide the necessary nutrients through nasogastric feedings or parenteral hyperalimentation.

Potassium and sodium are two important electrolytes which may need to be increased or decreased. Just as the need for protein varies, so does the need for potassium. Depending on the aged patient's particular problem or phase of illness, potassium will need to be increased or severely restricted. It is during the diuretic phase of acute renal failure that potassium is lost. Careful observation of serum potassium levels will indicate the amount of necessary potassium intake. Potassium replacement in all probability will be gradual. The nurse will realize that acute renal failure can become chronic renal failure. In the latter case potassium is not excreted. It is an easier intervention to provide potassium input than to remove it. Therefore, in chronic renal failure or uremia the amount of potassium administered should be restricted. Likewise, sodium levels are carefully assessed and usually restricted in uremia. Neither potassium nor sodium is excreted in severe renal abnormalities. The amount of sodium restriction may be rigid when the aged patient manifests signs of congestive heart failure or hypertension. Just as potassium is lost during the diuretic phase of acute renal failure, sodium is also lost. In this instance sodium is replaced. Besides assessment of serum potassium and sodium levels, assessment of urinary loss may also be noted. The nurse must observe the patient's BUN, creatinine, and electrolyte panel in relation to the amount of either dietary or parenteral intake of protein and electrolytes. The relationship between the two may be of help to the physician who assesses the day-to-day needs of the patients. Therefore, the nurse either assumes responsibility of supervising the aged patient's dietary intake or carefully instructs the team regarding the significance of accurate dietary measurement. The aged patient who returns home must be instructed regarding dietary needs and cautioned about use of salt substitutes. Since salt substitutes are low in sodium and high in potassium, the patient who has a tendency to retain potassium should avoid salt substitutes as well as juices containing potassium. A dietitian can be consulted in helping the patient cope with required dietary changes.

Spiritual nutrition may also be important to the patient. This is especially true for the patient with uremia. Spiritual nutrition should be provided before the patient becomes too confused or lethargic to derive comfort from it. As soon as possible a minister, priest, or rabbi should be contacted, provided the patient has given approval. Spiritual comfort may serve to ease the depressed or discouraged patient.

COMMUNICATION

Aged patients need to feel they can communicate their fears and concerns with someone in the environment. Those most frequently within their environment are nurses, who listen to their concerns or complaints and assess changes in their behavior. Aged patients may be concerned over the uncertainty of their renal status and the possible need of expensive therapy. The patient who lives alone and is without a family has particular needs. Male patients may be concerned over special diets that require personal attention. Such a patient may have previously eaten in restaurants both for the nutritional intake and the socialization it provided. Now he is forced to restrict his diet, prepare the food himself, and eat without the familiar socialization. Needless to say, the patient needs the nurse's and dietitian's support at this time. If the patient lives in a boardinghouse or hotel, special diets can be prepared by the chef, and meals can continue to be eaten with friends. It may be difficult, however, for the patient who lives alone to maintain a diet, particularly if the patient is on hemodialysis. If the patient does deviate from a restricted diet, the blood chemistry will reveal the deviation. The nurse can show the patient the changes in the BUN or electrolyte panel that indicate failure to follow the diet. Patients who faithfully follow all dietary restrictions also can be shown their blood chemistry panels and thus be encouraged by realizing they are helping themselves to maintain what little kidney function remains.

The aged male patient who is concerned about his impotence may want to communicate with a member of the health team and should be given an opportunity to be counseled. Whenever possible the wife should be included in counseling sessions. Before the aged impotent man seeks quick remedies for his problem, professional counseling should be provided.

As the renal patient's condition becomes more unstable or critical, the behavioral picture may change. The patient may be well oriented and alert one hour and disoriented or lethargic the next. All changes in behavior need to be further assessed and reported. The changes can reflect metabolic problems, blood gas changes, or electrolyte imbalance. Sudden behavioral changes should be attributed to the renal problems rather than to "old age." The nurse should communicate possible reasons for the patient's behavior to the family and should inform them that the behavior is a reflection of the disease. While the patient is in a confused state, the nurse must continually maintain open communication between the patient and the wires and tubes. The aged patient may accidently remove the cardioscope leads, Foley catheter, or IV tube, thus terminating communication of the various therapies. The nurse must constantly reality test during the renal patient's confused states.

AERATION

Psychological aeration has been discussed under other components of FANCAP. Environmental aeration is a field in which the nurse can intervene by protecting the patient from distressing factors within the environment, especially because of the uremic patient's lowered resistance to infection. The environment should be comfortable. The patient whose bed is close to the window may receive the sun's heat and have a tendency to perspire and will have greater than normal insensible loss of water. On the other hand, the environment should not be too cool. Frequently, nurses regulate patients' environment according to their own metabolic needs. If they are working hard, the environment may seem particularly warm, but not to the uremic patient. The patient in renal failure may actually have a reduced temperature. Harrington and Brener (1973) remark, "Hypothermia occurs in many patients with renal failure and is related to the degree of uremia—patients with more severe uremia tend to have lower temperatures. Some have a usual rectal temperature of 95°F or lower." The patient's temperature may not be a good parameter for assessing infection.

Pulmonary aeration is assessed according to the lungs' ability to compensate for metabolic acidosis. As was discussed under the component "Fluids," respirations may be rapid and deep (Kussmaul's respiration). The lungs become primary vehicles for stabilizing the body's pH. Because the lungs are significant in maintaining relatively stabile acid-base balance, they must be protected. Aged patients are susceptible to pneumonia, particularly hypostatic pneumonia associated with immobility. Diseased lungs can inhibit acid-base balance because they contribute to acidosis. The resulting factor is metabolic acidosis with uncompensating respiratory acidosis. If for some reason the pulmonary system is ineffective in restoring the body's pH to a more normal level, sodium bicarbonate should be administered. Respiratory acidosis associated with pathological conditions independent of renal disease may need to be assisted with a volume respirator. Such assistance invariably creates respiratory alkalosis, thus restoring to the lungs their compensatory ability.

PAIN

The aged patient may need help in coping with the psychological pain associated with the illness. Psychological pain cannot be alleviated with narcotics, analgesics, or tranquilizers. Such pain may originate because aged individuals feel their sense of personal integrity is being threatened. They are forced to alter or completely change their life-style. Change is not easy for individuals whose life-style has been patterned by repetition. Consequently, they need assistance in identifying those areas which need not change and areas in which change is mandatory. Psychological pain can be just as severe as physiological pain. The problem is that psychological pain is less easily recognized. The nurse may observe subtle changes in the patient's behavior unrelated to renal abnormalities. Such behavior includes depression, tearfulness, or quietness and may be expressed nonverbally. Physiological pain is usually expressed verbally.

Aged patients with urinary tract infection experience a burning sensation when they void. Such pain is uncomfortable and causes some concern. In between voiding patients may ignore the symptom. Their attention becomes more focused as they develop persistent lower back pain indicating renal involvement. The physiological pain is no longer ignored because the pain is now persistent. Probably the most excruciating pain is that associated with passing renal calculi. Patients may experience passage of a ureteral calculus (stone in the ureter) characterized by pain radiating down the ureter. In addition to excruciating pain, they may also experience nausea, diaphoresis, and vomiting. The pain may last a few minutes or several hours. If patients are able to tolerate fluids, nurses should attempt to keep them well hydrated. Hydration helps the stone to pass. Analgesics may also be needed to reduce the pain. Furthermore, nurses should strain the urine to note passage of stones.

Another physiological pain experienced by the patient with renal abnormalities is headache. The headache may be attributed to hypervolemia or hypertension, both of which are factors in renal failure. Analgesics may be contraindicated because of the kidneys' inability to excrete their constituents. Therefore, the treatment has to be symptomatic—reduction of blood pressure and elimination of edema. Pain, regardless of its origin, should be identified and alleviated whenever possible.

In conclusion, treatment and nursing care of the aged patient with renal abnormalities begins conservatively. Conservative treatment involves diet, medication, fluid restriction, and symptomatic management of uremic manifestations. The conservative approach may help individuals with renal insufficiency or acute renal failure. Such may not be the case with chronic renal failure or uremia. These pathological states require more aggressive therapy, such as peritoneal dialysis or hemodialysis. Because of the individual's age or other related problems, the latter means of treatment may not be possible. The goal is to prevent renal abnormalities from occurring. The best means of prevention is early detection. As nurses increase abilities in physical assessment and diagnosis, renal abnormalities in the aged will be assessed within the individual's own community. Community diagnostic centers will greatly enhance the diagnosis, treatment, and teaching of aged patients.

REFERENCES

Guyton, Arthur: *Textbook of Medical Physiology,* Saunders, Philadelphia, 1971, pp. 445–447.

Harrington, Joan, and Etta Brener: *Patient Care in Renal Failure,* Saunders, Philadelphia, 1973, pp. 51, 55, 66, 76.

Jaffe, Jack: Common lower urinary tract problems in older people, in *Working with Older People,* vol. IV, Department of Health, Education, and Welfare, 1971, pp. 141, 143–145.

Kahn, Alvin, and I. Snapper: Medical renal diseases in the aged, in *Working with Older People,* vol. IV, Department of Health, Education, and Welfare, 1971, pp. 131, 133–139.

Metheny, Norma, and W. D. Snively: *Nurse's Handbook of Fluid Balance,* Lippincott, Philadelphia, 1974, pp. 61, 134, 214.

Oliver, Jean: Urinary system, in Albert Lansing (ed.), *Cowdry's Problems of Aging,* Williams & Wilkins, St. Louis, 1952, pp. 631, 637, 645–647.

Shock, Nathan: Age changes in renal failure, in Albert Lansing (ed.), *Cowdry's Problems of Aging,* Williams & Wilkins, St. Louis, 1952, pp. 614, 629.

TWENTY

MUSCULO-SKELETAL PROBLEMS IN AGING

Ann Herbert Shanck

OLD MAN
For some reason I cannot explain
that old man was fascinating
for me to see
hobbling, so much wiser
than I
down the street
with his hunched hand
on the top of his cane.
Carol Staudacher

LEARNING OBJECTIVES

- Describe briefly the "normal" muscle complaints of the aging person.
- Differentiate between osteoarthritis, rheumatoid arthritis, osteoporosis, and gout on the basis of etiology, anatomy, and physiology.
- Differentiate between the pain experiences of osteoarthritis, rheumatoid arthritis, osteoporosis, and gout.
- Give a general description of the medical management of osteoarthritis, rheumatoid arthritis, osteoporosis, and gout.
- Identify causes of fractures in the elderly.
- Differentiate between intracapsular and extracapsular hip fractures.
- Discuss nursing implications for osteoarthritis, rheumatoid arthritis, osteoporosis, and gout.
- Discuss the role of the nurse as a consumer advocate when working with patients and/or clients with musculoskeletal disorders.

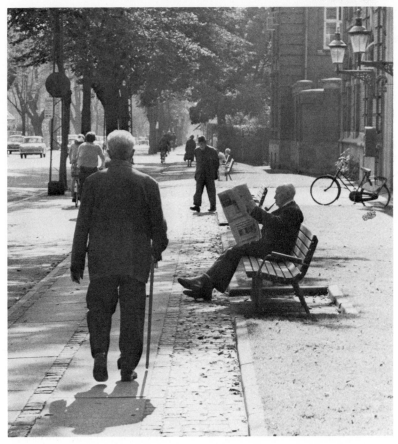

FIGURE 20-1 "For some reason I cannot explain/that old man was fascinating/for me to see . . ." (Carol Staudacher). (*Photo reprinted with permission of the World Health Organization. Photo by Erling Mandelmann.*)

Musculoskeletal system changes can significantly alter an older person's life-style by making many of the tasks of daily living more difficult. However, these changes need not be totally disabling with proper diagnosis and treatment.

This chapter will discuss muscle disorders, osteoarthritis, rheumatoid arthritis, osteoporosis, gout, and fractures along with their medical management as well as the implications for nursing.

MUSCLE DISORDERS

Skeletal muscles waste naturally, and there is general decrease in the muscle strength, endurance, and agility. This decrease in bulk is part of the general atrophy of organs and tissues; re-

generation is not active, and fibrous tissue replacement occurs. Atrophy of the small muscles of the hand make them appear thin and bony, and the leg and arm muscles become thin and flabby. There is surprisingly little weakness considering the degree of wasting.

There is a picture of general flexion when one views the posture of an aged person. The head and neck are held forward, the dorsal spine becomes gently kyphotic, upper limbs are bent at the wrists, and the hips and knees are slightly flexed. Changes in the vertebral column and in the intervertebral disks cause such changes, and there is ankylosis of ligaments and joints, shrinking and sclerosis of tendons and muscles, and degenerative changes in the central nervous system.

Muscle cramps become more bothersome with advancing age and are characterized by sustained involuntary and painful contractions of muscles. One muscle group of the calf, foot, thigh, hand, or hip is usually involved. The cramps occur after unusual muscle activity and especially at night. In most instances they occur in "normal" people and the reason is unknown. Paresthesias of the legs or "restless legs" may become more troublesome. Keeping the legs in motion can relieve the paresthesia. Lumbar osteoarthritis may compress nerve roots resulting in paresthesia, or it may occur without any cause (Grob, 1971).

OSTEOARTHRITIS

Osteoarthritis or degenerative joint disease is a noninflammatory disorder of the movable joints, which is characterized by deterioration and abrasion of articular cartilage and formation of new bone at the joint surfaces. It affects approximately 40 million people. Not much is known about the etiology. Some important systemic illnesses can initially produce part of or all the clinical picture of degenerative joint disease. Advancing age seems to be a predisposing factor in primary osteoarthritis. Secondary osteoarthritis, seen in younger people, is associated with trauma, infection, obesity, and occupational stresses, to mention a few causes.

The disease process affects the major weight-bearing joints—hips, knees, cervical, thoracic, and lumbar. Women, particularly, may develop Heberden's nodes. These are noted in the terminal interphalangeal joints of the fingers and help distinguish osteoarthritis from rheumatoid arthritis.

The clinical manifestations are local but cannot be correlated with the degree of joint changes found pathologically or radiologically. Weakness and immobility which may result from wasting are the only systemic signs. Pain, described as aching, is the main symptom which occurs on motion and weight bearing. Pain may increase before weather changes, as with other types of joint diseases. Stiffness on sitting or arising may occur for a short time, in contrast to rheumatoid arthritis in which the stiffness may persist for an hour or more. Pain is most pronounced after exercise and progresses during the day. When awake, the patient can splint the joint. At night he or she may be awakened with pain which occurs because the protective splinting is not present.

The knee joints are probably more frequently affected than any other joint. The quadriceps muscles may atrophy because of disuse due to pain. Overweight persons have an increased incidence of degenerative arthritis of the knees but not of the hips.

The most disabling site of the disease is the hip. Hip involvement is more common in women and occurs unilaterally in about half the patients. Motion produces pain which may be referred to the groin, buttocks, sciatic region, or inner aspect of the thigh or knee. Exostoses cause limitation of motion. The leg is often held in eversion, with the hip flexed and abducted. The gait is often shuffling and awkward. Severe pain can interfere with such activities as walking up and down stairs and getting out of a chair. The pathological changes in the femur also induce a tendency to fall.

Signs of inflammation are minimal except after trauma. Pain, muscle spasms, and contracture of capsule, fascia, or muscle incongruity of joint surfaces may cause limitation of joint motion. The flexion deformities of rheumatoid arthritis are much more severe. Muscle pain and soreness may be caused by abnormalities of posture and gait. The course is usually slow and progressive without characteristic exacerbations and remissions.

Osteoarthritis of the spine, spondylosis, is the commonest site of radiological change in men, and second to Heberden's nodes in women. Symptoms are usually mild to absent. A degeneration of the intervertebral disk occurs. If nerve root compression develops, there may be pain, distribution of which depends on the roots affected. Symptoms may become acute after such trauma as whiplash. Active or passive movement of the spine may aggravate pain and may be accompanied by muscle spasm. There could be sensory changes and signs of lower motor neuron lesion (muscle wasting and weakness) in the area innervated by the affected root.

Cervical arthritis may impair cerebral blood flow resulting in transient episodes of giddiness or syncope. Such episodes may occur at rest, on standing, or after rotation or extension of the neck, or less frequently during flexion. The patient may suddenly fall without loss of consciousness. A stroke may occur after movement or manipulation of the neck.

RHEUMATOID ARTHRITIS

Rheumatoid arthritis is a systemic disease of connective tissue in which joint inflammation is the predominant sign. The cause is unknown. In most patients the course of the disease is chronic and progressive and leads to characteristic deformities and disabilities. It usually begins between ages 20 and 60 with peaks around 35 to 45. It is three times more common in women than men. At least half of the 3.6 million Americans with the disease are 50 and above. The course in the elderly often progresses relentlessly despite all treatment. This may be explained by the diminished immune system of the aging client (Kolodny and Klipper, 1976).

The main lesion is inflammation of the synovial membrane with resulting erosion of the cartilage and bone. Adhesions also develop. The arthritis is usually polyarticular and involves small joints of hands and feet, whether or not major joints are also involved. The joints are usually involved symmetrically. The onset of the disease is usually insidious. The joints ache, especially on motion but also after rest. They become stiff after inactivity and especially on awakening.

The typical signs are best seen in proximal interphalangeal joints. There is a spindle-shaped appearance with soft-tissue swelling and atrophy of the contiguous muscle. Flexor contractions occur after a time. Metacarpophalangeal joint involvement leads to characteristic volar subluxation and ulnar deviation of the phalanges, and hand function is seriously impaired. Flexion contractures of hips and knees are also major causes of disability. The muscles of affected extremities may become severely weak and atrophied, much more so than would be expected from disuse alone.

Some systemic signs and symptoms include fatigue, malaise, slight fever, tachycardia, anorexia, weight loss, and mild or moderate anemia. The typical patient looks chronically ill.

The hallmark of rheumatoid arthritis is severe, painful morning stiffness, which does not go away in less than an hour or so; sometimes, if the client is not under treatment pain lasts for the entire day (Driscoll, 1975). Motion is limited because of the pain and stiffness. There is also gradual swelling, warmth, redness, and tenderness. These cardinal signs of inflammation differentiate rheumatoid arthritis from other arthralgias. Exacerbations and remissions are characteristic of this disease.

The American Rheumatism Association has systematized the criteria for diagnoses of rheumatoid arthritis. Eleven elements are given. These include morning stiffness, pain on motion or tenderness as observed in at least one joint, swelling in one or more joints, and symmetrical joint swelling. If these have been present continuously for 6 weeks or more, they are indicative of the disease. Other criteria include subcutaneous nodules, roentgenographic changes, a positive test for rheumatoid factor, poor mucin clot from synovial fluid, and histological changes in synovium and in nodules. The presence of 7 of these 11 findings warrants diagnosis of the classic disease, 5, that of definite disease, and 3, that of probable disease (Kolodny and Klipper, 1976).

GOUT

Gout is a metabolic disease with hereditary genetic transmission of unknown cause. It is shown by an increase in serum uric acid levels associated with recurrent attacks of acute arthritis of sudden onset and excruciating pain. Deposits of monosodium urate monohydrate may lead to tophaceous deposits in and around joints. Gout may lead to major renal disease, but if treated appropriately, it usually runs a mild course. The big toe is the most frequent site, but no joints are spared. Early recognition is important to prevent the damage of chronic gout.

Classically, acute gout may involve the great toe, ankle, knee, wrist, hip, and elbow. Attacks quickly come and go leaving the joint symptom-free. An acute attack shows a red-hot, incapacitated, immobilized, and excruciatingly painful joint.

OSTEOPOROSIS

The commonest of the metabolic bone diseases affecting the elderly is osteoporosis. It is characterized by a reduction in the quantity of bone, leading to an increased incidence of fracture resulting from minimal trauma. There is too little bone, but no alteration in its chemical composition. Women tend to lose bone faster than men, and on the average they begin to lose bone a decade earlier. This state occurs in approximately one-fourth of all elderly persons and most frequently in women between the ages of 50 and 70. It is an important cause of morbidity in the elderly.

There are many theories about the development of osteoporosis. Some of the causes advanced are: long-term inadequacies in diet, reduced absorptive efficiency of the aging digestive system, estrogen deficit, immobilization, long-term administration of high amounts of corticosteroids, and decreased activity.

The effects are most marked in the lumbar and thoracic spine, distal forearm, and neck of the femur. Vertebral collapse may result in loss of several inches in height and a marked kyphosis ("dowager's hump"). Such collapse may occur spontaneously or from trauma. Changes in the lumbar spine may be so excessive that the ribs lie on the ileum and the lung capacity is reduced. Jowsey (1977) states that osteoporosis, merely by definition, depends on the presence of a symptomatic fracture. Disease is not present because of a decrease in bone mass, although decreased bone mass is obviously the reason that fractures occur. The importance of the trauma in causing the fractures must not be underestimated. Although the trauma is often minimal, without it there is no fracture or symptoms.

The most frequent symptoms are pain in the back and the spine deformity. Pain usually results from the collapse of the vertebral bodies. These episodes often occur after sudden bending, lifting, or jumping movements which may have seemed trivial. Sometimes they are unrelated to trauma. Slight movements such as turning in bed can increase pain. Pain episodes last from a few days to several weeks, when patients can then resume their former activities. Some have minimal acute pain but have continuous deep nagging sensations in the fracture area brought about by sudden position changes or straining. Most have disappearance of or very little pain between episodes of vertebral body collapse. Others never have acute pain but complain of varying degrees of backache—often made worse by standing or moving suddenly. The course is not predictable, and there may be intervals of several years between fractures.

MEDICAL MANAGEMENT

According to Ehrlich (1973),

Arthritis is the culmination of insults upon a joint. Sometimes it is part of a generalized and systemic disease, as in rheumatoid arthritis. At other times, the problem is specifically localized, as in most instances of degenerative joint disease. There are probably as many causes for arthritis as there are arthritics. In analyzing some cases, more emphasis must be placed on physical and physiological alterations; in others, the emphasis must be on interpersonal relationships.

Those involved in the care of the arthritic person must understand that no drug will cure or prevent disability. Salicylates are useful drugs as analgesics and for anti-inflammatory action in any form of arthritis. In many patients it is the only drug needed.

Aspirin remains the drug of choice for rheumatoid arthritis. It is cheap, effective, reasonably well tolerated, and safe for long-term use. The patient should understand why aspirin is preferred. The therapeutic dose for an adult gives a serum level of 20 to 30 mg per 100 mL (3.6 to 5.4 g daily). This needs to be measured if no response to adequate dosage appears after 4 to 6 weeks.

The cause of failure must be determined. Side effects become obvious after a few days. Lack of efficacy can be established only after 4 to 6 weeks. Assuming dosage to be in the therapeutic range, lack of efficacy is rarely an indication for stopping aspirin. This is an indication for adding another agent.

Gastric discomfort and tinnitus are the major side effects. These may be avoided by

stopping therapy, then reintroducing aspirin at a slower rate of increase. Gastric discomfort may be lessened by taking frequent low doses with water, meals, milk, or alkali. Enteric-coated tablets are usually well absorbed and better tolerated but also are more expensive. Lack of compliance may account for an apparent aspirin failure. If serum level is less than 20 mg per 100 mL, the patient has probably not been taking the prescribed dose. If the level is in the therapeutic range, one can call the patient an "aspirin failure."

It is not within the realm of this discussion to detail the drug possibilities if aspirin therapy fails. Briefly, the nonsteroidal anti-inflammatory drugs (NSAID) may be tried next if aspirin fails, but, if unsuccessful, the remaining NSAID options should not be pursued.

For those who cannot tolerate aspirin, NSAIDs may be given. Four new ones in the United States are ibuprofen (Motrin), fenoprofen (Nalfon), tolmetin (Tolectin), and naproxen (Naprosyn). Indomethacin and phenylbutazone are the prototype NSAIDs. It is hoped that the newer agents will have fewer side effects.

When neither aspirin nor an NSAID works, a more active (and toxic) drug must be considered, e.g., gold and penicillamine. When these fail, the choice is among cytotoxic therapy, immunopotentiating agents, and systemic steroid therapy. Many rheumatologists believe that no group of drugs has been so misused as corticosteroids. The relief is dramatic and immediate, but the side effects are not worth the risk (Calin, 1978).

Psychological support cannot be overemphasized because of the pain and disability as well as the fact that an emotional upset can trigger an attack.

The primary objectives in rheumatoid arthritis are to inhibit inflammation and the symptoms of inflammation, to preserve function, to prevent joint deformities, and to restore function by repairing previous damage. Rest, physical therapy, and salicylates compose the basic treatment. This plan will be sufficient during most of the disease course for practically all patients. Both systemic and local rest help to resolve synovial inflammation.

A proper balance of rest and exercise should be part of the patient's daily program until joint and muscle functions have recovered. Then a regular program of active and passive exercises to maintain general muscle fitness and prevent atrophy should be performed within the limits of pain. Isometrics help to improve muscle strength and prevent atrophy. The exercise should be decreased, but not discontinued, if pain lasts more than an hour after exercise.

Heat and massage produce some symptomatic relief. Heat may be dry (electric pad, infrared, diathermy, or ultrasound) or moist. Massage should be gentle over joints but vigorous over muscles to help prevent atrophy.

Complete bed rest must be avoided in order to prevent flexion contractures which occur, as it is easier to flex an inflamed joint to ease pain and spasm while in bed. Position at rest is of utmost importance. Local articular rest and/or correction of deformities may be accomplished by well-fitted, lightweight splints or shells. Traction and sandbags may be useful in restoring or maintaining alignment as an alternative to splints. Canes, crutches, or other mechanical devices may be used when weight-bearing joints are involved. Bedboards along with firm mattresses are usually prescribed to reduce workload on muscles and to support the body. For the same reason a patient should have a firm chair. If the chair is high, this will assist the patient to rise without having to rock. Rocking chairs provide some activity even at rest.

Aspirin is the main analgesic for osteoarthritis but not at the near-toxic doses used for rheumatoid arthritis. The usual dosage is 600 mg, four times daily as needed. NSAIDs may be utilized. Systemic corticosteroids are not used, but intra-articular steroids can be used, especially in the knee. If indicated, the program should direct itself toward weight reduction in order to decrease stress on weight-bearing joints. A gradually intensified exercise program of isometric and range of motion exercises is important to maintain mobility and strong support around joints. Hot packs may relieve pain in sore muscles adjacent to osteoarthritic joints. Patients need to be reminded that there is no "cure" and improvement may not be immediately obvious.

The prevention and control of arthritis can fail despite comprehensive and supportive medical and nursing management. At this time re-

constructive surgery may be considered. Inglis (1973) feels that pain is the major indication for all reconstructive surgery in arthritis. Although motion, strength, and joint control are important facets in the evaluation of any surgical procedure, the reduction of pain ultimately signals the success or failure of surgery.

Commonly used surgical procedures are (1) synovectomy, the removal of diseased synovial membrane; (2) osteotomy, repositioning of joint surfaces to improve articulation and thus reduce trauma from friction; (3) cup arthroplasty, provision of an artificial joint usually of plastic or metal; (4) arthrodesis, fixation of a joint by fusing the joint surfaces; (5) total joint replacement arthroplasty, replacement of the joints by a prosthesis implanted in contacting bone.

Most total hip replacements in osteoarthritis are done to relieve pain, whereas in rheumatoid, this procedure is as important for correcting gait disturbance and limited range of motion as for pain relief (Feinstein and Habermann, 1977). Knee and hand replacements have been good. Recently experimental prostheses for shoulder, wrist, and elbow have been developed (Swezey, 1978).

There are many treatment regimens for osteoporosis because of the many possible mechanisms for its development. The criteria for effectiveness of therapy in well-established osteoporosis are few and poor. The basic approach is to alleviate pain with analgesics and to safeguard the patient against falls and other trauma. With no simple criteria to measure the effectiveness of therapy, physicians are obliged to follow a multifaceted approach. They choose a program to meet the needs of the individual and base its success on whether the patient responds, e.g., cessation of height loss and reduction of fracture incidents.

The efficacy of treatment aimed at strengthening bone is not ensured. Estrogen or testosterone is used along with supplementary calcium and vitamin D to facilitate absorption (Krane, 1977). Jowsey (1977) feels concurrent administration of fluoride and calcium is the most promising of the available therapeutic programs.

Colchicine is very effective for acute attacks of gout. Other drugs which lower blood levels of uric acid (probenecid, sulfin pyrazone) may be used. Diet restriction of foods high in purine might be helpful.

FRACTURES

Fractures among older persons do not always result from osteoporosis. Factors such as muscular weakness, impaired vision, reduced reaction times, and mental confusion all contribute to accidents, falls, and broken bones (Kart et al., 1978). Elderly women exhibit a higher rate of fractures than do elderly men. However, the usual cause of serious fractures in middle-aged and older adults relates more directly to bone loss than to the frequency of forceful accidents (Wylie, 1977).

The hip is a common site. Two main classifications of hip fracture are intracapsular and extracapsular. In both, the patient will complain of pain, the affected leg will be in external rotation, it will be shorter than the uninjured one, and the greater trochanter can be felt in the buttocks.

An intracapsular fracture occurs when the bone is broken inside the hip joint and capsule. An extracapsular fracture occurs outside the capsule to an area 2 inches below the lesser trochanter. Bone atrophy of the femoral neck may cause intracapsular fracture when the bone gives way and the individual falls or slips on a rug or waxed floor. These are examples of indirect violence to the hip. Complications occur from these fractures because of the limited blood supply and difficulty in getting accurate approximation and rigid immobilization of the fragments.

Direct violence, such as a fall directly onto the trochanter or when the leg is twisted, causes extracapsular fractures. The intertrochanteric region has a rich blood supply and union usually occurs without any difficulty.

Fortunately, with the advent of pins, nails, and prostheses, the care of the patient with a fractured hip is simplified and shortened. The preferred method of treatment is surgery. Rarely do we find the elderly patient strung up in traction for several weeks or months, with all the additional threats immobilization brings, not the least of which is sensory deprivation.

Major differences in care of the various types of hip surgery involve positioning in bed and the ambulation schedule. These treatments will vary according to the physician's orders. The pre- and postoperative care is the same as for any surgical patient with the inclusion of *special consideration for the geriatric patient, such as discriminate use of sedation and careful monitoring of fluids and electrolytes.*

Many of the management suggestions could include valuable preventives for hip fracture. The fear of falling and a resulting fracture immobilizes an old person both physically and socially. If a fracture does occur, the institution of an organized exercise program becomes essential for the immediate mobilization of the individual.

We protect the "feeble aged" from falling by fastening them in a chair or bed and then wonder at their inability to walk. Monteiro (1967) presents the possibility that although age, sex, race, and urbanization correlate with fracture incidence rates, other factors which bear a less direct but important relationship are socioeconomic status and social role. She also suggests that changes in social roles and abrupt hospitalization affect the patient's personality and chances of survival. She urges more research in this area.

IMPLICATIONS FOR NURSING

The collaboration of the incapacitated person, the nurse, the physician, and the family are needed to provide an understanding of the underlying nature of musculoskeletal diseases. I have indicated a number of ways that medical therapy prescribes a variety of measures to alleviate symptoms, and some might be implemented by nursing without a specific order. The implication for nursing in assisting the aged with musculoskeletal problems is a rehabilitative approach. Mitchell (1977) says rehabilitation is the process of restoring a person to his previous capabilities, or helping him make the most of his existing capabilities. *The person must participate if he is to make the most of his abilities, and this is where the nurse can play a large role.* Many nurses think that rehabilitation

has to be administered by selected people in selected places, but this is simply not so. Old people with these disorders often feel crippling is inevitable and irreversible, and the health team has an obligation to convince them otherwise.

There is probably no other area where the support of the nurse in the promotion of the patient's capabilities is more significant than in the management of this group of disorders. To assist older patients acquire the will, and to help them take the responsibility for their own growth, we use the nurse's technical know-how and scientific knowledge. Any suggestions for the actions of the nurse would naturally involve collaboration with the physician in the medical and surgical management of the patient and medical orders wherever needed or demanded. (See Figures 20-2 to 20-4.)

According to Mitchell (1977) the data to be assessed include:

1. Medical restrictions on activity
2. Musculoskeletal status
   a. General movement
   b. Muscle strength, tone, mass
   c. Range of joint motion
   d. Posture
   e. Handedness
   f. Deformities
   g. Abnormal innervation to muscles
3. Mobility
   a. Method of ambulation
   b. Gait
   c. Endurance

Assess the patient from the standpoint of functional ability and not from medical diagnosis or age. Storz (1972) has an excellent questionnaire.

We must review the patient's daily activities to see what potentially dangerous situations can be eliminated and what activities can be facilitated. We can provide many practical aids that are inexpensively made or bought to protect vulnerable joints (Hinshaw and Barrier, n.d.; Pigg, 1974; Independence Factory, n.d.).

Patients need to be encouraged to take an adequate diet, and the significance of the additives the physician may order should be stressed. Inappropriate use of vitamins should

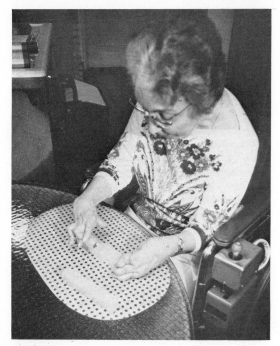

FIGURE 20-2 This woman has had arthritis for years but lives alone and manages independently. (*Courtesy of Anthony J. Skirlick, Jr.*)

be emphasized. Foods with high purine content should be avoided in gout, and forcing fluids is especially important to flush out uric acid salts. If obesity is a problem, help plan a reduction diet. The psychosocial aspects of eating are im-

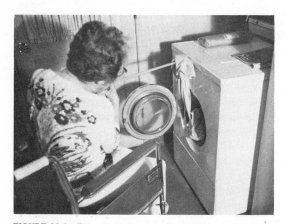

FIGURE 20-3 This photo shows how a stick is used to transfer washing and drying when arthritic hands have lost their strength and ability to grasp. (*Courtesy of Anthony J. Skirlick, Jr.*)

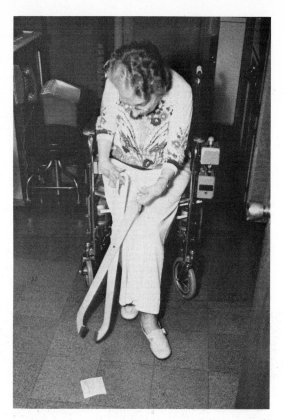

FIGURE 20-4 A scissorslike aid is used by this independent arthritic woman to pick up a piece of paper she has dropped. (*Courtesy of Anthony J. Skirlick, Jr.*)

portant, because since the aged are increasingly isolated, they probably do not spend enough on food, which is increasingly expensive.

Environmental intervention programs seem to reinforce high levels of activity.[1] McClanna-han's (1973) review of the literature describes many suggestions which would have an impact in deterring degenerative processes associated with aging. This researcher suggests that atten-

---

[1] Editor's note: A professional dog trainer has developed a program for crippled arthritic persons and others who are disabled to teach their dogs to perform certain critical tasks they are unable to do for themselves. Unlike Seeing-Eye dogs, which are trained by professionals, these Handi-Dogs can be trained by their arthritic owners. Dogs are taught to come, carry, and bark on command (Alamo Reeves, 5332 East Rosewood, Tucson, Arizona 85711).

tion to the design-for-living environments might lead to modification of "old" behavior. A few of the suggestions were handrails in dining halls and other areas besides corridors, changes in floor coverings to increase mobility, installation of ramps and wide doors, automatic door openers, levers instead of door knobs, simple folk dances to encourage locomotion as one type of recreational activity to use as therapy as well as for prosthetic effect of motor disabilities.

Surgical nursing requires different turning and positioning regimens for each type of surgical procedure, and every orthopedic surgeon has a preference. Orthopedic management is relatively new, and the nurse can help the patient realize that surgery is not an end stage measure. Some may feel that they are "too old" and do not realize that an instability of the knee may tax the heart more than the surgery done to correct the knee.

Exercise and rest have been emphasized. (See Figure 20-5.) The degree and amount depend upon the status of the patient. Sometimes these alone will reduce the need for pain medication. The patient should be assessed for ability to move the joints, because often our contact with this person is for some reason other than musculoskeletal disorder. Nurse and patient need to understand that overuse of either can be detrimental. The nurse can supervise full range of motion in unaffected joints and see that the patient moves the affected joint only to the point of resistance to pain. The nurse can help the patient achieve full range if he or she is unable.

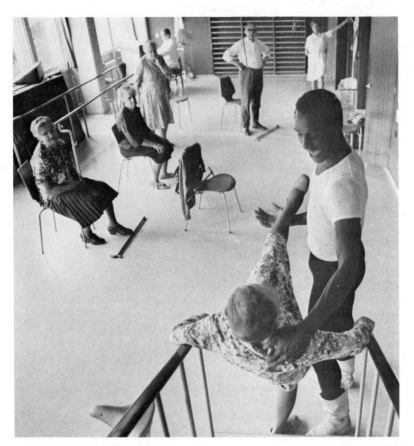

FIGURE 20-5   These old people, many of them over 80, take jazz ballet lessons twice a week. (*Reprinted with permission of the World Health Organization. Photo by Erling Mandelmann.*)

These movements also help to maintain muscle tone. When the individual cannot accomplish range of motion, the nurse may perform passive range of motion exercises. We might maximize the joint problems by poor positioning and body alignment or condoning too much bed rest or depriving the individuals of performing the activities of daily living.

To alleviate muscle atrophy which goes along with joint problems, isometric contractions can be demonstrated. Abdominal tightening, gluteal setting, quadriceps setting, resistive exercises, and foot circling are helpful. Deep breathing should be encouraged in arthritics because they have a tendency to breathe shallowly and develop a narrow, rounded chest which will lead to an increasing respiratory deficiency. In any exercise program individuals have to be carefully evaluated to see what they can tolerate. If they have pain and discomfort for too long a time after exercise, then there is probably joint overuse and they need to reduce exercise to a more tolerable level.

Be sure that splints are used if prescribed and that their use is properly demonstrated. Check out shoes because the elderly often scrimp on shoes. Well-made and well-fitted shoes are a potent therapeutic device for changing body alignment and providing balance. Neck collars can be made from rolled up newspapers, and these also must be worn properly. Sometimes sleeping on a Japanese pillow helps. Wearing stretch fit-one-size gloves to bed at night can combat the morning symptoms of swollen joints and morning stiffness. Caution patients *not* to wear them when the joint is acutely inflamed. Show osteoporotic patients how to take care of their backs; e.g., they should be cautioned not to pick up the grandchildren.

Convince them that there is nothing better than a regular exercise regimen for these disorders and for a general feeling of well-being. They should avoid unnecessary walking and stair-climbing during acute episodes and at the same time realize that excessive rest may cause stiffening and atrophy of cartilage and muscle. Poor body mechanics should be corrected as well as faulty work habits.

Drugs, especially the salicylates, are often prescribed. The individual does not often realize the importance of a regular regimen for taking salicylates, often taking them only when there is pain. Understanding the role of these drugs is important! The patient and/or client should know of the availability of other salicylates in the event that one kind does not work or produces side effects. The side effects of aspirin have been pointed out earlier, and the patient and/or client needs to be taught what they are. The significance of a drug history cannot be overemphasized. The elderly are vulnerable to quack remedies and cure-alls. They also have a tendency to self-dose, and their drugs may counteract each other.

If there is difficulty remembering when drugs are to be taken or recognizing the correct one, the nurse might help make up a drug calendar on which to mark the time for all drugs. Help the patient package the drugs for specified time periods, like a week; they could be put in sandwich bags, egg cartons, or ice cube trays. As one who has to bite the top of childproof aspirin bottles, imagine the challenge to arthritic fingers and poor eyesight! Patients should know that some companies sell regular-top bottles (for a price) or should be advised to transfer the pills into something else at home.

If estrogens are prescribed for osteoporosis, the female patient must understand the necessity for periodic breast examinations and Papanicolaou smears. She may be frightened by vaginal bleeding or stop taking the medication because she does not want to "menstruate" any more. She must realize that the estrogen may reduce the incidence of fractures, and with proper follow-up, these symptoms will be kept under control.

Psychosocial aspects of care cannot be overemphasized. There seems to be an emotional component in the course of rheumatoid arthritis, and the arthritic patient and/or client generally is very demanding and quite inflexible. There has to be improved communication among members of the health team, the individual, and the family in order to fully understand the treatment goals. We have to help the aging talk about what is bothering them; they may be worried about a radical change in life-style, fear of pain or of being an economic burden, or frustration at the relapses. The nurse must provide the spark of motivation toward restoration of function and maybe even survival. We cannot raise hope unduly!

Disability may also be imposed by society. Public buildings with great flights of stairs make it impossible for the elderly to get to the toilet. If they do make it, the door gets in the way, and it will be too narrow for the wheelchair or whatever appliance is being used. Chairs and toilet seats are too low; curbs and bus steps are too high. Thus life shrinks! Teamwork is important, and patients' efforts represent at least half the treatment program. *The aim is adaptation of patients to live with their musculoskeletal disorders, not to exist with them.*

Tribes of primitive people used to abandon their disabled; now we tend to place them in protective isolation (institutions of various sorts), bedrooms, or wheelchairs. Chronic crippling diseases do pose a tremendous economic burden by incapacitating the sufferers often while they are still consumers. Vignos (1973) feels we have our priorities wrong if we wish to improve the quality of life. More often than not, we find that the community is not even aware a problem exists.

I do not picture the nurse as necessarily having to perform any of or all these interventions solely in a hospital, patient's home, or care facility, but rather anywhere in the community where health teaching can be done. Old people can live in rundown tenement hotels, in too-large houses in the suburbs, and anywhere in between, and many do not go to physicians for various reasons. Many vegetate with these problems and live without hope.

By participating in community or consumer group activities, the nurse could effect change by teaching the elderly and their families prevention as well as how to adapt to deformities already present. For example, the average rheumatoid person waits 3 to 4 years before seeking treatment, and in that time unnecessary crippling will have taken place. Classes might be held under the auspices of adult education in senior centers, care facilities, and in the schools. Perhaps an in-service program for those working with the aged could be developed for continuing education credits. The program could be rotated through extended-care facilities according to geographic location, for the convenience of the staff. There are just too many being neglected and living without hope to wait until we might receive them as "patients." Let us orient society to our aging population, because preparation for successful aging must start in youth.

Health workers with the aged have a responsibility to aid their clients to take a look at their resources. We can help them remember how they may have coped in the past. Many of the aged wish to explore opportunities for activity but find themselves forced into idleness. We can help them view aging as still another challenge and to live fully with their physical incapacities until they die.

REFERENCES

Calin, Andrei: Rheumatoid arthritis, *AFP,* **18**(1):63–68, January 1978.

Driscoll, P. W.: Rheumatoid arthritis: Understanding it more fully, *Nursing '75,* **5**(12):27–35, December 1975.

Ehrlich, George: Introduction, in George Ehrlich (ed.), *Total Management of the Arthritic Patient,* Lippincott, Philadelphia, 1973, p. 2.

Feinstein, P. A., and E. T. Habermann: Selecting and preparing patients for total hip replacement, *Geriatrics,* **32**(7):91–96, July 1977.

Grob, David: Common disorders of muscles in the aged, in A. B. Chinn (ed.), *Working with Older People: A Guide to Practice,* vol. 4, *Clinical Aspects of Aging,* U.S. Public Health Service Publication 1459, Washington, 1971, pp. 156–162.

————: Prevalent joint disease in older persons, ibid., pp. 163–171.

Hinshaw, Edith S., and Dorothy Barrier: Physically handicapped (aids to self-help in homemaking, grooming, and clothing), pamphlet, North Carolina Agricultural Extension Service, Raleigh, N.C. (free), n.d.

Independence Factory: P.O. Box 597, Middletown, OH 45042 (non-profit volunteer organization).

Inglis, Allan E.: The surgery of arthritis, in George Ehrlich (ed.), *Total Management of the Arthritic Patient,* Lippincott, Philadelphia, 1973, pp. 61–109.

Jowsey, J.: Osteoporosis: Dealing with a crippling bone disease of the elderly, *Geriatrics,* **32**(7):41–50, July 1977.

Kart, C. S., et al.: *Aging and Health: Biologic and Social Perspectives,* Addison-Wesley, Menlo Park, Calif., 1978, pp. 44–59, 106–108.

Kolodny, A. L., and A. R. Klipper: Bone and joint diseases in the elderly, *Hospital Practice,* **11**(11):91–101, November 1976.

Krane, S. M.: Osteoporosis, in George W. Thorn et al. (eds.), *Harrison's Principles of Internal Medicine,* 8th ed., McGraw-Hill, New York, 1977, pp. 2028–2033.

McClannahan, Lynne: Therapeutic and prosthetic living environments for nursing home residents, *Gerontologist,* **13**(4):424–429, Winter 1973.

Mitchell, Pamela H.: *Concepts Basic to Nursing,* McGraw-Hill, New York, 1977, pp. 291, 332–334.

Monteiro, Lois A.: Hip fracture: A sociologist's viewpoint, *American Journal of Nursing,* **67**:1207–1210, June 1967.

Pigg, J.: 50 helpful hints for active arthritis patients, *Nursing 74,* **4**(7):39–41, July 1974.

Storz, Rita R.: The role of a professional nurse in a health maintenance program, *Nursing Clinics of North America,* **7**:207–223, June 1972.

Swezey, R. L.: *Arthritis: Rational Therapy and Rehabilitation,* Saunders, Philadelphia, 1978, pp. 1–20.

Vignos, Paul V.: Psychosocial problems in management of chronic arthritis, in George Ehrlich (ed.), *Total Management of the Arthritic Patient,* Lippincott, Philadelphia, 1973, pp. 111–128.

Wylie, C. M.: Hospitalization for fractures and bone loss, *Public Health Report,* **92**:33–35, January–February 1977.

OTHER RESOURCES

Arthritis Information Clearinghouse (AIC), P.O. Box 34427, Dept. N79, Bethesda, MD 20034, or call (301) 881-9411. This group was set up by the National Institute of Arthritis, Metabolism, and Digestive Diseases to "broker" the nationwide flow of arthritis information. The staff will lead you to the best audiovisual programs and pamphlets for your patients. A newsletter is being prepared.

The Stroke Patient, filmstrip with tapes. Concept Media, 1500 Adams Avenue, Costa Mesa, CA 92626.

Strokes, 16 mm/color/min. Short graphic description of physiology of strokes; includes brief description of poststroke residual. Request from local American Heart Association chapter.

TWENTY-ONE

FOOT PROBLEMS AND ASSESSMENT

Patricia Ann King

Of all exercises walking is the best.
Thomas Jefferson

LEARNING OBJECTIVES

- Delineate the physiological foot changes that occur with aging.
- Identify the nurse's role in promoting foot health.
- Describe at least four common foot problems of the elderly.
- Describe an assessment tool for systematically evaluating the condition of the lower extremities.
- Describe at least six treatment modalities that will promote foot welfare.

Portions of this chapter appeared in "Foot assessment of the elderly," *Journal of Gerontological Nursing,* 4(6):47–52, November–December 1978.

The foot is a forgotten part of the body. In the literature little attention was given to foot problems or to the significance of foot health. This situation has changed in recent years. Increasingly, documentation is being given to the importance of the foot as an organ for assessment and evaluation by members of the nursing and medical profession.

The foot is unlikely to be the cause of mortality, but it is often the cause of and site of morbidity, disability, and limitation of activity (Helfand, 1971b, p. 377). Foot problems are more likely to manifest themselves in the elderly population. Helfand's (1973) 5-year longitudinal survey of institutionalized elderly patients and his 3-year "Keep Them Walking" project (1968) of noninstitutionalized older citizens are landmark studies underscoring the high incidence of foot problems for this group.

Foot disability can lead to serious consequences for older persons. Once they are no longer able to ambulate freely, for whatever reason, their independence is curtailed, and their psychological well-being is affected. Feelings of helplessness may curtail rehabilitation (Helfand, 1970). Furthermore, their social life space may be confined, making them potential social isolates. Thus, the need for foot health for older persons is paramount.

Podogeriatrics is a term used to signify the caring for the aging foot. This chapter will focus on (1) the structure and function of the human foot, (2) foot disability in the aged, and (3) the nurse's role in podiatric care.

STRUCTURE AND FUNCTIONS OF THE HUMAN FOOT

The human foot has been defined as an "intricate mechanism that functions interdependently with other components of the locomotor system" (DuVries, 1959, p. 3). There are 26 bones, 107 ligaments, and 19 muscles in each foot. Kinetic and static functions are performed by the foot. When the foot acts to support the body in standing, it is performing a static function, while its action as a lever for propulsion during walking is a kinetic function (DuVries, 1959, p. 49; DuVries, 1973, p. 3).

The geriatric foot shows the effects of the "ravages of time, abetted by the static stresses imposed by weight-bearing and shoes" (Jahss, 1971, p. 327). The skin is atrophic, dry, and scaly with loss of hair and skin elasticity, while the nails appear striated and brittle (Helfand, 1967). Pain sensation is reduced and there is a diminished blood supply.

Of all the changes in the aging foot, the diminished blood supply is one of the most significant. Jahss (1971) assumes that there is marked circulatory impairment from arteriosclerosis in persons past 65 years and from arteriolosclerosis in diabetics by the time they are 45 years of age. The consequences which follow from this impairment may be severe, according to Jahss. Slight fissures in the skin of diabetics may lead to infection and gangrene. The same effects may follow for persons with advanced arterial insufficiency from minor trauma, a surgical procedure, or the application of a strong keratolytic agent.

The feet may provide valuable clues to a systemic disturbance. Riccitelli (1969, p. 205) states that the feet are often the site of many initial signs and symptoms, not only of peripheral vascular disorders but also of systemic diseases. For example, an ulcer on the foot that does not heal may be the first sign of diabetes. Wilkins (1967) calls attention to the digits of the extremities as being particularly vulnerable, both because they are situated at the periphery of the vascular tree and because they are often subjected to trauma and variable temperatures.

FOOT DISABILITY IN THE AGED

Riccitelli (1966) has classified the types of foot problems among older persons into five categories: mechanical, arthritic, circulatory, dermatologic, and neurotrophic. These disturbances may be associated with foot pain and disability. A model adapted from his classification scheme is shown in Figure 21-1.

MECHANICAL STRESSORS AND THE FEET

Helfand (1971b, p. 379) categorizes mechanical stressors into two types: macrotrauma and microtrauma. The former is due to a sudden injury

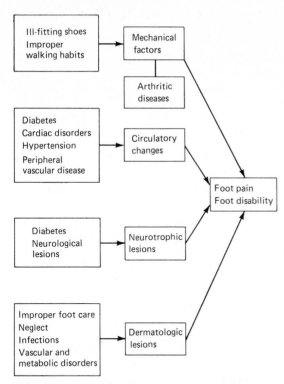

FIGURE 21-1 Causes of foot pain and disability. (*Adapted from M. L. Riccitelli, Foot problems of the aged and infirm, Journal of the American Geriatrics Society, 14(10):1058–1065, October 1966. Reprinted by permission.*)

resulting in fracture, while the latter results from a lifetime of stresses to the feet, such as poor stance and gait, poorly fitting shoes, or prolonged stretching of ligaments. According to Helfand (1967, p. 597), it is a myth that all foot problems are caused by poorly fitting shoes. He attributes the major cause of foot problems to microtrauma resulting from anatomic or pathomechanical changes. Hyperkeratotic lesions such as corns and calluses may be manifestations of these changes. Hallux valgus (displaced toe) and digitus flexus (hammertoe) are deformities that may lead to severe limitation of activity.

ARTHRITIC DISEASES AND THE FEET

Common joint diseases affecting the feet include: degenerative joint disease (osteoarthritis), rheumatoid arthritis, and gout. De-

generative joint disease is a noninflammatory disorder that progresses slowly from spur formation along the articular margins to marked deformities in the advanced stage (Riccitelli, 1966). Range of motion will be reduced at the involved joints. Rheumatoid arthritis, a chronic systemic disease, produces degenerative changes in the cartilage leading to deformity and limited mobility. In the foot the metatarsophalangeal joints are most likely to be involved. The toes may be cocked up or deformed. Gout, a metabolic disturbance in the skeletomuscular system, most commonly affects the great toe. The presence of hallux rigidus in an older person is highly suggestive of gout (Jahss, 1971, p. 328).

CIRCULATORY CHANGES, FOOT PAIN, AND DISABILITY

The disturbance of blood flow to the aging foot is usually a result of arteriosclerosis. The signs and symptoms of this disturbance are directly related to the degree of blood flow. The greater the deficiency of blood flow, the greater the circulatory disturbance, and the greater the manifestations of peripheral vascular disease (Wilkins, 1967, p. 724). Assessment of the lower extremities can yield valuable information on peripheral ischemia.

Intermittent claudication may be noted. It results when the tissues' metabolic demands exceed the available blood supply. Rest pain indicates a more severe tissue ischemia.

Diminished blood flow is revealed by (1) changes in skin color, skin temperature, and skin integrity, (2) absent or diminished pedal pulses, and (3) postural changes involving increased pallor on elevation and a delayed return to a pink color on dependency. *Skin color* may vary from red to reddish blue to marked pallor. It is an important indicator of blood flow. The more slowly the blood flows, the greater the oxygen loss and the more cyanotic the skin becomes (Fairbairn, et al., 1972). *Coldness of the extremities* is noteworthy when there are consistent differences between the extremities.

Skin changes reflecting tissue malnourishment include atrophy, dryness, fissures, shininess, thickened nails, absence of hair over the great toe, and thickened nails. When ulceration or gangrene develops, the terminal portions of the digits are the first to be involved (Juergens and Bernatz, 1972).

DERMATOLOGIC LESIONS OF THE FOOT

The aging foot is more susceptible to bacterial and fungous infections, to trauma, and to cold. Vascular and metabolic disturbances may be associated with pedal complications such as ulceration, chronic infection, calluses, corns, and plantar warts. Skin lesions may result from poorly fitting shoes, improper foot care, neglect, and infections (Riccitelli, 1966, p. 1064).

The presence of hyperkeratotic lesions (corns or calluses) at pressure points on the foot may cause considerable discomfort; they are potentially dangerous. If untreated, the built-up stratum corneum can exert pressure on the subcutaneous tissue resulting in necrosis and ulceration (Rakow and Friedman, 1969a and b).

Nail problems particularly troublesome in the aged are (1) onychocryptosis (ingrown toenail), (2) onychauxis (thickening of the nail plate), and (3) onychomycosis (fungous infection). An ingrown nail is one in which a nail segment penetrates the nail groove. It may result from improper cutting or external pressure. Thickened nails may result from arteriosclerosis or repeated trauma. Fungous nails characteristically are opaque, scaly, and hypertrophic and may be associated with a pungent odor and yellow striations. The course of treatment for the latter condition is long, and reinfection is likely.

NEUROTROPHIC LESIONS OF THE FOOT

These lesions may result from diabetes or a nervous system disorder. When sensation is diminished, as in diabetic neuropathy, the tissues are vulnerable to trauma. A trophic ulcer may develop at pressure points on the foot. This is a painless lesion usually associated with a callus and is likely to become infected. A neurological lesion may be the probable cause of a foot lesion when abnormal reflexes and changes in tactile or vibratory sensations in the foot are noted in a routine physical examination (Riccitelli, 1966). Helfand (1974) focused on a screening program

for pedal complications in diabetes. During a 10-week period, a random sample of diabetic patients attending a regularly scheduled clinic was evaluated by a podiatric team. Six and one-half percent of those screened had ulcerations with varying degrees of necrosis.

THE NURSE'S ROLE IN PODIATRIC CARE

Podiatrists have noted the importance of the nurse's role in foot care. Helfand (1971a) recommended that nurses become involved in assessing the feet. Simko (1974) urged nurses to play a more direct role in teaching, assisting with foot hygiene, and recognizing foot problems.

Nurses, too, have recognized this need. Bruck and Lambert's (1959) article on common foot disabilities appears to be the first in the nursing journals. It was their thesis that early attention to foot discomfort and irritation tends to prevent disabling deformities of the feet. Spencer (1970) pointed out the importance of foot health for the elderly and recommended the following roles for the nurse: (1) observing and recording foot problems, (2) making foot care part of the nursing care plan, (3) initiating communication with a podiatrist, and (4) including foot care requirements in discharge planning.

The roles the nurse can assume in foot health for the elderly can be identified as follows: (1) advocacy, (2) direct service, and (3) teaching.

ADVOCACY ROLE

Despite the gains made in recent years, the foot is still forgotten by many. Health care providers tend to ignore this part of the body in examinations and care. Older persons, themselves, tend to ignore their feet for several reasons: (1) they may be unable to care for them because of poor vision or an arthritic condition, (2) they have not been informed about the importance of foot care, and (3) they may have the attitude that foot pain and disability are parts of aging and nothing can be done about them. Thus, there is a need to alert these groups to the significance of foot health. This is where the advocacy role can be effective.

Nurses can speak for foot health maintenance for the elderly. There are opportunities in the community, the acute care setting, and the non–acute care setting. For instance, are there foot screening programs in the community for older citizens? If not, why not? A good example of what can be done was reported by Schank (1977) and Conrad (1977). Nursing students and faculty from the Marquette University College of Nursing worked with podiatrists in a foot education and screening program for the "well-elderly." The authors concluded that the program raised the level of community awareness in regard to foot health maintenance measures and recognition of treatable foot pathology.

Older persons may not know that some podiatric services are covered under the Medicare and Medicaid programs. Nurses can provide these people with information on the types of podiatry services available and the eligibility requirements by contacting the social security office or the state office of DHHS (formerly DHEW).

Specific services which an advocate for foot health can propose include the following:

1. Foot health maintenance instruction through continuing education and in-service programs.
2. Foot health teaching to nursing students and nonprofessional care givers in long-term care facilities.
3. Foot-screening clinics in long-term care facilities.
4. Foot-screening clinics in the community, possibly conducted by the county health department.

DIRECT-SERVICE ROLE: ASSESSMENT AND INTERVENTION

Assessment Anderson (1971) discusses foot assessment in relation to peripheral vascular diseases and advocates a foot inspection at the time of a patient's hospital admission and regularly after that. Fowler (1974) directs the nurse's attention to the "great right toe" as an impor-

tant body part to assess, since it may yield clues to systemic conditions.

Nursing assessment involves the gathering of information—subjective and objective—on the health status of the individual in order to make decisions relating to losses or potential losses in that status (Block, 1974). An observational instrument which is well defined, clearly understood, and systematically used facilitates the assessment process and provides the basis for sound nursing intervention. (See Figure 21-2.)

Martin and Smith (1969) designed an observational tool for assessing a diabetic patient's foot care practices. Hopp and Sundberg (1974) constructed a dryness scale for assessing the texture of the skin. King (1978) developed an observational instrument for assessing the lower extremities of the elderly client (Figure 21-2). Content validity was established and the tool was tested for reliability. The tool enables the assessor to (1) identify problems which should be referred to a physician or podiatrist and (2) recognize problems which require nursing intervention. There are four parts to the instrument. The first section involves a general assessment including items on mobility, gait disturbance, symmetry, foot hygiene, and foot wear. The second and third sections deal with a dermatologic and peripherovascular assessment, respectively, while the last section deals with an assessment for structural deformities.

In assessing gait, Wolanin's (1976) discussion is noteworthy. It is reprinted with permission from the author.

Gait Assessment The most revealing sign of impending mobility problems is shown by the gait of the elderly. The quick, springy, natural rhythmic step of earlier years changes to a slowed, measured, and unnatural gait, which may be a means of protecting the person from pain, loss of balance, or weakness. While not every gait problem can be corrected, many can be reduced; the pain and lack of safety may even be eliminated by means of prostheses or supports.

Each step is a dual act, with the body supported on one limb while the opposite limb swings forward from the pelvis, carrying the entire body through the swing phase; i.e., the foot

INSTRUCTIONS: For each item, circle the response in the appropriate column, unless directed otherwise. Clarification of items appears in the far-right column.

Patient number _____

Date _____

RN number _____

1. Mobility (check one)
   Walks with assistance ___ Walks with help of equipment ___
   Does not walk: Uses wheelchair __ Bedfast __

2. Ask the client, "Does the condition of your feet or legs
   limit your activity in any way?" YES NO
   If YES, describe _____

3. *Ask the client to walk approximately 10 ft.*
   Is there any gait disturbance? YES NO

4. *Remove the client's shoes and stockings.*
   Cleanliness of feet. Acceptable Unacceptable

5. Are the stockings a good fit? YES NO

6. Does the client usually wear well-fitting leather
   or (synthetic) shoes that cover his feet completely? YES NO

7. Does the client wear garters (circular)? YES NO

DERMATOLOGICAL ASSESSMENT

8. Skin lesions
   a. Fissure between the toes? YES NO
   b. Fissure on heel(s)? YES NO
   c. Excoriation on legs or feet? YES NO
   d. Corn(s) (Fig. 1)? YES NO
   e. Callus(es)? YES NO
   f. Plantar wart? YES NO
   g. Other, describe _____ YES NO

9. Itching on legs or feet? YES NO

10. Rash on legs or feet? YES NO

11. *Inspect pressure areas on the feet for localized
    areas of redness.*
    Are any present? YES NO
    If YES, which foot? Right Left

12. *Inspect legs, feet, and toes for localized
    swelling, warmth, tenderness, redness.*
    Is any present? YES NO
    If YES, specify location Rt. Leg Lt. Leg
    Rt. Foot Lt. Foot

13. Toenails
    a. Ingrown? YES NO
    b. Overgrown (long)? YES NO
    c. Thickened? YES NO
    d. Yellow discoloration? YES NO
    e. Black discoloration? YES NO

Fig. 1 Red, thickness

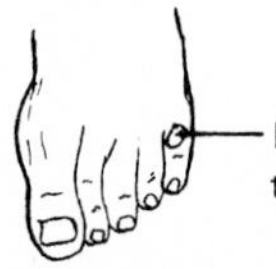

Corn: Painful, circular area of thickened skin, appearing on skin that is normally thin.

Callus: Thickened skin, occurring on skin that is normally thick, i.e., soles.

Ingrown toenail: A "tender overhanging nail fold" (Bates, 1974).

FIGURE 21-2 Nursing assessment of the lower extremity. [*Copyright 1978 by Patricia Ann King. Illustrations by Thomas A. King. The instructions and illustrations for palpating the pulses (Figures 2 and 3, Questions 16 and 17) are from Barbara Bates, A Guide to Physical Examination, J. B. Lippincott, Philadelphia, 1974. Figure 5 is from N. J. Giannestras, Foot Disorders, 1973, p. 65.*]

CIRCULATORY STATUS: FEET ONLY

14. Do the feet have any red, reddish blue, or bluish discoloration?	YES	NO
15. Is there any brownish discoloration around the ankles?	YES	NO
16. Is the dorsalis pedis present (Fig. 2)?	YES	NO
If NO, which foot?	Right	Left
17. Is the posterior tibial pulse present (Fig. 3)?	YES	NO
If NO, which foot?	Right	Left
18. Is the skin dry?	YES	NO

CIRCULATORY STATUS: BOTH FEET AND LEGS

19. Is edema present?	YES	NO
20. *Check the temperature of the legs and the feet with the backs of your fingers, comparing one extremity with the other.*		
Are the feet the same temperature?	YES	NO
21. Are the legs the same temperature?	YES	NO
22. Does the client have any pain in his legs or feet?	YES	NO
IF YES, describe _____		
23. *Inspect the legs, sides of ankles, soles, toes for ulceration.*		
Is any ulceration present?	YES	NO
If YES, specify location.	Rt. Leg	Lt. Leg
	Rt. Ft.	Lt. Ft.

STRUCTURAL DEFORMITIES

24. Hallux valgus (bunion) (Fig. 4)?	YES	NO
25. Hammer toes (Fig. 5)?	YES	NO
26. Overlapping digits?	YES	NO
27. *Ask the client to stand.*		
Are the legs the same relative size?	YES	NO
28. Are the legs the same relative length?	YES	NO
29. Are varicosities present?	YES	NO

Additional notes:

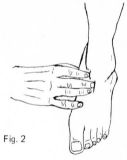

Fig. 2

Use three fingers on the dorsum of the foot, usually just lateral to the extensor tendon of the great toe.

Curve your fingers behind and slightly below the medial malleolus of the ankle.

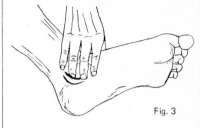

Fig. 3

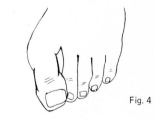

Fig. 4

Hallux valgus (outward deviation of great toe)

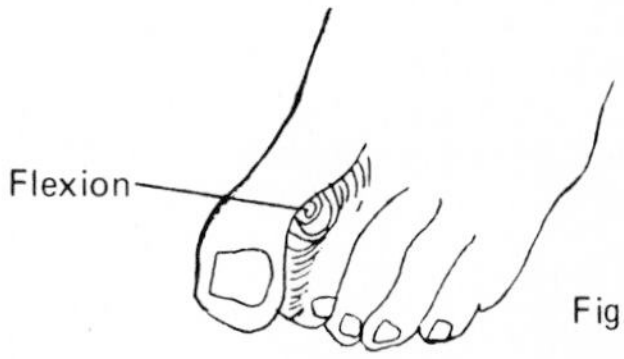

Flexion

Fig. 5

Hammer toe (flexion contracture)

strikes the ground at the heel and transmits the weight through to the toes as the swing foot becomes the stance foot. The arms swing in a coordinated movement which is symmetrical and rhythmic.

Antalgic gait. This gait is an adaptation to pain in any site from the lower back, the abdomen, hip or knee joint, calf, or foot. Usually the gait is changed to short steps on the affected side as the body endeavors to reduce the period of pain with each step. Most pain is exacerbated during weight bearing; the person shortens the stance phase and holds the limb in slight flexion. Podalgia, or foot pain, arises from foot problems plus misfitted shoes, and the protective gait can be diagnostic as to the site of the pain (heel, toe, etc.).

Short-leg gait. A contracture or ankylosis prevents full extension of hip or knee joint. During the stance phase the knee will be kept in flexion and the trunk will bend forward. A stiff knee requires a wide outward swing in order for the foot to clear the ground, and the person may lift himself or herself onto the toes of the stance foot while swinging the foot on the affected side. In flaccid hemiplegia the knee has a tendency for hyperextension to avoid buckling.

Foot deformities. The lack of elasticity, springiness, rhythm, or force in rolling off the foot from heel-strike to push-off leads to further observations: (1) deviation of the angle of the foot placement (toeing in or out), (2) walking on one or the other part of the foot, (3) unusual deviation in the width of the base (abducted gait), and (4) exaggerated outward rotation of the leg during the stance phase.

Paretic gaits. These are usually more easily seen in an attempt to walk rapidly, and they depend upon the group of muscles which are affected and how severely they are affected.

Quadriceps paralysis. If the knee gives way, the body tends to compensate by action of the gluteus and soleus muscles pushing the body forward so as to keep the line of gravity to the front of the knee. This is usually accomplished by marked trunk-swing forward, in advance for the knee.

Hip extensor paralysis. Normally the hip has reached its greatest flexion at heel-strike. To compensate for the paralyzed gluteus maximus, the pelvis is thrown into full extension on the involved side, and there is forward protrusion of the hip due to sudden backward motion of the trunk just after heel-strike.

Foot drop. The dorsiflexors provide the lift at toe-off phase so the foot can clear the ground. To compensate for foot drop, the knee must be raised much higher, which demands greater hip flexion, then the foot slap is heard as the foot strikes the ground.

Waddle gait. This gait usually is seen in weakness of the gluteus medius which is the principal abductor of the femur and is characterized by a drop and lag during the swing phase of the side opposite to the affected side.

Gait of incoordination. This gait is caused by lack of coordination (dyskinesia).

Festinating gait. The person moves with hurrying short steps, frequently on tiptoe, and with a forward position of the trunk (typical of parkinsonism).

Cerebral arteriosclerosis. This gait is characteristic of bilateral involvement and is manifested by extremely short steps.

Ataxic gait. This gait is caused by cerebellar lesions and is manifest by failure to maintain a rhythm, lack of measure in placement of foot, and inappropriate effort.

Observation of gait, plus an examination of the foot, may reveal the extent to which mobility may be regained, if appropriate measures are taken. These vary from hard sole, laced oxfords with a broad base heel, short and long leg braces, canes, hand rails, walkers. Every person's mobility status can be improved. While weak muscles may not be strengthened they can be augmented by numerous prosthetic devices and supporting measures including the relief of pain in arthritis, braces for weak joints, and hand rails for better support. (Kamenetz, 1972; Snyder and Baum, 1974)

Interventions   The objectives for podiatric care are as follows: (1) to maintain ambulation or maximum mobility, (2) to maintain structural integrity, (3) to prevent infection, and (4) to maintain comfort.

Temporary relief measures for some common foot problems have been discussed by Simko (1974). Conditions that should be referred to a podiatrist include ulcerations; overdeveloped, ingrown, and fungous nails; plantar warts; lesions; and hallux valgus. Common nursing problems are dry skin, elongated nails, limited mobility, and decubitus ulcers.

Dry Skin   Changes in the aging skin include a thinning of the epithelial and subcutaneous layers, a reduction in the number of sweat glands, and a stiffening of the collagen fibers in the dermis. As a result, the aging skin is dry, thin, and inelastic. Dryness can lead to fissure formation and infection. An experimental study by Hopp and Sundberg (1974) tested various foot care treatments on 60 men and women in two nursing homes. They concluded that the most economical and effective method of reducing dry skin was to use lotion only. The lotion used in the study was a mixture of lanolin and mineral oil.

Elongated Nails   Often older people are not able to care for their nails. Nurses can provide these people with the assistance they need. The equipment for nail care includes a nail nipper, curette, emery board, and emollient. The nails should be soaked (1) in warm water for 10 minutes or (2) with cotton that has been saturated with a commercial soaking agent for 3 minutes. A podiatrist can be consulted about the latter. Remove embedded loose material around cuticles and between the toes with a soft towel. Cut nails by clipping straight across. Do not cut into nail groove. File sharp edges with emery board. Apply emollient to soften cuticles.

Limited Mobility   Many neurological or musculoskeletal disorders such as stroke, parkinsonism, and arthritic lesions of the hip can limit mobility. When mobility is impaired, mechanical aids to ambulation are vital for maintaining independence. These include crutches, walker, cane, and wheelchair. The nurse's responsibility in this area is clearly stated in standard VIII of the *Standards for Geriatric Nursing Practice* (American Nurses' Association, 1973). It states, "The nurse assists older persons to obtain and utilize devices which help them attain a higher level of function and ensures that these devices are kept in good working order by the appropriate persons or agencies."

Once a device is obtained, proper instruction on its use must be given along with careful supervision. The nurse must be familiar with the four-point, three-point, and swing-through gaits (Lewis, 1976). In *walking with a cane* the person should advance the affected leg at the same time that the cane is advanced on the opposite side. In *using a walker* the person moves the walker forward, then moves the weak leg forward, followed by the strong leg. The toes should never be beyond the front legs of the walker. In *transferring,* the client moves the good side first toward the bed, wheelchair, or commode.

Devices need to be inspected at regular intervals. Flat tires or a missing foot pedal on a wheelchair are examples of faulty devices that require prompt attention.

Decubitus Ulcers   Whenever blood supply to an area is reduced, tissue requirements are compromised. A significant factor producing tissue ischemia is pressure. Prolonged pressure can lead to decubitation.

Older persons with limited mobility are more likely to develop decubitus ulcers. This problem is best treated by prevention. Constant vigilance and a consistent skin care protocol can be effective in preventing skin breakdown. Preventive measures include: (1) changing position frequently, (2) massaging bony prominences at regular intervals, (3) using protective devices such as heel guard, foot elevator, wheelchair cushion, or sheepskin, (4) using an air mattress or water bed for even distribution of body weight, (5) keeping skin dry and clean, (6) passive or active range of motion exercises, and (7) maintaining a nutritious diet.

TEACHING ROLE

The older adult has a right and need to participate in the learning situation (Pergrin and Wolanin, 1976). In our assessments we should determine the older persons' knowledge of foot care as well as their foot care practices before we make pronouncements. (See Figure 21-3.)

Roberts (1977), a podiatrist, offers three principles for foot health teaching for the older adult: (1) your feet are part of your total body, (2) do not accept any discomfort or disability with-

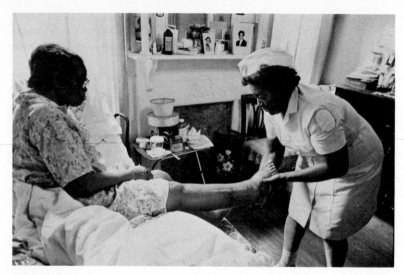

FIGURE 21-3 The nurse should determine the older person's knowledge of foot care, as well as the foot-care practices used. (*Courtesy of Harvey Finkle.*)

out investigating the cause and possible treatment, (3) use your body. These rules could be used effectively in a foot education program. For example, one can prepare a foot instruction guide incorporating them. One such guide is as follows.

Foot Care Instructions

1. You will promote good hygiene by:
   a. Washing your feet daily, using warm water and a mild soap. Dry carefully between the toes, since debris collected here may cause an infection.
   b. Wearing clean socks daily.
   c. Wearing an oxford or slip-on style shoe, made of leather, with round toes and broad 1- to 2-inch heels. Shoes should extend about $1\frac{1}{2}$ inches beyond longest toe. Before putting your shoes on, feel inside for any objects.
   d. Inspecting your feet regularly. If you are unable to do so, have someone else check them.
   e. Walking. This is the best exercise for you. If you are wheelchairbound:
      (1) Flex and extend your toes and ankles six times; do this several times a day.
      (2) Rotate your feet in a clockwise direction

six times and then in a counterclockwise direction six times; do this several times a day.
   (3) Be as active as possible.
   (4) Lie on your stomach (or on your back) for short periods of time to prevent hip and knee flexion.
   f. Softening dry skin with a vegetable shortening or a lotion containing lanolin and mineral oil.
   g. Trimming your toenails, straight across. If you are unable to do so, have someone else cut them.
2. In caring for your feet remember that:
   a. Harsh chemicals such as tincture of iodine and medicated plasters for corns should be avoided.
   b. Heating pads, hot water bottles, or ice packs should not be used on your legs or feet.
   c. Loosely fitting warm socks can be worn at night for cold feet.
   d. Sharp instruments such as knitting needles, knives, or razor blades should not be used on your feet.
   e. Practices such as wearing garters, sitting with legs crossed, and smoking should be avoided since they slow the circulation to the extremities.

3. In caring about your overall health, remember that:
   a. Systemic conditions can affect the feet. Conversely, foot problems can affect the body.
   b. Serious complications from foot problems can be prevented by seeking professional help early.
   c. Exercise can improve circulation.
   d. Foot health adds to the well-being of the individual.

This chapter has focused on the foot care needs of the elderly. The nurse, in a primary care role, can provide the elderly person with the necessary assistance in maintaining mobility, thus assuring independence.

REFERENCES

American Nurses' Association: *Standards of Geriatric Nursing Practice,* Kansas City, Mo., 1973.

Anderson, Helen C.: *Newton's Geriatric Nursing,* 5th ed., Mosby, St. Louis, 1971, pp. 102–104, 194–201.

Block, Doris: Some crucial terms in nursing: What do they really mean?, *Nursing Outlook,* **22**(11):689–694, November 1974.

Bruck, Helen O., and Claude N. Lambert: Common foot disabilities, *American Journal of Nursing,* **59**(11):1580–1583, November 1959.

Conrad, Doris: Foot education and screening programs for the elderly, *Journal of Gerontological Nursing,* **3**(6):10–15, November–December 1977.

DuVries, Henri L.: *Surgery of the Foot,* Mosby, St. Louis, 1973, p. 3.

———: *Surgery of the Foot,* Mosby, St. Louis, 1959, pp. 3 and 49.

Fairbairn, J. F. et al.: *Allen-Baker-Hines Peripheral Vascular Diseases,* 4th ed., Saunders, Philadelphia, 1972.

Fowler, Marsha D.: Behold the great right toe, *American Journal of Nursing,* **74**(10):1817–1819, October 1974.

Helfand, Arthur E.: At the foot of South Mountain, *Journal of American Podiatry Association* **63**(10):512–521, October 1973.

———: Hunting diabetics by foot, *Journal of the American Podiatry Association,* **64**(6):399–406, June 1974.

———: Keep them walking, *Journal of the American Podiatry Association,* **58**(3):117–127, March 1968.

———: Podiatric considerations for the aging patient, *Nursing Homes,* **20**:30–31, November 1971a.

———: Podiatry and the elderly patient, *Working with Older People: Clinical Aspects of Aging,* Department of Health, Education, and Welfare, Rockville, Md., **4**:377–388, July 1971b.

———: Podiatry: Essential nursing home care, *Nursing Homes,* **19**:35–36, May 1970.

———: Podiatry in a total geriatric health program: Common foot problems of the aged, *Journal of the American Geriatrics Society,* **15**(6):593–599, June 1967.

Hopp, Ruth Ann, and Sherrill Sundberg: The effects of soaking and lotion on dryness of the skin in the feet of the elderly patient, *Journal of the American Podiatry Association,* **64**(10):747–760, October 1974.

Jahss, Melvin H.: Geriatric aspects of the foot and ankle, in Isadore Rossman (ed.), *Clinical Geriatrics,* Lippincott, Philadelphia, 1971, pp. 327–328.

Juergens, J. L., and P. E. Bernatz: Arteriosclerosis obliterans, in J. F. Fairbairn et al. (eds.), *Allen-Baker-Hines Peripheral Vascular Diseases,* 4th ed., Saunders, Philadelphia, 1972.

Kamenetz, Herman L.: Clinical aspects of gait disturbances, *Clinical Review,* **3**(1):1–8, 1972.

King, Patricia A.: Foot assessment of the elderly, *Journal of Gerontological Nursing,* **4**(6):47–52, November–December 1978.

Lewis, LuVerne Wolff: *Fundamental Skills in Patient Care,* Lippincott, Philadelphia, 1976, pp. 255–257.

Martin, Elizabeth J., and Jane E. D. Smith: Diabetic foot care: Knowledge and practice, *ANA Clinical Sessions,* 1969, pp. 143–149.

Pergrin, Jessie V., and Mary Opal Wolanin: Positive health education for the elderly, paper given at the *9th International Conference on Health Education,* Ottawa, Aug. 31, 1976.

Rakow, Robert B., and Sandor A. Friedman: The significance of trophic foot changes, *Geriatrics,* **24**:135–139, May 1969a.

———: Peripheral vascular disease in the aged: Modern concepts and diagnostic techniques, *Journal of the American Geriatric Society,* **17**(2):205, February 1969b.

Riccitelli, M. L.: Foot problems of the aged and infirm, *Journal of the American Geriatric Society,* **14**(10):1058–1066, October 1966.

———: Peripheral vascular disease in the aged: Modern concepts and diagnostic techniques, *Journal of the American Geriatrics Society,* **17**(2):205–212, February 1969.

Roberts, Elizabeth H.: *On Your Feet,* Pyramid, New York, 1977, pp. 99–110.

Schank, Mary Jane: A survey of the well-elderly: Their foot problems, practices and needs, *Journal of Gerontological Nursing,* **3**(6):10–15, November–December 1977.

Simko, Michael V.: Foot welfare, in *Nursing and the*

Aging Patient, American Journal of Nursing, New York, 1974, pp. 62–66.

Snyder, Mariah, and Rebecca Baum: Assessing station and gait, *American Journal of Nursing,* **74**(7):1256–1257, July 1974.

Spencer, Marion G.: Podogeriatrics and the nurse, *ANA Clinical Sessions,* 1970, pp. 75–81.

Wilkins, Robert W.: Diseases of the peripheral vessels, *Cecil-Loeb Textbook of Medicine,* 12th ed., Saunders, Philadelphia, 1967.

Wolanin, Mary Opal: Nursing assessment, in Irene M. Burnside (ed.), *Nursing and the Aged,* McGraw-Hill, New York, 1976, pp. 410–412.

..

TWENTY-TWO

ASPECTS OF THE AGING GASTROINTESTINAL TRACT

June C. Abbey

Man does not live by bread alone,
But by faith, admiration, by sympathy.
Thomas Dunn English

LEARNING OBJECTIVES

- Describe digestive function changes.
- Describe esophageal problems that might occur in the elderly client.
- List three clinically important changes of gastric secretion in advancing age.
- List the difficulties encountered when studying the small bowel function of the aged person.
- List the three most common pancreatic disturbances in the aged.
- Describe symptoms of gallbladder disease.
- List the five main general difficulties which occur in intestinal disturbances.
- Discuss constipation in the aged client.

While the literature is replete with conditions that accompany aging, no disease condition can be found that is exclusive to the aged, and few from which the aged person is entirely free or immune. Nowhere is this more apparent than in the normal aging of the digestive processes. Many theories for and about aging exist. These are discussed elsewhere in Chapters 2 and 3 and more specifically to nutrition and metabolism in Chapter 23. While cellular and biochemical changes are interesting and informative, clinical application requires a focusing or selection of those theories of peculiar pertinence to digestion in general and the gastrointestinal tract in particular. The changes which dictate digestive modification are primarily those in (1) the nervous system—central, autonomic, and peripheral—and (2) the gastrointestinal system itself.

NERVOUS SYSTEM CHANGES

Whereas the electroencephalograms of healthy old subjects show only slowing of alpha-wave rhythm when contrasted to younger subjects, brain tissues do deteriorate with age. There is substantial evidence for a loss of neurons and a concomitant decrease in the weight of the brain most marked after the sixth decade. A significant reduction of cerebral blood flow and metabolism occurs with aging. Alterations of the sleep-wakefulness ratio and the ability to regulate body temperature suggest modification of hypothalamic function. Little evidence can be found, however, to demonstrate that the inability of the aged to cope with stress is a deficiency of the hypophyseal-adrenal axis, the main mediator of stress (Hall, 1973). Recently more and more studies investigate hypothalamic-pituitary control of aging (Everitt, 1973; Bender et al., 1970; Bellamy, 1968; Dilman, 1971). The hypothalamus, in addition to its role in sleep-wakefulness and temperature regulation, is important to (1) appetite and thirst; (2) control of diuresis and body fluid osmolarity; (3) expression of emotions such as rage and fear; (4) control of puberty, sexual activity, and lactation; (5) growth; (6) control of the thyroid and adrenal

cortex; and (7) control of the autonomic nervous system.

The control of the autonomic system over various organic functions appears labile and unpredictable. Parasympathetic and sympathetic ganglia morphologies probably contribute to changes in intestinal motility, thus causing constipation and intestinal paresis. By contrast loss of cortical inhibition presents the opposite picture of diarrhea or urinary incontinence. Elderly clients often exhibit orthostatic hypotension, a fact that reinforces the hypothesis of a defect in vasomotor and, therefore, autonomic control (Bristow et al., 1969).

Reduction of visceral sensitivity occurs and is easily demonstrated by the fact that the aged tolerate space-occupying lesions with little discomfort.

Investigators find a number of interesting related facts when comparing sensory with motor loss and latency. Sensory conduction velocity decreases at a faster rate than does motor, approximately 30 percent as contrasted to 15 percent between the ages of 20 and 95 years (LaFratta and Canestrari, 1966). This could account for both a diminished sensitivity and sluggish reflexes. If the sensing mechanism emits a delayed trigger, the motor reflex response will be slow and perhaps inaccurate. Most authorities concur that peripheral nerve conduction velocity decreases, but whether this is a reduction in the number of fibers or a change in properties, such as demyelination, is not definite (Hall, 1973, pp. 40–41; Sklar, 1971). Aging of the nervous system could, therefore, reasonably contribute to (1) inadequate motility with (2) delay in feedback mechanisms for both hormonal and enzymatic release; (3) diminished response to pain and intestinal sensations; and (4) decreased vasomotor response or shunting that normally accompanies exercise, ingestion, or strong emotion.

DIGESTIVE SYSTEM

Clinically speaking, changes in gerontological digestive function involve modifications of secretion, digestion-reduction, and simplification of foodstuffs, absorption, or motility. Any one or all of these processes can be affected by aging.

TEETH AND MOUTH

The digestive system begins with the mouth and teeth. With modern dental techniques the problem of the edentulous patient can be prevented at any age, and periodontitis presents a real threat for systemic infection to the aged. Etiology of the well-described progressive changes of aging is not known.

Currently a considerable amount of research attention is being given to the absorption of calcium by the elderly to determine the cause of both osteoporosis and periodontitis (Harper, 1978). Thinking involves two approaches. One group of investigators believes that a chronic long-term calcium deficiency causes both conditions which result from a long-term loss without replacement of calcium from both the long bones and the jaw. The other group of scientists feels that two separate disease processes exist: osteoporosis, a degenerative progressive disease, and periodontitis, a chronic infection of tooth lining and bone (Winick, 1978, p. 1971).

To other than the dentist, the root absorption and apical transparency of teeth look like receding gums. The grinding surfaces become worn down, and usually one or more teeth are missing. These changes, missing teeth, worn surfaces, and lessening of tooth support by the gums, require a diet containing softer foods. Existing teeth need the protection of oral hygiene, particularly in the lower jaw where the teeth acting as anchors for partial plates help immeasurably in chewing and breaking up food into smaller pieces. Bhaskar studied the oral mucosa of 785 elderly persons for changes relative to aging. He found sublingual mucosal vessel varicosities in 49 percent of the subjects. The mucosa of 21 percent contained white leukoplakias of which 12 percent were premalignant (Bhaskar, 1968).

Aged persons often complain of dry mouth. Mouth breathing and insufficient fluids with incipient dehydration contribute to the sensation. Studies show, however, a decrease in salivary gland secretion, with marked lessening of ptyalin and increased thickening of mucin. The saliva becomes alkaline rather than acidic. The reabsorption of sodium and potassium also diminishes. While it might be expected that these changes contribute to disorders of taste or smell, no relationship has been found.

Probably distortion of the perception of taste, due to medications, occurs in the older person more often than might be expected from the reports in the literature. Among the more commonly prescribed drugs for the aging and their side effect on taste are (1) insulin, which can decrease sensitivity to salty or sweet tastes; (2) antihyperlipemics, clofibrate or cholestyramine, which change taste acuity and (3) penicillin, which yields an aftertaste (Carson and Germican, 1976).

Disorders of taste and smell, other than a decline in the number of taste buds, as found by Arey, from 248 per papilla in children to 88 in subjects greater than 74 years, lack precise information (Arey et al., 1935). Simple gradual decline would seem unlikely to cause malnutrition, but foul tastes or smells could materially reduce food intake and the social pleasures of eating. Abnormal sensations of taste and smell frequently are associated with psychological disturbances, whether the subject is aged or young. It is well, however, to consider an underlying physiological problem, particularly if the onset is rapid. Congestive heart failure (Shafer, 1965), ischemia to the postcentral gyrus (Hughes, 1969), as well as the more common disturbances of upper respiratory or gastrointestinal infections, can cause gustatory and olfactory anomalies.

ESOPHAGUS

The esophagus, after years of functioning as a simple conduit for food with the normal subject hardly aware of its existence, becomes a most important concern for the elderly. While dysphagia is generally caused by conditions extrinsic to the gastrointestinal system and digestion such as pseudobulbar palsy or stroke due to cerebral vascular disease, or the compression-distortion of a bronchial tumor, the esophagus itself presents decrements in motility with aging (Kahn et al., 1977, p. 1053).

Distention of the lumen of the gastrointestinal tract normally causes peristalsis in rhythmic waves the entire length of the gut. The waves diminish in frequency along the tract such that the stomach shows more activity than the small intestine which has greater action than does the sluggish, slow-moving large bowel. Peristalsis consists of a wave of relaxation followed by a wave of constriction and depends largely on the integrity of innervation for synchronization and relaxation of the sphincters. These protect each preceding structure from reflux. The dependence of the tract on nervous tissue for regulation makes its rhythmicity vulnerable to aging; hence, studies have shown a decrease in the amount of esophageal peristalsis with asynchrony or aberrant waves, defects in sphincter relaxation with delays in emptying, and, therefore, dilatation of the esophagus (Soergel et al., 1964).

Dilatation and delay in emptying of the esophagus allow food particles to putrify, usually resulting in diffuse spasm, esophagitis, and gastric esophageal reflux. The common symptom of each of these is chest pain. With the aging patient, the incidence of cardiac and esophageal pain is common, and differentiation becomes a serious problem. Esophageal pain is generally related to posture, meals, and relief by antacids. It may produce severe substernal pain. Anticholinergic drugs often will help. Some authorities feel that gastric reflux is one of the most common causes of "heartburn." In fact, burning pain is characteristic of esophageal disturbance. The loss of an effective one-way valve mechanism at the gastroesophageal junction allows regurgitation of acid-peptic juices into the esophagus. Normally the stomach is protected by the presence of food and its own mucin, but the poorly protected esophageal mucosa becomes irritated and a burning feeling is felt. The feeling may be high in the throat or in the low retrosternal area. Chronic pulmonary disease and hoarseness can result from nocturnal regurgitation of gastric juices. Stooping, straining, or lying down usually accentuate the pain. Protracted gastroesophageal reflux often culminates in reflux esophagitis. This inflammation is generally accompanied by a localized superficial ulceration which may cause slow bleeding with subsequent anemia. Hiatal hernia frequently accompanies or predisposes to gastric reflux.

Hiatal hernia occurs when a portion of the stomach slips up through the diaphragmatic hiatus into the chest. Classification into sliding, rolling, or mixed type is based upon how much of the stomach moves up into the diaphragm. The most common, sliding type, designates movement of the junction of the esophagus above its usual position, thereby promoting reflux. In the rolling type (paraesophageal), the fundus of the stomach herniates up through the hiatus to lie above the diaphragm next to the esophagus. The junction remains in its normal position. The mixed type consists of both sliding and rolling types and is seen more than the paraesophageal hernia.

Symptoms of hiatal hernia are discomfort, belching, acid regurgitation, dysphagia or spasm, heartburn, and often chest pain localized over the lower sternum. Perhaps more suggestive of the condition is an elderly patient with frequent bouts of dyspepsia, whose "ulcer flares up after eating or going to bed." These people feel like vomiting without the accompanying nausea and occasionally complain of a "burning bile" taste. If ulceration occurs, the associated bleeding, however minimal, can cause anemia in the aged.

Despite the fact that esophagitis, ulceration, and stricture are serious complications, surgery is rarely considered and medical management is usually sufficient. While some studies report the incidence to be about 65 percent of all persons over 60, the occurrence is greater in obese women (McGinty, 1971). Weight reduction, using small, frequent feedings of a bland diet, is indicated. Clients eat better if meals are attractive and unhurried. Often raising both arms toward the ceiling to full extension will relieve the feeling of spasm, and the person will feel markedly more comfortable and be able to eat. This is particularly true if he or she has been hurried and tense. The client will feel better by avoiding stooping, bending, or lifting heavy loads and sleeping with the head of the bed elevated approximately 3 to 4 inches. Although antacids are useful, care is necessary to avoid overmedication which can cause metabolic alkalosis, chronic irritability, and tremors. In anemic patients iron therapy might be necessary. Surgery is reserved for rare cases of obstruction, strangulation, or intractable bleeding.

Unfortunately, there is a steady rise in the incidence of carcinoma of the esophagus with increasing age (Langman, 1971). The condition appears to be more common in males and in blacks. Protracted dysphagia and achalasia, wherein the gastroesophageal sphincter is stenotic or unable to relax, are the two most important symptoms. The person may initially have difficulty swallowing solid foods; later fluids present difficulties. Despite continued thirst, excessive salivation can occur. In the elderly, salivation is always a serious sign causing one to consider a cerebrovascular problem of the bulbar area or esophageal irritation and obstruction. As with most esophageal disturbances of the elderly, bleeding—either acute or chronic—presents the real threat of anemia.

Treatment depends upon the extent and location of the lesion and type of tumor. Squamous cell tumors respond rather well to radiotherapy; however, these lesions in the lower esophagus may require surgery. With the elderly, radiation might be palliative. As techniques improve, the seriousness of side effects should diminish. Currently, the condition causes considerable discomfort to the patient, frustration to staff, and sorrow to relatives.

STOMACH

Whereas the esophagus acts simply as a tube, the stomach enters actively into the process of digestion. The stomach secretes gastric juice, a combination of hydrochloric acid, pepsin, lipase, and mucin. Absorption, while more than that from the esophagus, is minimal. Water and water-soluble materials are hardly absorbed at all, even down high osmotic gradients. Little protein and carbohydrate absorption occurs. By contrast some fats and fat-soluble material are absorbed, which accounts for the rapid onset of response to ethyl alcohol ingestion. Organic acids such as aspirin (acetylsalicylic acid) which are water soluble in a high pH become fat soluble at a low pH. At pH 2, 95 percent can rapidly enter stomach mucosal cells. Large doses are toxic to mucosal cells and can cause severe damage and bleeding.

Fundamentally, there are three clinically important alterations of gastric secretions. Hyperacidity is rarely found in the older popula-

tion. Hypoacidity and achlorhydria increase in incidence with advancing age. In close association is the development of atrophic changes of the gastric mucosa (Fikry, 1965, pp. 216–217). The expected activity of drugs on the stomach, therefore, alters. Whether the increase in hydrochloric acid secretion caused by such drugs as caffeine, aminophylline, steroids, isoniazid, and reserpine is sufficient in the elderly to cause ulceration because of atrophic changes and diminished mucin secretion is idiosyncratic to each subject. Not enough is known to predict whether both mucin and hydrochloric acid formation decrease at the same or different rates.

Studies on diminished gastric secretions in aging disagree in quantity, quality, and rate of changes. This disconcerting lack of consensus probably results from different techniques over insufficient numbers rather than continued high-level function, for most authorities agree that there are progressive decrements in gastric secretions due to aging. This decrease appears to be proportional to age. Whatever the approximate year of onset, whether the second or fifth decade, secretions are lessened about 50 percent by the age of 70. More recent studies show approximately equal change in both sexes. The progressive change of gastric pH is also reflected in alteration of the bacterial composition of intestinal flora (Bertolini, 1969, pp. 624 and 633). In gastric atrophy there is a failure first of acid secretion, then of pepsinogen, and finally of the intrinsic factor necessary for vitamin B_{12} absorption.

Of the numerous specific types of gastric mucosal irritation and inflammation designated by the rubric of gastritis, three general types cause difficulty to the aging. The first, acute gastritis, results from specific injury or trauma to the mucosa. Bacterial toxins or organisms damage the gastric membrane. Food poisoning is an example of such a problem. More often seen, however, is the gastritis accompanying drug or alcohol ingestion. While this condition can be very painful, it is usually self-limiting and responds well to antacids and abstinence from the causative agents. The second type, chronic hypertrophic gastritis, is found upon gastroscopic examination when, despite normal barium x-ray studies, the patient continues to complain of burning, gnawing pain and dyspepsia. The rugae are prominent, stiff, and inflamed, but there is not appreciable effect on acid secretion. The third, chronic atrophic gastritis, includes any gastric inflammation from a mild superficial response through glandular involvement and decreased hydrochloric acid secretion to mucosal atrophy and complete absence of gastric glands (Leeming et al., 1973, p. 332). Glandular atrophy, in addition to causing achlorhydria, prevents formation of sufficient intrinsic factor, thereby promoting pernicious anemia due to insufficient vitamin B_{12} (cobalamin) absorption. The consequences are more fully developed in discussions of the hemodynamics of aging. Whether this condition is due to or enhanced by aging is not known. Pernicious and iron-deficiency anemias are associated with similar types of mucosal damage. The iron-deficiency or hypochromic anemia will respond to oral doses of vitamin C and iron. Ascorbic acid facilitates transport and absorption of the iron across gastrointestinal membranes.

Chronic pancreatitis and alcoholism have a high incidence of gastritis, as do viral hepatitis and abdominal radiation (Leeming et al., 1973). Symptomatology ranges from vague epigastric distress to acute painful flare-ups. Dilute hydrochloric acid in small doses is occasionally helpful.

Peptic ulcer, a general term denoting an ulceration of any area bathed by peptic juice, such as the lower esophagus, stomach, or duodenum, develops when the "aggressive factors" of gastric acid, pepsin secretion, local inflammation, and increased gastric stimulation overwhelm the "defensive factors" of mucosal resistance, mucosal blood flow, gastric mucus, and the inhibitory action of duodenal acidification, to erode the mucosa. The incidence of duodenal ulceration so exceeds that of the other sites that ordinarily peptic ulcer and duodenal ulcer are used synonymously by the lay person. There is a marked increase of duodenal ulcers in postmenopausal women, and Clarke's classic studies determined that individuals of blood type O of any age are more prone to develop ulcers (Clarke et al., 1959). Bleeding ulcers, whether gastric (stomach) or peptic (duodenal), should not be taken lightly and present a high incidence of fatal complications in the elderly. Larger ulcers occur in patients with the longest

history of symptoms. Oddly enough, gastric ulceration presents more generalized than specific symptoms. Vague upper abdominal pain or distress associated with weight loss, anorexia, epigastric distress, and vomiting is suspicious enough to warrant intensive investigation.

Although the incidence of stomach carcinoma has been decreasing, the tumor is still common, particularly among the elderly between the ages of 75 and 85. Persons with type A blood, males, or those who have a familial history of a parent with gastric malignancy and present symptoms should be thoroughly studied. The results of radical surgery are poor in the elderly with a 5-year survival rate of only 5 to 10 percent (Mine et al., 1970). Metastasis can involve the liver, lymph nodes, mediastinum, pancreas, and through the lymphatics it can spread to the lungs, bones, and the brain. Although intensive chemotherapy has so far been disappointing, some encouraging results have been obtained. Cytotoxic agents for palliation should afford a genuine likelihood of symptomatic relief for the patient and not be given primarily to assuage the frustration of helplessness experienced by the relatives and staff. Palliative treatment, by definition, must relieve, not transfer suffering to a different mode of equal or greater intensity of discomfort.

Gastric ulcers usually respond to a medical regimen and rarely require surgery. Bed rest alone is beneficial. With the elderly, however, the risks of immobility and imposed limitations probably outweigh the advantages, and allowing the person to ambulate while using drug therapy and diet to promote healing of the ulcer is probably preferable. Current opinion holds that a normal diet should be allowed, providing that food is avoided after the evening meal so as to reduce nocturnal acid secretion (Fordtran, 1973, p. 721).

In the event that medical treatment fails, surgical intervention is necessary because of the risk of fatal complications. Total or partial gastrectomies with a gastroduodenal anastomosis are hazardous procedures in the elderly. Even when the operation successfully treats the ulcer, a number of the patients develop one or more of a series of symptoms. The first, that of "dumping," ordinarily improves with time. *Dumping* refers to the rapid movement of food with a high osmotic power into the proximal gut. Owing to the osmotic pull, fluid builds up to drive the concentration toward equilibration. These activities are accompanied by tremors, postprandial sweating, weakness, nausea, and feelings of abdominal fullness and diarrhea. Patients presenting a history of psychological lability most often experience dumping; however, the phlegmatic personality is not immune. In most circumstances the patient can control the symptoms by limiting fluid intake with meals and avoiding foods that elicit the attack (Williams, 1971). The experience at best is frightening, and psychological support as well as dietary retraining is essential.

The second group of symptoms associated with gastric surgery is due to stenosis, obstruction, or regurgitation of bile and pancreatic juice into the remaining portion of the stomach. Revisional surgery may be necessary if there is copious vomiting of bile. Whenever the elderly person vomits a considerable amount of fluid, three problems are of concern: (1) fluid loss occurs quickly with the aged, and adequate replacement of electrolytes may be difficult; (2) diarrhea often accompanies vomiting; and (3) minimal absorption can take place (Williams, 1971). As with any digestive tract obstruction or stenosis, prompt evaluation and intervention are essential.

DUODENUM

As previously mentioned, duodenal ulcerations appear more frequently than gastric ulcers. They occur more often in men than women. Although the risk of developing a duodenal ulcer maintains a steady level throughout adulthood, with aging, epigastric tenderness may be less, owing to diminished pain sensation. To date successful medical management is problematical, and recurrence is frequent. Absorbent antacids are part of the usual therapy. Magnesium trisilicate or aluminum hydroxide can cause either diarrhea or constipation. A trade-off of aluminum hydroxide for the magnesium trisilicate often will control the diarrhea and vice versa. Occasionally a combination of each is given. The aim of treatment is to neutralize the acid secretion between meals; therefore, the

medication is given every 2 hours and at bedtime. It is not necessary to administer these after or with meals because the acid can act on the food. Small, frequent intake of nonirritating food can be effective. A totally bland diet is usually not necessary. Drug therapy in the aged presents some problems such as constipation or urinary retention with anticholinergics. If the patient has arthritis, substitute analgesics for aspirin or butazone may be necessary owing to the irritative action they can have on peptic ulcers. Hemorrhage may require emergency surgery. Elective surgery, by contrast, depends upon the possible risk of massive hemorrhage and the physical condition of the patient.

SMALL BOWEL

Studying small bowel function of the aged is fraught with difficulties because of (1) concomitant changes in other systems, (2) debilitation or disabilities both psychological and physiological of the patient population, (3) demands made by the test procedures on subject and staff, and (4) the paucity of authoritative research. This is particularly true in absorption studies. Absorption is the raison d'être of the gastrointestinal system; however, digestion must be complete before absorption can take place. The purpose of enzymes is to degrade complex molecules and macromolecules of foodstuffs into simpler compounds capable of being absorbed largely in the intestines.

Chewing begins the mechanical process in the mouth. The release of salivary amylase (ptyalin) has little relative importance because the food is in short contact with it before inactivation by the acid media of the stomach occurs. No absorption takes place in the mouth or esophagus.

The glands of the stomach secrete both pepsinogen and its activator, hydrochloric acid. Pepsin, activated pepsinogen, splits protein into smaller molecules (proteoses and peptones) but lacks the power to further degrade these products into amino acids for absorption. Whether gastric lipase is effective for hydrosis of fats is questionable, and pancreatic lipase (steapsin) is probably of greater effectiveness than either gastric intestinal lipase. Mucin protects the stomach lining from acid and enzymatic attack.

The vagus nerves and hormonal stimulation control gastric secretion in three so-called phases. Initially, the psychic or cephalic phase, that of awareness and anticipation brought on by either appetizing food or provocative odors, causes the secretion of gastric juices. By contrast, offensive foods, sights, or smells can significantly inhibit the gland's activity. The cephalic phase is abolished by sectioning of the vagi; therefore, it is entirely neurogenic and subject to the decrements of neurogenic aging. The second, or gastric, phase is initiated by both mechanical and chemical stimuli. Distention is the only effective mechanical stimulus. Interestingly, the intensity of stimulation by distention is proportional to the size of the meal. Secretagogues, chemicals which stimulate the release of the hormone gastrin, are extracts of meats and, to a lesser degree, of vegetables. Gastrin, in turn, causes the glands of the fundus to increase secretion. The intestinal, or third, phase elicits additional gastric secretion. After a significant amount of chyme reaches the intestine, enterogastrone, an "inhibitory" hormone, is formed in the intestinal mucosa by action of fat or fatty acids which inhibits both gastric secretion and movements of the stomach.

Pancreatic activity is also subject to both hormonal and neurological control. The two hormones involved, procreozymin and secretin, are made by the intestinal wall and activated by acid chyme. Secretin, upon reaching pancreatic cells after being absorbed into the general circulation, stimulates secretion of fluid and electrolytes by the pancreas into the duodenum. Pancreozymin promotes enzyme liberation. The neurological mechanism consists, simply speaking, of an antagonistic reflex relationship between vagal stimulation producing vasodilatation, and thereby increased pancreatic enzymes, balanced by sympathetic system excitation creating vasoconstriction and inhibition of secretory activity. The major enzymes are released as zymogens (inactive form) to be activated by other enzymes, or an appropriate change in pH. The enzymes are lipase, carboxypolypeptidase, amylase, ribonuclease, deoxyribonuclease, trypsin, and chymotrypsin. Pancreatic juice acts only in a neutral, slightly acid, or moderately alkaline medium. The juice contains alkaline salts, bicarbonates, and carbonates that "buffer" the acid chyme from the stomach.

Formed daily by the liver during the course of metabolism, bile salts contribute two important actions to digestion. These are (1) the emulsifying or detergent action on fat globules which decreases surface tension and allows intestinal tract agitation to break up the globules into minute droplets for the lipases to work upon; and (2) a hydrotropic function through which bile salt ions become attached to lipids. The electric charges of these ions increase the solubility of and promote the passage of lipids through the intestinal mucosa. Bile contains no enzymes. The secretion of bile by the liver is continuous, but it is stored in the gallbladder between meals or during periods of fasting. The gallbladder releases concentrated bile into the duodenum when stimulated by cholecystokinin. This hormone is extracted from the intestinal mucosa by the action of fats and acts specifically to cause contraction of the gallbladder muscle. Release requires coordination between hormonal stimulation and relaxation of the sphincter of Oddi.

In addition to copious amounts of mucus, the small intestine secretes several types of enzymes for the further breakdown or splitting of food substances into appropriate molecules. These are (1) a series of peptidases for splitting the polypeptides into amino acids; (2) the disaccharide to monosaccharide breakdown enzymes of sucrase, maltase, isomaltase, and lactase; and (3) lipase for changing neutral fats into glycerol and fatty acids. Control of amount and kind of enzymatic release results largely from local direct stimuli coupled with the intestinal intramural plexus which responds to stretching or distention.

No enzymes are secreted into the large intestine. Any further digestion is the result of bacterial flora continuing to digest cellulose sometimes to as much as 60 to 75 percent. Digestion of food is virtually complete prior to arrival of the chyme in the large intestine. Little or no food remains, therefore, to be absorbed from the large bowel.

ABSORPTION

The basic mechanisms of absorption are diffusion and active transport. Whereas diffusion is a simple process of movement of particles through digestive system membrane down the concentration difference, or with electrochemical gradient, active transport requires energy and a carrier agent. The substance can, therefore, move against the gradient or from an area of low concentration to that of high concentration. Although much is unknown about the mechanism of active transport, carriers are believed to (1) be either proteins or lipoproteins; (2) have specificity for certain substances; and (3) on occasion, as in the intestine, transport certain molecules through an entire cell layer. Almost all monosaccharides important to the body, amino acids, and amines, are actively transported. By contrast, the disaccharides such as sucrose and lactose are not actively transported at all.

As previously mentioned, no food absorption occurs proximal to the stomach. The thin mucous membrane beneath the tongue permits certain substances to be absorbed, such as medicines, but the quantity is minimal. Absorption of ordinary food products occurs primarily and virtually entirely in the small intestine.

Theoretically, because one digestive function appears to follow the other, each contributing to the further breakdown of food substances, any decrease in the activity of one portion of the gastrointestinal tract should be manifest in absorption or function of subsequent areas. The aged person would appear to be particularly vulnerable because of a tendency toward delay in peripheral nerve transmission and vasomotor response. In addition, there are the other contributory systemic changes of a progressive decrease in the size and permeability of capillary beds, as well as diminished elasticity of blood vessels and lungs which would lead one to expect changes in absorption (Bertolini, 1969, pp. 14–15). There are some changes due to aging related to the essential digestive enzymes.

Carbohydrates are absorbed in the form of monosaccharides after being hydrolyzed by amylases. The secretion of ptyalin (salivary amylase) remains relatively stable until the age of 60, when there is a rapid decrease. The pancreas undergoes atrophic evolution in old age with a reduction of exocrine cells for enzyme production. Related literature is sparse but suggests that the secretion of pancreatic enzymes decreases with age qualitatively (Meyer and Necheles, 1942). The decrement of pancreatic

amylase progresses slowly after the age of 20; however, this enzyme is so active it is apparently sufficient for digestion into old age (Bertolini, 1969, pp. 628 and 634). Information on intestinal maltase, lactase, and saccharase is limited and contradictory. While absorption rates of the monosaccharides differ, with glucose and galactose being absorbed faster, of more clinical importance is the need for vitamins B_1(thiamine), B_2 (riboflavin), B_6 (pyridoxine), and pantothenic acid in their absorption (Bertolini).

Lipids are emulsified by the action of bile and split into their components, glycerol, fatty acids, and sterols, by the lipases of the stomach, intestine, and pancreatic steapsin. The classic studies of Meyer and Necheles showed that although lipolytic activity experiences about a 20 percent reduction after the age of 20 to 30, the result is not very significant in limiting digestion of fats (Meyer and Necheles, 1942). Absorption of lipids slows with aging. Becker et al. (1950) found that the peak serum concentration of lipid occurred 7 hours after ingestion of a high-fat meal with aged subjects, rather than 3 hours as found in young adults.

Variation of pepsin production with aging is well recognized, and secretion diminishes by the sixth to eighth decade by approximately 65 percent of that found in the young adult. Even if the secretion were to remain normal, effective activity requires an acid medium, and loss of hydrochloric acid production is highly correlated with aging. Thus the first stage of secretion by either the pancreas or intestines, can contribute markedly to digestive and absorption impairment.

The reduction of pancreatic proteolytic enzyme activity begins at about 40 and progresses with age. Of these, trypsin is perhaps most important because of its specific action of splitting large polypeptides into smaller groups, the peptides. Each of the peptidases of the intestine has a singular peptide upon which it acts. The intestinal juice, by itself, cannot attack whole proteins; therefore, trypsin is essential for the partial initial breakdown of these complex molecules.

From the foregoing discussion, one is led to the belief that metabolism and absorption of fats and carbohydrates, although diminished, remain adequate. Proteins, however, can present difficulties, and any disturbance in the gastrointestinal tract will be reflected in their decreased absorption in the elderly.

In addition to foodstuffs and vitamins, the intestines absorb electrolytes and water. Sodium, the primary ion of extracellular fluid and an important contributor to the maintenance of blood volume, is absorbed both actively and passively. Whether active transport conserves chloride is in dispute. The phenomenon could easily be related to the absorption of sodium, that of a positive ion "dragging along" the negative chloride ion. Absorption of potassium and bicarbonate is effective, but again the exact mechanism is obscure. The gut is less permeable to polyvalent ions and, therefore, is a risk of deficiency. Calcium requires vitamin D for active transport and to increase membrane permeability for passive diffusion. The gut permeability is also much higher for the ferrous ion than for the ferric ion. Speculation relates this to the size of the hydrated trivalent ion as contrasted to that of the hydrated bivalent ion. Acidity of the gastric juice promotes reduction of ferric to the ferrous form, thereby affording a beginning explanation of the iron-deficiency anemias that accompany achlorhydria and gastric resections. Absorption of iron and phosphate compounds probably is both partly active and partly passive.

Water absorption is currently assumed to be a passive process (Horrobin, 1968, p. 274). The three methods suggested are (1) the hydrostatic pressure difference between the gut and the blood; (2) osmotic "pull" or "dragging" of ions such as hydrated sodium; and (3) osmotic equilibration wherein water can move in or out of the gut in response to its hyper- or hypotonicity in relationship to the blood (Horrobin). Absorption of ions or molecules into the blood would decrease the concentration within the lumen, and the water would follow into the blood. By contrast, the entrance of highly concentrated chyme containing fats, proteins, and carbohydrates would cause an influx of water into the intestine. The gut must absorb approximately 7 to 8 L of water a day to maintain this balance and ultimately the necessary fluid volume for circulation and temperature control.

Absorption depends upon the area that mucous membrane and villi present to the chyme in the intestine. A recent study of Warren et al. (1978) demonstrated a significant reduction in mucosal surface area in the older age group. Warren states the obvious when he says, "The reduction . . . could be nutritionally important where the intake of any nutrient is marginal . . ." (p. 850).

The elderly person, therefore, can be jeopardized by (1) too little water intake; (2) improper ingestion of highly concentrated foodstuffs such as sugar or salts; (3) inadequate active transport mechanisms for ionic and other molecule shifts into the bloodstream; and (4) gastrointestinal disturbances such as inflammation, irritation, or obstruction that lead to diarrhea or vomiting.

Bacterial flora of the intestine can change with aging owing to the decrement in quantity, and often quality, of enzymatic secretion. The reduction in enzymes increases the time required for digestion. Organisms, such as streptococci, which are normally inhibited by the gastric juice, can flourish. Normal saprophytes disappear. Such alteration can (1) decrease the amount of vitamin formation usually provided by the saprophytes, (2) change resistance of the intestinal tract, and (3) promote irritation or inflammation. The gradual decrease in the amount of feces is probably due to a reduction in caloric intake, rather than to any change due to aging.

Liver function primarily concerns itself with metabolic processes.

PANCREAS

The pancreas empties its largely basic and, therefore, buffering solutions into the duodenum. With aging there are structural changes in addition to the aforementioned enzymatic changes. Most marked are those of alveolar degeneration and obstruction of the ducts. As the pancreatic secretion is under hormonal as well as neurological control, this presents real difficulties, for release continues in response to intestinal formation of the hormones, and a blockage with back pressure can occur. Activation of the trypsinogen to trypsin can occur with subsequent recruitment of all the proteolytic enzymes in the ducts into digestive action on the pancreas itself, resulting in pancreatitis.

In the main, other than with acute pancreatitis, symptoms of pancreatic disease are vague and variable. Pain is the most frequently expressed symptom. With acute pancreatitis the patient can usually give an accurate history and description of location, duration, onset, and character; however, painless pancreatitis can and does occur. Rittenbury (1961) notes that approximately 12 percent of his patients over 60 did not complain of pain. In the elderly, the diminution of pain makes diagnosing pancreatitis difficult. When found, the pain is epigastric in the majority of patients and may radiate into the back or to the lower abdomen, although variations occur in the elderly. The pain can be confused with that of gallstones or biliary tract disease, particularly with old people who, according to Rittenbury, have a higher incidence of cholelithiasis. Usually abdominal tenderness and rigidity accompany the pain.

The three most common pancreatic disturbances evidenced by the aged are pancreatitis—acute or chronic—and carcinoma of the pancreas. The latter occurs predominantly in persons over 60 years of age (Brocklehurst, 1973). Surgery in the aged is usually reserved for the treatment of complications such as pancreatic abscess, gastric erosion, and obstruction. Anorexia, weight loss, and weakness are associated primarily with conditions existing over a period of time and, therefore, are found most often in chronic pancreatitis or carcinoma and are due to diminished intake and inadequate digestion. Nausea and vomiting accompany pancreatitis rather than an unobstructed carcinoma. Although weakness can be caused by severe nausea, vomiting, and fluid loss, in acute pancreatitis it is associated with potassium depletion. Persistent, progressive, painless jaundice classically describes pancreatic carcinoma. Jaundice also exists, however, in acute and chronic pancreatitis with biliary tract disturbance and, with increasing incidence, as iatrogenic side effects of tranquilizers and psychotropic drugs. One would expect diarrhea and steatorrhea with pancreatic disease due to irritation, inflammation, and a change in lipase secretion. Oddly enough, constipation is frequently found, and in chronic pancreatitis the elderly experience diarrhea less than any other age group (Hoffman et al., 1959). Diarrhea and steatorrhea were not even mentioned by Kalliomaki and Antila (1971) as problems in acute pancreatitis in patients where the median age was 63 years.

Both acute pancreatitis and carcinoma of the pancreas present disturbances in emotional or mental state. Carcinoma, normally with a relatively insidious onset, presents a change toward anxiety and depression. Some have a premonition of serious illness. Fras et al. (1967) state that these emotional corollaries existed in approximately three-fourths of the subjects in their study. Acute pancreatitis patients are critically ill, and their manifestations range from unconsciousness supposedly related to shock, cerebral ischemia, and hypokalemia, to severe disorientation or hallucinations. Pain can be sufficiently excruciating to cause collapse. The mechanism for the psychotic and emotional manifestations is not known. Acute pancreatitis of necessity requires hospitalization for replacement of fluids and electrolytes, e.g., potassium, transfusions if indicated, control of severe pain, a nasogastric tube with aspiration of the duodenum, laboratory studies, and expert clinical care to prevent or ameliorate shock. Chronic pancreatitis, although serious, can be managed between exacerbations at home if family members are aware of the importance of diet, replacement of pancreatic enzymes, and impact of anticholinergic medications and their timing. These people often have lingering and persistent pain which must be appreciated and not mistaken for malingering or imagined discomfort.

In acute pancreatitis and occasionally in carcinoma of the pancreas, blue or green areas of ecchymosis appear on the flanks or surrounding the umbilicus: these are extravasations of hemolyzed blood with beginning resolution. Carcinoma is associated with venous thrombosis and vascular occlusion; these can be particularly troublesome. The etiology appears to be an increase in serum trypsin (Straus, 1971, p. 198).

Although pancreatitis is associated with biliary tract disease, no relationship to vascular diseases has been noted. The converse, however, appears to be true with a rise in vascular disease in conjunction with pancreatitis (Leeming et al., 1973, p. 336).

GALLBLADDER

Changes in gallbladder function associated with aging relate to emptying rather than filling or concentrating bile. The bile is thicker, richer in cholesterol, and of smaller volume according to Bertolini (1969, p. 624). Biliary tract disease is common in the elderly, and the presence of gallstones increases with aging. McKeown's extensive autopsy studies show an incidence of 20 percent in persons over 70 years (1965, p. 165). Gallstones are more common in women than men. While cholelithiasis may be symptomless, particularly in the elderly, the risk of obstruction when gallstones enter the common or cystic ducts is real. Depending upon the size of the stones, the consistency of the bile, the amount of mucus, and the presence of inflammation, the passage of gallstones may be impeded or blocked entirely. Stasis, inflammation, or infection develop proximal to the stone with retrogressive cholecystitis and possibly pancreatitis or liver involvement due to ascending cholangitis.

The pressure of jaundice due to obstruction indicates the absence of bile in the intestine with a subsequent decrease in the amount of absorption of fat-soluble vitamins. Prior to surgery, a decrease in the quantity of vitamin K for prothrombin formation can lead to serious bleeding and clotting problems evidenced by a tendency of the patient to bruise easily. Jaundice can also be caused by hepatitis or drug intoxication such as phenothiazine ingestion (Eastwood, 1971).

Pain is the most important symptom of gallbladder disease. Nausea, vomiting, and fat intolerance often accompany biliary tract problems with or without stones or pain. The pain is found in the right upper quadrant just below the rib cage, the right scapular region, or occasionally the right shoulder.

As with all potentially obstructive conditions, two treatments are possible, either conservative medical management largely symptomatic or surgical removal of the gallbladder. Each has its proponents and arguments. Suffice it to say, a full-blown obstruction requires emergency surgery. The mortality as reported by Hyams (1973, p. 378) is less than 1 percent with patients younger than 60 years old; however the rate goes up to 7 percent in patients over 70 years. Most authorities suggest the conservative regimen for older patients. Hospitalization is dependent upon severity of symptoms, condition of the patient, and the risks of the required procedure. Medical treatment consists of a low-fat diet, antacids, and, where indicated, weight reduction.

INTESTINAL DISTURBANCES

The intestines, both large and small bowels, are susceptible to five main general difficulties: (1) mechanical obstruction, (2) paralytic obstruction, (3) vascular or hemorrhagic problems, (4) malabsorption, and (5) diverticulosis. Malabsorption primarily affects the small intestine, while diverticulosis is largely associated with the colon. As with other portions of the digestive tract, malignancy occurs more often in the elderly. Cancer of the colon and rectum are reported by Strauss (1971, p. 196) as being the second leading cause of death due to cancer in the aged. Brocklehurst (1973, p. 346) states that it is "the most common form of malignant disease in old age."

Intestinal obstruction from whichever cause, mechanical or paralytic, in the older person is a serious to critical condition requiring hospitalization with intensive treatment. The signs common to each are distention, constipation, and usually vomiting if the small intestine is involved. A colicky, cramping, severe pain suggests a mechanical source, whereas absence of pain heralds a paralysis or atony (Mitty, 1974). X-ray and barium studies confirm the diagnosis. A clear differentiation is essential because, while medical treatment will usually be attempted in paralysis, mechanical obstruction indicates prompt surgical intervention in order to save as much of the bowel as possible from ischemic strangulation. Subsequent perforation with peritonitis in any age group is a critical threat to life, but even more so in the elderly. Both etiologies lead to pallor, dehydration, shock, and abdominal tenderness. Fever, although present in both, more often is associated with paralytic obstruction and underlying infections, such as pneumonia, septicemia, and peritonitis.

Gases from digestive processes and the bacterial flora continue to form proximal to the obstruction, and the inflamed gut leaks plasma into the lumen. None of these can be absorbed because of the related pressures, inflammation, and ischemia. The developing distention, therefore, requires decompression by a Miller-Abbott tube and suctioning. As the suctioned fluids and electrolytes are lost to blood volume, they must be immediately replaced (Finkel, 1971). Potassium and sodium losses are most representative of the electrolytes. Acid-base disturbances can also be severe. Pancreatic secretions are rich in bicarbonate, and these can readily be lost to suctioning. Most patients, therefore, have a combination of acid-base, sodium, and potassium disturbances. The reader is referred to any standard textbook on fluids and electrolytes or gastroenterology for definitive clinical management. Should the decompression be unsuccessful in paralytic obstruction, surgery will be necessary. Even with adequate medical management, replacement therapy, and transfusion, the prognosis in elderly patients is always circumspect and the occurrence of complications is not rare (Rzepiela, 1973).

Resection of a portion of the intestinal tract in the elderly in order to remove a gangrenous portion and restore patency, as with younger populations, decreases the surface area necessary for absorption of both nutrients and water. Protein, fat, and vitamin absorption can be compromised. Such a decrement in the aged may mean the difference between being an "active senior citizen" and an "old invalid." It is imperative, therefore, to make accurate, early assessment of the seriousness of the condition and begin treatment.

Aging of the vasculature affects the digestive tract in a variety of ways (Droller, 1972). Atherosclerosis can narrow the lumen, compromise vasoconstriction or vasodilatation, and form plaques which precipitate thrombi or emboli. In addition, a decrease in cardiac output due to failure or shock contributes to a diminished or marginal blood flow to the intestines. The reduction of blood to supply nutrients to the bowel leads to tissue injury and necrosis of varying degree of the mucosa and intestinal wall. This results in coffee-ground vomitus if involving the stomach, tarry stools if the upper gastrointestinal tract is affected, and bright-red blood if the large bowel is affected. Ming (1965) states that the use of vasoconstrictors in shock probably contributes to the low-flow state.

Occlusion or rupture of a large intra-abdominal vessel usually involves the superior mesenteric or aortic arteries; however, large veins can also be involved. Involvement of large vessels dictates the seriousness of the condition. The onset of pain, shock, and, when involving the colon, loose stools with red blood or clots in each of these situations is dramatic and precipitous. The prognosis is grave despite emergency surgical intervention. If extensive resection of gut is required, the specter of malabsorption is always present.

CONSTIPATION

The two problems of most concern to the greatest number of elderly patients, and to those people involved with the intimate care of the older person are, however, constipation and fecal incontinence. To discuss either one, it would be ideal to have rigid research studies clearly differentiating the degree of motility changes encountered by aging, the effects of specific drugs, and the alterations in the physiology of defecation. To date no satisfactory method or tool has been devised to measure the assumed decrements accurately. Some pertinent findings have been established that could have bearing on the problems. A selection of the more obvious is:

1. While motility increases during and after food ingestion, propulsiveness occurs in the physically active but not the resting patient.
2. The gastrocolic reflex, heretofore related to the ingestion of food into the stomach, causing increased colonic activity, appears to be more an effect of the entrance of chyme into the small intestine (Holdstock et al., 1970; Holdstock and Misiewicz, 1970).
3. There is a defecation center in the medulla, the diencephalon, and cerebral cortex which controls and coordinates this activity.
4. Mass distention of the rectum arouses the defecation reflex which then involves both voluntary and involuntary muscles. If the reflex is inhibited, the rectum relaxes.
5. Stretching of the rectal wall initially causes increased anal contractility followed by relaxation.
6. Voluntary contraction of the external sphincter can be maintained only for a minute (Brocklehurst, 1973, p. 349).

7. The amount of feces decreases with age (Bertolini, 1969).
8. Anatomic changes accompanying aging of the large bowel are atrophy of the mucosa and muscle layers, abnormality of the intestinal glands, arteriolar sclerosis, and delay in peripheral nerve transmission.

An articulating summation of the foregoing suggests that activity and exercise would promote large bowel propulsion and, therefore, be helpful in amelioration of constipation. In view of the complicated interaction and coordination by voluntary and involuntary centers, one would expect difficulty in control and evacuation following any central nervous system assault, such as a cerebrovascular accident. If the external sphincter can be voluntarily contracted for only a minute, the slow-moving aged person, who needs greater time for almost any activity, should have quick, unobstructed access to the commode or toilet.

According to Brocklehurst (1973, p. 352), although old people worry about constipation, there is no evidence to support the contention that constipation is a function of aging. The definition of constipation can include either insufficient feces or hard, dry stools causing pain on defecation. There is a possibility that elderly people develop an idiopathic megacolon. In institutionalized elderly, constipation appears to be a contributing cause of megacolon through gross large bowel distention and accompanying diarrhea and fecal incontinence. Volvulus can develop secondarily to the megacolon and is highly associated with institutionalized over the age of 70.

Almost all elderly people are concerned about their bowels and use a laxative which not only causes evacuation but also has a predictable, known, and, therefore, controlled, effective time and action. This allows for a modicum of planning of daily activities, visits, and chores. Constipation with impaction occurs most readily in immobilized or inactive patients who do not have adequate water intake and who do not change position and use their abdominal muscles sufficiently. Mentally confused old patients may disregard or not feel a distended rectum and, therefore, develop constipation. The essential part of treatment is a respect for the client's concern. This, coupled with careful examination and recording of the factors associated with the condition, will allow for diet modification to include sufficient fluids, bulk, and appropriate foods such as fresh fruit and vegetables to promote motility and propulsion. Weaning from the nighttime laxative may not be possible after years of dependency, and compromise is often the best course with the elderly client.

Chronic constipation can cause fecal impactions in which the stool may be soft or hard. A hard fecolith can be caused by decrease in motility and advancement in the large bowel of the feces. Because of the slow movement, more and more water is absorbed by the intestine. After softening with a small retention enema of detergent or wetting solutions, a follow-up enema should be given. Large enemas, no matter of what solution, should be avoided in the elderly because the sudden distention of the colon can cause mild shock. Perforation of the large colon or diverticula is also a possibility. The manual removal of a fecal impaction is often necessary in the aged person.

FECAL INCONTINENCE

Fecal incontinence is a real care problem with the aged, and while not a threat to physical survival, in the fully aware, mentally normal elderly it can be an exquisitely sensitive source of embarrassment. It can be caused by any of the following:

1. Fecal impaction or gross constipation, with overflow of the formed stool or mucous diarrhea due to mucosal irritation
2. Neurological anomalies with loss of synchronization of control mechanisms and decrease in inhibition of rectal contractions, hence an increased inhibition of the rectal sphincter leading to leakage (Brocklehurst, 1973, p. 358)
3. As a side effect of an underlying disease condition of the colon, rectum, or anus, such as carcinoma, colitis, diabetic neuropathy, or hemorrhoids

Treatment is directed at the underlying cause. In the event the condition is neurological, scheduling of bowel movements is possible by careful habit training and reinforcement, and where indicated, to create constipation by mild agents such as kaopectate and then institute bowel control (Agate, 1971, p. 468).

The incidence of diverticulosis markedly increases with aging. Atrophy of the intestinal wall is felt to be a factor contributing to its development. It is uncommon in regions of the world where a high-residue, less refined diet is eaten. Inflammation or diverticulitis occurs particularly in men. The onset is usually sudden, with spasm, rebound tenderness, and signs of local peritonitis. Conservative treatment of bed rest, parenteral fluids, nothing by mouth, and antibiotics most often is sufficient.

Formerly maintenance therapy utilized a low-residue diet; more recently Painter and his colleagues have reported considerable success with medical management through the use of bran as a well-tolerated, inexpensive, effective means of increasing roughage and decreasing symptomatology of diverticular disease (Painter et al., 1972; Salter, 1973). Recurrent attacks are frequent.

SUMMARY

Digestive disorders of the aged are, for the most part, poorly studied and understood. Practicality has had a great deal to do with this situation. Elderly people have low energy levels; they cannot tolerate long procedures; they take more time to accomplish tasks; sometimes they are forgetful, and oftentimes, starving for attention, they skew the test results. Measurement tools need perfecting and simplifying if they are to be used with the aged and infirmed. Despite all the drawbacks, however, it is apparent that risks for digestive disorders evolve out of four areas:

1. Obstruction, whether mechanical or paralytic
2. Absorption problems of decreased intake, lessened intestinal surface area, diminished enzymatic activity or secretion, curtailed motility or propulsion
3. Vascular pathologies, ischemia, hypovolemia, anemia, atherosclerotic changes, limited supportive cardiac output, and changes in capillary beds
4. Neurological changes due to aging

Knowledge and vigilance in these areas can materially contribute to the care and welfare of the aging individual.

REFERENCES

Agate, J.: Special hazards of illness in later life, in I. Rossman (ed.), *Clinical Geriatrics,* Lippincott, Philadelphia, 1971, pp. 461–472.

Arey, L. B., M. J. Tremaine, F. L. Monzingo: The numerical and topographical relations of taste buds to human circumvallate papillae throughout the life span, *Anatomical Record,* **64:**9–35, December 1935.

Becker, G. H., J. Meyer, and H. Necheles: Fat absorption in young and old age, *Gastroenterology,* **14:**80–92, January 1950.

Bellamy, D.: Long-term action of prenisolone phosphate on a strain of short-lived mice, *Experimental Gerontology,* **3:**327–333, December 1968.

Bender, A. D., C. G. Kormendy, and R. Powell: Pharmacological control of aging, *Experimental Gerontology,* **5:**97–129, July 1970.

Bertolini, A. M.: *Gerontologic Metabolism,* Charles C Thomas, Springfield, Ill., 1969.

Bhaskar, S. N.: Oral lesions in the aged population, *Geriatrics,* **23:**137–149, October 1968.

Bristow, V. A., et al.: Diminished baroreflex sensitivity in high blood pressure and ageing man, *Journal of Physiology,* **202:**45P–46P, February 1969.

Brocklehurst, J. C.: The large bowel, in J. C. Brocklehurst (ed.), *Textbook of Geriatric Medicine and Gerontology,* Churchill Livingstone, Edinburgh, 1973, pp. 346–363.

Carson, J. A., and A. Germican: Disease—Medication relations in altered taste sensitivity, *Journal of American Dietary Association,* **68**(6):550–553, June 1976.

Clarke, C. A., et al: Secretion of blood group antigens and peptic ulcer, *British Medical Journal,* (1):603–607, March 7, 1959.

Dilman, V. M.: Age-associated elevation of hypothalamic threshold to feedback control, and its role in development, ageing and disease, *Lancet,* **1:**1211–1219, June 12, 1971.

Droller, H.: Atheromatous disease of the vessels supplying the gut, *Age and Ageing,* **1:**162–167, August 1972.

Eastwood, H. D. H.: Causes of jaundice in the elderly: A survey of diagnosis and investigation, *Gerontologia Clinica,* **13**(1,2):69–81, 1971.

Everitt, A. V.: The hypothalamic-pituitary control of ageing and age-related pathology, *Experimental Gerontology,* **8:**265–277, October 1973.

Fikry, M. E.: Gastric secretory functions in the aged, *Gerontologia Clinica,* **7:**216–226, 1965.

Finkel, R. M.: Renal and electrolyte disorders associated with intestinal diseases, *Hospital Medicine,* **7**:109–119, June 1971.

Fordtran, J. S.: "Reduction of acidity by diet, antacids and anticholinergic agents" in M. H. Sleisenger and J. S. Fordtran (eds.), *Gastrointestinal Disease,* Saunders, Philadelphia, 1973, pp. 718–742.

Fras, I., E. M. Litin and J. S. Pearson: Comparison of psychiatric symptoms in carcinoma of the pancreas with those in some other intra-abdominal neoplasms, *American Journal of Psychiatry,* **123**: 1553–1562, June 1967.

Hall, D. A.: Metabolic and structural aspects of aging, in J. C. Brocklehurst (ed.), *Textbook of Geriatric Medicine and Gerontology,* Churchill Livingstone, Edinburgh, 1973, pp. 426–435.

Harper, A. E.: Recommended dietary allowances for the elderly, *Geriatrics,* **33**(5):73–75 and 79–80, May 1978.

Hoffman, E., E. Perez, and V. Somera: Acute pancreatitis in the upper age groups, *Gastroenterology,* **36**:675–685, May 1959.

Holdstock, D. J., and J. J. Misiewicz: Factors controlling colonic motility: Colonic pressures and transit after meals in patients with total gastrectomy, pernicious anemia or duodenal ulcer, *Gut,* **11**:100–110, February 1970.

——— et al.: Propulsion (mass movements) in the human colon and its relationship to meals and somatic activity, *Gut,* **11**:91–99, February 1970.

Horrobin, D. F.: *Medical Physiology and Biochemistry,* Williams & Wilkins, Baltimore, 1968.

Hughes, G.: Changes in taste sensitivity with advancing age, *Gerontologia Clinica,* **11**(4):224, 1969.

Hyams, D. E.: The liver and biliary system in J. C. Brocklehurst (ed.), *Textbook of Geriatric Medicine and Gerontology,* Churchill Livingstone, Edinburgh, 1973, pp. 364–383.

Kahn, T. A., et al.: Esophageal motility in the elderly, *Digestive Diseases,* **22**(12):1049–1054, December 1977.

Kalliomaki, J. L., and L. E. Antila: Problems in acute pancreatitis, *Journal of American Geriatrics Society,* **195**:517–525, June 1971.

LaFratta, C. W., and R. E. Canestrari: A comparison of sensory and motor nerve conduction velocities as related to age, *Archives of Physical Medicine and Rehabilitation,* **47**:286–290, May 1966.

Langman, M. J.: Epidemiology of cancer of esophagus and stomach, *British Journal of Surgery,* **58**: 792–793, October 1971.

Leeming, J. T., S. P. G. Webster and I. W. Dymock: The upper gastrointestinal tract, small bowel and exocrine pancreas, in J. C. Brocklehurst (ed.), *Textbook of Geriatric Medicine and Gerontology,* Churchill Livingstone, Edinburgh, 1973, pp. 321–346.

McGinty, M. D.: Hiatal hernia, *Hospital Medicine,* **7**:133–143, April 1971.

McKeown, F.: *Pathology of the Aged,* Butterworth, London, 1965.

Meyer, J., and H. Necheles: Studies in old age IV. The clinical significance of salivary, gastric, and pancreatic secretion in the aged, *American Journal of Digestive Diseases,* **9**:157–159, May 1942.

Mine, M., et al.: End results of gastrectomy for gastric cancer; effect of extensive lymph node dissection, *Surgery,* **68**:753–758, November 1970.

Ming, S. C.: Hemorrhagic necrosis of the gastrointestinal tract and its relation to cardiovascular status, *Circulation,* **32**(9):322–341, September 1965.

Mitty, W. F.: A guide to differential diagnosis and management of abdominal pain in the elderly patient, *Hospital Medicine,* **10**(6):52–67, June 1974.

Painter, N. S., A. Z. Almeida and K. W. Colebourne: Unprocessed bran in treatment of diverticular disease of the colon, *British Medical Journal,* **2**: 137–140, April 15, 1972.

Rittenbury, M.: Pancreatitis in the elderly patient, *American Surgeon,* **27**(7):475–494, July 1961.

Rzepiela, E.: Early postoperative complications of acute abdominal diseases in elderly patients, *Gerontologia Clinica,* **15**(2):92–112, 1973.

Salter, R. H.: Some aspects of diverticular disease of the colon, *Age and Ageing,* **2**:225–229, November 1973.

Shafer, J.: Dysgeusia in the elderly, *Lancet,* **1**(7376):83–84, Jan. 9, 1965.

Sklar, M.: Gastrointestinal diseases in the aged, in A. B. Chinn (ed.), *Working with Older People: A Guide to Practice, vol. IV, Clinical Aspects of Aging,* Government Printing Office, PHS Pub. No. 1459, Washington, July 1971, pp. 124–130.

Soergel, K. H., F. F. Zboralski and J. R. Amberg: Presbyesophagus: Esophageal mobility in nonagenarians, *Journal of Clinical Investigation,* **43**: 1472–1479, July 1964.

Straus, B.: Disorders of the digestive system, in I. Rossman (ed.), *Clinical Geriatrics,* Lippincott, Philadelphia, 1971, pp. 183–202.

Warren, P. M., M. A. Pepperman and R. D. Montgomery: Age changes in small-intestinal mucosa, *Lancet,* **2**(8094):849–850, Oct. 14, 1978.

Williams, J. A.: The effects of gastric operations, *Annals of the Royal College of Surgeons of England,* **48**:54–62, January 1971.

Winick, M.: Nutrition and aging, *New York Journal of Medicine,* **78**(12):1970–1971, October 1978.

TWENTY-THREE

NUTRITION AND THE ELDERLY

Barbara A. Moehrlin
Mary Opal Wolanin
Irene Mortenson Burnside

There are not specialty diets, only special people.
Madge L. Myers

LEARNING OBJECTIVES

- List five physiological parameters which influence the nutrition of the elderly.
- List four psychosocial parameters associated with nutrition and the elderly.
- Identify three special problems related to nutrition in the elderly.
- Describe three interventions in the special problems.
- Identify three feeding problems in the elderly.
- List two interventions in each feeding problem identified.
- Define malnutrition.
- Identify malnutritional states in the elderly.
- List steps for prevention of malnutrition.
- Plan a nutrition education program for the elderly.
- List five steps to include in a nutritional evaluation.

The authors are especially grateful to Doris Constenius, R.D., for carefully reviewing this chapter.

• Complete a nutritional assessment on an elderly client.

_____

This chapter about nutrition and the older person is divided into four sections. The first is an overview of the literature after 1970. The overview is subdivided into four categories: (1) the physiological aspects of nutrition and aging, (2) the psychosocial aspects of nutrition and aging, (3) special problems related to nutrition and the elderly, and (4) assessment of the nutritional status of an elderly client. The second section covers nursing intervention and psychosocial aspects of nutrition and discusses one county's experiences in a Title III nutrition program. The third section discusses special feeding problems nurses may encounter. The fourth section is a set of questions to help health professionals assess the nutritional status of elderly clients.

Concern for the nutritional status of the elderly has increased during the last decade and was expressed at the White House Conference on Food, Nutrition, and Health in 1969, during the 1971 White House Conference on Aging, and also at the Post–White House Conference in 1973. The conferences recognized that the elderly form a high-risk group which is a prime target for nutritional problems and deficiencies, and that malnutrition is widespread among the aging population (WCFNH, 1969; White House Conference on Aging, 1971; Post–White House Conference on Aging, 1973).

In 1977 Butler (1977, pp. 3–4) listed the following areas which the National Institute on Aging (NIA) research program hoped to expand the nutritional knowledge base:

1. What constitutes an adequate diet for the older person, focusing on the changes that occur with age in the need for nutrients
2. What older people eat
3. The factors that affect eating habits — economic, behavioral, and physiological
4. Changes in the physiology of digestion with age
5. The assimilation of nutrients into the body tissues in the older person

6. Risk factors for pathology in middle and old age correlated with nutritional status
7. Topics of special significance, such as the interaction of nutritional variables and drugs

Recently a special report on aging was issued by the Department of Health, Education, and Welfare, the Public Health Service, the National Institutes of Health, and the National Institute on Aging (1979, pp. 6–7). This report includes a section on nutrition and aging requesting research with emphasis in the following areas:

1. Epidemiologic and clinical research on the relationship between aging, nutritional status, dietary intake, and health status
2. Effects of specific diseases on nutritional status and interactions of nutrients with therapeutic agents, surgical procedures, or preventive regimens
3. Effects of aging on nutrient requirements and utilization, digestion, absorption, and metabolism
4. Basic and clinical nutrition studies on the interrelationships between aging and:
   a. Factors which may regulate changes in lean body mass, body composition, energy balance, regulation of metabolic processes, and disease susceptibility
   b. The effects of nutritional deficiencies on long-term health and longevity
5. Effects of nutrition on age-related mental changes

It can readily be seen that awareness of the importance of nutrition in aging, health, and disease has increased significantly. Most authors (Dickman, 1979; National Dairy Council, 1977; Lewis, 1978; Watkins, 1975) agree that nutrition for the elderly includes more than an adequate diet. Physiological, psychosocial, economic, and cultural aspects of aging must also be included. Good nutrition may be the difference between the active, productive older person and the "rocking chair" client with the "tea and toast" syndrome who has multiple disabilities and requires unlimited resources. NIA continues to emphasize the importance of proper nutrition saying, "Nutrition is the cornerstone of preventive medicine—adequate diet throughout life,

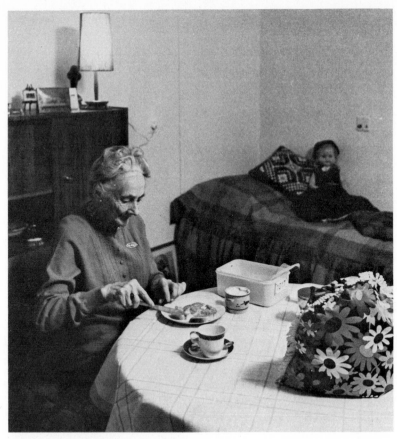

FIGURE 23-1 Eating alone is a pervasive problem in the elderly living in the community. The "tea and toast syndrome" is common, as can be seen in this photograph. (*World Health Organization. Photo by E. Schwab.*)

including the later years, is an effective means to maintain good health and minimize degenerative changes in old age" (*Geriatrics,* Editorial, 1978) (see Figure 23-1).

OVERVIEW OF THE LITERATURE

PHYSIOLOGICAL ASPECTS OF NUTRITION AND AGING

The physiological parameters which influence the nutrition of the elderly are of two types: hereditary and environmental. Lifetime eating habits act as an environmental influence which in turn affects the biological process of aging

and the development of chronic disease (Lewis, 1978) (see Figure 23-2).

O'Hanlon and Kohrs (1978) have summarized several dietary surveys which assessed the nutritional intake of older Americans. The methods used for the collection of data in these studies included food records, 24-hour recalls, and diet histories. Most of the surveys used the recommended dietary (or daily) allowances (RDAs; see below) as the standard for measuring the adequacy of the participants' dietary intake and took into consideration the RDA tables for people over 51 years of age. The authors summarized the conclusions of these surveys for use by researchers, educators, and other persons interested in nutritional status of the elderly.

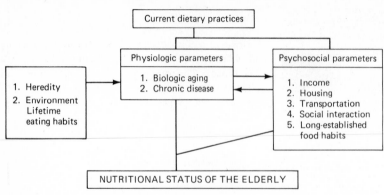

FIGURE 23-2 Factors influencing the nutritional status of the elderly. (*From Clara M. Lewis, Nutritional Considerations for the Elderly, F. A. Davis, Philadelphia, 1978, p. 2.*)

Conclusions were as follows: (1) calories and calcium are the nutrients most often below standard, (2) calcium intake is particularly deficient in women, (3) and protein and niacin are the nutrients frequently found to be in good supply.

Though the above surveys were extensive, Butler (1977) testified that these national studies were inadequate both in methodologies and sampling procedures in terms of the elderly population. He cited one of the surveys that did not collect data on anyone over age 74 and others that did not include samples of persons who were malnourished or in institutions. Additionally, he stated that the studies which required participants to estimate and recall food intake were misleading in regard to older people and that, overall, not enough elderly people were surveyed (p. 9).

AGING OF BODY ORGANS

Aging of the body organs involved in food intake and/or utilization may have a negative effect on nutritional status (Lewis, 1978). The aging process is the result of diminished organ function due to cell loss and decreased metabolism in the remaining cells. Krehl (1974) discussed nutritional components that may be involved in the process of aging and reviewed theories on causes of aging. One such theory involves the concept of the effects of free radicals and their effect on cell membranes. He stated, "These membrane changes adversely affect the flow of

nutrients into and out of the cell and may be a factor in increasing cell death associated with aging" (p. 66).

Krehl also pointed out that the research around vitamin E is still debatable. He notes that vitamin E, because of its role in protection against excessive oxidation of cellular lipids, is recommended to prevent atherosclerosis. The amount of vitamin E needed, however, has not been determined.

Vitamin C is another nutrient that is being researched in regard to the aging process, according to Krehl. Both Krehl (1974) and Albanese (1976) agree that vitamin C may exert a protective role because of its ability to act as a synergist to vitamin E in minimizing peroxidation and at the same time to behave as an aqueous free-radical trap.

Schlenker (1978) reported that atrophy of the papillae in the tongue may be another example of an age-related process. The number of taste buds in the papillae is reduced owing to continued wear throughout the years; hence the ability to distinguish tastes—salt, sweet, sour, and bitter—is notably reduced. However, the sensitivity to sweet is often retained, which may account for the preference of "sweets" by some older people (Lewis, 1978) (see Figure 23-3).

One longitudinal study in Michigan found that one-third of the women had papillae atrophy. An evaluation of their nutrient intake revealed that those with papillae atrophy had significantly lower intake of vitamin C (Barrows and Schlenker, 1978). The wearing of dentures

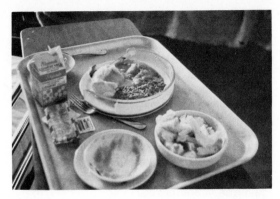

FIGURE 23-3 When institutionalized patients are left to feed themselves, they will often eat the dessert and drink the milk and leave all else on the tray, as can be seen in this photograph. (*Courtesy of Anthony J. Skirlick, Jr.*)

also seems to be associated with papillae atrophy since 71 percent of the subjects in the above study wore dentures. Difficulty in swallowing due to decreased secretion of saliva and diminished neuromuscular control of swallowing also occurs with aging and may contribute to dry tongue and reduced taste sensation in the elderly (Goldman, 1979).

Investigations of age-related changes in smell and taste discussed in the 1979 Special Report on Aging concluded that "diets of the elderly may improve with better understanding of how taste and smell of food and nutrients are affected by normal aging and age-related diseases, and of how food palatability can improve with salt and sugar substitutes and other taste- and flavor-enhancing substances" (p. 17).

The elderly need the same kind of balanced diet as any other age group. The components of

a balanced diet are: (1) enough calories for energy but not enough to lead to overweight, (2) essential amino acids, (3) essential fatty acids, (4) vitamins, (5) essential elements, (6) fiber, and (7) water. *The only age-related differences are that the elderly usually need fewer calories and, because they have a higher drug (medicine) intake than other age groups, are likely to have more nutrition-related problems* (Dickman, 1979, p. 74) (see Figure 23-4).

In 1943 the Food and Nutrition Board of the National Academy of Sciences—National Research Council established a set of guidelines recommending nutrient values necessary to maintain a healthy and adequate diet. The RDAs are the amounts of 15 vitamins and minerals plus protein and calories estimated to be needed for both sexes throughout the life cycle. Consumption of these allowances will maintain good nutrition in essentially all healthy persons in the United States under current living conditions. They are designed to afford a margin of safety above average physiological requirements in the population. The RDAs have been revised several times as new research data have become available (National Academy of Sciences, 1974, p. 2).

In 1974, and more recently in 1980, the RDAs were modified, and additional tables were provided for persons over age 51 years (see Table 23-1). Weg (1978), however, voices continued concern that "these values, estimated to exceed the requirements for most persons, and developed with the 'reference' person (healthy, young, active) as the base, do not relate to the individuality and heightened differences among older persons. . . . The 51+ years values for nutrients

Peanuts / *Charles Schulz*

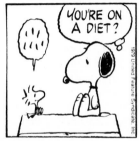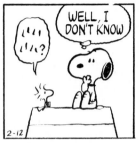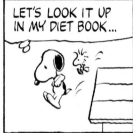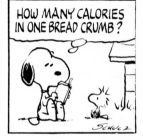

FIGURE 23-4 *Copyright 1979, United Feature Syndicate, Inc.*

TABLE 23-1
RECOMMENDED DIETARY ALLOWANCES

	Age	Female	Male
Calories, kcal	51–75	1800	2400
	76+	1600	2050
Protein, g	51+	44	56
Vitamin A, μ RE	51+	800	1000
Vitamin E, mg α TE	51+	8	10
Ascorbic acid, mg	51+	60	60
Niacin, mg	51+	13	16
Riboflavin, mg	51+	1.2	1.4
Thiamine, mg	51+	1.0	1.2
Calcium, mg	51+	800	800
Iron, mg	51+	10	10

NOTES: RE = retinol equivalent; TE = tocopherol equivalent.

SOURCE: *Recommended Dietary Allowances,* 9th ed, 1980 (in press). Reproduced by permission of the National Academy of Sciences, Washington, D.C.

do not consider the differentiation that occurs within a large group" (pp. 125–126). Krehl (1974) recommends that the RDAs should provide a guideline which will prescribe individualized dietary recommendations.

PSYCHOSOCIAL ASPECTS OF NUTRITION AND AGING

Lewis (1978) outlines the "psychosocial parameters that influence current dietary practices and subsequent nutritional status: (1) income, (2) housing, (3) transportation, (4) social interaction, and (5) long-established food habits. These factors affect either the availability or the acceptability of food" (p. 5). The reader is referred to the diagram in Figure 23-2.

The President's 1970 Task Force on Aging stated, "The lonely older person who finds going to the store too great a burden; the older person who is nutritionally ignorant; the chronically ill older person unable to prepare a hot meal—are all part of the problem" (p. 48). Butler (1975) agreed with the task force and reiterated that "one's food habits may serve one well or badly in old age. Quite apart from malnutrition due to limited incomes, one sees nutritional inadequacy in the diets of older people resulting from poor habits, misinformation, grief and loneliness" (p. 365). One of the immediate goals to be included in a national policy on aging recommended by Butler (1975) is goal 3, elimination of malnutrition and poverty among the elderly. To accomplish this goal, he further recommends immediate reform of the social security system, income taxes, and retirement and pension plans.

To alleviate some of the nutritional problems of the elderly, particularly those due to inadequate income and physical disability, two programs have been developed: the food stamp program, initiated through a congressional act of 1964, and Meals-on-Wheels, established in the 1950s and 1960s and run largely by voluntary organizations. Food stamps, although used by many older persons, nevertheless have been denied to many because of the difficulty in transportation to sites where stamps are sold, long waiting lines to buy the stamps, and degrading treatment by both workers in the stamp program and grocery store employees. This program also did not meet the needs of the homebound, very poor, disabled, isolated, or those with ethnic food preferences (National Dairy Council, 1977). In 1974 the Senate Select Committee on Nutrition and Human Needs reported that only 27 percent of older people eligible for food stamps were receiving them (Butler, 1975).

Meals-on-Wheels programs which provide one or two meals per day for the homebound are also inadequate in number, serving only a small portion of eligible persons. These meals have been provided in the past by voluntary organizations such as home health agencies. More recently the National Meals-on-Wheels Act of 1977 was passed. Its primary intent is to provide federally funded hot meals to homebound, blind, and disabled elderly who cannot go to the Title III nutrition sites. *One author cautions that although Meals-on-Wheels is a valid and necessary service, we need to know whether the meal has been eaten.* Another question to be asked is whether participation in this kind of program increases the older person's isolation and loneliness (Flynn, 1978).

Brickner (1978) provides a detailed account on how to set up a Meals-on-Wheels program including (1) choosing a site for cooking and packaging of food, (2) staffing patterns, (3) delivery, and (4) financing. He also describes how to write a Title VII (now Title III) proposal and includes a question guide to follow.

Congress passed legislation in 1972 which established a nutrition program authorized by Title VII of the Older Americans Act. This program (NPOA) is designed to serve those individuals who are over 60 years and their spouses (regardless of age) who do not eat adequately because they cannot afford to do so, lack the mobility to shop, lack the skill and/or facilities to cook properly, or lack the incentive to eat alone. This program's primary aim is to serve meals in congregate sites. It provides Meals-on-Wheels only secondarily.

The NPOA sites started serving meals in September 1973, and by mid-1976 there were almost 850 programs nationwide. The average number of meals served per day during 1976 was over 250,000 (AOA Fact Sheet, DHEW, 1976).

Title VII of the Older Americans Act was amended in 1979 and is now known as Title III (Hessing, 1979).

Bikson and Goodchilds (1978) prepared a paper, *Old and Alone,* for an American Psychological Association symposium and presented data which showed that "married couples and single women typically eat at home, and that a disproportionately small number of single men eat at home" (p. 11). Additionally, the authors found that "older single men do not eat at home because they do not know how to prepare food for themselves; it is likely that for the duration of their married lives a spouse had responsibility for arranging meals" (p. 12).

Other psychosocial aspects of nutrition and the elderly include education. Shannon and Smiciklas-Wright (1979) report that older people tend to follow dietary practices common where they live and prior habits established when they were young. These habits are influenced by (1) background, (2) religion, (3) and socioeconomic

class as well as reduced mobility and social isolation. As a result of these factors, older people's diets are not only uninteresting but also deficient of nutrients.

The elderly were not privy to the nutrition and health education that is prevalent in today's schools and in the media. As a result the NPOA mandated an educational component in its program. Shannon and Smiciklas-Wright (1979) point out that the eating patterns of older people have long been established. They advise that educational programs in nutrition should not stress drastic changes in food habits, but rather should use current eating patterns to the best benefit. The nutrition staff of the Florida Division of Health (1973) prepared material on 10 topics (with outlines) that they found beneficial and interesting to older audiences:

- Food for Health
- How Food Became You
- Food—What's in It for You?
- One or Two Can Eat Well Too
- Stretching the Food Dollar
- Food and Special Needs of the Older Adult
- Food Facts—and Fads
- Taking Care of Food Safely
- Eating Out
- Where to Turn for Help with Food, Nutrition and Diet

The staff advises that each session should be planned for about one hour and include informal group discussion, films, food demonstrations, and nutrition games. Finally, they recommend serving nutritious refreshments to promote sociability and informality.

SPECIAL PROBLEMS IN NUTRITION AND THE ELDERLY

The literature describes several disorders relating to nutrition and the elderly which may be due to chronic diseases and/or deficiencies.

MALNUTRITION

Todhunter and Darby (1978) discuss *malnutrition* and define it as "the term used to describe not only pathologic states that arise from a dietary deficiency of essential nutrients or calorie excess but also for any significant deviation in dietary pattern that may result in an undesirable risk factor or that can be detected by physical examination or biochemical or physiologic tests" (p. 51).

Krehl (1974) states that malnutrition is a complex problem which is not only physical but also a combination of psychosocial and economic factors. He proposes that the term *latent* (or *hidden*) *nutritional deficiency* be used instead of *malnutrition* to apply to a broader spectrum of aberrant nutritional problems. Butler (1975) reports that malnutrition can be responsible for reversible organic brain syndrome which, if left untreated, can become irreversible.

The term *malnutrition* applies to problems with both under- and overnutrition, and nutrient deficiencies and imbalances. Garetz (1976) is concerned with breaking the dangerous cycle of depression and faulty nutrition; both overeating and undereating may be due to an underlying problem of depression. The mechanism involved in overnutrition is that the person overeats to cope with depression, becoming obese which may lead to a loss of self-esteem and/or the development of chronic diseases. Garetz lists the following reasons for overeating and overweight in the aged: (1) to ward off anxiety, depression, loneliness; (2) social isolation; (3) poverty; (4) to compensate for reduction of sexual and interpersonal relationships; (5) reduction in activity and basal metabolism rate; and (6) proneness to overweight (genetic and learned) (p. 75).

A better understanding of patterns of food selection and good intake is needed to study lifelong obesity and that which occurs with advancing age. Although obesity is often considered a disease needing treatment, there is "evidence from 17 population studies showing that mortality is lower among the elderly who are mildly or moderately overweight, perhaps because they are protected against certain diseases or can withstand illness better" (Andres, 1979).

Garetz (1976) states that undernutrition also may be caused by several factors: (1) ignorance about nutrition; (2) social isolation; (3) depression; (4) psychotic conditions; (5) alcoholism; (6) poverty; (7) medical diseases and medications that impair appetite and absorption, storage, and utilization of food; (8) decreased mobility; and (9) dental problems (p. 74). Garetz concludes that "poverty, social isolation and depression are common factors in both undernutrition and overeating in aged persons" (p. 75).

ANEMIAS

Anemias are another common disorder in the aged. Flynn (1978) asserts that "anemia and aging do not go hand-in-hand" but are common especially in low-income and chronically ill persons. Dietary anemia due to iron deficiency usually occurs over a period of time and may present rather vague symptoms or even more often may be asymptomatic. Flynn (p. 22) describes the causes of dietary-related iron-deficiency anemia:

1. Income below levels to buy adequate food
2. Inability to prepare food because of physical disability
3. Eating foods low in dietary iron
4. Anorexia due to grief response
5. New dentures
6. Dislike of cooking and eating alone

Krehl (1974) reports that an elderly person may have a combination of nutritional anemias at the same time. Macrocytic anemias are due to deficiencies of folic acid and/or vitamin B_{12}. Folate deficiencies are seen in people who eat very little, follow fad diets, or are alcoholics and often coincide with ascorbic acid deficiencies. Vitamin B_{12} deficiencies may be due to pernicious anemia or result from following a strict vegetarian diet (Todhunter and Darby, 1978).

FLUID IMBALANCE

Water is an essential component of nutrition and composes about 70 percent of a person's total body weight. Albanese (1976) reported that a person of average weight, aged 65 to 90 years, must drink or get from food 1.3 quarts of water daily to maintain a normal fluid balance. According-ing to Albanese, "maintenance of fluid balance is essential to distribution of nutriments to the ultimate cellular units, elimination of wastes, and innumerable physiochemical processes" (p. 8). The elderly are particularly susceptible to fluid imbalance, which is frequently accompanied by electrolyte imbalance, acidosis, or alkalosis. Some common problems which can cause fluid imbalance are: (1) dehydration, (2) edema, (3) water intoxication, (4) constipation, (5) diarrhea, and (6) diaphoresis (Kee, 1973).

Dietary fiber is another essential component for maintenance of proper bowel function. The elderly are particularly prone to constipation because intestinal muscle tone diminishes with age (National Dairy Council, 1977). Dietary fiber is also of value in controlling obesity by acting as a filler and reducing caloric intake (Dickman, 1979).

VITAMIN DEFICIENCIES

Vitamin B_{12} and folic acid deficiencies are likely to be associated with symptoms of dementia (Cameron et al., 1977). Dickman (1979) lists four major factors that contribute to vitamin deficiencies: (1) an inadequate diet (especially in vitamin C since many older persons forego eating fruits and vegetables), (2) incomplete digestion or absorption, (3) loss of vitamins by processing or storage of foods, and (4) destruction by cooking and short-term warming before serving (p. 78).

Hypovitaminosis can cause reversible organic brain syndromes (Butler, 1975). Both Severinghaus (1972) and Krehl (1974) are in favor of the use of regular vitamin supplements by the elderly, especially those who do not choose the proper foods or whose living conditions make proper choices difficult. However, Krehl cautions against excessive use or overdose of vitamins A and D which can prove to be dangerous when accumulated in the body.

Diabetes, hypertension, cardiovascular diseases, and osteoporosis are influenced by nutrition. Overweight persons risk an increased incidence of these diseases. The most frequently occurring problem among obese persons is maturity-onset diabetes, which often can be controlled with diet alone (Todhunter and Darby, 1978).

Table 23-2 is a summary of the signs and symptoms to watch for in the conditions of dehydration, edema, and water intoxication (Kee, 1973). (See Figure 23-5.) Constipation, diarrhea, and diaphoresis are also important to assess.

Sodium-restricted diets have long been an accepted method of treatment for patients with cardiovascular problems and hypertension. When diuretics are used, sodium and potassium levels must be carefully monitored (Todhunter and Darby, 1978).

OSTEOPOROSIS

Osteoporosis is a major problem, especially in elderly women, and is due to multiple deficiencies, namely, insufficient amounts of calcium in the daily diet, a decrease in the production of sex hormones, and a lack of physical exercise. Albanese (1976) reports that intestinal malabsorption syndromes will reduce calcium availability in the face of adequate intake. He

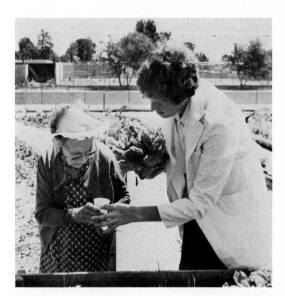

FIGURE 23-5 Adequate hydration is essential for maximum body functioning. Many elderly suffer the effects of dehydration which can result in confusional states. When one is working with the elderly, one must be alert to clinical signs of dehydration, thirst being a major reliable indication. (*Courtesy of Anthony J. Skirlick, Jr.*)

TABLE 23-2
SIGNS AND SYMPTOMS OF FLUID IMBALANCE

Condition	Signs and Symptoms	Condition	Signs and Symptoms
Dehydration	Dryness of lips, conjunctiva, and mucosa		Cyanosis
	Decreased skin turgor		Moist rales in the lung
	Increased thirst (may not always be present)		Neck vein or sublingual vein engorgement
	Elevated temperature (low grade)		Increased central venous pressure (CVP)
	Increased pulse		Localized edema
	Fullness of tongue (furrowed in advanced stages)	Water intoxication	Nausea and vomiting
	Sunken eyeballs		Diaphoresis
	Low blood pressure		Mental changes
	Decreased urine output	Constipation	Immobility
	Nausea and vomiting		Straining during bowel movement
	Decreased appetite		Opiates, iatrogenic, drugs (especially, antacids, diuretics, analgesics, tranquilizers)
	Weight loss		
	Confusion and agitation		Depressive state
	Recent diarrhea		Diarrhea (due to fecal impaction)
	Hyperventilating		Cramping
	Large amounts of sputum		Nausea
	Fluid/food intake decreased		Urinary incontinence
	Altered lab studies show:		Headaches
	Decreased urine chloride (below 50 meq)	Diarrhea	Frequent liquid stools
	Specific gravity above 1.030		Cramping
	Elevated serum sodium or protein		Fever
	Elevated hemoglobin, hematocrit, BUN		Increased carbohydrate, protein diet (tube feeding)
			Viral or bacterial infection
	Possible decubiti from dehydration	Diaphoresis	Fever
Edema	Dyspnea		Excessive heat in room (e.g., too many blankets, hot sun from a window)
	Constant irritated cough		

SOURCES: Ann Boylan and Bernard Marbach, Dehydration: subtle, sinister . . . preventable, *R.N.,* 42(8):37–41, August 1979; Joyce L. Kee, Fluid imbalance in elderly patients, *Nursing '73,* 3(4):40–43, April 1973.

further advises that vitamin D increases calcium absorption and that vitamin C is essential for biosynthesis of collagen—bone protein (p. 8).

Research advances reported in the 1979 *Special Report on Aging* link osteoporosis and vitamin K, saying, "The effects of osteoporosis . . . may be arrested with adequate vitamin K intake. . . . Institute grantees have discovered that when an individual experiences vitamin K deficiency, the resulting decrease in the protein osteocalcin causes calcium loss in bone. This calcium loss, in turn, causes a decrease in the amount and strength of bone tissue in old people, making affected bones weak, porous and highly susceptible to fracture" (p. 12).

Severinghaus (1972) emphasizes that prevention of osteoporosis must begin at least in the middle years, if not in youth. Milk and dairy products should be especially encouraged in the diet. Watkins (1975) reports that long-term studies show that once fractures occur, the process of osteoporosis cannot be reversed but can only be slowed by intake of supplemental calcium.

ALCOHOLISM AND DRUGS

Alcoholism has been cited in almost every resource as having an especially devastating effect on the nutritional status of the elderly, especially for men. In addition to damaging vital body organs (e.g., the liver), chronic alcoholism often leads to multiple vitamin deficiencies (i.e., folic acid and ascorbic acid) and/or obesity (Krehl, 1974).

Butler (1975) warns that "there are also dangers in the casual prescription of alcohol for older people to help them sleep, improve their appetite and add to their sociability. Alcohol blunts reaction time, impairs coordination and fuzzes mental abilities especially memory. Serious falls and misjudgments can result" (p. 363).

A multitude of drugs can cause nutritional deficiencies, specifically vitamin deficiencies and malabsorption of vitamins and other elements, particularly calcium, even when there is an adequate diet. Some common offenders are aspirin, anticonvulsants, indomethacin, Coumadin anticoagulants, isoniazid, prednisone, mineral oil, KCl, and methotrexate (Dickman, 1979).

Butler (1977) advocates investigation of the "possible synergistic effect of a borderline nutrient intake with prolonged drug therapy" (p. 8). Once the relationship between the drug and the specific nutrient deficiency is figured out, Dickman (1979) recommends that either the drug or the diet be changed. If changing the medication is not practical, increasing dietary vitamins or adding supplemental vitamins is advised.

DENTAL STATUS

Older people's dental status may significantly influence their nutritional status, so much so that it can lead to malnutrition. Todhunter and Darby (1978) note that although new dental caries in the elderly decrease, gingival and periodontal diseases and frequent loss of teeth are common. "Poor teeth and poorly fitted dentures can make chewing difficult," according to Williams (1978). She continues that "a denture can

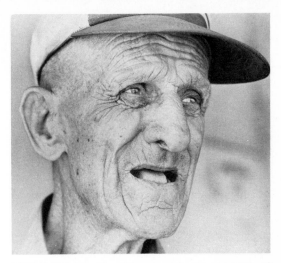

FIGURE 23-6 Toothless old man needs diet containing soft foods. (*Courtesy of Jim Wisdom.*)

only be as successful as the health of the tissue on which it rests" (p. 196). Flynn (1978) reports that "anemia and weight loss may also be related to ill-fitting dentures (or their absence). The soft diet of tea, milk, crackers, soup and toast often accompanies this condition" (p. 22) (see Figure 23-6).

ASSESSMENT OF THE NUTRITIONAL STATUS OF THE ELDERLY

Weg (1978) states, "Physicians and other health professionals (i.e., nurses) who attend older persons, both in communities and institutions, must also suffer the ignorance of their own deficient education in nutrition and aging" (p. 134). She continues on a more hopeful note, however, saying that updated nutritional knowledge is available for those who need and want it and that we all can change both in our thinking and in our practices.

A nutritional assessment is as important as any other part of a person's total evaluation. Krehl (1974, pp. 63–64) outlines five steps to include during a nutritional evaluation:

1. Observing the general appearance of the individual
2. Taking a detailed medical, personal, and social history

3. Taking a careful dietary history, either abbreviated or detailed, depending on the circumstances
4. Making a thorough physical examination
5. Obtaining pertinent laboratory measurements

Weir et al. (1978) affirm that body weight is the most useful single observation for assessment of the nutritional status. However, the authors admit that this might provide problems in terms of current guides, height, body frame, skin fold thickness, and individual interpretations. Additionally, aging changes and fluid retention must also be taken into consideration.

Krehl (1974) indicates that neurological findings and examination of the skin, eyes, and oral cavity including the tongue, lips, gums, and teeth are also very important. Todhunter and Darby (1978) favor the diet history which should provide data about food patterns, food resources and attitudes (likes and dislikes), and the kinds of dietary supplements that are taken. Flynn (1978) also discusses the assessment parameters related to dietary history:

> Assessing food intake requires a broad nutritional survey. Availability of the food, transportation to food stores, adequate resources, ability and interest in preparing food, combined with general health status all need consideration. Heavy bundles, distances from stores, and flights of stairs may inhibit food shopping. Some elderly are fearful of being robbed and thrown to the ground. News of such incidents travel quickly among the elderly in a community and creates fear of going out. (p. 21)

NURSING INTERVENTION IN PSYCHOSOCIAL ASPECTS OF NUTRITION

SYMBOLISM OF FOOD

The symbolism of food to the elderly client is often ignored by health professionals. Williams (1978) points out that milk has more psychological meaning than any other food and discusses sex-related attitudes. Masculine meanings are associated with foods such as meat and bread. Eggs are nutritionally as good as meat (in fact better for ideal amino acid combustion), but eggs never quite substitute for meat. Vegetables and fruits carry feminine meanings, especially fruits. The same author points out that "food habits are among the oldest and most entrenched aspects of many cultures" (p. 134). Foods popular in one culture may repulse someone of a different culture. Religious aspects of a culture also control the acceptability of food, as one author (IB) learned in one Malaysian household where hamburgers were forbidden "because they contained ham."

Jewish food patterns are often rigidly adhered to in Jewish long-term care facilities, but Japanese, Italian, Greek, and Mexican food patterns need special consideration, too. The nurse will need to study cultural practices of each individual to determine what needs changing in the diet and what should be left intact.

JAPANESE CULTURE

At one Japanese Senior Center in a small, renovated house in California, 30 to 40 elderly Japanese usually attend daily programs. On the day that a Japanese meal is prepared, the attendance goes up to 60. The food is prepared by a volunteer who had special education in Tokyo. Chopsticks are always used. Donations are 75 cents per person for a Japanese lunch. A sample Japanese menu served is shown in Table 23-3.

In Japan, September 15 is a special day called "Respect Elder Day." Those over 75 years of age in Japan receive extra money. One current issue of a Japanese journal (*Nutrition and Cooking,* 1979) includes photographs of food and recipes which would appeal to the older Japanese. Watanabe (1979) uses this journal as a resource for planning, cooking, and serving meals for senior citizens once a week.

SOCIALIZATION

Socialization factors are also an important aspect of nutrition. No one enjoys eating alone all the time. Eating is considered an occasion for both social and psychological communication. Going shopping for food can also be an impor-

TABLE 23-3
SAMPLE JAPANESE MENU

Japanese	American	Nutritive Value
Garnish:		
Daicon	Shredded radish	Fiber
Kaiso	Seaweed	Vitamin A Calcium Iron
Sashimi	Raw fish*	High in protein, vitamins B₁ and B₂, calcium
Dengaku	Tofu (bean curd)	Same as above
Kyuri	Salad (cucumber)	
Akowa	Rice with bread	Carbohydrate
Ocha	Green tea	Fluid intake

* Very expensive, so used on special occasions such as Respect Elder Day.

tant time to socialize with friends, especially if one walks to and from the grocery store. Many older people fall into the "tea and toast" syndrome when they have to eat alone. Fixing adequate meals for one or sometimes even two is "too much bother." Lewis (1978) suggests that isolation is linked to nutrition and may lead to malnutrition. People who are lonely may become even more indifferent and, therefore, fail to reach out to anyone at all. People who live alone are particularly at risk of malnutrition, especially those who have recently lost a spouse (Garetz, 1976). These facts apply to older people living in both the community and institutions. Recognizing the need for socialization, many institutions encourage eating in community dining rooms and have even encouraged participation by families and other visitors. Some institutions have conveniently located facilities (i.e., microwave ovens and refrigerators) so people can get something to eat or drink at any time. (People with pacemakers should not use microwave ovens.)

The community nutrition projects funded under Title III have also taken the need for socialization into consideration and have specified that this need be one of the conditions of eligibility for the program. The following is one experience in working with a Title III nutrition site.

EXAMPLE OF GROUP FEEDING

Title III nutrition sites are prime target areas for community health nursing services to reach the aged. This is evidenced by the experiences of nurses in one large county in northern California. In February 1974, 13 nutrition sites in 7 target areas were established in the county. Over 950 meals per day were provided as well as a Meals-on-Wheels program. Sites were placed throughout the community utilizing ethnic centers, churches, previously established senior centers, and public buildings. To date, there are a total of 25 sites with two Meals-on-Wheels programs that serve 2225 daily meals.

The program operators recently summarized the program's success: "It is successful, not only because the carefully balanced nutritional meal ensures that low income seniors eat well, but also because the opportunity to socialize with their peers serves as a focal point in the lives of many elderly people" (Senior Nutrition and Service Program, 1977).

One senior citizen wrote, praising the program, "I like the program because my health problems will not allow me to stand long enough to cook or go shopping for food. For one who lives alone and cannot move about much, it is an enormous lift. The many different types of people supply a daily interest as do the various programs (music, slides, lectures). I am sure it delays senility." Another said, "I never eat vegetables at home, but I eat them here." And still another said, "I don't eat on the days I don't come here."

HOUSING

Inadequate or substandard housing often affects the nutritional status of the elderly. It is estimated that 30 percent of older people in the United States live in unsatisfactory housing. Those people who live at or below the poverty level have even greater problems due to lack of hot and/or running water, central heating, and inside toilets. This type of substandard housing is found most often in rural areas of the South (Harbert and Ginsberg, 1979).

As a result many older people may not have the incentive, strength, or energy to cook when they lack proper facilities or have to spend the greater part of their incomes for housing. Many older persons live in single-room housing—hotels, boarding or rooming houses—which have no cooking facilities, space for food storage, or refrigeration. Such a lack limits the kind and amount of food that can be bought and consumed. These persons should be encouraged to attend the Title III nutrition sites. People on supplemental security income (SSI) may be eligible for a restaurant or meals allowance. They should check with their Social Security Administration office. Other possible alternatives include using an electric coil to heat liquids; hot plates, toaster ovens, and crock pots to cook canned, frozen, or convenience foods or one-dish meals; canned milk which will keep without refrigeration for 2 or 3 days after it has been opened; individual servings of canned juices; fresh fruits and vegetables (purchased in small amounts); peanut butter and cold or instant hot cereals. These suggestions may not be suitable alternatives for those persons who have low incomes or are on special diets (i.e., low sodium). Safety factors and fire regulations must also be taken into consideration.

The nurse or other health professional can refer the person who needs improved housing to the local housing authority. Many government-subsidized housing units are available to the elderly. However, long waiting lists may make this kind of housing seem "out of reach" or impossible to obtain—perseverance is necessary! One such local housing project for the elderly recently took 300 applications in 2 days for 120 available units. Other types of housing including some retirement homes, senior housing projects or high-rise apartments, and board and care homes provide one to three meals per day on the premises. Although this is a desirable alternative, even many of these places do not provide the individualized or special diets that are frequently needed by older people.

TRANSPORTATION

Many people in their seventies, eighties, and nineties no longer drive a vehicle because they are either unable to pass a driver's license test or unable to afford a car. Lack of transportation makes grocery buying difficult for the elderly living at home. Taxis are usually prohibitive in cost; however, some counties do subsidize transportation by taxi to physicians' offices, grocery stores, or nutrition sites. Vans are also made available in some areas for picking up persons going to nutrition sites. This is crucial in rural areas, if there are no support systems.

Some older persons have resorted to bicycles, and a three-wheeler with a basket helps them bring their purchases home. Active oldsters who can walk to the store are often afraid of being mugged, as stated earlier by Flynn (1978).

Nurses may frequently find themselves in the role of advocate for clients, or encouraging them to solve their problems of lack of transportation. This may become an even greater problem as gasoline becomes scarcer.

INCOME

The escalation of inflation has raised havoc with elderly persons on fixed incomes. With increased rents and costs of transportation or gasoline, aged people are often forced to economize by reducing both the quality and the quantity of food intake.

Nader (1978) described a food advisory service (FAS) begun in California in 1975 which serves over 7000 elderly. Food is bought directly from wholesalers and grocers, then distributed to 85 community centers. The project began when two women, Pat Coats and Sandi Piccini, were horrified to read in a newspaper that senior citizens were eating dog food. The elderly participate in running the markets of FAS, and a "dialogue and friendliness develops out of the purchasing process." Nurses will need to know about such community resources in the aged person's community.

Lewis (1978, p. 30) makes the excellent point to "encourage the elderly to feel that *money spent for food is well spent* in terms of physical and emotional health; describe physical or emotional symptoms that may result from nutritional deficiency." The "Other Resources" at the end of this chapter may be helpful to some readers who teach the aged.

NUTRITION SITES FOR THE ELDERLY

Special consideration for the ethnic needs of the older people were considered when the nutrition sites were established. There were one kosher, one black, one Japanese-American, two Filipino-American, and four Mexican-American nutrition sites. Most of the sites also have a variety of community resources available to them including transportation, public health nursing services, and social services.

One author, Barbara A. Moehrlin, has been involved in a special senior health program at 4 of the 25 nutrition sites. Public health nurses are there prior to mealtimes from one to four times a week. Nursing services available at the four sites include:

1. Health assessment clinics which offer individuals some basic health tests such as blood tests for iron, blood pressure checks, and overall health evaluation.
2. Individual counseling sessions (a public health nurse will provide an opportunity for senior citizens to discuss their health problems on a continuing basis).
3. Educational programs held periodically cover health topics of interest and importance to senior citizens. Topics include nutrition, chronic diseases, safety, etc.
4. Special health screening clinics are offered periodically. Senior citizens can receive dental and hearing evaluation and chronic disease testing.
5. Special self-help groups to guide senior citizens in preventing health problems which might result from loneliness, stress, overweight, etc.
6. Information and referral is given to the oldster who needs other community resources and services such as Department of Social Services, district public health nurses, and private physicians.

Nutrition education is also an integral and ongoing part of the nursing services. A variety of nutrition education programs have been tried and proved successful:

- Individual counseling by public health nurses regarding weight loss, special diets, iron-rich foods, and special nutrients (i.e., potassium, sodium, cholesterol). All are a standard part of teaching in each visit to the nurse. Diet histories and 24-hour recalls are used for special problems.
- Slide-tape presentations on nutritional topics (with a Caremate projector, which can be used by individuals or small groups while they are waiting to see the nurse). Two slide-tapes for nutrition programs have been developed by the health department's nutritionist on "Iron, Anemia and You" and "Salt in Your Diet." After watching these programs, clients can ask questions of a nurse or a community worker, who is also present and trained in basic nutrition.
- A community worker trained in basic nutrition presents a display of food models depicting a nutrition problem or question to those persons who are waiting to see the nurse. (An example is a display of foods high and low in calories. The viewer is asked to choose which of two foods is high or low in calories, i.e., which product is higher in calories—butter or jelly?
- Pamphlets are available during counseling or teaching. Two large-print pamphlets were designed by the health department's nutritionist on proper nutrition for the elderly and potassium-rich foods. The pamphlets are easy to read and understood by the older people.

Public health nurses at these nutritional sites have been instrumental in identifying health and psychosocial problems, and to help select appropriate interventions to solve problems and guide the elderly in maintaining or improving their state of health. See Figure 23-7, which depicts a typical meal being served at one of the sites.

SPECIAL PROBLEMS REGARDING NUTRITION AND THE AGED

INTRAVENOUS FEEDINGS

Confusion states are common problems with hospitalized old patients who may require intravenous feedings. They do not understand what is happening to them and may attempt to pull out the intravenous needle. Usually the staff

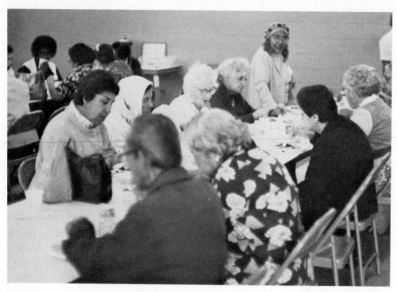

FIGURE 23-7 The importance of the nutrition sites for socializing and for camaraderie during the noon meal must be emphasized. Instructors can utilize the sites as settings in which to teach students to observe social interaction, eating patterns, cultural habits, and educational programs. (*Courtesy of Anthony J. Skirlick, Jr.*)

quickly restrains them, causing further agitation as they struggle to free themselves. When the intravenous feeding was started, the aged patient was not told what would happen. This tends to be especially true with the hard-of-hearing and confused aged. We sometimes assume that if an elderly person is disoriented, he or she will not understand anyway, and so we do not bother to explain what we plan to do and why it is necessary.

The presence of another person can reduce anxiety, and it would be helpful to find a "sitter" to stay at the bedside while the intravenous feeding is given. In a nursing home setting, another resident who is alert may even offer to do this.

Feeding can be a problem for both the old person and the one doing the feeding. Generally, a nurses' aide, a relative, or a home health aide does the feeding. There are instances in which an elderly person has been fed too fast, or the wrong diet has been given, for example, hard fried liver to a patient with difficulty swallowing, who subsequently choked to death.

Nurse's aides often feed several residents at one time, and there is no doubt they do have some extremely trying patients to handle. It can

be a tiresome and tedious daily affair to feed someone who is a very slow eater, has to go to the bathroom during the meal, refuses to eat, or spits out food (see Figure 23-8).

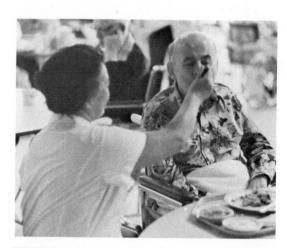

FIGURE 23-8 Feeding patients is often done hurriedly and with impatience. Individuals assigned this task are labeled "feeders" in many facilities. Often an aide can be seen feeding two or more persons simultaneously. In-service education about feeding patients is important, especially about feeding individuals with swallowing problems. (*Courtesy of Anthony J. Skirlick, Jr.*)

If a patient is very regressed, how much tolerance and patience can the aide be expected to muster? Older persons who have Alzheimer's disease may no longer "know how to eat." Such individuals seem to be finicky eaters, but they may actually have feeding apraxia, which is an inability to manipulate their hands and the utensils appropriately for eating. Observation and guidance while eating, careful food selection, and behavior modification can help such persons to eat more independently (Blass, 1979).

REFUSAL TO EAT

It is also possible that the person doing the feeding can experience guilt feelings. If one urges food or medicine to an individual who is begging to die and does not want to eat, one can feel strong emotions. One private-duty nurse was told by the physician and relatives to get food into the patient, even though the patient held her teeth tightly together and refused to let the nurse feed her. The relatives scolded both patient and nurse because she did not eat. She had willed herself to die, but to spare herself and the nurse the embarrassing scoldings of relatives, she ate minimal amounts and detested every minute and every bite. While the person in the home setting who refuses to eat can be permitted to do so, present federal regulations do not permit such behavior in institutions. (See the film *Gramp* listed in "Other Resources" at the end of the chapter; also see Jury and Jury, 1976.)

NUTRITIONAL PROBLEMS AND MENTAL ILLNESS

Another difficult person to feed is the individual with mental illness. A paranoid person may feel that the food is being poisoned and can frighten staff members with grandiose delusions, sarcasm, and/or accusations. In-service education is needed to explain the dynamics of paranoia to staff members, as well as handling the nutrition problem. Weinberg (1970) described the defense mechanism of projection: everyone is taking everything away from them, and so they feel people are stealing from them and are "out to get them."

Depressed individuals, as the woman described above, also eat poorly and complain of no appetite. One must consider the reasons an aged person is not eating; if a depressive state is responsible, a sustained effort should be made to intervene in the depression. Persons who have suffered a stroke often become depressed.

VIGNETTE 1

One elderly man who had had a stroke was fiercely independent and refused to be fed. He had to use his left hand, which was awkward for him, and he was uncoordinated. He made a big mess with food all over his bed linen, occasionally jabbed himself in the face with the fork, and became increasingly depressed. An astute nurse sat down with him one day to talk about his problems, and he related the depression and the eating difficulties. This is the plan they worked out together. A drawsheet was put across the front of him at mealtime so that, if he spilled, the entire top linen did not have to be changed. Changing the bed linen had been humiliating to him. He was given a spoon instead of a fork, and food that he really liked and that was easier to manage (for example, more finger foods). The nurse was astounded at the change in the patient after the new approach had been implemented.

INDIVIDUALS WITH DEMENTIA

The profusion of elderly with dementia also creates nutritional problems because they forget to eat, they take medicines incorrectly, they leave burners on, and they become hazardous at times. The day to day care of these persons is largely the responsibility of nurse's aides and/or home health aides and relatives.

VIGNETTE 2

One nurse's aide improved the feeding routine of four confused old women in her charge. Every morning she dressed them neatly, applied makeup, and put jewelry on them because they would be going to lunch. She was undaunted even when one of the old ladies picked up an earring and ate it!

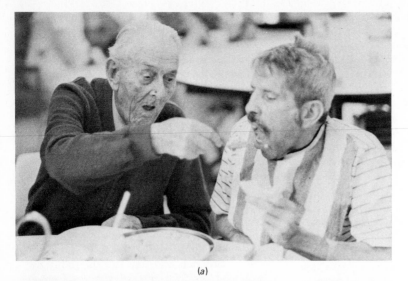

(a)

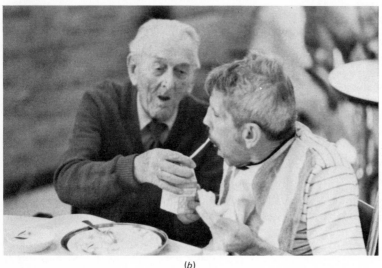

(b)

FIGURE 23-9 We would do well to encourage the buddy system in institutions more than we do. The intent expression of the older helper can be seen in this photograph. And the fact that the older person is needed by a younger person is an important aspect of this relationship, too. (*Courtesy of Anthony J. Skirlick, Jr.*)

The aide assigned one woman to be the hostess, which also helped improve the social atmosphere and communication. When the women improved and were moved to another wing, they requested to go back to their original ward "for lunch with friends."

The problems of nutrition in nursing homes have been studied. The findings of one study conducted in a nursing home are as follows (Benedict, 1975):

- The majority of the patients had a diagnosis of cerebrovascular accident or hip fracture (femur); some had carcinoma.
- The patients were never checked to develop a feeding list.
- The patients' trays were often placed out of their reach.
- Approximately 20 percent of the patients who could feed themselves needed help in setting up the tray or cutting their food.
- Sixty percent of the patients needed to be fed.

Some patients were found to be mentally unable to feed themselves although they were physically capable (see Figure 23-9).

- Forty percent stated that the food was cold when they received it.
- Approximately 10 percent of the patients stated that they did not like the food they were being served.
- Most of the patients were on a general diet. Some were receiving modified diets.
- General dietary staff, sometimes student help, served the trays.
- The serving personnel's attitude and appearance varied by individual.
- Although all meals were involved, the dinner tray was most often left uneaten (see Figure 23-3).
- Meals were sometimes interrupted by therapy or treatments.
- Some patients received medications which could be upsetting to the digestion just before mealtime.
- Patients were sometimes upset when families visited around mealtimes.
- Although some patients were overinclined to talk at mealtimes, it did not appear to affect their eating.

SUGGESTIONS FOR INTERVENTIONS IN FEEDING PROBLEMS

1. Attend to the sensory losses, especially when there is hemianopsia (half of the visual field is gone, usually owing to stroke) because persons so affected cannot see half of the food on the tray. (See Chapter 33 for a discussion of hemianopsia.)
2. Explain procedures to the confused elderly, those suffering from dementia, for example.
3. Help the person with Alzheimer's disease to learn to eat; use behavior modification strategies (Blass, 1979).
4. Improve in-service education about nutrition and feeding the aged.
5. Intervene in states of paranoia and depression.
6. Cater to dietary wishes whenever possible, especially with foods symbolically important for cultural or religious reasons.

7. Encourage the elderly to help one another (see Figure 23-9).
8. Learn about the resources available in the community, e.g., Meals-on-Wheels, Friendly Visitors.

ASSESSMENT OF NUTRITIONAL STATUS

Nutritional assessment of elderly persons is important in order to determine their specific dietary needs. The following lists describe the specific problems of high-risk persons whose nutritional needs may not be met.

Psychosocial Problems

- Those on very low income
- Those who abuse alcohol and other central nervous system depressant drugs
- Those who have had recent bereavements (grief work, depression)
- Those on a low-sodium diet
- Those who live alone or are lonely
- Older persons removed from their cultural diet pattern
- Those who are confused, forgetful, and disoriented
- Those who are working toward an intentional or subintentional death

Mechanical Problems

- Persons with loss of mobility and strength
- Persons with neurological deficits, or arthritic conditions which prevent hand and/or arm coordination, especially on the dominant side, or who have dysphagia or loss of tongue strength
- Persons with visual problems
- Persons who must be fed
- Persons with diminished vision or no vision
- Persons with decubiti
- Persons with loss of chewing ability (edentulous or teeth in poor repair)
- Persons with respiratory problems
- Persons on many pharmaceuticals, especially drugs which dry the mouth, such as tranquilizers and diuretics, or which nauseate
- Persons who undergo surgery or other events

which involve withholding oral feedings and replacement by intravenous infusion

Many of the elderly fall into several of the high-risk categories simultaneously, and these become the very high risk persons predicted for nutritional inadequacy.

This third component for survival subsumes a knowledge of the psychosocial and cultural background of nutrition as well as the physiological and mechanical problems which are peculiarly those of the aging. *Food in those persons who make up the plurality of cultures in the United States has a value which is greater than nutritional needs. It furnishes a means of marking the great turning points in life and sharing intimate moments of family and friendship, and it is a status symbol indicating class* (Weg, 1978). Of all these, it is the absence of a social event which makes the lonely malnutrition of the solitary elderly person more poignant. One of the first objectives which should confront the nurse making an assessment is that of defining the relationships which retain the social event of daily foods or their lack. *The person who eats alone should be suspected of marginal nutrition, and this fact should lead to observation and inspection for further signs.*

The second objective should be to consider how the person obtained food—income level and strength for buying and preparation. Again, doubtful circumstances should lead to examination for marginal or frank nutritional deficits.

Nurses' knowledge of the nutritional needs of all people plus knowledge of pharmacology will lead them to special observations of the older person on special medication. There is evidence that many commonly prescribed drugs for the elderly increase vitamin C requirements: aspirin, barbiturates, paraldelhyde, phenytoin. Some anesthetics require ascorbate for detoxification and excretion, a substance which is not stored and must be replenished daily; vitamin C depletion can occur within 40 days in normal human subjects on an ascorbate-free diet (Butterworth, 1974). Folate tends to occur in the same foods as vitamin C, and a deficiency of ascorbate should be followed by assessment for anemia. Other medications are nauseating or uncomfortable.

The loss of potassium from patients taking diuretics poses a threat in securing and keeping sufficient quantity of this electrolyte. Potassium requires daily replenishing, since it is not stored in the body. It, too, is found in foods and fruits which are fresh and contain vitamin C, or in relatively expensive foods. The older person on a limited diet which requires little preparation, such as snack foods, is a candidate for potassium deficiency, especially if deprived of food for any time (e.g., by nausea and vomiting). Surgery followed by intravenous feeding consisting of glucose in distilled water, and diagnostic tests which require purging and bowel preparation, also can lead to potassium deficiency.

The question is, "How is this person getting a daily quantity of vitamin C and a daily replenishment of potassium?"

After reviewing the psychosocial and economic aspects which lead to nutritional deficiency, the nurse should review the mechanical process by which food is ingested.

1. Do neurological or arthritic changes make hand movements or self-feeding difficult or impossible? Does limited vision prevent seeing food?
2. Does the mouth have mechanical ability to bite, chew, moisten, and swallow:
   a. Are there at least two adequate opposing incisors for biting?
   b. Are there at least two adequate opposing molars for chewing?
   c. Is periodontal disease present? Do teeth have enough gum support to be firm or are they loose?
   d. If teeth have been removed, have they been replaced adequately with either bridgework or dentures?
   e. Inspection under the denture should indicate whether decubiti exist which prevent chewing with comfort.
   f. Is the tongue strong enough to clean around the teeth?
   g. Is moisture present in the mouth (inspect under the tongue) for moistening food for swallowing?
   h. Is there any neurological problem which prevents coordinated swallowing? (Suspicion is raised by inability to close lips tightly, or if tongue is pulled slightly to one side on protrusion.)

Offering the client a drink of water gives a clue as to the ease of swallowing. Drooling is a sign of general neurological deficiency in the tongue-use swallowing process.

The simple process of weight determination leads to many indications of nutritional deficiency. Butterworth (1974) states that Prevost in a review of 80 medical-surgical hospitalized patients selected on the basis of 2 weeks or more hospitalization found that body height was not recorded in 56 percent of cases, body weight in 23 percent of cases, and not recorded regularly in 43 percent of the cases. Of those whose records could be analyzed, weight loss occurred in 61 percent and averaged 5 kg. Hospitalized patients were not allowed food by mouth for an average of 3.1 days. Anemia was present in 37 percent on admission, and another 16 percent developed anemia during hospitalization. Many meals were replaced with intravenous feedings of glucose 5 and 10%. Patients had sophisticated diagnostic studies, complex drug programs, and highly specialized surgical management, but no nutritional management as such. On the basis of the above, it is evident that failure to make base-line height and weight measurements is a quintessential failure in nutritional observation. Medical records indicate that elderly persons are more likely to be hospitalized (Bliss et al., 1967), so that becomes a crucial point for assessment.

A history of weight loss is usually correlated with the appearance of the skin which appears to hang loosely over the structures that have lost subcutaneous tissue. The skin of the elderly does not have the rich blood supply which gives color to youth and young adulthood, but the lack of redness of the mucosa leads to a yellowing-gray appearance usually associated with age but which may actually be a part of anemia. Age need not be colored gray.

The mouth is an index of adequate nutrition. Vitamin deficiency is followed by cheilosis (a pathological condition with reddened lips and fissures at the angles); swelling and reddening of the tongue; loss of papilla; and reddened spongy gums, with loss of tissue. The feet serve as another index of nutrition from a circulatory standpoint: shiny dry hairless skin denotes poor nutrition.

Minimum physical inspection and observations of the aging patient should include:

- Assessment of the ability to bite, chew, and swallow.
- Check for hydration (see hydration assessment under "Fluids").
- Testing for involvement of the cranial nerves (Judge and Zuidema, 1968).
- Cranial nerve VII (facial): Drooping of the mouth. Testing for taste on the anterior two-thirds of the tongue on the weak side of the face.
- Cranial nerves IX and X (glossopharyngeal and vagus): Loss of gag reflex, paralysis of pharynx and palate and perhaps of larynx.
- Cranial nerve XII (hypoglossal): Unilateral tongue weakness, with a pull toward the weak side by the protruded tongue and a pull toward the unaffected side when it is resting in the mouth. Fasciculations of the tongue.
- Weight change over time (recent weight loss or gain).
- Foot inspection for condition of skin and loss of sensory ability.
- Color and condition of mucosa as seen through lips, fingernails, and the mouth, particularly the gums.
- Physical correlates of depression.
- The laboratory findings related to nutrition should be correlated with the clinical picture presented by the patient. If hospitalized or in an institution, the intake record should be evaluated for (1) intravenous fluid as replacement of normal nutrition and (2) antibiotic administration for change in the intestinal flora which might affect assimilation of vitamins.

Base-Line Information

- Weight, height; history of weight loss or gain.
- Skin condition: Dry, scaly, flaccid, wrinkled, degree of turgor and tension, and sensation; response to tactile stimuli (Gosnell, 1973).
- Pattern of eating: Needs to be coaxed or assisted; picks at food and leaves major portion; eats some foods from each of the basic four groups (Gosnell, 1973).
- Tube-fed.
- Recent dietary disturbances: surgery, diagnostic tests, or personal crises.
- Evidence of involvement of cranial nerves VII, IX, and XII.

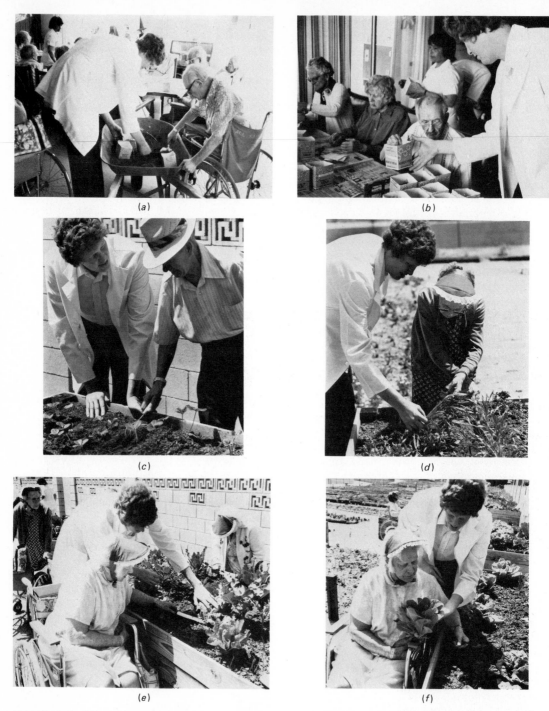

FIGURE 23-10 This photographic essay on nutrition shows a group of elderly residents of Reseda Convalescent Hospital in Southern California who are growing a garden. Sequentially, the essay depicts planting the seeds, harvesting, and delivering the crop to the dietitian, who is shown preparing the greens for a salad. The final reward can be seen in the last photograph—the gardener is eating the freshly harvested greens. (*Courtesy of Anthony J. Skirlick, Jr.*)

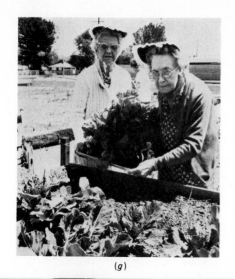

(g)

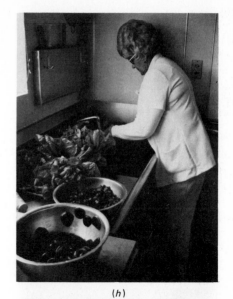

(h)

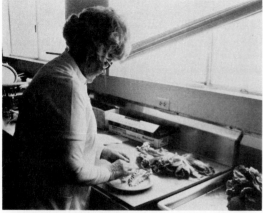

(i)

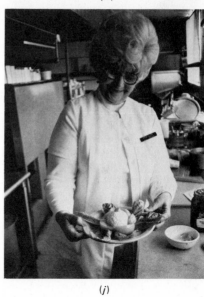

(j)

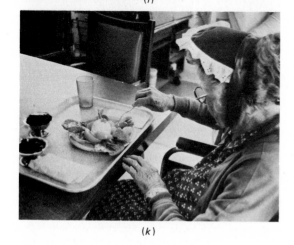

(k)

- Vital signs.
- Psychosocial: Socioeconomic status—income level and living conditions; language and/or cultural barriers; special diet which differs markedly from usual cultural pattern (low sodium, diabetic, or low residue). Recent changes in life, e.g., losses.

Worthington (1979, p. 161) developed the following questions to help health professionals provide complete nutritional assessments of their clients:

1. What are the clients' physical limitations?
2. Are they able to plan for their food needs?
3. Do they know what their food needs are?
4. Are they physically able to shop for food?
5. Do they have a convenient means of transportation?
6. Can they handle food themselves and get it back to their residences?
7. If they have special nutritional needs or limitations, are they able to read and understand labels on food packages?
8. Do they understand their condition and needs well enough to follow dietary directions?
9. If they cannot shop for food themselves, what other options are open to them?
10. What are their housing arrangements?
11. Do they live alone or with others?
12. If they cannot take care of themselves, will those with whom they live take over this responsibility?
13. What facilities are available for food storage, refrigeration, preparation, cleanup, and garbage disposal?
14. Are clients able to use facilities to prepare an adequate diet?
15. What kinds of utensils are available?
16. Have the utensils been rearranged to be within easy reach?
17. Is there a pleasant place to eat comfortably?
18. Are there enough dishes and tableware for attractiveness and sanitation?
19. Do clients have someone with whom to eat?
20. What are the clients' usual eating patterns?
21. Are there eating patterns?
22. Are there foods which are disliked or do not agree with the clients?
23. Have any dietary limitations been prescribed?
24. What food items are eaten in a representative day (24-hour recall)?

Psychosocial considerations include socioeconomic status—income level and living conditions; language and/or cultural barriers; special diet which differs from usual cultural pattern (low sodium, diabetic, or low residue); recent changes in life (e.g., losses).

The photographic essay in Figure 23-10 depicts how the cultivating of food can be implemented in an institution. Special gardens were made by building trays off the ground so people in wheel chairs could slide under them. The process offered these advantages: conforms with life style (always enjoyed gardening), provides exercise, increases the feeling of being needed, allows for more social interaction, and permits long-established food patterns to be continued as the residents plant and grow vegetables they like.

REFERENCES

Albanese, Anthony A.: Nutrition and health of the elderly, *Nutrition News,* **39**(2):5–8, April 1976.

Andres, Reubin: Quoted in a letter from Information Office, National Institute on Aging, July 30, 1979.

AOA Fact Sheet: National Nutrition Program for Older Americans, DHEW Publication no. (OHD) 76-20230, April 1976.

Barrows, Charles, and Eleanor Schlenker: *Nutrition and Aging,* DHEW Publication no. (NIH) 78-1409, 1978.

Benedict, Sharon: *Medical Care Evaluation Studies for Utilization Review in Skilled Nursing Facilities,* Hospital Utilization Project, Pittsburgh, PA, June 1975.

Bikson, T., and J. Goodchilds: Old and alone, Paper for the Symposium on Family Patterns: Social Myth and Social Policy, presented at a meeting of the American Psychological Association, Toronto, August 1978.

Blass, John: Quoted in letter from Information Office, National Institute on Aging, July 30, 1979.

Bliss, M. R., et al.: Preventing pressure sores in hospitals: Controlled trial of a large-celled ripple mattress, *British Medical Journal,* **1**:393–394, Feb. 18, 1967.

Boylan, Ann, and Bernard Marbach: Dehydration: subtle, sinister . . . preventable, *R.N.,* **42**(8):37–41, August 1979.

Brickner, Philip: *Home Health Care for the Aged,* Appleton-Century-Crofts, New York, 1978.

Butler, R.: *Nutrition and Aging,* Testimony before the Senate Select Committee on Nutrition and Human Needs, Department of Health, Education, and Welfare, Rockville, Md., Sept. 23, 1977.

———: *Why Survive?,* Harper & Row, New York, 1975.

Butterworth, Charles E., Jr.: The skeleton in the hospital closet, *Nutrition Today,* March/April 1974.

Cameron, Ian, et al.: Assessing and managing dementia, *Patient Care,* Nov. 30, 1977, pp. 90– 116.

Dickman, Sherman R.: Nutrition, in Adina M. Reinhardt and Mildred D. Quinn (eds.), *Current Practice in Gerontological Nursing,* Mosby, St. Louis, 1979.

Florida Division of Health: *Food for Health for the Older Adult,* In-step Project, Division of Aging, August 1973.

Flynn, Kathleen, T.: Iron deficiency among the elderly, *Nurse Practitioner,* December 1978, pp. 20– 24.

Garetz, Floyd K.: Breaking the dangerous cycle of depression and faulty nutrition, *Geriatrics,* **31**(6):73– 75, June 1976.

Geriatrics: Editorial, September 1978.

Goldman, Ralph: Decline in organ function with aging, in Isadore Rossman (ed.), *Clinical Geriatrics,* 2d ed., Lippincott, Philadelphia, 1979.

Gosnell, Davina J.: An assessment tool to identify pressure sores, *Nursing Research,* **22**(1):55– 59, January/February 1973.

Harbert, Anita S., and Leon H. Ginsberg: *Human Services for Older Adults,* Wadsworth, Belmont, Calif., 1979.

Hessing, Joel P.: Older American Act of 1965 as amended, 1978, a summary of the federal regulations, Aging services development, California Department of Aging, Training Branch, October 17, 1979.

Howard, Rosanne Beatrice, and Nancie Harvey Herbold: *Nutrition in Clinical Care,* McGraw-Hill, New York, 1978.

Judge, Richard D., and George D. Zuidema: *Physical Diagnosis: Physiologic Approach to Clinical Examination,* 2d ed., Little, Brown, Boston, 1968.

Jury, Mark, and Dan Jury: *Gramp,* Grossman, New York, 1976.

Kee, Joyce L.: Fluid imbalance in elderly patients, *Nursing '73,* **3**(4):40– 43, April 1973.

Krehl, Willard A.: The influence of nutritional environment on aging, *Geriatrics,* **29**(5):65– 76, May 1974.

Lewis, Clara: *Nutritional Consideration for Elderly,* Davis, Philadelphia, 1978.

MacHudis, Morris: Dentistry for the elderly, in William Reichel (ed.), *Clinical Aspects of Aging,* Williams & Wilkins, Baltimore, 1978, p. 422.

Nader, Ralph: Helping elderly people buy good food at low cost, *San Jose Mercury News,* San Jose, Calif., Dec. 25, 1978, p. 7B.

National Academy of Sciences: Recommended dietary allowances, National Research Council, Food and Nutrition Board, Washington, 1974.

National Dairy Council: Nutrition of the elderly, *Dairy Council Digest,* **48**(1):1– 6, January/February 1977.

National Institute on Aging, Information Office: Nutrition, behavior and the life cycle, Workshop, DHEW, Bethesda, Md., June 1979.

Nutrition and Cooking, Keiro-No-hi, Women's University of Nutrition, **45**(9):26– 27 and 199, September 1979.

O'Hanlon, Pauline, and Mary Bess Kohrs: Dietary studies of older Americans, *American Journal of Clinical Nutrition,* **(31)**:1257– 1269, July 1978.

Post-White House Conference on Aging Reports, Government Printing Office, Washington, 1973.

Robertson, H.: Dentures: Their significance in psychogeriatric nursing, *Nursing Mirror,* **36**:42– 43, Feb. 6, 1970.

Santa Clara County Department of Social Services: The senior nutrition and service program of Santa Clara county, unpublished report, 1977.

Schlenker, Eleanor D.: Effective nutrition states on human life span, in *Nutrition and Aging,* DHEW Publication no. (NIH) 78-1409, Rockville, Md., 1978.

Severinghaus, Elmer L.: Nutritional problems after fifty, *Nutrition News,* **43**(5):1– 5, February 1972.

Shannon, B., and H. Smiciklas-Wright: Nutrition education in relation to the needs of the elderly, *Journal of Nutrition Education,* **11**(2):85– 89, April/June, 1979.

Todhunter, E. Neige, and William J. Darby: Guidelines for maintaining adequate nutrition in old age, *Geriatrics,* **33**(6):49– 57, June 1978.

Toward a Brighter Future for the Elderly, report of the President's Task Force on Aging, Washington, April 1970.

Watanabe, Miyo T.: Personal communication, 1979.

Watkins, Donald M.: Nutrition for the elderly of today and tomorrow, *Nutrition News,* **38**(2):5– 8, April 1975.

Weg, Ruth B.: *Nutrition and the Later Years,* Andrus Gerontology Center, University of Southern California, Los Angeles, 1978.

Weinberg, Jack: "Psychiatric Aspects of Aging," lecture, Andrus Gerontology Summer Institute, Los Angeles, June 1970.

Weir, D., et al.: Recognition and management of the nutritional problems of the elderly, in W. Reichel (ed.), *Clinical Aspects of Aging,* Williams & Wilkins, Baltimore, 1978.

White House Conference on Aging: Food, nutrition, and health, Government Printing Office, Washington, 1969.

———: Food, nutrition, and health, 1971, Government Printing Office, Washington, 1971.

Williams, Sue Rodwell: *Essentials of Nutrition and Diet Therapy,* Mosby, St. Louis, 1978.

Worthington, Bonnie: Nutrition, in Doris Carnevali and Maxine Patrick (eds.), *Nursing Management for the Elderly,* Lippincott, Philadelphia, 1979.

OTHER RESOURCES

FILMS

Calories: Enough Is Enough, 12 min/color/1975/16 mm. Producer: Journal Films, Inc., 930 Pitner Avenue, Evanston, IL 60202.

Gramp: A Man Ages and Dies, 16 min/16 mm/b&w. An old man with dementia takes out his teeth and refuses to eat; 3 weeks later he dies. Mass Media, Ministries, 2116 Charles Street, Baltimore, MD 21218.

Help Yourself to Better Health, 16 min/color/16 mm. Available from: Film Department, Society for Nutrition Education, 2140 Shattuck Avenue, Suite 1110, Berkeley, CA 94704. Handout booklet, *A Guide for Food and Nutrition in Later Years.*

NUTRITION GAMES (Florida Division of Health, 1973)

Nutrition games can be used as teaching tools and to increase involvement of an audience. As teaching tools, they can replace part of a discussion, or they can be used for a social hour. Examples are *Nutrition Bingo* or *Food-O, Food Monopoly Game,* Nutrition crossword puzzles, and Nutrition Card Games, e.g., *Yummy Rummy, Menu Rummy, Checkstand, The Supermarket Game.* Many of these games were prepared for youngsters, but they could be adapted for seniors, e.g., *The Nutrition Game, The Calorie Game.* Available from Games that Teach, Graphics Company, P.O. Box 331, Urbana, IL 61801. A useful reference is: *Teach Nutrition with Games,* available from Nutrition Education Service Center, Montclair State College, Upper Montclair, N.J.

PAMPHLETS

Beek, Charles R.: Laxatives: What Does Regular Mean?, *FDA Consumer,* DHEW Publication (FDA) 76-30-03, May 1975.

Bohan, M., et al.: *Food without Fuss for Senior Adults,* University of Florida, Cooperative Extension Service.

Community Service Society: *Meals for One with Quantities for One or Two,* Community Service Society, 105 East 22nd Street, New York, NY 10010.

Eating Right for Less, Consumers Union, Mount Vernon, N.Y., 1976.

Florida Division of Health, P.O. Box 210, Jacksonville, Florida: *Need Iron? Eat It.*

———: *You Can Eat and Enjoy It.*

General Mills: *Meal Planning for the Golden Years,* Minneapolis, Minn., 1966.

A Guide for Food and Nutrition and Later Years, Society for Nutrition Education and AARP, NRTA, Berkeley, Calif., 1976.

King, Charles Glen, with George Britt: *Food Hints for Mature People,* Public Affairs Pamphlet, no. 336, 381 Park Avenue South, New York 10016, 1971, $0.25 each (discounts on quantity orders).

Metropolitan Life Insurance Company, 1 Madison Avenue, New York, 10010: *Four Steps to Weight Control.*

———: *New Metropolitan Cookbook.*

National Dairy Council, Chicago 60606: *Foods I Remember.*

———: *To Your Health in Your Second Fifty Years.*

Santa Clara County Health Department 2220 Moorpark Avenue, San Jose, CA 95128: *Iron* (also available in Spanish).

———: *Nutrition in the Golden Years.*

———: *Potassium Rich Foods.*

———: *Why Is Calcium Important?*

Simko, Margaret D., and Karen Colitz: *Nutrition and Aging: A Selected Annotated Bibliography,* DHEW, Administration on Aging (SRS) 73-20237, 1973.

U.S. Department of Agriculture: *Food Guide for Older Folks,* Home and Garden Bulletin, no. 17, Government Printing Office, Washington, 20402, 1974, $0.20.

Your Retirement Food Guide, American Association of Retired Persons and National Retired Teachers Association, 215 Long Beach Blvd., Long Beach, CA 90802.

TWENTY-FOUR

DRUGS AND
THE AGED

Ronald C. Kayne

The secret of the care of the patient is in *caring* for
the patient.
F. W. Peabody

LEARNING OBJECTIVES

- Cite the incidence of hospital admissions due
  to adverse drug effects.
- Cite three physiological variables which may
  change with age and affect a patient's response to an administered drug.
- Name three patient settings in which medication errors may be expected to occur.
- Define delirium.
- Identify seven mechanisms which can give rise
  to delirium in the aged.
- Identify seven classes of drugs which may be
  associated with drug-induced delirium in the
  aged.

This chapter deals with drugs, their use by the elderly, and some of the consequences thereof. Its purpose is to broaden the reader's perspective to include the patient's mental as well as physical response to drugs. It is not intended to provide a detailed description of all individual drugs of potential use by the elderly. Such information is readily available in nursing pharmacology texts and the nursing, pharmacy, and medical literature, and is well beyond the scope of this chapter. Nor is it intended to capsulate into a few pages all the pharmacological and therapeutic principles necessary for nurses to responsibly assume their duties as geriatric patient care providers. Rather, it is an attempt to provide a basis for an understanding of a few specific, but not uncommon, problems associated with the use of drugs in the elderly, so that the patient's needs may be better met.

DRUGS: AN OVERVIEW

The elderly ambulatory or hospitalized patient often uses drugs on a routine and long-term basis. The elderly constitute roughly 10 percent of the population but account for approximately 25 percent of the drugs used. This higher utilization of drugs may contribute to the problems associated with drugs in the aged. We tend to regard the use of drugs in the elderly as commonplace, expected, and without risk (Brady, 1973). Although no one can deny the benefits that drugs afford the elderly, we need to develop an appreciation of the risks involved in the use of drugs; no drug is devoid of toxicity, and useful, potent drugs can cause morbidity and mortality (Smith and Melmon, 1972).

Adverse reactions to drugs pose a serious health problem for the aged. *Three to five percent of all hospital admissions are a consequence of adverse drug reactions* (Hurwitz, 1969a; Miller, 1973; Caranasos et al., 1974), *and there are proportionately more drug-induced illnesses leading to hospitalization for patients over 61 years of age than for those under 61* (Caranasos et al., 1974). Of all hospitalized patients 10 to 30 percent have a drug reaction (Seidl et al., 1966; Hurwitz and Wade, 1969; Hoddinott et al., 1967), and such adverse reactions occur more often in the elderly than in the younger adult age groups (Hurwitz, 1969b). It has been estimated that

one-seventh of all hospital days is devoted to the care of drug reactions, at a cost annually of $3 billion (Task Force on Prescription Drugs, 1969).

This chapter addresses itself to the apparent vulnerability of the elderly to adverse drug reactions and the frequently nonspecific, often misleading, and obscure presentation of such adverse reactions. A nonspecific *failure to thrive,* characterized by an insidious and progressive physical deterioration, deteriorating social competence, loss of appetite, and diminishing concentration, has been described in the elderly as being due to, among other causes, the adverse effects of drugs (Hodkinson, 1973a).

Mental disturbances due to drugs are not uncommon (McCarron and McCormick, 1967). Patients over 60 years of age, as opposed to those under 60, have a higher incidence of adverse drug reactions (Hurwitz, 1969b), the first signs of which may be a change in mental status. Advanced age is reported to be a predisposing factor in the development of delirium in response to etiologic factors, such as sensory deprivation or the physiological stress associated with physical illnesses, including those that are drug-induced (Lipowski, 1967).

In the elderly, changes in behavior and mental status are all too frequently attributed to the patient's age, "senility," or a functional disorder, e.g., depression, and an underlying adverse drug reaction or other physical disorder goes unrecognized and unreported. The possibility of a change in mental status or the sudden appearance of mental symptoms as being caused by conscientiously prescribed and administered drugs needs constantly to be borne in mind. This chapter will attempt to provide a basis for an understanding of the many psychiatric, behavioral, and physical, often nonspecific, manifestations attributable to the adverse effects of drugs used in the elderly.

FACTORS INFLUENCING THE INCIDENCE OF ADVERSE DRUG REACTIONS

EFFECTS OF AGE ON DRUG DISPOSITION

Age appears to affect the mechanisms responsible for drug disposition. The onset, intensity, and duration of a patient's response to an administered drug is dependent upon individual variations in the degree and rate of (1) absorption from the site of administration, (2) distribution within the body, (3) metabolism, and (4) elimination of the drug from the body. There is increasing evidence that the distribution, metabolism, and elimination of drugs change with age, often resulting in a greater concentration of drug at its site of activity or a longer persistence of drug activity in the elderly, as opposed to the younger adult (Wade, 1972), with a commensurate risk of drug-induced disease.

Superimposed on these variables are differences due to the consequences of disease, often multiple in the elderly, and to the concurrent administration of other drugs, often multiple and long-term in the elderly. Disease or drug-induced changes in the mechanisms for drug disposition may influence the degree or rate of absorption, distribution, metabolism, or elimination of yet other drugs in a regimen, e.g., the impaired oral absorption of tetracycline in the presence of aluminum, magnesium, or calcium antacids, or the ability of phenobarbital to stimulate the hepatic metabolism of the oral anticoagulant, sodium warfarin (see Table 24-1).

Elderly patients may manifest signs of toxicity to what may be considered usual adult doses, especially of those drugs whose elimination from the body is dependent upon excretion by the kidney (Ewy et al., 1969). The latter is due to decreased renal function in the elderly, independent of any underlying renal disease (Friedman et al., 1972), as demonstrated by a decreased creatinine clearance per kilogram body weight in the presence of unaltered serum creatinine values (Siersbaek-Nielsen et al., 1971); i.e., the elderly, even those with normal serum creatinine concentrations, generally have diminished renal function (creatinine clearance).

In the absence of any underlying liver disease, the metabolic and excretory functional capacity of the liver generally remains within a normal range despite the anatomic and physiological changes associated with aging (Goldman, 1971).

When drugs which are predominantly excreted by the kidney, i.e., gentamycin, digoxin, nitrofurantoin, etc., are administered to elderly patients, their impaired ability to eliminate the drug from the body dictates consideration of an

TABLE 24-1
NONPROPRIETARY NAMES AND TRADEMARKS OF DRUGS

Generic Name	Trademark
Amitriptyline	Elavil
Benztropine	Cogentin
Chlordiazepoxide	Librium
Chlorpromazine	Thorazine
Chlorpropamide	Diabinese
Diazepam	Valium
Digoxin	Lanoxin
Diphenhydramine	Benadryl
Ethacrynic acid	Edecrin
Furosemide	Lasix
Gentamicin	Garamycin
Glutethimide	Doriden
Guanethidine	Ismelin
Haloperidol	Haldol
Hydrochlorothiazide	Esidrix, HydroDiuril
Imipramine	Tofranil
Methyldopa	Aldomet
Nitrofurantoin	Furadantin, Macrodantin
Pentazocine	Talwin
Phenformin	DBI-TD, Meltrol
Propantheline bromide	Pro-Banthine
Reserpine	Serpasil
Sodium warfarin	Coumadin
Thioridazine	Mellaril
Tolbutamide	Orinase
Trihexyphenidyl	Artane

individualized, often less frequent or reduced, dosage regimen, lest accumulation of the drug occur with resultant exaggerated or adverse effects.

MEDICATION ERRORS

Elderly patients frequently have multiple chronic disease states that require long-term, multiple drug therapy. Errors of omission or commission in the self-administration of medication in ambulant patients, resulting in erratic dosage or overdosage, are not uncommon (Blackwell, 1972; Stewart and Cluff, 1972), the first sign of which may be an adverse drug reaction, e.g.,

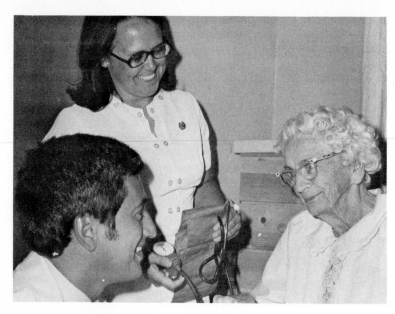

FIGURE 24-1 A nurse-pharmacist team checking the status of an elderly nursing home resident who is in her nineties. (*Courtesy of Will Patton.*)

changes in mental status. In a recent study of ambulant patients, a lack of comprehension of the directions for proper usage of medication correlated well with noncompliance, and patients 65 years of age and over had the lowest comprehension level (Boyd et al., 1974). In another study, 59 percent of an elderly, chronically ill outpatient population made errors in the self-administration of prescribed medications, and 26 percent committed medication errors considered to be potentially serious (Schwartz et al., 1962). The aged patient may continue to take a medication long after a rational need for the drug has disappeared or may discontinue the use of a prescribed drug even though its continued use is essential to the preservation of well-being (Brady, 1973). However, the occurrence of medication errors is not limited to the self-administration of medications in outpatient populations. A significant incidence of medication errors has reportedly been associated with the administration of prescribed drugs in acute-illness hospitals: for every six doses of medication administered in an acute hospital setting, one medication error was reported to have occurred (Baker et al., 1966).

Limited published data exist on medication error rates in nursing homes. A 1970 General Accounting Office audit entitled "Continuing Problems in Providing Nursing Home Care and Prescribed Drugs Under the Medicaid Program in California" reviewed 1 month's medical records of 106 patients in 14 nursing homes and revealed that 311 medication doses were administered in quantities in excess of those prescribed and 1210 prescribed doses that were not administered at all. A California Regional Medical Program—Area V developmental project reported a medication error rate of 14 percent in two Los Angeles County skilled nursing facilities, and a 32-percent error rate in a third such facility. Monitoring of drugs contributed to a significant reduction in the incidence of medication errors (Kayne et al., 1973).

DRUG-INDUCED DELIRIUM

THE DEMENTIAS: A REVIEW

The dementias are psychiatric disorders caused by or associated with impairment of brain function, reflecting either irreversible loss or dysfunction of brain cells. Three forms of dementia can be differentiated: (1) senile dementia of the Alzheimer type in the elderly and Alzheimer's

DRUG EXPERIENCE REPORT *(In confidence)*	Form Approved OMB No. 57-R0071

PATIENT INITIALS *(Optional)*   **AGE**   **SEX**   ☐ M   ☐ F   **DATE OF REACTION ONSET**

SUSPECTED REACTION(S) *(We have particular interest in serious, rare and unusual reactions.)*

SUSPECTED DRUG(S); TRADE/GENERIC NAME *(Manufacturer's name, if possible)*

DISORDER OR REASON FOR USE OF DRUG(S) *(Optional)*   **ROUTE**   **TOTAL DAILY DOSE**   **DATES OF ADMINISTRATION**

OTHER DRUGS TAKEN CONCOMITANTLY

COMMENTS *(Optional)* eg. **OUTCOME & LABORATORY DATA**

PHYSICIAN'S NAME, ADDRESS, AND ZIP CODE   **PROFESSIONAL TITLE**

FORM FD 1639a (6/74)   PREVIOUS EDITION MAY BE USED.

FIGURE 24-2 The Food and Drug Administration conducts an advance drug experience reporting program which solicits information relating to suspected adverse drug reactions.

disease in the presenium; (2) multiinfarct or cerebrovascular dementia; and (3) delirium when dementia is secondary to some other cause and reflects potentially reversible brain dysfunction. Differentiation of mental dysfunction as being due to senile dementia or delirium is important, since delirium is so much more amenable to treatment and potentially reversible (Agate, 1970; Libow, 1973).

Delirium is a psychiatric disorder due to a physical condition which causes cerebral dysfunction (McCarron and McCormick, 1967). The psychiatric dysfunction is characterized by disorientation to person, place, or time; memory impairment for both remote and recent past; impairment of intellectual function and judgment; and, commonly, lability of affect (Butler, 1971; Verwoerdt, 1971). The patient with delirium may present with a history of sudden onset of fluctuating disturbances of awareness or consciousness, from mild disorientation to stupor or coma.

There is no direct relationship between the cause of delirium and the degree of impaired mental functional capacity. The patient may present with less than all manifestations of the syndrome. Deficits in orientation, memory, intellectual function, and affect may be less than uniformly apparent (Goldfarb, 1973); one or more of the symptoms may predominate. *Psychiatric manifestations may be more prominent than signs and symptoms of the underlying illness* (McCarron and McCormick, 1967).

The terms *acute brain syndrome, acute confusional state, toxic psychosis,* and *clouding of consciousness* appear frequently in the literature and are used to describe reversible organic psychiatric disorders or their components

(Lipowski, 1967); they are referred to here as *delirium*.

Loss of the special senses, i.e., impairment of hearing or vision, in the aged may give rise to a loss of independence and to social isolation which are associated with sensory deprivation, a cause of perceptual disturbances (Nicholson, 1974). Delirium may be superimposed upon, may coexist with, or may complicate a preexisting perceptual disturbance, senile or multiinfarct dementia (Hodkinson, 1973b), functional disorder, or a hallucinatory phenomenon associated with drug intoxication or drug withdrawal (Goldfarb, 1973).

Although some acute confusional states may be part of a chronic progressive deterioration of brain cells, often they reflect a syndrome which is the result of some specific treatable disorder (Gurian, 1973). In a study involving elderly first-admission patients to a psychiatric screening ward in a metropolitan general hospital, almost half were hospitalized as a result of delirium. Of these, 13 percent had delirium syndromes only, without any evidence of senile or multiinfarct dementia, and 33 percent had delirium superimposed upon senile or vascular dementia (Epstein and Simon, 1967).

Delirium may be demonstrated as being caused by cerebral dysfunction by identifying an adverse drug reaction, systemic disease, pulmonary or cardiac insufficiency, or some other condition which interferes with normal cerebral function. Pneumonia, left ventricular failure, and acute or chronic urinary tract infections associate highly with acute confusional states in the elderly (Hodkinson, 1973b). (See Chapter 14 for additional information regarding dementias.)

Prompt recognition and treatment of the underlying physical disorder will resolve the psychiatric manifestations and restore the patient's previous state of health.

MECHANISMS PRODUCING DRUG-RELATED DELIRIUM

Important mechanisms in the production of acute and reversible mental changes in the aged, which may occur during drug therapy as a result of *excessive, therapeutic, or inadequate dosage,* include the following:

1. Abrupt reduction in cerebral blood flow, due to acute hypotension or diminished cardiac output, occurring secondary to congestive heart failure or cardiac arrhythmias
2. Reduced arterial oxygenation secondary to anemia, pneumonia, or chronic obstructive pulmonary disease
3. Reduced glucose utilization by the brain, due to hypoglycemia
4. Increased intracranial pressure secondary to space-occupying lesions, e.g., subdural hematomas
5. Nutritional deficiencies due to inadequate intake, malabsorption syndromes, or alcoholism
6. Disturbances in the metabolic environment of brain cells secondary to fluid or electrolyte imbalances, acidosis, hypothyroidism, hyperthyroidism, diabetic coma, azotemia and uremia, or liver disease
7. Any febrile state

DRUGS FREQUENTLY ASSOCIATED WITH DELIRIUM

DRUGS WITH ANTICHOLINERGIC (ATROPINE-LIKE) ACTIVITY

Dose-dependent, phenothiazine-induced acute confusional states have been reported and have been observed to occur more readily in the aged (Shepherd, Lader, and Lader, 1972). In a study of 236 elderly patients admitted to a psychogeriatric service, at least 37 (16 percent) presented with mental disorders that were directly attributable to psychotropic drugs (Learoyd, 1972). Confused mental states may occur in the elderly during phenothiazine therapy, especially if administered concurrently with other drugs possessing intrinsic anticholinergic activity. The naturally occurring belladonna alkaloids, i.e., atropine and scopolamine; the antipsychotic drugs, such as chlorpromazine, thioridazine, haloperidol, etc.; the tricyclic antidepressants, e.g., amitriptyline, imipramine, etc.; the antiparkinsonian agents, e.g., trihexyphenidyl, benztropine, diphenhydramine, etc.; the synthetic anticholinergics used to treat peptic ulcer disease, e.g., propantheline bromide; and antihistamines used in over-the-counter sleep and cold preparations, all possess atropine-like activity. When administered in usual adult doses, either alone or particularly in combination (Janowsky et al., 1972), these drugs may cause delirium characterized by disorientation, impairment of immediate memory, agitation, delusions, visual or auditory hallucinations, or aimless picking or grasping at bedclothes, intravenous tubing, or nonexistent objects (Greenblatt and Shader, 1973). Changes in mental status and behavior are more variable and unpredictable than the peripheral effects of anticholinergic toxicity, i.e., dry skin and mucous membranes, tachycardia, blurred vision, constipation, or urinary retention, and are not uncommon.

Elderly patients appear to be especially vulnerable to the deliriant effects of many anticholinergic drugs used to treat parkinsonism and depression (Hollister, 1973). Estimates of the prevalence of acute mental symptoms induced by atropine-like drugs used in the treatment of parkinsonism range from 19 to 30 percent (Greenblatt and Shader, 1973). Elderly patients, especially, are susceptible to trihexyphenidyl-induced mental disturbances (Stephens, 1967). Confusional states secondary to the therapeutic use of tricyclic antidepressants occur with increased frequency in older age groups (Davies et al., 1971).

In a patient with preexisting chronic brain syndrome or functional disorder, the first response to an aggravated or worsened confused state is often to increase the use of a prescribed tranquilizer. The patient may require less drug therapy, not more.

ALCOHOL AND OTHER CENTRAL NERVOUS SYSTEM DEPRESSANTS

Acute or chronic alcoholism may be associated with delirium in elderly patients. In a study of 71 elderly patients admitted to a psychiatric screening ward with delirium, 51 were associated with alcohol abuse (Epstein and Simon, 1967). Acute changes in mental functional capacity are associated with the alcohol withdrawal syndromes, i.e., delirium tremens (O'Toole, 1972). Hypoglycemia secondary to chronic depletion of carbohydrate stores (Dun-

dee et al., 1972), vitamin deficiencies, and dehydration and electrolyte imbalances are not uncommon findings in alcohol abusers, and may contribute to acute changes in mental status. Chronic alcoholism is a common cause of thiamine (vitamin B_1) deficiency, which may be associated clinically with memory and cognitive defects, and peripheral neuropathy characterized by severe lower extremity pain, paresthesia, and muscle tenderness and weakness.

In addition to alcohol, other drugs with primary CNS activity commonly used in the elderly patient and associated with reversible mental symptoms include the barbiturates, the nonbarbiturate antianxiety agents and sedative hypnotics, e.g., chlordiazepoxide, diazepam, glutethamide (Zivin and Shalowitz, 1962), etc., the nonnarcotic analgesics pentazocine and the salicylates (VanDam, 1972), and the narcotic analgesics.

A 7 to 10 percent incidence of bizarre perceptual disturbances, such as visual and auditory hallucinations, delusions, euphoria, feelings of depersonalization, panic, and thought disorders, have been reported following the parenteral or oral administration of usual therapeutic doses of the nonnarcotic analgesic pentazocine (Wood et al., 1974). Interestingly, it has been reported that pentazocine, as well as morphine, affords a higher degree of pain relief in the elderly. This may be related to a decreased amount of nervous tissue or decreased pain sensitivity of this tissue with aging (Bellville et al., 1971).

Paradoxical excitement may occur with the nighttime, as well as the daytime, administration of sedative-hypnotic drugs, although the decrease in sensory cues that occurs with darkness may be a contributory factor. Night nurses may find that they need to observe carefully elderly patients that have been given sedative-hypnotics; those patients who have to get up during the night to go to the bathroom may become confused and have difficulty orienting themselves and are accident-prone while in this state. Nighttime hypnotics may further impair brain function in an elderly patient with preexisting impaired mental functional capacity and may have some residual effect on the patient's cognitive functioning the following day, i.e., a less alert, less interacting patient (Pfeiffer,

1973). The use of these drugs would best be avoided whenever other measures can be used safely and efficaciously.

Central nervous system depressants, including the antipsychotic agents and the tricyclic antidepressants, when administered in usual adult doses, either alone or particularly if given concomitantly, may cause oversedation in elderly patients. The elderly appear to be particularly vulnerable to the sedative effects of chlordiazepoxide and diazepam. "Drowsiness is not a side-effect of sedative drugs; it is a characteristic of their use" (Weatherall, 1965). Drug-induced immobility can adversely affect the cardiovascular, respiratory, gastrointestinal, urinary, and musculoskeletal system, and metabolic and psychosocial equilibrium (Olson et al., 1967). Chest infections, i.e., pneumonia, often a terminal event in elderly patients, may be precipitated by the immobility of the tranquilized, oversedated patient and give rise to changes in mental status (Hodkinson, 1973b). Drug-induced immobility may lead to perceptual changes, dehydration, or decubitus ulcer formation with resultant infection, all three potentially giving rise to changes in mental status.

DRUGS ASSOCIATED WITH ORTHOSTATIC HYPOTENSION

Normally upon standing, gravitational forces result in a shift of blood from the head and upper parts of the body to a pooling of blood in the abdomen and legs. But before this shortage of blood can result in a clinically significant fall in systemic blood pressure, several compensatory reflex mechanisms restore the status quo. These compensatory reflex adjustments are so effective that in a healthy young adult the systemic arterial pressure is lowered only transiently upon standing.

Compensatory mechanisms are not so efficient in the elderly; hence postural hypotension in the elderly is not uncommon. In a study of 494 relatively healthy persons living at home, aged 65 or over, the frequency of orthostatic falls in blood pressure increased with age (Caird et al., 1973). There is considerable frequency of postural hypotension in the elderly, especially in the presence of cerebrovascular disease (Gross,

1970) and in patients recovering from illnesses associated with periods of immobility, e.g., stroke, congestive heart failure (Nicholson, 1974).

Drugs with potential hypotensive effects that interfere with or compromise the compensatory reflex mechanisms responsible for maintaining adequate systemic blood pressure upon standing may contribute to postural hypotension. The reduction of cerebral blood flow secondary to marked postural hypotension, associated with the clinical use of the antipsychotic, tricyclic antidepressants, or the sympatholytic antihypertensive agents, i.e., guanethidine, reserpine, and methyldopa, especially if administered concurrently, may be sufficient to precipitate cerebral ischemia resulting in changes in mentation, dizziness, or syncope. Elderly patients with impaired motor function due to parkinsonism, unstable knees from osteoarthritis, or neurological deficits, e.g., hemiplegia or hemiparesis, are particularly vulnerable to falls and resultant trauma, such as subdural hematomas and fractured hips, secondary to orthostatic hypotension.

Elderly patients receiving the above drugs should be cautioned against rising too rapidly or, if appropriate, protected from doing so. This is especially important in the morning, following a hot bath, or for those patients who have to get up once or more during the night to urinate, e.g., elderly males with benign prostatic hypertrophy. Such patients should arise from bed in stages over several minutes, with assistance if appropriate; they should arise slowly from a lying to a sitting position, then dangle their legs over the side of the bed, and then finally stand up. If the patient complains of dizziness or transient feelings of faintness upon standing, and postural hypotension is suspected, it can easily be confirmed by recording the blood pressure in lying, sitting, and standing positions. Taking blood pressure only in the lying down position can be dangerously deceptive and a disservice to the patient.

DIGITALIS

Digitalis Toxicity Digitalis toxicity is one of the most common of the serious drug-induced diseases (Nies, 1972; Hurwitz and Wade, 1969).

In two recent epidemiologic, prospective studies of patients receiving digitalis, signs and symptoms of toxicity were reported in 23 percent (Beller et al., 1971) and 18.4 percent (Shapiro et al., 1969). Mortality attributable to cardiac toxicity reportedly ranges from 3 to 21 percent of those intoxicated (Smith and Haber, 1973). In a third such study, 19.8 percent of 192 patients demonstrated signs of toxicity; in the 70 to 79 age group it was 28.8 percent, and in the 80 to 89 age group, 25 percent (Hurwitz and Wade, 1969). Another investigator reported that patients 65 years of age or older associated with a greater than twofold risk of adverse reactions to digoxin, as compared with all other patients (Duhme et al., 1974). Equal doses of digoxin result in higher serum levels in the old (Ewy et al., 1969). However, it appears uncertain whether age per se is responsible for the apparent prevalence of digitalis toxicity in the elderly, beyond the extent to which it correlates with advanced heart disease, reduced lean body mass, and impaired renal excretion (Mason, 1974; Beller et al., 1971).

The excretion of digoxin is dependent upon kidney function; thus the diminished renal function associated with aging allows excessive accumulation of digoxin and places the patient at a greater risk of developing toxicity, unless the dosage is reduced appropriately. The apparent susceptibility of the elderly to digoxin toxicity is probably, at least in part, related to the diminished renal function associated with aging.

Manifestations of Digitalis Toxicity The digitalis-toxic patient may complain of headache, dizziness, or disturbances of vision; may present belligerent, disoriented, or hallucinating; may complain of fatigue or weakness; may appear apathetic or depressed; or may complain of a poor appetite, nausea, vomiting, or abdominal discomfort. Neurological or gastrointestinal symptoms may be a concomitant or impending sign of cardiac toxicity.

In a study of 179 digitalis-toxic patients, 95 percent complained of acute fatigue. In 82 percent, muscular strength was diminished to the point that there was difficulty in walking and in raising the arms. Mental disturbances were present in 65 percent. These included bad dreams, agitation, drowsiness, syncope, pseudohalluci-

nations, and delirium. One patient was directly admitted to a mental hospital; 95 percent complained of visual disturbances. Gastrointestinal symptoms were present in about 80 percent of the patients; 65 percent complained of abdominal pain (Lely and van Enter, 1972).

Unfortunately, digitalis-induced cardiac rhythm disturbances may precede gastrointestinal or neurological signs of toxicity: a serious or fatal arrhythmia may be the initial manifestation of digitalis toxicity.

Worsening of congestive heart failure is recognized as a not infrequent sign of digitalis toxicity (Stafford, 1972). Changes in mental status may be observable signs of decreased cerebral perfusion due to diminished cardiac output occurring secondary to digitalis-induced cardiac arrhythmias or worsening cardiac failure.

DIURETICS

Dehydration Diuretics, including furosemide, ethacrynic acid, and the thiazides, e.g., hydrochlorothiazide, may cause marked dehydration and electrolyte disturbances in elderly patients, resulting in impaired mental functional capacity. Dehydration may be suspected in patients when the skin turgor is decreased or the mucous membranes are dry. However, loss of subcutaneous fat and atrophic epidermal changes in many elderly patients makes the usual observations for skin turgor useless. Moistness is misleading if the patient is a chronic mouth breather; the mucous membranes of the mouth may be chronically dry. *Turgidity, or fullness of the tongue, is a constant and reliable sign; a shrunken, furrowed tongue is a reliable sign of dehydration, but usually represents an advanced stage of the disorder* (Lapides et al., 1965).

A very reliable clinical indication of dehydration is thirst; however, evidence of thirst may be obscure in elderly debilitated patients if the perception of thirst is impaired, or if the patients have difficulty in making their needs known, and water is not accessible. Dehydration without complicating infection may cause a significant fever in elderly patients; however, this is not always the case. Hypotension or a scanty and concentrated urine may also present as evidence of significant fluid depletion. Other common sources of fluid and electrolyte loss in the elderly, which may contribute to states of imbalance, include excessive perspiration, expectoration of copious amounts of sputum, vomiting, diarrhea, excessive use of laxatives, inadequate fluid intake, excessive urination associated with uncontrolled diabetes mellitus, and hyperventilation which in some elderly patients may cause a significant loss of water via the lungs.

Hyponatremia Sodium depletion secondary to diuretic therapy may give rise to hyponatremia (Schulze, 1973), especially during periods of excessive salt restriction. If the serum sodium concentration is low, water shifts into the cells; the cells may become overhydrated, and their function impaired. In the brain, this is associated with a clouding of sensorium. Dizziness and headaches may be prominent (Weiner and Epstein, 1970). Depression characterized by weakness, apathy, agitation, anorexia, and insomnia may be an early sign of chronic hyponatremia (Lewis, 1971). A psychosis characterized by disorientation to person, place, and time; confused rambling speech; and frequent drowsiness were associated with a low-sodium syndrome in a 72-year-old female (Burnell and Foster, 1972). Correction of serum sodium concentration was accompanied by resolution of all psychiatric symptoms.

Hypokalemia Values for serum potassium concentrations in healthy elderly persons aged 60 or older ranged between 3.5 and 5.5 meq/L (Priddle et al., 1970; Leask et al., 1973). In a study of 1000 consecutive admissions to a geriatric unit, serum potassium concentrations on admission were reported below 3.5 meq/L in 12 percent of the females and 8.8 percent of the males. Forty percent of the 104 cases of hypokalemia were secondary to iatrogenic causes (Judge, 1968).

Depletion of body potassium stores, as evidenced by hypokalemia, has been reported to occur in the elderly in diverse clinical situations and may frequently be due to multiple contributory factors, not the least of which is diuretic therapy, particularly in the presence of concomitant dietary salt restriction (Schwartz et al., 1968). The clinical use of diuretics is associated with potassium loss progressing, in the absence

of adequate potassium supplementation, to depletion of body potassium stores. The following factors may contribute to the development of hypokalemia in the elderly: (1) an inadequate dietary intake of potassium or intravenous infusions of potassium-free solutions; (2) excessive gastrointestinal loss due to intestinal or biliary fistulous drainage, protracted vomiting, diarrhea, nasogastric suction, excessive use of laxatives (Cummings et al., 1974), or enemas; or (3) hyperaldosteronism secondary to congestive heart failure or hepatic cirrhosis with ascites.

Changes in mental status and behavior, anorexia, complaints of vague gastrointestinal discomfort, and prominent muscle weakness progressing to the point of compromised ambulation are findings associated with severe potassium depletion. Muscle weakness associated with hypokalemia may be most prominent in the legs (Weiner and Epstein, 1970). In a study of 50 hypokalemic patients the following clinical manifestations and their respective incidences were observed: muscle weakness, 90 percent; anorexia, nausea, or vomiting, 84 percent; impaired mentation, 81 percent; abnormal respiratory pattern, 64 percent; and hypoactive bowel sounds, 52 percent (Surawicz, 1968).

Potassium depletion is particularly serious in the patient receiving concurrent digitalis, because hypokalemia predisposes to digitalis toxicity. In one series, 9 percent of patients taking digitalis alone demonstrated evidence of toxicity, while 24 percent of patients taking digitalis with diuretics showed toxicity (Hurwitz and Wade, 1969).

RESERPINE

Reserpine, alone or in combination with other drugs, is widely used in the treatment of hypertension. Mental depression associated with the use of reserpine, in some cases accompanied by marked agitation (agitated depression), may be insidious in onset and include suicidal tendencies. The risk of developing mental depression during reserpine therapy increases with age (Parker and Murphy, 1961).

Some of the depressions associated with reserpine may be secondary to hyponatremia induced by diuretic-reserpine combinations. The concomitant use of tricyclic antidepressants may even further complicate this state by producing dry mouth, with subsequent increases in fluid progressing to water intoxication (Lewis, (1971).

INSULIN AND THE ORAL HYPOGLYCEMICS

Insulin and the oral hypoglycemic agents, the sulfonylureas, e.g., tolbutamide, chlorpropamide, etc., especially in the presence of diminished caloric intake, excessive exercise, or resolution of an infectious process, may induce marked hypoglycemia with resultant acute mental changes. The onset of severe hypoglycemia in the aged may be unheralded by the signs and symptoms of increased sympathetic nervous system activity; tachycardia, tachypnea, or diaphoresis may not occur. The patient may become comatose without warning. Episodes of bizarre behavior, slurring of speech, disorientation, confusion, somnolence, or inability to be easily aroused should always be viewed with extreme suspicion in the elderly diabetic patient receiving insulin or oral hypoglycemic agents (Rifkin and Ross, 1971). In addition, chlorpropamide has been associated with inappropriate ADH secretion progressing to water intoxication (Weissman et al., 1971) which may give rise to changes in mentation. Phenformin, a nonsulfonylurea oral hypoglycemic agent, has been implicated in the occurrence of lactic acidosis, in patients with renal impairment or states of tissue anoxia, e.g., congestive heart failure, chronic obstructive pulmonary disease, etc., early signs of which may be changes in states of awareness or consciousness.

Drugs commonly used in the aged, e.g., digoxin, diuretics, antihypertensives, analgesics, sedative-hypnotics, antipsychotics, insulin, and oral hypoglycemics, may induce behavioral, as well as physical, adverse effects. In the aged, changes in behavior and mental status are all too frequently attributed to the patient's age, to senility, or to a functional disorder. Consideration of the vulnerability of the aged to adverse drug reactions and recognition that changes in mental status and behavior may be drug-induced are essential to professional nursing assessments.

REFERENCES

Agate, J.: *The Practice of Geriatrics,* 2d ed., Charles C Thomas, Springfield, Ill., 1970, pp. 361–365.

Baker, K. N., W. W. Kimbrough, and W. M. Heller: *A Study of Medication Errors in a Hospital,* University of Arkansas Press, Fayetteville, 1966.

Beller, G. A., et al.: Digitalis intoxication: A prospective clinical study with serum level correlations, *New England Journal of Medicine,* **284:**989–997, 1971.

Bellville, J. W., et al.: Influence of age on pain relief from analgesics, *Journal of the American Medical Association,* **217:**1835–1841, 1971.

Blackwell, B.: The drug defaulter, *Clinical Pharmacological Theories,* **13:**841–848, 1972.

Boyd, J. R., et al.: Drug defaulting, II: Analysis of noncompliance patterns, *American Journal of Hospital Pharmacy,* **31:**485–491, 1974.

Brady, E. S.: Drugs and the elderly, in R. H. Davis (ed.), *Drugs and the Elderly,* Andrus Gerontology Center, University of Southern California, Los Angeles, 1973, pp. 2–3.

Burnell, G. M., and T. A. Foster: Psychosis with low sodium syndrome, *American Journal of Psychiatry,* **128:**1313–1314, 1972.

Butler, R. N.: Clinical psychiatry in late life, in I. Rossman (ed.), *Clinical Geriatrics,* Lippincott, Philadelphia, 1971, pp. 443–444.

Caird, F. I., G. R. Andrews, and R. D. Kennedy: Effect of posture on blood pressure in the elderly, *British Heart Journal,* **35:**527, 1973.

Caranasos, G. J., R. B. Stewar, and L. E. Cluff: Drug-induced illness leading to hospitalization, *Journal of the American Medical Association,* **228:**713–717, 1974.

Cummings, J. H., et al.: Laxative-induced diarrhea: A continuing clinical problem, *British Medical Journal,* **1:**537–541, 1974.

Davies, R. K., et al.: Confusional episodes and antidepressant medication, *American Journal of Psychiatry,* **128:**95–99, 1971.

Duhme, D. W., D. J. Greenblatt, and J. Koch-Weser: Reduction of digoxin toxicity associated with measurement of serum levels, *Annals of Internal Medicine,* **80:**516–519, 1974.

Dundee, J. W., et al.: Effects of rapid infusion of ethanol on some factors controlling blood sugar levels in man, *Quarterly Journal of Studies on Alcohol,* **33:**722–733, 1972.

Epstein, L. J., and A. Simon: Organic brain syndrome in the elderly, *Geriatrics,* **22:**145–150, 1967.

Ewy, G. A., et al.: Digoxin metabolism in the elderly, *Circulation,* **39:**449–453, 1969.

Friedman, S. A., et al.: Functional defects in the aging kidney, *Annals of Internal Medicine,* **76:**41–45, 1972.

Goldfarb, A. I.: Integrated psychiatric services for the aged, *Bulletin of the New York Academy of Medicine,* **49:**1070–1083, 1973.

Goldman, R.: Decline in organ function with aging, in I. Rossman (ed.), *Clinical Geriatrics,* Lippincott, Philadelphia, 1971, p. 35.

Greenblatt, D. J., and R. I. Shader: Drug therapy: Anticholinergics, *New England Journal of Medicine,* **288:**1215–1219, 1973.

Gross, M.: The effect of posture on subjects with cerebrovascular disease, *Quarterly Journal of Medicine,* **39:**485–491, 1970.

Gurian, B. S.: Psychogeriatrics, *Bulletin of the New York Academy of Medicine,* **49:**1119–1123, 1973.

Hoddinott, B. C., et al.: Drug reactions and errors in administration on a medical ward, *Canadian Medical Association Journal,* **97:**1001–1006, 1967.

Hodkinson, H. M.: Medicine in old age: Non-specific presentation of illness, *British Medical Journal,* **4:**94–96, 1973a.

————: Mental impairment in the elderly, *Journal of the Royal College of Physicians of London,* **7:**305–317, 1973b.

Hollister, L. E.: *Clinical Use of Psychotherapeutic Drugs,* Charles C Thomas, Springfield, Ill., 1973, p. 154.

Hurwitz, N.: Admissions to hospital due to drugs, *British Medical Journal,* **1:**539–540, 1969a.

————: Predisposing factors in adverse reactions to drugs, *British Medical Journal,* **1:**536–539, 1969b.

————, and O. L. Wade: Intensive hospital monitoring of adverse reactions to drugs, *British Medical Journal,* **1:**531–536, 1969.

Janowsky, D. S., et al.: Combined anticholinergic agents and atropine-like delirium, *American Journal of Psychiatry,* **129:**360–361, 1972.

Judge, T. G.: Hypokalemia in the elderly, *Gerontologia Clinica,* **10:**102–107, 1968.

Kayne, R. C., A. Cheung, and M. M. McCarron: Acute brain syndrome in an elderly patient, *Drug Intelligence and Clinical Pharmacy,* **8:**476, 1973.

————, ————, and ————: Monitoring of drug therapy of long-term care patients, presented at the Second Annual Scientific Session, Western Division of the American Geriatrics Society, Los Angeles, Calif., Oct. 2, 1973.

Lapides, J., R. B. Bourne, and L. R. MacLean: Clinical signs of dehydration and extracellular fluid loss, *Journal of the American Medical Association,* **191:**413–415, 1965.

Learoyd, B. M.: Psychotropic drugs and the elderly patient, *Medical Journal of Australia,* **1:**1131–1133, 1972.

Leask, R. G. S., G. R. Andrews, and F. I. Caird: Normal values for sixteen blood constituents in the elderly, *Age and Ageing,* **2:**14–23, 1973.

Lely, A. H., and C. H. J. van Enter: Non-cardiac symptoms of digitalis intoxication, *American Heart Journal,* **83:**149–152, 1972.

Lewis, W. H.: Iatrogenic psychotic depressive reaction in hypertensive patients, *American Journal of Psychiatry,* **127:**1416–1417, 1971.

Libow, L. S.: Pseudo-senility: Acute and reversible organic brain syndromes, *Journal of the American Geriatrics Society,* **21:**112–120, 1973.

Lipowski, Z. J.: Delirium, clouding of consciousness and confusion, *Journal of Nervous and Mental Disease,* **145:**227–255, 1967.

McCarron, M. M., and R. A. McCormick: *Acute Organic Disorder Accompanied by Mental Symptoms,* Department of Mental Hygiene, Sacramento, Calif., 1967.

Mason, D. T.: Digitalis pharmacology and therapeutics: Recent advances, *Annals of Internal Medicine,* **80:**520–530, 1974.

Miller, R. R.: Hospital admissions due to adverse drug reactions: A report from the Boston Collaborative Drug Surveillance Program, *Clinical Pharmacology and Therapeutics,* **14:**142–143, 1973.

Nicholson, W. J.: Medicine in old age: Disturbances of the special senses and other functions, *British Medical Journal,* **1:**33–35, 1974.

Nies, A. S.: Cardiovascular disorders, in K. L. Melmon and H. F. Morrelli (eds.), *Clinical Pharmacology: Basic Principles in Therapeutics,* Macmillan, New York, 1972, p. 190.

Olson, E. V., et al.: The hazards of immobility, *American Journal of Nursing,* **67:**781–796, 1967.

O'Toole, V. Q.: Alcoholic liver disease: Delirium tremens, *Drug Intelligence and Clinical Pharmacy,* **6:**314–317, 1972.

Parker, J. M., and C. W. Murphy: Reserpine: A comparison of chronic toxicity in animals with clinical toxicity, *Canadian Medical Association Journal,* **84:**1177–1180, 1961.

Peabody, F. W.: Care of the patient, *Journal of the American Medical Association,* **88**(12):877–882, March 19, 1927.

Pfeiffer, E.: Use of drugs which influence behavior in the elderly: Promises, pitfalls, and perspectives, in R. H. Davis (ed.), *Drugs and the Elderly,* Andrus Gerontology Center, University of Southern California, Los Angeles, 1973, p. 43–44.

Priddle, W. W., S. F. Liu, and D. J. Breithaupt: Management of hypertension: Further sodium and potassium studies, *Journal of the American Geriatrics Society,* **18:**861–892, 1970.

Rifkin, H., and H. Ross: Diabetes in the elderly, in I. Rossman (ed.), *Clinical Geriatrics,* Lippincott, Philadelphia, 1971, p. 402.

Schulze, B.: Metabolic complications of hydrochloro-thiazide therapy, *Drug Intelligence and Clinical Pharmacy*, **7:**501–510, 1973.

Schwartz, D., et al.: Medication errors made by elderly, chronically ill patients, *American Journal of Public Health*, **52:**2018–20209, 1962.

Schwartz, W. B., C. van Ypersele de Strihou, and J. P. Kassirer: Medical progress: Role of anions in metabolic alkalosis and potassium deficiency, *New England Journal of Medicine*, **279:**630–638, 1968.

Seidl, L. G., et al.: Studies on the epidemiology of adverse drug reactions, III. Reactions in patients on a general medical service, *Johns Hopkins Hospital Bulletin*, **119:**229–315, 1966.

Shapiro, S., et al.: The epidemiology of digoxin: A study in three Boston hospitals, *Journal of Chronic Diseases*, **22:**361–371, 1969.

Shepherd, M., M. Lader, and S. Lader: Major tranquilizers, in L. Meyler and A. Herxheimer (eds.), *Side Effects of Drugs: A Survey of Unwanted Effects of Drugs Reported in 1968–1971*, vol. VII, Excerpta Medica, Amsterdam, 1972, p. 72.

Siersbaek-Nielsen, K., et al.: Rapid evaluation of creatinine clearance, *Lancet*, **1:**1133–1134, 1971.

Smith, T. W., and E. Haber: Medical progress: Digitalis (fourth of four parts), *New England Journal of Medicine*, **289:**945, 1125–1128, 1973.

Smith, W. M., and K. L. Melmon: Drug choice in disease, in K. L. Melmon and H. F. Morrelli (eds.), *Clinical Pharmacology: Basic Principles in Therapeutics*, Macmillan, New York, 1972, p. 5.

Stafford, A.: Drugs acting on the heart, in L. Meyler and A. Herxheimer (eds.), *Side Effects of Drugs: A Survey of Unwanted Effects of Drugs Reported in 1968–1971*, vol. VII, Excerpta Medica, Amsterdam, 1972, p. 272.

Stephens, D. A.: Psychotic effects of benzhexol hydrochloride (Artane), *British Journal of Psychiatry*, **113:**213–218, 1967.

Stewart, R. B., and L. E. Cluff: A review of medication errors and compliance in ambulant patients, *Clinical Pharmacology and Therapeutics*, **13:**463–468, 1972.

Surawicz, B.: The role of potassium in cardiovascular therapy, *Medical Clinics of North America*, **52:**1103–1113, 1968.

Task Force on Prescription Drugs: Final report, U.S. Department of Health, Education, and Welfare, 1969.

VanDam, L. D.: Drug therapy: Analgetic drugs—the mild analgetics, *New England Journal of Medicine*, **286:**20–23, 1972.

Verwoerdt, A.: Clinical geropsychiatry, in A. B. Chinn (ed.), *Working with Older People, vol. IV: Clinical Aspects of Aging*, U.S. Department of Health, Education, and Welfare, 1971, p. 67.

Wade, O. L.: Drug therapy in the elderly, *Age and Ageing*, **1:**65, 1972.

Weatherall, M.: Side-effects, *British Medical Journal*, **1:**1174–1176, 1965.

Weiner, M., and F. H. Epstein: Signs and symptoms of electrolyte disorders, *Yale Journal of Biology and Medicine*, **43:**76–109, 1970.

Weissman, P. N., L. Shenkman, and R. I. Gregerman: Chlorpropamide hyponatremia: drug-induced inappropriate ADH activity, *New England Journal of Medicine*, **284:**65–71, 1971.

Wood, A. J. J., et al.: Medicines evaluation and monitoring group: Central nervous system effects of pentazocine, *British Medical Journal*, **1:**305–307, 1974.

Zivin, I., and M. D. Shalowitz: Acute toxic reaction to prolonged glutethimide administration, *New England Journal of Medicine*, **266:**496–498, 1962.

TWENTY-FIVE

NORMAL AGING CHANGES IN THE REPRODUCTIVE SYSTEM

Ruth B. Weg

So, lively brisk old man
Do not let sadness come over you;
For all your white hairs
You can still be a lover.
Goethe

LEARNING OBJECTIVES

- Discuss the role of sex and sexuality in old age.
- Examine sexual changes in the male, both physical and psychological.
- Identify the four stages of intercourse and the progressive changes found in the elderly.
- Identify in detail the six stages of the climactic period in a woman's life.
- Identify changes in the four stages of intercourse in a woman's life.
- Evaluate sexual dysfunction in the elderly.

HISTORICAL AND CULTURAL PERSPECTIVES

Normal aging remains a difficult concept to incorporate into the thinking of society at large and researchers and practitioners in the field. The legacy of cross-sectional studies comparing college youth to ill, institutionalized elderly found the older person to have marginal percentages of youthful capacities. Therefore, aging became associated not only with a decline in function of organ systems, but also with disease. The view of aging as a pathological condition was evident in a *Newsweek* article (1973). However, results of updated longitudinal investigations indicate that the decrements are gradual and not as extensive as earlier thought (Shock, 1973). What is perhaps most significant is that for the majority of older people even the summation of decline in more than one system leaves them able to cope with the demands of everyday living.

There is, however, one organ system that stands apart from the others. Changes with time in the reproductive system and the potential for success or failure as a sexual partner may represent a fearsome and ego-damaging trauma. Reproductive decline suggests the end of productive life, and the culture still largely equates sexual performance with manliness or womanliness. Any recognizable loss or dysfunction in this capacity may be construed as a step closer to death, as well as the awesome image of asexuality.

The equation of sex with death, sex with life—particularly with long life—or both is an oft-repeated theme in the history of thought concerning longevity. In the fascination of rejuvenation from primitive to modern times, there has been an exploration from the gamut of magic and sorcery with potions and elixirs through folklore remedies of plant and animal tissues to the claim for Gerovital H₃, a procaine solution (Aslan, 1972). Most frequently, the measure of youth and potential for immortality were sexual capacity and performance (Trimmer, 1970).

In the biblical days of King David of Israel, the ministrations and body warmth of a young virgin were the final treatment to help revive the aging, ill king. Throughout history, aging males have sought aphrodisiacs or sex stimulants to extend the "manliness" of sexual potency. First recorded recipes were allegedly found on a Babylonian cuneiform tablet, from about 800 B.C. In China, between 350 and 250 B.C., prevailing Taoist concern over longevity led to elaborate techniques to augment and conserve body "essence" or semen (Gruman, 1966). Dr. E. Steinach, in 1920, picked up on this concept and suggested that tying off sperm ducts (vasa deferentia) would provide an internal accumulation of sex hormones and make the individual young again. Plants, such as orchids, sweet potatoes, mandrake, and countless others, had been recommended as sexual rejuvenants (Trimmer, 1970). Animal products for rejuvenation, including the use of partridge brains and Chinese bird's-nest soup, reached a peak with the use of sex glands, their extracts or both, by Dr. C. E. Brown-Séquard, a French scientist. Using himself as the experimental animal in 1889, he injected the extracts from testes of guinea pigs. But his Parisian colleagues scoffed at his claim that three injections had turned the clock back 30 years. After World War I, the insertion of slices of chimpanzee testes in the bursae of male patients ushered in the vogue of "monkey gland" grafting as rejuvenation treatment. The sex hormone and cell therapy of today had their experimental origins in the nineteenth century (Guillerme, 1963).

SEXUALITY AND THE WHOLE PERSON

The importance of sex and sexuality for society is obvious. Procreation ensures the continuance of the human race. Sexual differentiation is the substrate for relationships between man and woman and the structural patterns of family. Expression of sexuality is a composite of prenatal developmental and postnatal learning experiences superimposed on a definite, inherent sexuality. It is, therefore, inescapable that in human sexuality, as in so many other aspects of behavior, people are extremely flexible, and sexual behavior covers a wide spectrum.

The sex hormones involved in the development of reproductive structure and function from conception through old age stimulate sexual attraction and activity. These same hormones affect other developmental processes, such as protein synthesis, salt and water balance, bone growth and resorption, cardiovascular function, and possibly the immune surveillance mechanisms. Usually, every human being is provided with all the natural biological equipment for reproduction and sexual interactions. But human sexuality is more than the reproductive system, hormones, and sexual intercourse; it connotes the capacity for involvement in all of life that grows from the fact that there are two sexes.

The total personality participates in the complexities of sexual behavior and is not separable in practice from the anatomy and physiology involved. For the individual, the acts of intimacy and warmth associated with sexuality have a significance beyond the pleasurable release of sexual tension. As a reaffirmation of the connection with other of life's functions, it is an important assertion and commitment of self. Psychologists and psychiatrists see some danger in the preoccupation with sexual technique and the resulting depersonalization of sex. Dr. Rollo May (1969) states, "Sex becomes a meaningless aside, a 'cul-de-sac' when looked upon as an isolated human function."

SEXUALITY IN OLD AGE

In a somewhat magical and strange mood, society at large has viewed older people as sexually inert, disinterested, and dysfunctional. Many younger people appear anxious and embarrassed about the idea that older people (especially parents) may still be seeking the intimacy, pleasure, and tenderness of sexual expression more appropriately reserved for youth. Mores and practices of the culture have led to certain assumptions and attitudes: Desire in the middle-aged and aged is null, and if by some aberration, desire is still present, the frailties of aging prevent lovemaking and may even cause it to be dangerous! Moreover, aging leaves one physically unattractive and sexually undesirable. The terrible consequences of negative attitudes may be realized in the self-fulfilling prophecy among middle-aged and older people. Susceptible to the created image, many face the middle and older years with fear and acquiescence.

Older men are often arbitrarily seen, by the public and professionals alike, as somehow sexually impaired (Masters and Johnson, 1970). The apprehension of becoming old is commingled with fear of loss of sexual adequacy and is a common preoccupation of men in middle and later years. Nevertheless, men appear to fare somewhat better than women. Witness the plaudits for older men who remain sexually involved at whatever level; e.g., a late marriage is seen as a sign of vitality. There is a widespread acceptance of the 50-year-old man who chooses a new friend or wife of 28. The young woman's response, erotically and romantically to a man who could be her father, is considered normal. Unfortunately, only a minority of older men are in a position to have this choice. When status, job, and power have been left behind, the identification of male vigor with achievement is difficult. Loss of confidence and depreciating self-image may lead to difficulty, if not impotency, in sexual relations.

Many people are revolted by the thought of an old woman making love with a young man. "That old women are repulsive is one of the most profound esthetic and erotic feelings in our culture" (Sontag, 1972). An analytical view identifies the youth as a victim of the oedipal complex. Marriage of an older woman to a younger man is a break with a fierce taboo. The kindest evaluation of older women assigns them to yet a third sex—the neuters of society. A developmental cycle is completed from "young and sexy" to "mature and exciting" and finally from 50 on into the anonymity of the sexually unseen (Butler and Lewis, 1973).

ROLE OF SEX AND SEXUALITY IN LATER LIFE

Yet the need for intimacy and love, as with other human needs for dignity, self-concept, involvement, and intellectual growth, begins very early in the human body and continues all through life. These needs and wants are not banished from human personality and behavior in the middle or late years, at age 50 or 65. On the contrary, the reality of an "intimate other" may be more critical in these older years when life space has diminished and meaningful relationships are fewer, as friends and relatives move away or die (Lowenthal et al., 1967). Roles as citizen, worker, and active parent may be lost or less structured as power and influence slowly disappear. Recently an article suggested that the expression of the sensual and sexual needs of the aged could be considered an important deterrent to suicide (Leviton, 1973).

There is increased agreement among those who study sexual responses among older people that sex and sexuality can provide important psychological and physiological outlets as the years advance. Frank (1961) identified the opportunity for sexual relations as an important primary source of psychological reinforcement for some older people. This, he suggested, was particularly true for men at a time when they face loss of the prestige and self-confidence that accompanies their narrowing work world. For women, the need becomes critical when they fear a diminution of attractiveness and desirability following menopause. "What people need and want is intimacy and authentic love" (May, 1969).

Studies, beginning with the now classic works of Kinsey et al. (1948, 1953) on sexual behavior in the human male and female and continuing with the significant work of Masters and Johnson (1966, 1970) and others (Pfeiffer and Davis, 1972) have amply documented that sexual interest and activity may persist through the ninth decade of life. While it is true that sexual interest and activity decrease with the advancing years, cessation is most often found to be a function of decline of physical health of one or both of the partners.

Upon comparison of the sex urge in youth and old age, there remains a remarkable constancy of sexual drives throughout life. Older men are generally more active than women, but this difference may be more apparent than real. Women who are old today formed their attitudes and practices related to sexual activity during the Victorian period. Mores and morality at that time dictated the woman's primary sexual role as procreative, and interest in sex beyond that was improper. Today, there are more older women than men and most older women are widowed. Between 65 and 74 years, women outnumber men by 130 to 100. This ratio climbs to 166 women to 100 men after 75 years. The absence of a capable, socially sanctioned mate is a forceful inhibiting factor (Pfeiffer and Davis, 1972).

Fortunately, the picture is not entirely homogeneous; in keeping with the reality not all old people are alike in their appearance, needs, or behavior. Honest, open expressions of feelings, needs, and wants on the part of younger people have made it possible for older persons to reach out—to touch and be touched without benefit of marriage vows.

SEXUALITY FOR OLDER MEN AND WOMEN: BEHAVIOR AND PHYSIOLOGY

Loss of sexual vigor should be no greater than loss of other physical capabilities (Rubin, 1965; Masters and Johnson, 1970). Rather, impotency before advanced age (between 80 and 90 years) often appears to be a function of psychological problems rather than physical incapacities. The misconception that loss of fertility associated with the decrease in sex hormones is causally related to depressed libido and basic competence is easily refuted by data from clinical evidence (Masters and Johnson, 1970; Pfeiffer and Davis, 1972). Age does not necessarily alter performance nor eliminate the quality of satisfaction and pleasure of sexual gratification (Greenblatt and Leng, 1972). Sexual interest and capacity extend into old age (Kinsey et al., 1948, 1953; Masters and Johnson, 1966; Pfeiffer and Davis, 1972; Rubin, 1965).

Longitudinal studies are those that provide the most satisfactory information about changes with time of an individual's capacities. Such an investigation over a 6-year period was reported by the Duke Center for the Study of Aging and Human Development. Primarily white, middle- and upper-class men and women were tested and interviewed for a 2-day period at appropriate intervals. They found a larger number of variables influenced current sexual behavior of men as compared with women. Increased age, antihypertensive drugs, declining health, and anxiety over examination had a measurable negative effect. Past enjoyment, interest, and frequency, the three indicators of early sexual life function correlated positively with present interests and activity among men and women. For women, however, current interest and activity were more dependent upon marital status. This confirmed previous observations that, among elderly women today, the presence of an interested, able mate is not always enough. Optimally, he also needs to be her marriage partner. Contemporary mores still provide greater opportunities for older men to engage in extramarital or nonmarital sex. Cessation of sexual relations was reported by 14 percent of the males and 40 percent of the females. Women attributed cessation to mates, and the men confirmed this statement. This reemphasizes earlier findings that the pattern of marital coitus (particularly among middle-aged and aged) is typically controlled by the husband's desire and his aging, rather than by the wife's loss of interest or capacity (Masters and Johnson, 1970).

Conclusions from this investigation draw attention to concepts basic to sexuality in the lives of the now elderly and thus to the development of sexual patterns all through life. The data demonstrate the essentially interactional nature of sexuality in the dependence of woman's activity on man's desire; in the apparent decline of sex interest in older women as protection or defense, frequently against the aloneness of widowhood; the wide range of individual differences; and the most important factor in determining sexual interest and activity in the old—a lifelong enjoyment and participation.

In their controversial report on an 11-year scientific inquiry into physiology of sex among nearly 800 men and women, Masters and Johnson (1970) added a qualifying note to the measured and observed active involvement in sexuality: there was a decrease in the intensity and rapidity of response.

Commonalities between men and women as reproductive and sexual human beings exist, but are often ignored. Changes in hormones affect older men and women alike in alteration of sleep patterns, weight gain, receding hair growth, and loss of hair color and genital tissue. Children know sexuality as a generalized body response, and in "the primary sexual response

of the adult male and female, there is no differentiation between man and woman . . . "; the basic qualities of orgasm are "the same for male and female" (Toszak, 1969). However, it is equally useful to look at men and women separately for the particular physiological changes and especially as they bring these capacities into meaningful relationships.

THE MALE: ANATOMY AND PHYSIOLOGY

At ages 60, 70, and 80, the male reproductive system is measurably different in form and function from what it was at 20, 30, and 50. But as with other aspects of normal aging, reduced function does not mean absence of capacity.

Rubin (1964) found that half the men, 75 to 92, reported continued sexual intercourse. Another investigation revealed the average frequency of coitus for the majority of men over age 65 is four times a month. Masturbation is a recurrent practice among 25 percent of them (Tarail, 1962).

Physical Changes Hormone (testosterone) production continues into old age. Though testosterone in men is available at a higher level for a longer period than estrogen in women, the concentration is increasingly inadequate and affects the genital tissues. A gradual decline in sexual energy, muscle strength, and viable spermatozoa result from this hormone depletion. The testes become smaller and less firm; testicular tubules (that produce spermatozoa) thicken and begin a degenerative process which finally inhibits the production of spermatozoa. As the prostate gland enlarges, its contractions become weaker. There is a reduction in volume and viscosity of seminal fluid so that the force of ejaculation decreases. No one of these changes is major, but together they are responsible for some real and apparent changes in the total expression of sexuality.

As Sexual Partner There is a recognizable difference in sexual responsiveness and activity. At the Reproductive Biology Research Foundation in St. Louis, Masters and Johnson (1970), using clinical observation and interviews, have documented for the first time the significant aging changes in the physiology of the sex act.

Frequency of intercourse, intensity of sensation, speed of attaining erection, and force of ejaculation are all reduced. To a greater or lesser degree (a function of individual differences), each of the four phases of intercourse depart from the youthful pattern.

1. *Excitement phase.* Excitement builds more slowly. Intensity and duration of sex flush and involuntary spasms are diminished. Erection, longer to attain, has stimulated little testicular elevation or scrotal sac vasocongestion.
2. *Plateau phase.* The plateau phase usually lasts longer than during youth, with minimal vascular engorgement of testes. Increase in penile circumference is marked by absence or reduction of preejaculatory fluid emission.
3. *Orgasmic phase.* The orgasmic phase is usually of shorter duration and may have a reduced or totally missing first stage or ejaculatory demand. In most younger males the entire ejaculatory process is divided into two well-recognized stages: the first ejaculatory inevitability is brief (2 to 4 seconds) in which control is very difficult; the second marks the expulsion of the seminal fluid bolus through the full length of the penis and may be complete within one or two contractions, as contrasted with four or more at a younger age.
4. *Resolution phase.* The refractory period in the aging male may be extended from the 2 minutes of the younger male to 12 to 24 hours. In the older man, the loss of erection and return of the penis to a flaccid state may take a few seconds compared to youth's minutes or hours.

Although most males over 60 engage in intercourse once or twice a week, the capacity to enjoy sex more frequently is greater and depends upon appropriate stimulation to erection. Natural delays in achieving erection are accompanied by the capacity to maintain the erection without reaching orgasm. This reduction in ejaculatory demand is appropriate to the slower excitation response in the older woman, and serves to enhance the possibility of increased arousal and orgasm to the greater satisfaction of both.

Other factors unrelated to physiological capacities or health may also modify the sexual patterns of older men (either reduction of sexual activity or increase of extramarital sex), related more to the quality of the relationship with mate; e.g., a marriage partner for 30 years is often cited as a reasonable basis of boredom for the male. Without renewed efforts at maintaining the total excitement in a fully shared involved life, such boredom is understandable.

THE FEMALE: ANATOMY AND PHYSIOLOGY

Physiologically, the older woman need experience little sexual difficulty. If moderate good health, a positive attitude toward sex, and an available effective sexual partner prevail, sexual activity can extend until the very late years (until 90). Nevertheless, certain myths and stereotypes that have surrounded the menopause persist into aging: the end to sexual desire and attractiveness culminating in defeminization, the inevitability of depression, involutional melancholia, and even insanity. These myths have been repeatedly refuted by physicians, psychologists, psychiatrists, and practitioners and researchers alike (Deutsch, 1945; Benedek, 1959; Neugarten, 1968; Masters and Johnson, 1970). According to Masters and Johnson (1966), "There is no time limit drawn by advancing years to female sexuality." They found significant sexual capacity and effective sexual performance among 61 menopausal and postmenopausal women, aged 40 to 78 years.

However, cultural expectations and early role models compounded by ignorance may lead to severe psychological reactions. In a society where so much is measured by the yardstick of youth, its unlined beauty, vigor, and performance, anxieties mount over attractiveness, the empty nest, and the evaluation of career, community involvement, and marriage.

There is no inevitability about major physical or psychological crises, premenopausal, during menopause, or postmenopausal. Statistical morbidity and mortality data demonstrate that long years of good health remain (Brotman,

1973). Each female will live through a highly individualized pattern. Freed from fear of pregnancy and care of children, some may seek new sexual partners with interest, while others look forward to the end of the sexual involvement which may have provided limited pleasure and gratification.

The Climacteric This total period begins in many women when they are in their forties and ordinarily may span 10 to 20 years. It is characterized by a sequence of phases: reduced fertility; irregular or absent menses; blood vessel instability; and anatomic atrophy. The phases will vary in degree and extent, depending upon the individual's rate of change.

1. A decrease in likelihood of pregnancy develops. The remaining follicles are least susceptible to stimulation by pituitary gonadotropins.
2. Estrogen concentration and activity decrease in proportion to the decrease in follicular maturation and in corpora lutea formation. The reduced amount of estrogen is insufficient to stimulate uterine lining to the former premenstrual proliferated state. Secondary sex characteristics and other metabolic processes (protein synthesis, bone formation, salt and water balance, reciprocal hormonal interaction with other glands) are maintained at a reasonably homeostatic level for some time (often until late sixties).
3. The onset of menopause occurs during the 2- to 3-year period of irregular menses prior to total cessation of menstruation. There may be irregular bleeding which is usually correctable by dilation and curettage, if necessary. Statistics indicate 25 to 30 percent of postmenopausal bleeding may be due to malignancy, but between 70 and 75 percent of all bleeding will cease without medical or surgical intervention. Other complaints that may be noted during this period include palpitation, irritability, anxiety, depression, loss of appetite, insomnia, and headache. They are relatively infrequent and do not involve enough women to be called "characteristic of menopause."
4. Upon follicle exhaustion, the primary estrogen source is gone. Although the adrenal glands synthesize hormones that are metabolized to female sex hormones, progressive diminution may lead to loss of support to vascular and genital tissues. For some women, a common transitory discomfort is the "hot flash," or "flush," a troublesome, periodic dilatation of small blood vessels. The flush involves heat, sweat, and patchy redness starting on the chest and extending to neck and face. It is equally significant that many women complete the climacteric and never experience the flush.

   There is a difference of opinion concerning the etiology of the vascular instability, but it may be due to the increased secretion of pituitary gonadotropin without the moderating, reciprocal effect of the estrogen/progesterone ratio.
5. Finally, between the ages of 60 and 70, the continued sex steroid "starvation" results in atrophy of the uterus and vagina and involution of related genital tissues. Mild regression of secondary sex characteristics may occur.
   a. Skin elasticity decreases; glandular tissue and tone diminish, causing ligaments to relax so that breast and other area contours are less firm.
   b. There is a loss of vulvar substance, the mons pubis flattens and labia majora are less full.
   c. Vaginal mucosa thins and decreases in length with the disappearance of the rugal pattern. Estrogen-deficient vaginitis may be present.
   d. Cervix, corpus uteri, and ovaries shrink at times to prepubertal size.
   e. Portions of the urinary tract, the urethra, and bladder frequently suffer similar atrophy.
   f. Bartholin glands that lubricate vagina may decrease with age.
   g. There is a modest reduction in the size of the clitoris, the covering labia minora or hood atrophies along with the mons fatty tissue. For the clitoris, there is "no objective evidence to date to suggest any appreciable loss in sensate focus" (Masters and Johnson, 1970).
6. Possible pathological diseases that frequently accompany aging have been linked

to estrogen deficiency. There is a statistical rise in atherosclerotic changes in the coronary blood vessels in postmenopausal women and in younger women after removal of ovaries (Davis, Jones, and Jarolem, 1961; Higano, Robinson, and Cohen, 1963). Moreover, estrogen-treated women without ovaries experience fewer coronary accidents. However, the cause and effect is not quite that singular or direct. Although the causes of atherosclerosis and any consequent coronary accidents are not clear, female sex hormones seem to be part of the enzymatic machinery in the metabolism of fats and proteins. Beyond that, heredity, total diet, exercise, and stressful life-styles have also been implicated (Seyle, 1970, 1973; Newton and Morgan, 1968).

Osteoporosis, the leaching out of calcium, with a measurable loss of bone substance, leads to diminished height, instability in maintenance of normal posture, ease of fracture, and often acute pain. Some estrogen-treated women and men are stabilized, others do not respond (Bartter, 1973). There is research that indicates exercise and lifelong dietary habits may be more important than estrogen in maintenance of bone structure (Lutwak, 1969). Good results have been reported with greater calcium intake which increases retention of protein and activation of osteoblasts. Another factor, genetic in origin, may be the porosity of the bone. It is conceivable that those with less porous bones may be more susceptible to any estrogen-primed alteration in calcium metabolism. Finally, if estrogen were solely responsible, estrogen therapy should inhibit and even reverse the progress of osteoporosis in men. Such is not the case. Studies are then equivocal and would require continued pursuit of a more exact molecular mechanism leading to a predictive or preventive therapy.

As Sexual Partners As with older men, both neuronal (decrease in rate of responsivity) and hormonal (steroid starvation) factors combine to effect the recognizable changes in anatomy and function of older women as sexual partners.

The act of coitus may prove unsatisfying and even painful to some postmenopausal women. The thinning vaginal walls and decreased lubrication may make penetration difficult. If cracking of vaginal walls has occurred, there may be some bleeding and pain. Under hormonal deprivation, uterine contractions, as part of the female orgasm, may also cause pain. Burning and frequency of urination after sex may also occur, since the atrophic bladder and urethra are more susceptible to irritation and not protected by the thinning vagina. With advancing years, the intensity of physiological reactions and duration of anatomic and physiological response to effective stimulation are decreased through all four phases of the cycle.

1. *Excitement phase.* Lubrication time is increased from a matter of 15 to 30 seconds to as much as 5 minutes. This is comparable with the involution of the aging male in whom erective delay is a natural fact of aging. Involuntary expansion potential of the vagina is reduced in reaction time and extent. This is especially notable since the vaginal canal of younger women can expand to accommodate a baby's head. The purplish hue of vasocongestion in the younger woman changes to pink.

2. *Plateau phase.* Involuntary uterine elevation is reduced. There is a lack of the deep sex skin coloration in the labia minora, so predictive of impending orgasm. The labia majora do not elevate and flatten against the perineum as in younger women, and may hang limply in folds around the vaginal opening. The clitoral response includes the elevation and flattening on the anterior border of the symphysis, similar to younger women.

3. *Orgasmic phase.* Duration of orgasm is considerably reduced between ages 50 and 70 years. Uterine contractibility from fundus to midzone to lower segment may be similar to that of younger women, but rather than rhythmic, may be spastic and pain-inducing. The contractions are fewer, from 3 to 5 down to 1 or 2. Vaginal orgasmic platform of outer one-third is still initiated within 8-second intervals, but contractions are reduced from 8 to 12 to 4 to 5 times.

4. *Resolution phase.* Rapid resolution, as with older men, is characteristic of female sex steroid imbalance. Pelvic viscera return to

prestimulatory state, uterus to nonelevated position, and the moderately expanded vaginal canal collapses. If any labia minora color change is present, it is faint, and its disappearance is initiated even before orgasm is reached.

These normal anatomic and physiological modulations of the female reproductive system are not experienced either in part or all by all women at the same time. Moreover, these changes do not alter the fact that, in most reports since Kinsey et al. (1953), there is no falling off in sexual arousability with rising age. Frequently there is an increase. The inference for a lifetime of sexuality is clear from the fact that for women regularity of sexual stimulation and activity will overcome the effect of sex steroid inadequacy or starvation. Reportedly, the pattern of masturbatory release of sexual tension is increased in women after menopause through the sixth and seventh decade, and in men after 65.

The functional separation of fertility and libido is best revealed in the high level of sexual desire and activity reported by women after hysterectomies (Post, 1967). Menopausal and postmenopausal women maintain the multiorgasmic capacity of their younger years (Kinsey et al., 1953; Masters and Johnson, 1970; Toszak, 1969). Nevertheless, menopausal and older women who have chosen to use their energies for homemaking and mothering may experience greater difficulty coping with the symptoms of these midlife physiological changes (Neugarten, 1968; Rutherford and Rutherford, 1966). Those women who have been able to combine the homemaker and worker roles (outside the home) would appear to be largely free of most of the psychological and physical responses that were said to be inevitable (Glass and Kase, 1970; Gorney and Cox, 1973).

BASES FOR DYSFUNCTION

If, indeed, the normal aging of the reproductive system leaves older men and women with active interest and capacity, what are the factors that contribute to the dysfunctional, sexless, impotent image of the over 65? They tend to be the same factors that would affect sexuality and the whole person at any age: disease and surgery of the urogenital system, other systemic diseases, and lastly but closely interlaced with the aforementioned and societal attitudes, emotional disturbance.

Declining level of general health and current practice in treatment of the complaints of older patients have led to widespread drug abuse (Townsend, 1971; Lamy and Kitler, 1971). Alcohol, marijuana, and tranquilizers (e.g., chlorpromazine, reserpine) weaken erection and delay ejaculation. Unabated use may lead to impotency. Anemia, diabetes, fatigue, malnutrition, and a variety of metabolic abnormalities at any stage of life—untreated—may inhibit desire, abort arousal and sexual climax, and logically influence the entire physical and affective quality of living. Overeating and consequent obesity may substitute for sexual desire, have serious consequences for cardiovascular health, and be particularly damaging for the self-image.

With advancing age, there is the increased possibility of one or more chronic diseases which alone or in combination may have secondary physiological effects on the reproductive system and modify sexual expression, either directly or indirectly. The major source of difficulty is fear on the part of the older person that any sexual involvement will exacerbate an illness, even lead to death (Masters and Johnson, 1970; Rubin, 1966).

During sexual intercourse, heart rate, blood pressure, and oxygen consumption increase at levels comparable to moderate rather than strenuous exercise. As such, sexual activity, rather than being a threat to health, may be both therapeutic and preventive; e.g., there is an increase in adrenal corticosteroids which relieves some of the symptoms of arthritis, and the sense of well-being reduces physical and emotional tensions. For the sake of an estimate of 1 percent sudden coronary death after intercourse (Butler and Lewis, 1973), the unique benefits of human warmth and sexuality are lost to many. Only extreme coronary pathological disease need call for abstinence. As in youth, pain and malaise effectively suppress libido and magnify the aging, already declining, capacity.

Perhaps the most direct effects are those that derive from dysfunction or surgery of the urogenital system. Pelvic surgery has signaled an end to effective sexual activity for large numbers of older men and women. Clinical data suggest that although prostatectomies and hysterectomies appear to depress desire and capacity for climax, they are not inevitable physiological consequences of the surgery (Finkle and Moyers, 1960). The suggestion that emotion (fear of inadequacy, concern with sexless image) is more important than the surgery is more than reasonable. More than 80 percent of patients who had undergone prostatectomies and 70 percent of women with hysterectomies retain potency and coital enjoyment (Patterson and Craig, 1963). There are men and women who have low sex drives, and such surgery may be a welcome excuse for cessation.

The interactions of stress, hormonal activity, and general health and aging may be explored by measurable criteria (Seyle, 1970). It is common knowledge that ovulation may be inhibited by other systemic illness as well as by strong emotional experiences, e.g., anguish, fear, and anxiety. Clinical data have accumulated to suggest that thought and affect can be parents to a physiological change in youth and aging (Osofsky and Seidenberg, 1970; Brod et al., 1959; Weiss, 1972; Rahe et al., 1970).

These correlations between psyche and physiology reinforce the interdependence of all body systems and put into sharper focus the importance of societal attitudes and ambient support for older people. As with all other organ systems, normal aging of the reproductive system brings decreased efficiency and increased time for responsivity and tissue changes of internal and external genitalia. There is no question of the decrease in fertility—few people over 65 retain the drive for more progeny! Unlike other organ systems, the human reproductive apparatus has a function beyond childbearing. It is integrated as a major means of interpersonal communication, involving the warmth and satisfaction unique to body contact. Among older people, the basic human needs for intimacy, love, achievement, and self-concept are at greater risk at a time of life that augers so many other losses—those of friends, relatives, job status, active parenting, and decision making. Compounding the shrinking functional world, the older man and woman face society's image of "neuter" and nonperson. Fiction had been elevated to fact, and myth to reality, by constant repetition so that older people have accepted their "third sex" fate and professionals have acted accordingly.

With the increasing numbers of older, healthier, more aware persons (growing in greater proportion to younger groups), demands for their fair share of life's offerings and a capacity for living more fully have been activated. Longitudinal studies have belied the mythology. Sensitive, supportive response from professionals and the society will potentiate what capacities older persons retain, rather than concentrate on the deficiencies.

IMPLICATIONS FOR THE HELPING PROFESSIONS: WHAT CAN BE DONE

Suggestions for interventions by the nursing and other helping professions indicated by Burnside (1973) are excellent (see Chapter 32). While all of them are appropriate sequelae to this chapter, the following are in the nature of additions:

1. That they (the helping professions) join with gerontologists in calling for departments of geriatrics in nursing schools, medical schools, and hospitals (Libow et al., 1972).
2. That gynecological and other medical textbooks in use be evaluated and culled to delete the myths related to aging men and women (Scully and Bart, 1973); e.g., in most texts, men are said to set the sexual pace for marital coitus, but nowhere is the multiorgasmic nature of women mentioned.
3. That sex education be instituted for middle and old age (as well as for youth) so that older people may understand and accommodate to extend and use what capacities exist.
4. That sexuality be appropriately seen as a function of commonalities and differences, thereby appreciating the quality of a relationship and focusing on the person, not a performance.
5. That the need for affect and sexual expression (outside of intercourse) be recognized as essential to being and feeling alive; that they be

nurtured especially in older people for the mental and physical well-being that ensues.

6. That continued effort be made (and for the society at large) for greater acceptance of alternate life-styles that could ameliorate the alienation of those who are single, alone, and old.

7. That although there may be no substitute for another human in the fullest pleasure of sexual expression, masturbation may be a necessary outlet for sexual release and maintenance of genital tissue readiness.

8. That serious consideration be given to replacement-estrogen therapy for women as a viable alternative to psychotherapy and sedation in the prevention and/or treatment of the emotional and physiological changes that accompany middle and old age (Masters and Johnson, 1970; Schleyer-Saunders, 1971; Sheffery, Wilson and Walsh, 1969). Phenobarbital or thioridazine (Mellaril) will not alter the skeletal, genital, and muscular tissue changes. While psychotherapy may alleviate or prevent a serious depression, only estrogen replacement can affect the metabolic apparatus directly.

The specter of cancer with hormone therapy has not developed as earlier anticipated (Rhoades, 1965; Glass and Kase, 1970). More than 90 percent of uterine cancers are in women over 40 years, and breast cancer also increases with age, when estrogen stores are low: 1.8 percent before 30, 75 percent develop over 40 (Leis, 1967).

Estrogen in combination with testosterone does retard the tissue changes and other physiological symptomatology associated with the climacteric (Masters and Johnson, 1970); many of the common complaints can be completely avoided with replacement therapy (Rogers, 1969).

I will close with what I feel is the uniquely human striving of us all, men and women alike—young and old:

Tho' much is taken, much abides; and tho'
We are not now that strength which in old days
Moved earth and heaven; that which we are, we
* are;*

One equal temper of heroic hearts,
Made weak by time and fate, but strong in will
To strive, to seek, to find, and not to yield.

Alfred, Lord Tennyson
Ulysses

REFERENCES

Aslan, A.: Principles of drug therapy, in *Proceedings of the 9th International Congress of Gerontology: Symposia Reports,* **2:**115–118, 1972.

Bartter, F. C.: Bones as a target organ: Toward a better definition of osteoporosis, *Perspectives in Biology and Medicine,* **16:**215–231, Winter 1973.

Benedek, T.: Sexual functions in women and their disturbance, in S. Arieti (ed.), *American Handbook of Psychiatry,* Basic Books, New York, 1959.

Brod, I., et al.: Circulatory changes underlying blood pressure elevation during acute emotional stress (mental arithmetic) in normotensive and hypertensive subjects, *Clinical Science,* **18:**269–279, 1959.

Brotman, H.: The aging: Who and where, *Perspectives in Aging,* **11**(1):8–12, January–February 1973.

Burnside, Irene: Sexuality and aging, *Medical Arts and Sciences,* **27**(3):13–27, 1973.

Butler, Robert, and M. Lewis: *Aging and Mental Health,* Mosby, St. Louis, 1973.

Davis, M. E., R. J. Jones, and C. Jarolem: Long term estrogen substitution and atherosclerosis, *American Journal of Obstetrics and Gynecology,* **82:**1003–1018, 1961.

Deutsch, H.: *The Psychology of Women,* Grune & Stratton, New York, 1945.

Finkle, A., and T. Moyers: Sexual potency in aging males: IV. Status of private patients before and after prostatectomy, *Journal of Urology,* **84:**152–157, 1960.

Frank, L.: *The Conduct of Sex,* Morrow, New York, 1961.

Glass, R., and N. Kase: *Women's Choice: A Guide to Contraception, Fertility, Abortion and Menopause,* Basic Books, New York, 1970.

Gorney, S., and C. Cox: *After Forty,* Dial, New York, 1973.

Greenblatt, R., and J. Leng: Factors influencing sexual behavior, *Journal of the American Geriatrics Society,* **20**(2):49–54, 1972.

Gruman, G. J.: History of ideas about the prolongation of life, *Transactions of the American Philosophical Society,* **56**(p. 9), 1966.

Guillerme, J.: *Longevity,* Walker, New York, 1963.

Higano, N., R. Robinson, and W. Cohen: Increased incidence of cardiovascular disease in castrated women: Two year follow up studies, *New England Journal of Medicine,* **268**:1123–1125, 1963.

Kinsey, A. C., W. B. Pomeroy, and C. I. Martin: *Sexual Behavior in the Human Male,* Saunders, Philadelphia, 1948.

——, ——, ——, and P. H. Gebhard: *Sexual Behavior in the Human Female,* Saunders, Philadelphia, 1953.

Lamy, P., and M. Kitler: Drugs and the geriatric patient, *Journal of the American Geriatrics Society,* **19**(1):23–33, 1971.

Leis, H.: *Medical World News,* **8**:63–70, 1967.

Leviton, Dan: The significance of sexuality as a deterrent to suicide among the aged, *Omega,* **4**(2):163–174, Summer 1973.

Libow, L., et al.: *Educational Symposium 1972,* Gerontological Society Meetings, Puerto Rico.

Lowenthal, M., et al.: *Aging and Mental Disorder in San Francisco,* Jossey-Bass, San Francisco, 1967.

Lutwak, L.: Symposium on osteoporosis: Nutritional aspects of osteoporosis, *Journal of the American Geriatrics Society,* **17**(2):115–119, 1969.

Masters, W. H., and V. Johnson: *Human Sexual Inadequacy,* Little, Brown, Boston, 1970, p. 337–338.

——, and ——: *Human Sexual Responses,* Little, Brown, Boston, 1966, p. 247.

May, R.: *Love and Will,* Norton, New York, 1969.

Neugarten, B. (ed.): *Middle Age and Aging,* University of Chicago Press, Chicago, 1968.

Newsweek, Can aging be cured? April 16, 1973, pp. 56–66.

Newton, H. F., and D. B. Morgan: Osteoporosis: Disease or senescense, *Lancet,* **1**:232–233, February 3, 1968.

Osofsky, F., and R. Seidenberg: Is female menopause depression inevitable? *Journal of Obstetrics and Gynecology,* **36**(4):611–615, 1970.

Patterson, R. M., and J. B. Craig: Misconceptions concerning the psychological effects of hysterectomy, *American Journal of Obstetrics and Gynecology,* **85**:105–111, 1963.

Pfeiffer, E., and G. Davis: Determinants of sexual behavior in the elderly, *Journal of American Geriatrics Society,* **20**(4):151–158, 1972.

Post, F.: Sex and its problems, *Practitioner,* **199**:377–382, 1967.

Rahe, R. H., J. Mahan, Jr., and R. J. Arthur: Prediction of near future health change from subjects preceding life changes, *Journal of Psychosomatic Research,* **14**:401–406, 1970.

Rhoades, F. P.: The menopause: A deficiency disease, *Michigan Medicine,* **64**:410–412, 1965.

Rogers, J.: Estrogens in the menopause and postmenopause, *New England Journal of Medicine,* **280**:364–367, 1969.

Rubin, I.: Common sex myths, *Sexology,* **32**:512–514, 1966.

——: Sex after 40 and after 70, in Ruth Brecher and E. Brecher (eds.), *An Analysis of Human Sexual Response,* New American Library, New York, 1966.

——: Sex needs after 65, *Sexology,* **30**:709–711, 1964.

——: *Sexual Life after Sixty,* Basic Books, New York, 1965.

Rutherford, R., and J. Rutherford: Menopause: Feat or defeat? *Psychosomatics,* **7**:89–93, 1966.

Schleyer-Saunders, E.: Results of hormone implants in the treatment of the climacteric, *Journal of American Geriatrics Society,* **19**(2):114–121, 1971.

Scully, D., and P. Bart: A funny thing happened on the way to the orifice: Women in gynecology textbooks, *American Journal of Sociology,* **78**(4):1045–1050, 1973.

Seyle, H. A.: Homeostasis and heterosis, *Perspectives in Biology and Medicine,* **16**(3):441–445, 1973.

——: Stress and aging, *Journal of American Geriatrics Society,* **18**(9):669–690, 1970.

Sheffery, J. B., T. A. Wilson, and J. C. Walsh: Double-blind cross-over study comparing chlordiazepoxide, conjugated estrogens, combined chlordiazepoxide and conjugated estrogens and placebo in treatment of the menopause, *Medical Annals of the District of Columbia,* **38**:433–436, 1969.

Shock, N.: *Biomedical Science: Prospects in Aging. Presentation to Convocation,* Andrus Gerontology Center, University of Southern California, February 1973.

Sontag, S.: The double standard of aging, *Saturday Review,* pp. 29–38, September 23, 1972.

Tarail, M.: Sex over 65, *Sexology,* **28**:440–442, 1962.

Toszak, B.: The human continuum, in B. Toszak and T. Toszak (eds.), *Masculine/Feminine,* Harper & Row, New York, 1969, p. 305.

Townsend, C.: *Old Age: The Last Segregation,* Grossman Publishers, New York, 1971.

Trimmer, E. J.: *Rejuvenation,* Barnes, Cranbury, N.J., 1970.

Weiss, J. M.: *Psychological factors in stress and disease, Scientific American,* **226**(8):104–113, June 1972.

TWENTY-SIX

ASSESSMENT OF OLDER CLIENTS' SEXUAL HEALTH

Virgil Parsons

Love is the salt of life; a higher taste
It gives to pleasure, and then makes it last.
George V. Buckingham

LEARNING OBJECTIVES

- Define and describe sexual health care.
- Explain the "who," "when," and "where" of sexual health assessment.
- Identify and describe at least five factors which influence present sexual interest and activity in older persons.
- Explain three methods for assessment of older clients' sexual health status.
- Outline a plan for using information from sexual health assessment in intervention and evaluation of nursing care.

Sexual health care has become an accepted part of total health care, and nursing personnel have a responsibility to promote sexual health when providing care and services. Unfortunately, many nurses have not had the educational experiences needed to acquire the knowledge and skills to provide care for clients with sexual concerns. This is particularly true in the nursing care of older people where many nurses and other health care providers seem to ascribe to the prevalent assumptions that:

(1) Old people do not have sexual desire; (2) they could not make love even if they did want to; (3) they are too fragile physically and it might hurt them; (4) they are physically unattractive and therefore sexually undesirable; (5) anyway, the whole notion is shameful and decidedly perverse. (Butler and Lewis, 1977, p. 112)

Recent evidence indicates disagreement with the above assumptions. A 65-year-old man wrote to Ann Landers expressing concern and stating, "I don't feel like an old fool. Although I'm not the man I was 35 years ago, I still have a lot of pep and am far from dead sexually" (Landers, 1977, p. 21). Another item, of dubious distinction, reports that a 64-year-old man was found guilty of attempted rape (*San Jose Mercury,* 1977). These and similar incidents suggest that older people's awareness of their sexuality is increasing and they will expect and demand appropriate sexual health care from health care professionals.

SEXUAL HEALTH CARE

According to Mace, Bannerman, and Burton (1974, p. 10), sexual health care refers to those interventions which are aimed at assisting people to conduct their sexual lives successfully, that is, to achieve positive sexual health. The concept of sexual health includes three basic elements:

1. A capacity to enjoy and control sexual and reproductive behavior in accordance with a social and personal ethic

2. Freedom from fear, shame, guilt, false beliefs, and other psychological factors inhibiting sexual response and impairing sexual relationships
3. Freedom from organic disorders, diseases, and deficiencies that interfere with sexual and reproductive functions

The skills required for sexual health care are not so very different from the skills needed for comprehensive nursing care. Nurses generally should be able to:

1. Use the nursing process of assessment, planning, implementation, and evaluation to promote positive sexual health
2. Provide education and counseling in sexuality
3. Make referrals to appropriate sources for sexual problems needing intervention beyond nurses' ability

In order to provide sexual health care, nurses need a broad knowledge base in the biopsychosocial aspects of sexuality and must have objective, accepting attitudes. Cooperation and collaboration with other health care providers will enhance effective sexual health care.

ASSESSMENT

Sexual health care is often given a low priority in nursing care services to older clients. Many factors contribute to minimizing the importance of sexuality. Sometimes, nurses are not comfortable with their own sexuality and thus feel uncomfortable about dealing with clients' sexual behavior and functioning. Nurses often must cope with lack of knowledge and negative attitudes of colleagues, administrators, clients' families, and even physicians. Frequently, the hindrance to initiating sexual health care is simply the nurses' anxiety and embarrassment about discussing clients' sexuality during assessment. Common questions of nurses are:

1. Which clients need sexual health assessment?
2. Where should sexual health assessment be done?

3. When is the best time for sexual health assessment?
4. What exactly should be assessed?
5. How does one go about assessing the sexual health status of clients?
6. What does one do with the information obtained through sexual health assessment?

WHO, WHERE, WHEN?

These questions can be answered fairly easily. To some extent, the sexual health status of *all* clients should be ascertained. This premise applies to clients in all clinical settings, even where the presenting problem does not seem to directly affect sexuality. The exact location will be described when the "how" of sexual health assessment is discussed.

In response to the question of "when," the best response is—as soon as possible. Common sense is the best guide, but anytime a full health assessment is done, sexuality should be one of the areas asked about. Even when the immediate problem precludes asking clients about their sexual health, as soon as the situation is appropriate, nurses should gather this information.

WHAT?

Assessments of sexual health should include questions about clients' sexuality which determine the current status of sexual functioning and distinguish causes of sexual problems or dysfunction. Effort should also be made to assess the quality of clients' interpersonal relationships, as well as situations with sexual partners, which have bearing on health status. Nursing personnel should think of sexuality in a broad context, one that encompasses the total identity of the individual (see Figure 26-1).

"Sex" is just one of the parts that make up the meaning of sexuality. True sexuality means more than just the love act between two people; it comprises the sharing part of humanness, the humanness which belongs to each one of us, whether we are young or old. It has to do with our feelings about ourselves as total persons, with feelings about our masculinity or our femininity. Sexuality includes those intangible ties that bind— love, trust, empathy, companionship, touch, tenderness and affection. And, ultimately,

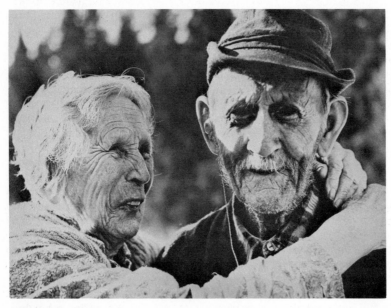

FIGURE 26-1 "Sexuality . . . comprises the sharing part of humanness, the humanness which belongs to each one of us, whether we are young or old" (Fox et al., 1978, p. 16). (*A. S. Norsk Telegrambyra.*)

sexuality deals with who we are, how we see ourselves, and how others see us. (Fox, 1978, p. 16)

More information on what to consider when assessing older clients' sexual health is provided by Friedman's (1978, 1979) excellent summary of factors influencing sexual expression in aging persons. She describes a system of variables which influence present sexual interest and activity in older persons. These variables include: (1) demographic factors, such as age and marital status, (2) value systems, such as degree of religiosity, (3) knowledge of sexuality and changing sexual function, (4) prior patterns of sexual expression, (5) social and economic resources, (6) physical health, and (7) emotional health. Research studies regarding sexuality of the aging person have been sparse and inconclusive, but they have illuminated these factors which may affect sexual expression in older persons. Friedman's information, along with Weg's thorough summary of changes in the aging person's reproductive system (Chapter 25 in this book), provides a knowledge base for determining the "what" of assessing older clients' sexual health.

HOW?

The most frequent question regarding sexual health assessment of older clients is "how." Nurses commonly ask:

1. How do I introduce the topic of sexuality?
2. How do I ask the questions?
3. How do I handle my own anxiety?
4. How do I handle clients' embarrassment or discomfort?

Some of the concern behind these questions is based on the mistaken idea that older clients do not care and/or do not want to talk about sexuality. Burnside (1979), Runciman (1975), and Steffl (1978) describe this idea as largely a myth, and their assertions are supported by research studies (Brower and Tanner, 1979; Wasow and Loeb, 1975). When given the opportunity, older people seek information and want to learn about sexuality and sexual behavior.

Two basic premises are essential for effectively carrying out a sexual health assessment with an older client. First, nurses must recognize and accept each client as a sexual being with sexuality as an integral part of his or her total identity. Secondly, nurses should consider that sexual health, along with all other aspects of health, is a legitimate concern of health care providers. Every client deserves that nurses understand and believe these two premises.

Also basic to sexual health assessment is the requirement that nurses use the same interpersonal concepts and skills that apply to all nursing (Parsons and Sanford, 1979). Much of the assessment is done through interviewing; providing support, active listening, and use of feedback all serve to assist the nurse to obtain needed information and to establish a working relationship with the client. The assurance of trust and provision of privacy are essential. Physical privacy, i.e., conducting the interview in a place where the nurse and client will not be interrupted, should be augmented by a guarantee of confidentiality (Woods, 1979, p. 77).

Sexuality should be introduced early in the nurse-client relationship to reinforce the belief that sexual health is an appropriate component of the client's health. Terminology and language should be mutually understood by the nurse and client, and the nurse should check whether terms are clear to the client. Seldom will it be necessary to use "street language" as the mode of communication, but nurses should be familiar with a variety of words used for sexual behavior and functioning. Nurses should convey attitudes of acceptance and objectivity during the interview and offer to discuss potential concerns with the client should they occur.

Very often, a sexual health assessment can be accomplished by one or a few questions in the overall health history. A simple question such as "Has anything lately interfered with your sexuality or sexual functioning?" may be all that is needed. Woods (1979, p. 79) lists three questions for a "brief sexual history" which can be integrated with a health history.

1. Has anything (illness, surgery) interfered with your being a (mother/wife, father/husband)?
2. Has anything (heart attack, injury) changed

the way you feel about yourself as a (man, woman)?

3. Has anything (disease, physical changes) changed your ability to function sexually?

These brief questions encourage clients to express and explore sexual concerns, and many clients will proceed to state their concerns about sexual identity, roles, and functioning without further prompting.

When a client does describe a specific problem, the nurse should shift to a format for completing a "sexual-problem history" (Annon, 1976, pp. 76–77). The following questions are based on Annon's guidelines.

1. Description of current problem.
   a. Can you describe the problem?
   b. Tell me about the problem.
2. Onset and course of the problem.
   a. When did the problem begin?
   b. Was the onset gradual or sudden?
   c. Over time, has the problem changed, increased, decreased?
3. Client's concept of cause and maintenance of problem.
   a. What do you think caused the problem?
   b. What maintains the condition or problem?
4. Past treatment and outcome.
   a. Have you had a medical evaluation of the problem?
   b. Have you received any professional help for the problem?
   c. What have been the results of these efforts?
5. Current expectations and goals.
   a. What would you like to have done for the problem?
   b. What do you hope will be done about the problem?

This exploration of a problem can be brief, but the nurse should make sure that enough time is allowed to gain adequate information. If the questioning must be very brief, follow-up is essential for assuring the client that the problem is a concern of health care planning.

A full sexual history is not often necessary, but nurses should be aware of this form of assessment. These interviews progress from less sensitive issues to more sensitive ones. Also, a life-cycle approach is used, exploring the client's childhood and psychosexual development and education with progression to current sexual behavior and practices. The full sexual history is beyond the skill of most nurses, and appropriate referral should be made if it is deemed necessary. Green (1975, pp. 9–19), Semmons and Semmons (1978, pp. 27–43), and Woods (1979, pp. 75–94) are sources for outlines of a full sexual history.

Sexual health assessment interviews and questions should always be integrated with other sources of information about the client's health status. Physical examinations, diagnostic laboratory procedures, as well as information about medications used, all assist in determining the client's current sexual health status.

In addition to knowledge and guidelines for sexual health assessment, it is often helpful for nurses to carry out a learning exercise which simulates sexual health assessment and serves to increase their awareness of attitudes and level of comfort in talking about sexuality. This activity should be done several times, first with a person with whom the nurse feels fairly comfortable. It is useful to ask the questions of another nurse and then to reverse roles of interviewer and client, so that both participants get practice in sexual health assessment. The following are questions for a sexual history interview:

1. What was your parents' attitude toward sex, nudity, and touching?
2. How would you rate or describe your parents' sexual adjustment?
3. What is the effect of your parents' sexual adjustment on your sexuality and present sexual functioning?
4. What physical traits do you like in a person of the opposite sex?
5. What physical traits do you like in a person of the same sex?
6. Describe one thing that sexually excites you or "turns you on." Describe one thing that "turns you off."
7. How would you rate or describe your present sexuality? What about it would you like to change?
8. What is one thing you would like to tell a present or past partner about your relation-

ship (sexual and otherwise) that you were (or are) afraid to tell him or her?
9. What is it like—how does it feel—to ask and answer these questions?

This learning activity can be carried out with willing clients once nurses have reached a point where they feel at ease talking with clients about sexual behavior and functioning. Sexual health assessment, like any skill, requires continued practice for proficiency.

AFTER ASSESSMENT

Sexual health assessment is only the first step in integrating sexual health care into the nursing process. Based on sexual health assessment data, intervention should be aimed at any health problem which interferes with sexuality and sexual functioning. Teaching and counseling are interventions that are in the specific realm of nursing care and practice. Also, nurses can be instrumental in decreasing the isolation of long-term care settings by increasing clients' interaction with persons of the opposite sex, encouraging clients' interest in their personal appearance, and providing activities which give clients the impetus to seek interpersonal interaction.

Evaluation of sexual health intervention should be planned around goals that are mutually chosen by clients and nurses. Clients are the best judge of whether interventions have been appropriate, adequate, and realistic to meet their goals. Nurses will need to seek verbal expression of satisfaction by clients to evaluate whether nursing interventions have been helpful.

SUMMARY

Sexual health should be a focus for the nursing and health care of all older clients. To accomplish this, nurses must become proficient in assessment of clients' sexual health and use this assessment as a beginning point to end the suffering that clients feel when their sexuality is negated or ignored. As Krizinofski (1973, p. 679) states:

Including sexuality in comprehensive care is culturally and socially the function of nursing. In the care of aged patients and patients with long-term illnesses in nursing homes or health related facilities, the challenge to create a fully human environment is uniquely nursing's challenge.

REFERENCES

Annon, J. S.: *Behavioral Treatment of Sexual Problems,* Harper & Row, New York, 1976.

Brower, H. T., and L. A. Tanner: A study of older adults attending a program on human sexuality: A pilot study, *Nursing Research,* **28**(1):36–39, January 1979.

Buckingham, George V.: *Book of Familiar Quotations,* Ottenheimer, Publishers, New York, 1955, p. 144.

Burnside, I. M.: Psychosocial caring: Touch, sexuality, and cultural aspects, in I. M. Burnside, P. Ebersole, and H. E. Monea (eds.), *Psychosocial Caring throughout the Life Span,* McGraw-Hill, New York, 1979.

Butler, R. M., and M. I. Lewis: *Aging and Mental Health,* Mosby, St. Louis, 1977.

Fox, N., et al.: Sexuality among the aging, *Journal of Practical Nursing,* **41**:16–18, August 1978.

Friedman, J. S.: Factors influencing sexual expression in aging persons: A review of the literature, *Journal of Psychiatric Nursing and Mental Health Services,* **16**(7)34–47, July 1978.

———: Sexuality in older persons: Implications for nursing practice, *Nursing Forum,* **18**(1):92–101, January 1979.

Green, R.: Taking a sexual history, in R. Green (ed.), *Human Sexuality: A Health Practitioner's Text,* Williams & Wilkins, Baltimore, 1975.

Krizinofski, M. T.: Human sexuality and nursing practice, *Nursing Clinics of North America,* **8**(4):673–681, December 1973.

Landers, A.: Annie's reply requires more space than her column allows, *San Jose Mercury,* 21, Nov. 30, 1977.

Mace, D. R., R. H. O. Bannerman, and J. Burton: *The Teaching of Human Sexuality in Schools for Health Professionals,* World Health Organization, Geneva, 1974.

Parsons, V., and N. Sanford: *Interpersonal Interaction in Nursing,* Addison-Wesley, Menlo Park, Calif., 1979.

Runciman, A.: Problems older clients present in counseling about sexuality, in I. Burnside (ed.), *Sexuality and Aging,* Andrus Gerontology Center, University of Southern California Press, Los Angeles, 1975.

San Jose Mercury: Nine-year term for attack, 13, Nov. 28, 1977.

Semmons, J. P., and F. J. Semmons: The sexual history and physical examination, in M. U. Barnard, B. J. Clancy, and K. E. Krantz (eds.), *Human Sexuality for Health Professionals,* Saunders, Philadelphia, 1978.

Steffl, B. M.: Sexuality and aging: Implications for nurses and other health professionals, in R. L. Solnick (ed.), *Sexuality and Aging,* Andrus Gerontology Center, University of Southern California Press, Los Angeles, 1978.

Wasow, M., and M. B. Loeb: Sexuality in nursing homes, in I. Burnside (ed.), *Sexuality and Aging,* Andrus Gerontology Center, University of Southern California Press, Los Angeles, 1975.

Woods, N. F.: *Human Sexuality in Health and Illness,* Mosby, St. Louis, 1979.

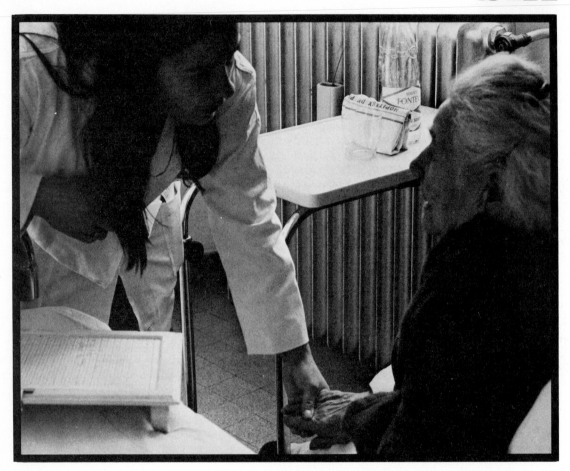

SIX

E. Schwab, reprinted with permission of the World Health Organization.

ASSESSMENT OF THE ELDERLY CLIENT

Aging is not a disease.

Anonymous

Is there such a thing as an impartial history? And
what is history? The written representation of past
events. But what is an event. . . . It is a notable fact.
Now, how is the historian to discriminate whether a
fact is notable or not? He decides this arbitrarily,
according to his character and idiosyncrasy, at his
own taste and fancy—in a word, as an artist. . . .

Anatole France
"The Garden of Epicurus"

TWENTY-SEVEN

THE NURSING ASSESSMENT

Mary Opal Wolanin

. . . the last is the greatest treason:
To do the right deed for the wrong reason.
T. S. Eliot

LEARNING OBJECTIVES

- Identify variations of the nursing process which care of the elderly necessitates.
- Identify "high-risk elderly" in making assessments and in planning nursing care.
- Differentiate between the holistic functional approach and other forms of assessment.
- Implement the systems approach when assessing the elderly in their social and physical environment.
- Demonstrate knowledge of the aging process to alter the usual assessment patterns.
- Analyze multiple health problems of the aged during the designing of a nursing diagnosis.

Chapter 27, "The Nursing Assessment," and Chapter 28, "Nursing Intervention and Evaluation," will be concerned with the use of the nursing process with the elderly client in any setting. There are specific assessments in other chapters, and these two chapters will not contain the same kind of material but will look at the nursing process as a guide to professional nursing care. The nursing process with the elderly person involves all the familiar components of the problem-solving approach: data gathering, problem definition, specific data gathering, interpretation, analysis and recognition of recurrent patterns, developing a working hypothesis or diagnosis, and finally organizing a treatment plan with implementation and evaluation.

EVALUATION

Although the nursing process begins with an initial hypothesis which guides the data gathering that is the assessment, this chapter will start with evaluation as the beginning of the nursing process. It has always been the final action and often is omitted entirely. In fact there is no consensus as to what is being evaluated—the nursing process or the client outcomes. It is necessary to look at the interaction of three different factors which lead to any outcome—the nursing process, the setting with its assets and limitations, and finally, the interaction of all these factors on client outcomes. It is easy to say, "We will look at client outcomes in our evaluation," but the intrinsic interaction of the other factors will not be ignored. In order to make an evaluation, the very origins of the word must be considered. *Evaluation* is based on *values,* and at some point the hard question must be asked and answered, "Whose values?" For the purposes of this chapter, evaluation will be based on the nurse-client interaction, which consists of the nursing process and its contributions to the welfare of the client. This means that definite goals have to be set for nursing to achieve with the client. It also requires certain standards of nursing care that are specific enough for nurses to know how independently they can function in making the necessary judgments.

Standards are the reasonable expectations of nursing performance; unfortunately, they are usually stated in general or even ambiguous terms which can be interpreted variously by different people in different settings. An example is the geriatric nursing standard that "the nurse supports and promotes normal physiological functioning of the older person." In one institution this might be interpreted as feeding, bathing, and getting a client around in a wheelchair. In a second it might be interpreted as maintaining adequate nutritional status, assisting with self-care, developing good hygiene including skin and mouth care, and maintaining the highest mobility and activity the client's condition is capable of sustaining. In still another, the relief of anxiety might be a crucial part of promoting normal physiological status. With such flexible standards the nurse must know the framework within which to work and must test it often. This is *process* which can be evaluated as *process* and depends upon the values of the nurses giving care and upon the resources (structure) of the setting (Wolanin, 1975).

Structure (resources or the setting) and process are fairly easily observed. They have traditionally been used by licensing agencies for judging the care of institutionalized clients. Client outcomes are much more difficult to measure because:

1. Goals have not been definitely stated. Baseline data are rarely available. Client outcomes are measured as an afterthought and consist of self-report on the part of either the nurse or the client. The question "Was the care appropriate?" may not have been either asked or answered because no one had really looked at the needs of the client.
2. Present systems of using records in auditing may be limited to what the nurse recorded as important and even to the nurse's ability as a creative writer.
3. The end product (client outcome) is not necessarily dependent upon nursing care. There are times when recovery may be as much the result of what was not done as of what was done (benign neglect?).

For the client who has been subjected to routine or automatic care, the end product—recovery—may not be related to the nursing care but to some other factor such as being removed from a stressful environment—a result which could have been achieved as well in a hotel.

The position taken in this chapter is that deliberative nursing action (Orlando, 1961) is that which is based on a philosophy, guided by a systematic assessment, has goals set by the nurse interacting with the client (negotiating or even contracting), and results in moving the client to the best level of health. For the elderly person this may mean toward a peaceful death, a goal which both client and nurse might agree is the most important outcome in the closing days of life. Throughout the steps of the nursing process, preparation is made for evaluation. The nursing process is a period of learning for both the nurse and client. Only by evaluating does one know whether any new knowledge has been added to the nursing repertoire. Only by evaluating against certain base-line criteria can the nurse or client know that change has occurred.

THE NURSING CARE EQUATION

In the elderly person the process takes on added dimensions at each step. Data gathering is much broader in scope—the elderly, by definition, have begun to demonstrate the psychosocial and physiological changes which accompany aging, and many have additional problems which are residues of a life with physical and emotional stresses. Intervention, properly planned and implemented, may contribute to increasing the independence and participation of elderly persons as they finish their lines. Problems which are not recognized or treated may lead to a diminished existence on a physical or emotional level. Accurate base-line data are essential; mutual planning and validation can lead to a trusting relationship, and disuse can be prevented or detected early enough to intervene.

The nursing process is continuous as new data are added daily. With the elderly, diminished capacity is expected, but no one is all sick, no one is sick all the time, and conditions change from day to day. Aging is not illness, but illness tends to increase aging.

The nursing process is based on the nursing-care equation

$$x + y = z$$

where x = the unknown, the elderly person who is diminished by problems of aging or health

y = the nursing service needed to assist the aging person to function adequately in the environment

z = a person who is able to function adequately in the environment (z is a constant)

Or the equation can be stated:

Elderly person with remaining resources + nursing care to complement or supplement the elderly person's resources = person able to function adequately in the environment

This equation arises from Henderson's definition of nursing as a process which assists the patient who lacks the strength, the will, or the knowledge to return to health and independence, or to a peaceful death (Henderson, 1964).

The x in the equation is based on an adequate assessment of the elderly person with full appreciation of the resources which remain; y is estimated after analysis and interpretation based on nursing knowledge. It is a plan which will not diminish the elderly person by taking away any remaining abilities. It prescribes only the *quantity and quality of nursing care* needed out of a vast repertoire of nursing skills. The symbol y is based on relationship and fails if the end point is not a person who can function within the requirements of the environment. This may vary from the intensive care unit (minimum requirements of the elderly person) to the person's home, where he or she may need only a sense of self which must be maintained through a relationship with another.

But if x, the unknown, is the starting point of the equation, what does x represent when translated into human terms? It is a human being with some assets or resources which enable him or her to function, and only by exact assessment of those resources can we make an estimate of the amount of *y*, or nursing care, that is adequate in quantity and quality. We use the systems approach with the properties or attributes given by Putt (1978, p. 2):

- Nature: *Systems can be real or conceptual.*
- Structure: The arrangement of the component parts.
- Process: Functioning of the system with exchanges of energy, matter, and information.
- Order: All systems have an interlocking hierarchy and can be divided into subsystems and the parts manipulated.
- Wholeness of the unit with interdependence of variables: *Changing one part can affect the whole system.*
- Exchange of energies: All systems have potential for increasing their order of complexity through exchanging energies or increasing disorder or disruption by dissipation of energy.
- Change with time: Most systems decay through time or increase and grow toward a higher level of organization.
- Degree of openness: *Open systems exchange energies in form of materials or information or both.*
- Degree of stability: Systems may be adaptive or stable. Adaptation is related to learning. Stability is equated with nonadaptation. Self-correction via feedback—return of information to system.

DEFINING THE INITIAL PROBLEM

Nurses are not sought by the elderly until some loss threatens a change in their usual life-style; the nurse is not expected to alter that life-style, but to assist in adaptation to physical or emotional changes which interfere with the aging person's ability to manage. But working with disabilities, or losses in ability, of necessity forces adapting to a changing life-style, whether within one's own home or, at the extreme, in an institution where choices are highly restricted. The principle on which nurses must plan care is that the elderly person does not come asking to find a new life-style, or even a greatly altered one, but asks that those who are in the helping professions recognize and honor his or her way of life while assisting in making alterations required by lack of the person's own resources. *Nursing's task, then, in working with the elderly, is to determine how far the aging person wishes to have someone else take over some tasks, and to what extent the client can keep control.* Too often, when asking for a little help, the elderly person is forced to take the whole package.

ASSESSMENT

The literature review leads to confusion regarding the many uses of the word *assessment*. Different nursing and medical authors use it to represent various parts of the process of determining the client's problems. The usual problem-solving approach involves data gathering through observations, definition of the problems, gathering specific information focused on the problem, and analysis of the findings (Carrieri and Sitzman, 1971). For some authors the analysis is termed *assessment;* this is particularly true in the problem-oriented approach which is being widely used at present. The SOAP process involves having a defined problem, adding subjective and objective observations regarding the client and that problem, then making an "assessment" (Weed, 1971; Griffith, 1971; Corbus et al., 1977).

Little and Carnevali (1969) use the term *assessment* as it will be used in this chapter—in relation to data gathering at any point in the nursing process. Analysis and data gathering go hand in hand. Analysis of datum A leads to the need to observe for datum B, and the two together lead to preliminary analysis. It is doubtful that one can gather pure data in isolation without making a running analysis. At each step in the nursing process assessment is made; the evaluation of care given, and its effect, are based on an assessment of the client's response. In summary, then, assessment in this context refers to the process of observing and gathering data.

Traditionally the health history and physical examination have been done by the physician, and the nursing history tended to be developed through listening, exploring, and observation. The data base for the elderly may or may not include the health history and physical examination done by the physician, but it must include a wide range of observations such as physical assessment and history taking by the nurse. The rapidly expanding role of nurses, especially in the geriatric field, frequently makes them the primary care agent; in many instances, the nursing intervention may well be the preventive one which will lead to health maintenance, so that the curative role of the physician need not be sought. Since this data-gathering role is so immense in the elderly, and since it includes so many facets which are not included in the usual physical examination, this area will receive a great deal of emphasis in this section.

If the assessment has been thorough, the resources of the client should stand out against a picture of the whole person. The lost resources are the nurse's problem to supplement and complement with knowledge, strength, and will.

A secondary benefit of the systematic and whole-person-oriented assessment is the establishment of a base line for many parameters which must of necessity change with further aging, illness, or recovery. This base line, written in objective terms using data which are measurable, often offers the only opportunity for detecting small changes that may indicate grave psychophysical interruptions in being.

Assessment of the elderly focuses on three areas: (1) the person as a physiological and social being, (2) the person's physical and social environment, and, finally, (3) the interaction of the elderly person with the environment. No assessment of the elderly person is complete without considering these three areas. For the third, it is necessary to look at the older person where he or she lives.

VIGNETTE 1

Mrs. B. told the nurse she dreaded having her grandchildren visit her. On exploration, the nurse learned that it was not the noise, which the grandmother enjoyed for a short time, or their rowdy affection, which she craved, but the fact that they left the furniture in new positions. Mrs. B. was able to control her environment and live with her decreasing sight as long as no one changed the arrangement of one article in her house, but her knees were black and blue after stumbling into rearranged furniture, and at times she fell. When she was moved to the hospital for diagnostic work-up she was panic-stricken and bedbound, for she did not know "where anything was."

Perhaps the most crucial interaction the elderly make is with their social environment. *As contacts become fewer, it is important that those which remain be intensified and meaningful.* The physical environment may add to or detract from the elderly person's life: added light may enable the person with decreasing vision to use that which remains to the maximum, or a cane may assist in maintaining equilibrium.

STANDARDS: GERONTOLOGICAL NURSING PRACTICE

The Standards of Gerontological Nursing Practice are based on the premise that knowledge and theories of the aging process, when applied to nursing practice, will improve the care of the aged. In the practice of gerontological nursing, the nurse must continually question the assumptions upon which gerontological nursing practice is based, retaining those which are valid and searching for and utilizing new knowledge.

The Standards are stated according to a systematic approach to nursing practice—the assessment of the health status of older adults, the plan of nursing actions, the implementation of the plan, and the evaluation. These specific divisions are not intended to imply that practice consists of a series of discrete steps, taken in strict sequence, beginning with assessment and ending with evaluation. The processes described are used concurrently and recurrently. Assessment, for example, frequently continues during implementation; similarly, evaluation dictates reassessment, replanning, and the implementation of the new nursing actions. (Standards: Gerontological Nursing Practice, ANA, 1976, p. 4)

The standards subsume a background knowledge of the present practice of nursing in general, and of the present knowledge concerning gerontology and geriatric nursing. Within the simply stated standards lies a wide range of behavior by nurses which leads to the next steps in the nursing process. These behaviors involve the listening, observing, exploration, and inspection which make up the assessment.

THE CLIENT'S PARTNERSHIP IN ASSESSMENT

Assessment has traditionally been a nursing function, but for the elderly person it is a cooperative function in which the person is an active participant in a process which depends on willing collaboration. Every individual has little secrets, which for reasons best known to him or her must be protected from prying eyes. With the elderly a long life has developed many areas of secrecy, some of shame and embarrassment which cannot be disclosed without threat to self-esteem and integrity. The sharing of information always threatens the disclosure of some of these painful areas; therefore, the assessment must be open and conducted without arousing suspicion of the older person. If there is a need for information, it should be explained. Information which is already available through other sources should not be asked for, nor should unneeded information, or information which cannot be used. This means that an "eyeball" assessment should be made before asking the client to assist with a detailed assessment. The older person who walks briskly to the water cooler for a drink probably answers the question, "How does this person meet survival needs and needs to be safe in a hostile environment?" The assessment process is reduced by the observations which are obvious. On the other hand, such an independent person does not usually ask for nursing care.

FUNCTIONAL ASSESSMENT OF THE ELDERLY PERSON

A number of assessment schemes have been devised. One is the Erickson "head to toe" assessment in which the client is assessed literally from the head down.[1] Other assessments follow

---

[1] Developed at the University of Washington by Roberta Erickson.

systems, with various physiological systems assessed separately. Chapters 21, 23, 26, 29, 30, 31, 32 describe special assessments. Wolanin and Phillips (1980) have developed tools for assessment of the physiological status, interaction with the social and physical environment, special sensory assessment tools, and a tool for developing a sense of the life history of the client. Lantz has developed a tool for an assessment for the beginning of individualized care (Lantz, 1976). Many more have been and are being developed. Each has been created for use in a particular setting by nurses with a known level of competency and skills. Nurses must be comfortable with the assessment tool they use or they will not use the tool creatively. Instead forms become ends in themselves rather than means to ends. Unimaginative routine use of any tool tends to depersonalize the client.

Because each of the assessment schemes mentioned above tends to follow the medical model of disease orientation, the *functional assessment* is proposed here. It looks at clients where they are and their struggle to maintain themselves as whole persons in their environment—independent as far as possible, but accepting help from care givers to supplement their failing resources. It tries to answer the question, "How does this aging person function as a human being?" instead of "How does this diabetic manage self-care?" or "How can we restore function to the hemiplegic left side?" The conceptual framework is holistic—people with fewer and fewer resources attempting to live in their world. Nurses' assessments must be accurate for the nursing diagnosis indicates what must be done to assist the elderly to attain their best state of being.

FANCAPES ASSESSMENT

Assessment is based on the perceptual principle that we see what we look for. In systematic assessment the effort is made to look widely and not only to see the present but to have a knowledge of consequences of some of the phenomena observed and to reduce the possibility of missing data. This requires awareness of high-risk conditions which have the potential of

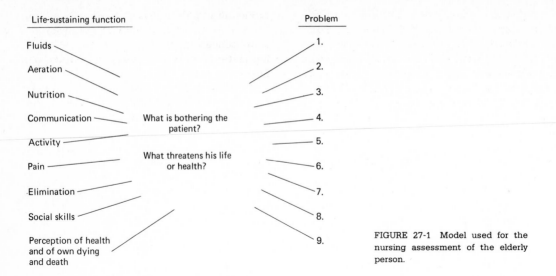

Life-sustaining function	Problem

Fluids

Aeration

Nutrition

Communication

Activity

Pain

Elimination

Social skills

Perception of health and of own dying and death

What is bothering the patient?

What threatens his life or health?

1.
2.
3.
4.
5.
6.
7.
8.
9.

FIGURE 27-1 Model used for the nursing assessment of the elderly person.

becoming problem areas. In the assessment guide below, the assumption is made that each professional nurse has a particular style of assessing. No checklist as such is offered, for checklists have a way of becoming carved in stone and stultifying innovation. Geriatric nurses must look far beyond any checklist, for the perfect list has not yet been created, and they must be able to use their experience to broaden their base of observations. It is assumed that physical assessment skills beyond the basic nursing skills will be integrated into the usual nursing observations.

The overall framework for this functional assessment is based on June Abbey's[2] FAN-CAPES (*f*luids, *a*eration, *n*utrition, *c*ommunication, *a*ctivity, *p*ain, *e*limination, and *s*ocialization or *s*ocial skills). To this the author has added the clients' perception of their own health status and the place of dying and death in their lives. The assessment attempts in each category of

function to ask the two following questions: (1) What is bothering the client? (subjective data), (2) What interferes with the client's health or threatens his or her life? (objective data) (Weed, 1971). Such an assessment should result in a comprehensive view of the way the person functions in the environment (see Figure 27-1).

FLUIDS

Does this person get enough fluids to maintain body processes? High-risk persons include:

- The confused and disoriented.
- Those with neurological deficits, visual problems, or arthritis which prevent ingestion for mechanical reasons.
- Those on large doses of tranquilizers.
- Those who require feeding, tube feedings, or intravenous infusion.
- Alert persons who are incontinent and frequently restrict their fluids.
- Depressed persons; those in crisis or in grief work.
- Those suffering iatrogenic dehydration, as for diagnostic tests or surgery. For the marginally dehydrated, withholding fluids can lead to rapid dehydration.
- Elderly persons on diuretic regimens.
- Elderly persons in high ambient temperatures, especially in areas of hot winds.

[2] The author is indebted to June Abbey, University of Utah, Salt Lake City, for this acronym which forms a simple checklist of systems of functions in the human being. It was first used in 1969 and 1970. Professor Abbey's doctoral dissertation is "FANCAP: A Useful Tool for Teaching Clinical Nursing," University of California, Berkeley, 1977. The reader will note the addition of *E* and *S* to FANCAP.

Adequate intake of fluids for body processes, a vital survival need, is based on a feedback system which is usually recognized as thirst. Oversedation or mechanical problems may prevent this feedback system from responding properly. Fluids may simply not be accessible to chair or bedbound persons, and lack of mobility may make such persons dependent on others to recognize and maintain their fluid intake. Dehydration may come about over a long time in such cases, but when a critical point is reached, it is only second to the need for aeration for survival. Rapid dehydration is reached in any situation preventing fluid intake or involving loss of body fluid through vomiting, diarrhea, diuresis, or burns. The aging person who has a subclinical state of chronic fluid deficit is vulnerable, and remediable action should be taken before an acute situation exists.

Assessment includes the appearance of the elderly person: the dryness of the lips and conjunctiva, the thickness of speech which occurs with a dry mouth. Skin can rarely be used as a criterion because dryness often occurs from other causes. But the loss of fluid in the periorbital areas leads to an appearance of "sunken eyeballs."

Inspection and Observation

- Amount of moisture in mouth, critical area being under the tongue (note medications which leave mouth dry)
- Concentration of urine quantity, color, and specific gravity
- Mushiness of eyeballs when pressed gently between thumb and finger over the eyelid
- Tenting of skin over back of hand (a fold of skin remaining when skin is picked up between examiner's thumb and forefinger)
- Prescribed medications: tranquilizers, diuretics, and sedatives
- Restriction of fluid for reasons of diagnostic tests, pathology, or surgery
- Mechanical ability to express thirst, or to obtain own fluid
- Ability to swallow

Base-Line Information

- Evidence of saliva under tongue, skin turgor, eyeball tension

- Intake and output of fluids
- Urinalysis or appearance of urine which indicates concentration
- Estimate of person's ability to obtain own fluids:
  - Mechanical (neuromuscular): Joint and visual impediments
  - Psychosocial: Depression, confusion, crisis state, and grief
- Medications which dehydrate or lead to dehydration by sedating
- Conjunctival moisture
- Periorbital hydration

AERATION

How does the client perform gas exchange? Does dyspnea interfere with the ability to function? High-risk persons are those who:

- Are bedfast or immobile
- Have congestive heart failure
- Have emphysematous disease
- Have a pulmonary infection
- Have problems in swallowing or coughing
- Have a weakness in the chest muscles
- Make sudden change in altitude
- Are kyphotic with the chest cage rigid and altered in its dimensions and expansion
- Are anemic, i.e., lack red blood cells or hemoglobin for oxygen transport

Oxygen is the first necessity of life at any age. The dramatic episodes, when need for oxygen becomes critical, are found in the aging person as in all persons and are as important to recognize. Sudden obstruction of the airway is always an emergency, and food lodged in the windpipe is being increasingly blamed in sudden deaths while eating. The elderly who have weakness in the muscles used for swallowing are particularly vulnerable. But in the elderly, the effects of aging, disease, and environmental factors, such as smoking and industrial fumes, may lead to a more chronic and insidious loss of ability to perform gaseous exchange. Chebotarev et al. (1974) made observations on 308 essentially healthy subjects 20 to 90 years of age. The elderly and old subjects showed diminished vital lung capacity, at the expense of all its component volumes: increased residual volume, decreased ventilation effectiveness, decreased bronchial patency, bronchospasm, decreased filling of the lung with blood, reduced elasticity and increased rigidity of pulmonary vessels, and disturbed uniformity of pulmonary ventilation. Arterial blood oxygen saturation was reduced. For the nurse, then, the essential question is: Does this person have adequate gaseous exchange?

Oxygen lack is not a cumulative response; it is usually situational and expressed by dyspnea on exertion. Base-line information must include the amount of exertion which does not cause dyspnea. Unfortunately, this is measured by having clients reach the point of dyspnea and subtracting. Can the clients speak entire phrases without stopping to "catch a breath"? Have they limited their speech to short sentences and phrases only? Can they walk across a level surface, and how far? Can they climb steps, and how many? This estimation of oxygen need takes a little observation but is paramount in planning care and detecting change.

Part of the health assessment of the elderly person includes the drugs which maintain health. (See Chapter 24, "Drugs and the Aged.") Digoxin is the sixth most frequently prescribed drug for the elderly, and heart disease is the third-ranking problem (17 in 100 persons) according to a 1966 task force study (Lofholm, 1973). This frequency alerts the nurse to the need to assess the cardiorespiratory status of the client and to maintain careful records. Especially important are inspection and observation. Inspection is the carefully planned systematic examination which uses physical examination and instruments such as the stethoscope and other monitoring devices. (See Chapter 18, "Cardiopulmonary Abnormalities in Aging.")

Inspection and Observation

- Resting pattern of breathing and resting rate of respiration
- Dyspnea on exertion—talking, movement
- Auscultation of the chest for chest sounds
- Cough and ability to cough
- Depth of respiration
- Edema in abdominal area, dependent areas, and measurement of abdominal girth
- Appearance of any cyanosis

- Ability to lie flat
- Maintenance medications and emergency medications
- Ability to blow out a candle, a simple test of respiratory function
- Drugs which depress the respiratory centers
- Kyphosis
- All laboratory studies

Base-Line Information

- Rate and pattern of respiration at rest and on various degrees of exertion during activity appropriate to life-style and needs of the client
- Chest sounds
- Observation of cough and swallowing
- Medications for maintenance and for emergency: reaction and efficacy
- Medications which depress the respiratory center
- Changes in chest cage: kyphosis—rigidity

NUTRITION

How does this client meet nutritional needs? High-risk persons are those with specific problems and whose nutritional needs may not be met. (See Chapter 23 for a further discussion of nutrition assessment.)

COMMUNICATION

Can this person communicate sufficiently to meet physical needs? Sufficiently to have a meaningful relationship with another? High-risk persons are those who have:

1. Mechanical problems
   a. Aphasia, both receptive and expressive
   b. Neurological deficits (parkinsonism, multiple sclerosis)
   c. Laryngectomy
   d. Oversedation
   e. Dehydration
   f. Recent blindness or deafness
2. Psychosocial and cultural problems
   a. Depression
   b. Confusion
   c. Language barriers
   d. Cultural barriers (age is a cultural barrier)
   e. Crisis state

After the survival needs of air, fluids, and nutrition, the need to communicate is the most important in the human hierarchy. It probably forms the thin line that separates the person from the nonperson. Self-esteem is based on meaningful communication on a verbal and nonverbal level (Kazmierczak, 1975, p. 21). Intangibles, such as trust, are part of communication, and the continuous process of self-identity depends on them. The original assessment must include an estimate of the elderly person's ability to communicate which is stated clearly in the base-line information of the record.

Inspection and Observation

1. Mechanical
   a. Hearing acuity and prosthesis, if any
   b. Quality of voice: weakness or hoarseness
   c. Visual acuity and prosthesis, if any
   d. Ability to read and write
   e. Mouth inspection (presence of teeth; tongue strength)
   f. Dyspnea
2. Psychosocial
   a. Response to verbal communication
   b. Alertness or depression
   c. Evidence of confusion, disorientation or incoherence
   d. Language barriers

Base-line information includes all the above plus an estimate of the clients' ability to maintain their hearing aids or to clean their glasses.

ACTIVITY

What prevents this person from taking responsibility for self-care needs? What prevents the activity which is necessary to maintain his or her physiology? High-risk persons are those elderly who have:

- Osteoarthritis and other arthritic conditions.
- Neurological deficits.
- Fractures.
- Feet with arthritic spurs, calluses, plantar warts, elongated toenails, and other deformities. (Every person over the age of 60 is suspect for some foot problem. See Chapter 21, "Foot Problems and Assessment.")
- Malnutrition.

- Neuropathies (diabetic or pernicious anemia, alcoholism).
- Diminished vision.
- Apathy or depression.

The first question to ask oneself is, Does this person use his or her body to the fullest extent possible? Major limitations in the face of comparatively minor disability are more frequently the result of withdrawal or depression. The next question is, Can this person manage the activities of daily living? Storz (1972) has listed five categories of daily living:

1. Self-care, including bathing, toileting, grooming, and dressing
2. Mobility, including sitting, standing, walking, climbing stairs, dialing a phone, picking up objects from the floor, writing with a pencil, opening doors
3. Eating, including managing food on a plate, shopping, and preparing food
4. Housekeeping, including making a bed, washing dishes, cleaning the refrigerator and bathroom, and vacuuming carpets
5. Behavioral disabilities, including wandering, panic, and signs of deterioration such as incontinence and poor self-care

The second question is usually related (after depression) to loss of functioning in some part of the skeletal and/or neurological system. Three important variables enter into assessment; two are recency of loss of function and dominance of the affected side. The greatest disabilities are those which involve disruption of learned patterns of coordination, such as use of the hands and use of the lower extremities in standing and walking (Wolanin, 1974). The third variable relates to cumulation of motor losses. One loss at a time, with assistance in adaptation before the next loss, may prevent the devastation which occurs with cumulative losses without adequate time lapses. How fast has this person lost mobility? A massive stroke is a sudden event, after which the person may be faced with a loss of the dominant side and the ability to communicate. How many motor losses have occurred? How fast?

Motor losses form a hierarchy, with the greatest loss being that of speech and swallowing, followed by loss of the use of the dominant hand, the dominant arm and shoulder, the dominant leg and foot, the nondominant hand, the nondominant arm and shoulder, and the nondominant leg and foot. Since losses rarely occur in single motor units, losses are invariably multiple and complex.

Gait Problems The most revealing sign of impending or established mobility problems is shown by the loss of the springy step of youth and its replacement by the wide-based shuffling gait of the elderly. See Chapter 21 for more on gait assessment.

Osteoporosis Osteoporosis is an important problem of older persons, men as well as women. Approximately 25 percent of all white women over the age of 60 have spinal compression fractures due to osteoporosis, and the risk of hip fractures is at least 20 percent by the age of 90. Coupled with this fact is that one-sixth of all hip fracture patients die within 3 months of injury (Heaney, 1973). Of those who do not die, this event may be the fork in the road which leads to future immobility and possible institutionalization. All skeletal bones are affected by osteoporosis, and a history of fracture is an indication that the process has occurred. Fractures of the forearm, the ribs, and the hip are the most common. (See Chapters 3 and 20 for further discussions of osteoporosis.)

Kyphosis, which is the mark of the compression fracture, leads to a gait change which frequently is noted by a wider base and head-down walking position. The center of gravity has been changed with the new alignment of the spine; the greater the kyphosis, the greater the alteration from the earlier posture. The kyphosis may be so great that the lower ribs will rest on the pelvis. Inspection reveals this problem, and history alerts. Mobility assessment is preventive as well as descriptive. Recognition of osteoporosis should set into motion safety precautions which may prevent fractures.

Inspection and Observation Check for a history of losses and note sequences of losses. Motor abilities are shown by:

- Strength of dominant hand in clasping.
- Ability to oppose thumb and forefinger or another finger (writing, eating).
- Wrist motion, which must be sufficient to handle tools for eating.
- Coordinated movements of both hands for work.
- Strength of shoulder muscles (ability to raise arms in purposeful activity such as combing or shampooing hair).
- Resistance force of biceps and triceps in lifting.
- Ability to turn head from side to side. Note angle of turn.
- Quadriceps strength as shown by walking or tightening when lying supine.
- Ability to rise from chair, bed, or toilet.
- Use of assistive devices: walker, wheelchair, crutches, cane, braces.
- Swallowing ability (see "Nutrition" above).
- Nutritional assessment and history.
- Foot condition (stress and pressure areas indicated by callus formation, spurs, ulcers, and varicosities).
- Loss of sensation.
- Ability to turn body in bed.
- Gait assessment.
- Pain with walking.

Base-Line Information

- Function as shown by normal extremities or parts
- Degree of loss of function in any joint as shown by angle of extension and flexion; pedal pulses; varicosities
- Description of condition of feet and legs, including sensory ability
- Pedal pulses; anterior tibial pulses; varicosities
- Pressure areas; skeletal changes which impede walking
- Gait and use of prosthesis
- Dominant-hand function
- Ability to perform activities of daily living

PAIN

Is this person in discomfort or pain? Does the pain interfere with the ability to function? Does lack of pain prevent safety? High-risk persons in relation to pain include:

- Diabetic patients with neuropathy (pain is a warning of danger)
- Those with neurological deficits involving loss of sensation or pain
- Aphasics who cannot express pain
- The overtranquilized, sedated, or comatose person
- Persons in personal crisis, anxiety, and fear
- Those with long-term disabilities such as arthritis

Human experiences described as painful seem to have three factors: (1) a breach in the protective barrier or wholesomeness of the person, (2) a signal that warns of danger, (3) an unpleasantness (McCaffery, 1972). Pain may not only be physical according to the above conceptualization, but may include the painful affects, or emotional experiences such as grief and mourning, fear, anxiety, and guilt (McCaffery, 1972). The person in crisis or panic because of being unable to cope with a threatening situation is in pain. For the older person with reduced resources, threatening situations loom large. Coping mechanisms which operated smoothly in earlier years may fail. Such a person may be completely disorganized in thought and actions and present bizarre behavior. Early recognition of both panic states and situations leading to panic states can lead to crisis intervention which can prevent permanent damage.

Pain is primary. Until it is relieved, no person functions adequately. But pain in the elderly takes on changed characteristics. It may be a myth that the elderly do not feel pain with the same intensity as the younger person, but the elderly endure pressure from sitting or lying, and even from fractures of bones, with an equanimity which deserves research. Two questions must be asked: Do elderly persons perceive themselves as having pain or discomfort? Does the external appearance of the client lead to the assumption that a painful condition exists? The diabetic who does not feel the pebble in a shoe or a wrinkled stocking sole may quickly develop an ulcer without being aware.

Pressure sores develop which would appear to cause pain, yet the patient does not complain.

On the other hand, pain is personal and cannot be validated except through testimony and certain physiological and physical signs. Some older persons use pain as a means of getting the recognition not given to them unless they complain. This represents mental pain.

Inspection and Observation

1. Physical pressure, discomfort, and pain
   a. Signs of pressure over bony prominences, especially the sacroiliac tuberosities, acetabula, heels, and feet
   b. Patient's perception of the pain
   c. Customary mode of relieving pain
   d. External examination of any area pinpointed as painful by patient
   e. Joint stiffness or guarding of joints
   f. Presence of decubiti
2. Mental pain or discomfort
   a. Disorganization of thoughts and incoherent speech
   b. History of recent loss
   c. Inability to concentrate on answers
   d. Overt symptoms of anxiety

Base-Line Information

- Description of pain: location, frequency, intensity and actions which bring relief
- Alteration of normal skin appearance or of normal conformation of the musculoskeletal system; presence of swelling
- Areas of reduced sensory perception
- Objective signs of mental pain: the elderly person's statement of the condition

ELIMINATION

Is this person able to care for elimination needs without assistance? High-risk persons who may have problems in this area include those with:

Urinary Problems

- Older women with cystocele (especially women who have borne children)
- Older men with prostate problems

- Persons with urinary tract infections
- Persons with diabetes or other neurological deficits
- Persons with reduced mobility (arthritic or neurological deficit)
- Persons who are forgetful, confused, and disoriented
- Posttransurethral resection in men
- Patients with renal insufficiency or bladder infections

Bowel Problems

- Persons with hemorrhoids
- Persons who have always taken laxatives
- Persons with reduced food intake
- Persons with change in diet (less fresh fruit and vegetables)
- The confused and disoriented person
- The dehydrated person

A study made of older persons who were institutionalized, rather than kept in their own homes where a spouse or relative could care for them, found that the deciding factor was usually incontinence. Aberrant behavior such as confusion and poor judgment could be tolerated, but incontinence of urine and feces were not (Underwood, 1973). Problems with elimination are cited, with the problem of confusion, as being the two most common ones of the aged; in some respects, they determine the line at which the aged decide they have lost control over their lives.

Elimination is an hourly and daily necessity. The inability of natural systems to function requires intervention, and various intrusive procedures are used to aid defecation and bladder emptying. These very procedures are the warning signs to the elderly that their resources are failing or have failed and that they are dependent on others for this most basic self-care. Self-respect is highly correlated with ability to control one's excretions.

VIGNETTE 2

The retired oil company executive had surgery which required indwelling catheter and bladder irrigations. Although he had private-duty nurses and privacy, his one conclusion from the entire process was,

"They will never get my pants off me again."

A thorough nursing assessment guide for urinary continence management can be found in Table 36-1, and so it will not be covered in this chapter.

Regarding defecation, the assessment questions should center around how the person maintains a lifetime pattern of elimination and what barriers prevent it.

Mechanical Problems

- Is the elderly person alert enough to take care of toileting needs (overmedicated)?
- What is the pattern of voiding and defecation?
- Are there signs of impaction, diarrhea, or hemorrhoids?
- Are there assistive devices such as colostomy appliances?
- If the client is confined to a wheelchair, has he or she mastered transfer to the toilet or commode?

Social Problems

- Does the client speak the same language as the care giver, both from the standpoint of language itself and of colloquialisms?
- Is the client frightened and insecure with relocation and/or other stress?
- Have drugs been given which alter either voiding patterns or intestinal peristalsis?
- Does the elderly person require privacy which is not available in the present setting?
- Is the client confused and disoriented?
- What terminology does the client use for defecating?

Inspection and Observation

- Rectal inspection (digital examination, if indicated).
- What is the usual bowel and bladder routine for this person?
- What methods does the client use for bowel regulation?
- Medication profile.
- State of alertness and orientation.
- Mobility.

- Character of stools.
- Assistive devices or surgical alterations.
- Ability to care for own toileting.
- Evidence of concern about elimination.
- Blood urea nitrogen (BUN) and creatinine clearance tests, if available.

Base-Line Information

- Bowel pattern: methods patient uses to regulate function
- Assistive devices (colostomy)
- Client's evidence of concern over elimination
- Estimate of person's ability to care for own toileting
- Estimate of ability to care for assistive devices
- Incontinence of urine or stool
- Output in relation to intake

SOCIALIZATION OR SOCIAL SKILLS

Can this person negotiate a way through the "system"? Is this person able to give and receive love and friendship? Is there a meaningful person in his or her life? High-risk persons are those who have:

- Neurological deficits which prevent mobility and/or verbal communication
- Depression
- Hearing and visual deficits
- Loss of mobility
- Relocation from a familiar setting to an unfamiliar one
- Altered life-style which they have not chosen
- Loss of sexual orientation (the homosexual male in the all-female environment of the nursing home or hospital)

Relationships with other humans and pets separate the person from the nonperson. Bennett and Nahemow (1972) studied the socialization and social adjustments in five residential settings for the elderly which they graded as total institutions after Goffman (1961) in diminishing order: state hospital, nursing home, home for the aged (institution), home for the aged (apartments), and a public housing project. Socialization was inversely related to the totality

of the institution. This was not related to social adjustment. Goldfarb (1972) describes the decreased life expectancy of the elderly who enter homes for the aged. The findings were that once older persons become acclimated to an institution and regain a sense of security, they should not be transferred again. The problem of relocation is usually one in which questions asked at the beginning of this subsection must be answered negatively, but it need not be (Wolanin, 1978). Loss of significant relationships which are not replaced, inability to acquire socialization into the system, and decreased opportunities to practice social skills can lead to lack of self-esteem and confidence. Behavioral changes involve aggression and withdrawal.

With the recognition that at least 10 percent of our population has a sexual orientation as homosexual persons, grave problems of lack of understanding arise from a critical and often judgmental health care system. Elderly persons without a family are often denied access to the caring person in their life. Institutional staff tend to be female from the front office back. Is there a broad acceptance of differing life-styles so that the loving relationships which have been developed over the years can be continued? Are ties respected? In the highly sex-segregated occupational field of caring for the aged, this fact deserves careful consideration. Almost no studies have been done in this field, but nurses should begin to observe the special needs that will assist the aging homosexual during the final stages of life. (See "Assessment" in Chapter 26.)

Inspection and Observation

- What is the ability to interact with the care giver on a give-and-take level?
- What sensory deficits make socialization difficult or impossible?
- Is the elderly person confused (sensory overload)?
- Is the elderly person withdrawn and depressed?
- What is the history of the person's life-style?
- What is known of the person's life history? To what extent have illness or incapacity removed the person from his or her life history?
- Is the client able to interact with the peer group?

- Who is the peer group?
- What is the history of recent losses (especially losses which diminish a positive self-concept)?

Base-Line Information

- What is the social orientation (family, work, church, other)?
- What is the mobility status?
- What sensory losses prevent interaction?
- Who is the "family" of this person—man, woman, pet?
- What are the responses to culturally approved gestures of friendship such as a handshake, greeting, or request for help?

DYING AND DEATH

Does this person see his or her health status as life-threatening? Is this person concerned with preparation for death at this time or with dying? High-risk elderly persons include:

- The elderly person who is alone and who has lost family and friends through death.
- The elderly person with changes in body function marked either by pain or weakness, or by change in body structure (Esberger, 1978, p. 37).
- The elderly person who has evidence of terminal illness.
- The person working toward a self-determined death either by intentional or subconscious means. This area is well discussed by Burnside in Chapter 12, "Suicide in the Aged Person" and is also covered in Chapter 39, "The Dying Aged Person."

Observation   Does the patient show signs of thinking of dying and death and wishing to discuss them? Which of these four questions is being asked:

1. Is this my approaching death?
2. Will I be cared for during my dying?
3. What is it like to die?
4. Will you be honest with me?

Is this person talking of dying?

Base-Line Information

- The client's covert or overt references to death.
- The client's relationship with at least one other trusted person: family, friend, or a staff member.
- Preparations, if any, which a person has made for death.
- The patient's self-assessment of health.
- Is there evidence that this person is taking means to determine the time and place of death either by intentional or subconscious acts?

ASSESSMENT OF THE ENVIRONMENT

Many elderly persons live in the same home and the same neighborhood in which they have always lived, but others have been forced to find new and strange surroundings, such as retirement villages, special housing for the aged, boarding homes, homes with other members of the family, and finally a special residence for protective care such as a nursing home.

VIGNETTE 3
   The 89-year-old woman surveyed the city apartment in which she lived after two moves from the Kansas farm which she had operated herself, riding cultivators and planting and harvesting wheat and corn. "Every time I move I lose something," she summed it all up.

Actually she had lost something before each move, and the loss had forced the change to a more protective and easier environment, but each change in location brings losses of the familiar and often results in loss of control over the aging person's life-style. Sommer (1973) described "hard architecture" of airports, nursing homes, hospitals, etc., as "designed to be strong and resistant to human imprint." To the inhabitant, it seems impervious, impersonal, and inorganic—built so the user cannot deface or destroy. Passive adjustment and psychological withdrawal are encouraged.

In assessing the space around the person, the first questions should be: To what extent does it represent this person and his or her lifestyle, and what is a compromise with a socioeconomic system which the person cannot change? What in the surroundings maintains the elderly person's identity? Are clothes those of his or her selection? Is there one memento that links the person to history, or was the past sacrificed to the restricted space of the present (Allekian, 1973) or to the institutional need to reduce clutter? The environment should be thought of as extending as far as the person who is being assessed needs to go. If that person has banking, food-stamp-buying, grocery-shopping, laundry, and transportation needs, these become inhibiting factors in maintaining independence when the community is planned for the younger person who is mobile and can make rapid adaptations. The fine print of the inserts in medical preparations or on Medicare blanks reduces the ability to control one's own life. As shoulder strength decreases, carrying a bag of groceries in the arms changes to using a shopping bag and decreasing the weight of the contents. Curbs and high bus steps decrease mobility.

The assessment of the environment should answer two questions:

1. What in the environment reduces a person's ability to function as a human being?
2. What can be changed to increase the capacity of the older person to maintain or increase functional ability and control?

The environment should be assessed in relation to the variables of architectural features, furniture arrangement, lighting, ventilation and climate control, and location and design of sleeping, eating, and recreational spaces. Chapters 31 and 32 will include some of the salient points to be assessed.

The Wheelchair For the incapacitated elderly person the wheelchair is "home," and it deserves a special assessment. It has a surface which provides the least possible friction when it is being moved. Is the floor covered with a surfacing that interferes with movement: shag rugs or several varying textures or colors of covering? Are various sizes of chairs available—a chair for the tiny person as well as for the tall? Are chairs deep-cushioned, requiring increased leverage for rising? Are chair arms spaced so as to give maximum leverage when the arms are used? All chairs should be fitted to the user.

VIGNETTE 4

The nursing home administrator spoke with authority: "I buy only one size of wheelchair. After all, it is only transportation." The student who was studying wheelchairs and their occupants was astounded. "Doesn't he realize these people live in their wheelchairs?"

Wheelchairs can fit as well as a well-designed shoe and increase function, or by their inhibiting design retard the mobility of the older person. The height of the arm may provide rest and leverage or may be too high in relation to the skeletal dimensions of the occupant.

The acute angle of the knee caused when a long-legged person is forced into a short leg space leads to impeded circulation and edema. The older person sleeping with the head pushed forward on the chest indicates a lack of total-body support. Beds are for rest and sleeping; a wheelchair should be designed to allow for greater activity and mobility. The tiny, frail, 75-pound woman may be more comfortable in a child's wheelchair in which the width of the seat and the proportions more nearly fit her own skeletal conformation.

Fitzgerald (1975) and Snyder (1975) have each looked at the wheelchair as an extension of the person which must be fitted exactly, with Snyder calling it "living space" and Fitzgerald referring to wheelchairs as "ambulation without legs."

Social Environment In assessing the social environment, the relationship of family and staff to the individual outweighs even physical arrangements in importance. Such books as Curtin's *Nobody Ever Died of Old Age* (1972) and Mendelsohn's *Tender Loving Greed* (1974) emphasize the necessity of the older person's maintaining relationships with other people. Both demonstrate that in any setting the older person needs at least one caring person who offers love and who will receive love when it is offered. While nurses recognize these needs, they often do not act upon them (Putnam, 1973).

Human Interaction   Some of the real tragedies of the aged occur when those who have shared their lives pass beyond sharing, either through death or distance. Life history gives identity to the individual, and the aged need someone who knew them as persons throughout their life-span in order to capitalize on the events which gave the greatest pleasure and self-esteem. Scrapbooks, pictures, and reminiscence help. (See Chapter 8 for more on reminiscing.) Human interaction is the real key, provided it is empathic and meaningful. Part of the reality is human, and the responses of other humans are the mirror in which each person defines body image and identity. *Professional helpers have the process of human identity in their hands, shaping it from moment to moment, for identity is a continuing process, never finished.* Many chapters in this book stress the quality of human interaction in the environment of the elderly.

ASSESSMENT OF ABILITY TO ADAPT TO ENVIRONMENT

Looking at people *in their environments* constitutes a relatively new approach to the study of the biopsychosocial person. Much research has blotted out the environmental component (Patnaik et al., 1974), but it can no longer be disregarded for a person is an open system, continuous with the environment rather than contiguous to it (Putt, 1978).

The *environment* is the reality with which people live and through which they view their world. The systematic approach to assessment which uses the framework of humans functioning in their environment should lead to answering the following questions about elderly individuals. This outline offers a means to planning how to meet the needs which the elderly cannot meet themselves.

1. How does this person meet survival needs—aeration, hydration, nutrition, and elimination?

   a. To what extent is he or she dependent upon others for assistance?

2. How does this person meet needs to be safe in a hostile environment? (It is assumed that any environment furnishes some threat to the individual—thermal, traumatic, and/or deprivation of necessary life components and human interaction and support.)

   a. What are the person's physical and social activity range and communication skill?

3. How does this person meet the need to feel confident as a person—maintain self-esteem?

   a. Can the person negotiate his or her way through the social world?

   b. Does the person have communication ability to relate to others?

4. How does this person relate to others; can this person give and accept love?

   a. Is it necessary for the person to withdraw into a fantasy life and reminiscence in order to people the world?

5. Is death a part of his or her daily thinking? Is this person making preparations for closing out his or her life?

   a. To what extent does this person need others to assist in readiness for a "good death"?

   b. What is this person's perception of his or her health?

Sensoriperceptual Contact with Environment   Everyone is limited by perceptual abilities which, in turn, are limited by the sensory organs. Few who are aging escape diminished vision, hearing, taste, smell, touch, and/or equilibrium (Timiras, 1972). Some failing sense organs can be extended by means of prostheses in order to retain contact with the real world, but when touch, taste, and smell are blunted, they become losses. One of the first questions any person working with the aging should try to answer is the extent to which they can sense the real world. (See Chapters 33 and 34 for discussions of senses, blindness, and sensory deprivation.)

In *Standards for Geriatric Nursing Practice* (1970), Standard VIII states, "The nurse together with the older person designs, changes or adapts the physical and psychosocial environment to meet his needs within the limitations imposed by the situation." And as Standard IX reminds the practitioner, "The nurse assists older persons to obtain and utilize devices which help them attain a higher level of function and ensures that these devices are kept in good working order by appropriate persons or agencies."

In assessing the adaptation of the environment to the person, and the person to the environment, a highly individualized process takes place, requiring many different skills. Essentially the first is recognizing the problem as existing on two levels: sensory deprivation and sensory overload (Chodil and Williams, 1970; Downs, 1974). Sensory deprivation becomes greater as increasing numbers of sensory systems are involved. (See Chapter 34 regarding sensory deprivation.) The person with limited vision and hearing is at greater risk than the person with total loss of one but relatively good functioning of the other. Each successive loss has a multiplier effect on ability to keep in touch with reality rather than an additive effect. If this reality includes other persons, interaction proceeds on each person's version of reality. The person with the limited sensoriperceptual apparatus, responding to what is very real to him or her, presents a picture of bizarre and confused behavior to the care giver, which may result in the label "confused and disoriented." Is the older person "confused and disoriented" or reacting to the only reality he or she knows? There can be no answer unless the sensoriperceptual limitations are taken into account (Wolanin and Phillips 1980).

Rapid changes in reality orientation are found in younger persons (Downs, 1974) under sensory deprivation research conditions, but they are everyday occurrences within institutional walls, or with persons having sensoriperceptual loss.

THE NURSING DIAGNOSIS

The nursing diagnosis is a statement of the conclusions of the nurse who has assessed the functioning ability of the patient, the barriers and assets in the environment, and finally the patient's interaction with the social and physical environment. It is based on the systematic collection of facts which are analysed according to nursing's own conceptual framework: in this case, the whole of human beings in their world. The collection of facts is dependent upon the skill, knowledge, and attitudes of the nurse. Attitudes relate positively to behaviors, and what nurses believe about using assessment and about working with the elderly will color what they see and their conclusions. Nursing is not such an exact science that two nurses can take the same data base and reach the same conclusions. But the nursing process is the best guide to nursing practice at this time when the standards used are based on consensus of the best nurses we now have.

The medical diagnosis will be a disease entity which will be included in the nursing assessment and will add one more framework on which to build data collection. For example, for the patient with the medical diagnosis of "diabetes mellitus, adult onset type," the nursing diagnosis will describe to what extent the patient knows the meaning of the diagnosis and its implications. There will be a clear statement about the ability to see his world around him—the knowledge that diabetic retinopathy may be a problem. The nurse will include a statement about the ability to carry out therapeutic self-care and the teaching needs in relation to monitoring the condition and planning and preparing a prescribed diet. The condition of the feet will have been assessed, and the statement will include the ability of the patient to see his or her feet and the teaching needs for patient and family in relation to foot care. The nurse will also include a statement as to whether there is a neuropathy which results in incontinence or sexual problems. The nursing diagnosis will contain the nurse's estimate of what a nurse needs to do to enable this patient to live in his or her own world with this disease.

The medical treatment will consist of regular monitoring of the effect of the prescribed treatment. The nursing intervention will be designed to ensure that the patient can function to the highest level as a human being even with diabetes. The goals are different—the nurse's goal is to assist the patient to live life to its fullest as far as nursing intervention can help. A good nursing diagnosis is prescriptive as well as descriptive. The nearly blind diabetic person must be supplied a world in which to function with little vision. Such a person will require teaching, and the nursing staff and family will require alteration in their approach to care. If the person is incontinent, the physical and social implications become central to planning for his or her functioning.

SUMMARY

The nursing process has been used as an approach to giving nursing care with a systematic assessment built around the functions of humans living in their world. The functional assessment is built around the FANCAPES framework devised by June Abbey and based on Maslow's hierarchy of human needs.

Emphasis has been placed on the predictive abilities of the nurse. The concept of high-risk elderly is used to alert and to place into motion the preventive measures which prediction allows. The conclusions which are drawn from the assessment and analysis of its findings are stated in the nursing diagnosis.

REFERENCES

Allekian, Constance I.: Intrusions of territory and personal space, *Nursing Research,* **22**(3):237–237, May–June, 1973.

Bennett, Ruth, and Lucille Nahemow: Socialization and social adjustment in five residential settings for the aged, in Donald P. Kent et al. (eds.), *Research, Planning and Action for the Elderly,* Behavioral Publications, New York, 1972, pp. 514–525.

Carrieri, Virginia K., and Judith Sitzman: Component of the nursing process, *Nursing Clinics of North America,* **6**(1):115–124, March 1971.

Chebotarev, D. F., O. V. Korkushko, and L. A. Ivanov: Mechanisms of hypoxemia in the elderly, *Journal of Gerontology,* **29**(4):393–400, July 1974.

Chodil, Judith, and Barbara Williams: The concept of sensory deprivation, *Nursing Clinics of North America,* **5**:453–465, 1970.

Corbus, H. F., et al.: The problem-oriented medical record in long term care facilities. A teaching method, *Journal of Gerontological Nursing,* **3**(4):24–29, July–August 1977.

Curtin, Sharon: *Nobody Ever Died of Old Age,* Monthly Press Book, Little, Brown, Boston, 1972.

Downs, Florence S.: Bed rest and sensory disturbances, *American Journal of Nursing,* **74**(3):434–438, March 1974.

Esberger, Karen: Body image, *Journal of Gerontological Nursing,* **4**(4):35–38, July–August 1978.

Fitzgerald, Alice M.: Ambulation without legs, *Journal of Gerontological Nursing,* **1**(3):12–16, July–August 1975.

Goffman, Erving: *Asylums,* Anchor Books, Doubleday, Garden City, N.Y., 1961.

Goldfarb, Alvin I.: Death rate of relocated nursing home residents, in Donald P. Kent (ed.), *Research, Planning and Action for the Elderly,* Behavioral Publications, New York, 1972.

Griffith, Elizabeth W.: Nursing process: A patient with respiratory dysfunction, *Nursing Clinics of North America,* **6**(1):145–154, March 1971.

Heaney, Robert P.: Menopausal effects on calcium homeostasis and skeletal metabolism, in Kenneth J. Ryan and Don C. Gibson (eds.), *Menopause and Aging,* Department of Health, Education, and Welfare, Publication (NIH) 73-319, 1973.

Henderson, Virginia: The nature of nursing: V, *American Journal of Nursing,* **64**(8):62–68, August 1964.

Kazmierczak, Frances G., et al.: Communication problems encountered when caring for the elderly, *Journal of Gerontological Nursing,* **1**(1):21–27, March–April 1975.

Lantz, John: Assessment: A beginning to individualized care, *Journal of Gerontological Nursing,* **2**(6):34–40, November–December 1976.

Little, Dolores E., and Doris Carnevali: *Nursing Care Planning,* Lippincott, Philadelphia, 1969.

Lofholm, Paul: Self-medication by the elderly, in Richard H. Davis (ed.), *Drugs and the Elderly,* Andrus Gerontology Center, University of Southern California, Los Angeles, 1973.

McCaffery, Margo: *Nursing Management of the Patient with Pain,* Lippincott, Philadelphia, 1972.

Maslow, Abraham: *Toward a Psychology of Being,* Van Nostrand, Princeton, N.J., 1962.

Mendelsohn, Mary Adelaide: *Tender Loving Greed,* Knopf, New York, 1974.

Orlando, Ida J.: *The Dynamic Nurse-Patient Relationship,* Little, Brown, Boston, 1961.

Patnaik, Beverly, et al.: Behavioral adaptation to change in institutional residence, *Gerontologist,* **14**(4):305–307, August 1974.

Putnam, Phyllis A.: Nurse awareness and psychosocial function in the aged, *Gerontologist,* **13**(2):63–166, 1973.

Putt, Arlene M.: *General Systems Theory Applied to Nursing,* Little, Brown, Boston, 1978.

Snyder, Lorraine Hiatt: Living environments, Geriatric wheel chairs and older person's rehabilitation, *Journal of Gerontological Nursing,* **1**(5):17–25, November–December 1975.

Sommer, Robert: *Tight Places: Hard Architecture and How to Humanize It,* Prentice-Hall, Englewood Cliffs, N.J., 1973.

Standards for Geriatric Nursing Practice, American Journal of Nursing, 1970 (pamphlet).

Standards: Gerontological Nursing Practice, American Nurses' Association, Kansas City, Mo., 1976, p. 4.

Storz, Rita R.: The role of a professional nurse in a health maintenance program, *Nursing Clinics of North America,* **7**(2):207–223, June 1972.

Timiras, P. S.: *Developmental Physiology and Aging,* University of California Press, Berkeley, 1972.

Underwood, Billye: Evaluation of the area wide project: Tucson, Arizona, unpublished study at the Pima Council of Aging, Tucson, 1973.

Weed, L. L.: *Medical Records, Medical Education and Patient Care,* Year Book, Chicago, 1971.

Wolanin, Mary Opal: Process criterion vs. impact criterion to measure quality of care in nursing homes, *Proceedings of the First North American Symposium on Long Term Care,* Toronto, July 27–31, 1975. Published by American College of Nursing Home Administrators, Washington.

———: Rehabilitation in non-life threatening conditions, in Victor Christopherson, Pearl Parvin Coulter, and Mary Opal Wolanin (eds.), *Rehabilitation Nursing,* McGraw-Hill, New York, 1974.

———: Relocation of the elderly, *Journal of Gerontological Nursing,* **4**(3):47–50, May–June 1978.

——— **and Linda F. Phillips:** *Confusion and the Elderly,* Mosby, St. Louis, 1980.

TWENTY-EIGHT

NURSING INTERVENTION AND EVALUATION

Mary Opal Wolanin

At least once in a lifetime everyone is called upon to muster all that he knows in the solution of a single problem.
Oliver Wendell Holmes

LEARNING OBJECTIVES

- Analyze the goal-setting process and the evaluation of care as related to performance of objectives.
- Describe why prediction is an expert nursing skill.
- List examples of prediction which increase preventive nursing intervention.
- Analyze critically the evaluation criteria commonly used in nursing the elderly.
- Describe special approaches needed to evaluate nursing care of the aged.

The previous chapter was devoted to the assessment of the individual, the environment, and the individual's interaction with that environment. Assessment is continuous, but at some point a nursing diagnosis is made which is a concise statement identifying the client's problems. It is not a summary of all the abnormalities, for in a functional assessment, the premise is *that only those areas in which the client cannot function are properly those of a helping person.*

There are many abnormalities which do not interfere with function, or which have been compensated sufficiently to offer no problem. Medical, social, and other professions, however, which have made estimates of the person's ability to function offer additional data that must be considered with the nursing assessment and add to it immeasurably. This is *shared assessment.* The physician's plan of treatment may include certain portions which the client cannot perform alone (therapeutic self-care), and this treatment is often relegated to the nurse, among other care givers.

The team approach has been stressed over and over with nurses because nursing is one professional category with access to the client. For the older person who is often perplexed by the sheer number of short and often superficial professional contacts, many prove iatrogenic. *Instead, as problems multiply, contacts with helpers should be reduced to a minimum until the client can negotiate a way through social interactions with many personalities again. For the weak and the frail, this is essential.*

McCauley and Anderson (1974) describe the problems with the team approach in the management of the patient with stroke. After a feasibility study, a nurse was chosen as "therapist" with team support. The patient interacted with one nurse; the nurse interacted with the therapeutic team. A well-designed study found that the nurse-therapist relationship with patients was as effective, as shown by recovery criteria, as care given by 13 disciplines in a rehabilitation setting. Designation of one nurse as primary nurse has been demonstrated as economically and therapeutically effective by Manthey et al. (1970); its more recent evaluation by Ciske (1974) points out the advantages when responsibility and accountability for nursing

care are placed in one nurse. *For planning and implementing patient care, or care of the aging person, it is believed that primary nursing care is the most advantageous due to the fact that interacting personnel can be kept to a minimum until and at such a time as they can assist the therapeutic process.*

GOALS

The primary-care nurse and the elderly patient develop the problem list together in a process which is open and contractual. For the nurse it may be necessary to sacrifice some points of view in relation to the autonomy that nurses often feel. Planning with the older person is not a discrete interaction for a short event in a long life. It must be a highly predictive interaction in which there is input from each side for clarification and cooperation. Goal setting as prediction offers the nurse a chance to validate the aging person's viewpoint toward the future. Nursing action may be integral to health maintenance or restoration, and to prevention of disabilities resulting from disuse and nonuse; finally, it may serve only as a biopsychosocial support system to an elderly person who is completing the life cycle. Goals must be shared in order to be attained. In *Standards for Geriatric Nursing Practice* (1970), geriatric nursing Standard I states, "The nurse demonstrates an appreciation of the heritage, values and wisdom of older persons."

At the time goals are set, evaluation comes into play. A definite plan toward meeting realistic goals results in a list of nursing actions which should achieve those goals. These actions are highly specific and form a nursing-care plan which can be checked for effectiveness in reaching short-range goals or in predicting outcomes in long-range goals.

Goal setting demands knowledge and experience in caring for older people in order that the multiplicity of problems can be given proper priorities as people move from one stage of recovery to another. At no time is the older person one who can wait until later for some attention to be paid to problems of secondary and tertiary significance. In the acute stage, the remainder of life may seem of little importance in relation to the lifesaving effort needed. For the older person life-saving without life preservation may have a hollow sound. Each loss of function is diminishing.

The multiplicity of problems of the resident in long-term care indicates that such care (used by only about 5 percent of the elderly population at any time) is related to physical and psychosocial losses which can no longer be handled in the family or community. Up to the point of changing to long-term care, however, there are years in which the older person manages quite well with some assistance. However, the stress of acute illness requires the nurse in an acute care unit to treat persons having many complex problems. The nurse in the acute care unit should look at the elderly patients not as short-term events (the 5-day hospitalization), but as people who will be discharged into an environment with which they will be less able to cope. In the acute care unit goals for functioning for the rest of life must be addressed in discharge planning.

VIGNETTE

The elderly man had a ruptured appendix. The operation was a success, tubes came out of three different areas of his body, and antibiotics were conquering the fever. His visitor approached the head nurse, "How long will he be here?" "We usually have people ready to go home in five days, at most a week." "Has he told you he lives in a motel?" A discharge plan was started which took into consideration that the patient lived alone and had no one to help him. The planning to help an elderly man cope with his future with a recently incised abdomen was harder than the plan to care for him in the hospital where nursing care was highly specialized.

Goals should be congruent with the patient's present and potential physical capabilities and behavioral patterns. They must include:

- Maintenance or restoration of mobility or activity
- Maintenance or restoration of contact with reality
- Maintenance of social skills and a meaningful relationship with at least one other person

It is suggested that primary nursing care as defined by Manthey (1970) leads to such action.

PREDICTION

One of professional nursing's greatest contributions to the older person should be prediction. Prediction is based on experience and research. The decision to take certain actions is based on the knowledge of consequences and that risk taking has a strong theoretical base. One of the goals in the care of the older person in the acute care unit is to minimize the risk of confusion in the orthopedic and surgical ward by predicting which variables will lead to confusion. Plans can be made for prevention. Wolanin and Holloway (1980) have listed the predictors for confusion. In the future more of these predictors will be used in planning nursing care. One goal is to *prevent disability*. Nursing is now at the point where we can predict—and when we can predict, we can prevent.

NURSING ACTIONS— IMPLEMENTATION

A goal is the end state toward which nursing action is directed. Nursing actions must be spelled out specifically and assigned to a definite person for accomplishment; then accountability must be demanded. The development of flowsheets or algorithms makes it possible to record the parameters of observations for an individual with many problems. They allow the observation of cause and effect relationships, or the associated relationships which lead to change in condition. *The multiplicity of problems in the elderly demands determination of priorities, but the low end of the priority list demands utmost concern with the risks and losses which may occur by placing it at less than major priority.* Priorities involve prediction based on knowledge and constant reassessment.

Nursing actions include not only priorities but a logical sequence toward attaining goals. According to "Medical-Surgical Nursing Standards of Practice" (1974), the nursing actions must specify:

- What is to be done
- How to do it
- When to do it
- Where to do it
- Who is to do it

The plan is communicated *to the patient and the family* and to all health personnel who may be involved.

IMPLEMENTATION

Implementation of the planned nursing actions is a dyadic process in which patient reaction and interaction make evaluation and reassessment necessary at each step. *Careful documentation and record keeping assist in maintaining continuous and consistent care toward achievement of goals.*

Throughout the process the nurse has the responsibility of maintaining the involvement of the patient and his or her family, for nursing the older person contributes to the future of the patient, short or long as it may be, and the contribution may be positive or negative. *The functional outcome of the person's illness should be stated as clearly as therapeutic outcome.* One does not recover from a fractured hip if the ability to react appropriately to one's reality is destroyed. Mobility and contact with reality are paramount both for physiological function and maintaining self-esteem. Geriatric nursing Standard V states, "The nurse supports and promotes normal physiologic functioning of the older person." At the same time, geriatric nursing Standard VI reminds the practitioner, "The nurse protects aged persons from injury, infection and excessive stress and supports them through the multiplicity of stressful experiences to which they are subjected" (*Standards for Geriatric Nursing Practice,* 1970).

EVALUATION

If goals are stated in terms of outcomes, evaluation of care becomes a matter of estimating their attainment (Taylor, 1974). *However, the reasons for nonattainment of goals may make evaluation*

one of the most important parts of the nursing process. Evaluation is a learning process, and, unless done, one may repeat a mistake over and over while ignoring the fact that two events occurring at the same time are related as to cause and effect. Geriatric nursing practice depends upon research. Evaluation is the first level of observation for developing a body of geriatric nursing knowledge which is based on sound principles of nursing care.

Performance-based criteria are a method of big business that nursing has adopted rather uncritically. There are parts of evaluation which can best be done by using performance criteria. The assumption, however, is made that we have exact nursing objectives and that the multiple variables which are the human interaction can be ignored. If an error is made on an objective or a performance criterion, it may be impossible for anyone to reach it. Errors may not be pinpointed as to their origin. Blame falls on the shoulders of people who do not achieve the objectives, often because the objectives are unrealistic. Evaluation is still largely a matter of values. The humanistic approach must take into consideration all the many aspects of performance evaluation: Whose performance? Whose standards? And under what circumstances? This is not to excuse poor nursing. It is to place evaluation in its true light. Are the science and art of evaluation such that we can make performance criteria and employ them without careful evaluation of our use?

Although assessment has been carefully done and realistic goals set with the patient, or with the staff and family, it is necessary at frequent intervals to recheck goals through time. Additional information will change the goals. If this sounds as if it were an argument against evaluation, it is not. It is an argument for watching the state of the art of evaluation and to not adapt any scheme offered by business or industry to our very human elderly patients. Evaluate nursing and patient outcomes within the nursing framework. We must devise our own evaluation techniques within a humanistic framework (Lamonica, 1979).

How does one evaluate the progress of an older person? By the 20-year-old's standards? By ideals, hopes, and dreams? The care of the elderly patient is a learning process for care givers, and the need for research and experience is great.

REFERENCES

Ciske, Karen: Primary nursing evaluation, *American Journal of Nursing,* **74**(8):1436–1438, August 1974.

Lamonica, Elaine L.: *The Nursing Process—A Humanistic Approach,* Addison-Wesley, Reading, Mass., 1979.

McCauley, Cecilia, and Albert D. Anderson: The nurse as a primary therapist in the management of the patient with stroke, *Cardiovascular Nursing,* **10**(2):1–6, March–April 1974.

Manthey, Marie, et al.: Primary nursing: A return to the concept of "my nurse" and "my patient," *Nursing Forum,* **9**(1):65–83, 1970.

Medical-surgical nursing standards of practice, *The American Nurse,* July 1974, p. 22.

Standards for Geriatric Nursing Practice, American Journal of Nursing, 1970 (pamphlet).

Taylor, Joyce Waterman: Measuring the outcomes of nursing care, *Nursing Clinics of North America,* **9**(2):337–348, June 1974.

Wolanin, Mary Opal, and Janet Holloway: Relocation confusion: Intervention for prevention, in Irene Mortenson Burnside (ed.), *Psychosocial Nursing Care of the Aged,* 2d ed., McGraw-Hill, New York, 1980.

TWENTY-NINE

PHYSICAL ASSESSMENT OF THE AGED: DIFFERENTIATING NORMAL AND ABNORMAL CHANGE

Dorothy Rinehart Blake

Was man weiss, man seht.[1]
Goethe

---

[1] What one knows, one sees.

LEARNING OBJECTIVES

- Describe the normal changes of aging apparent on physical examination.
- Describe some changes which are definitely abnormal.
- Explain how the normal changes of aging make the older person more vulnerable to the effects of any disease or stress.
- List the common signs and symptoms with which the very old respond to many disease processes.
- Identify health maintenance measures pertinent to the aged.

Describe some specific interventions useful in alleviating problems secondary to normal aging.

PURPOSE OF THIS CHAPTER[2]

As multicellular animals we have a finite, genetically determined life-span. The best health care will not prolong that span indefinitely. We can attempt to maintain good health by nurturing, not abusing, our bodies and by the early detection and treatment of disease. The detection of abnormal changes assumes an understanding of the common, normal changes of aging. This chapter will emphasize normal changes. The person doing the physical assessment can use the subsequent information in the context of a client's present health or symptoms, present diseases and treatment, and past health problems.

OVERALL DECLINE OF ORGAN FUNCTION

The organs and systems show a declining function with aging. This well-documented fact will not be repeated in the description of each system. Decline in function and reserve makes the body more susceptible to death from the stress of any disease, but this decline is a normal aspect of aging. Death is a normal outcome of even healthy aging.

Healthy aged people should feel healthy even though they lack the endurance of youth. If they do not feel healthy, a psychological or physical cause is likely to be present. I recall an account of a very old woman who asked to be admitted to a hospital because she was very tired. She died the next day; no specific disease was found. Perhaps in such instances, fatigue is a symptom of healthy aging; most often it is not.

---

[2] It is assumed that the student nurse will have had a basic course in physical assessment before studying this chapter (*IB*).

CHANGES IN THE BODY'S REACTION TO DISEASE

Detection of disease in the elderly is made more difficult by the body's more muted response to disease. The classic pictures of illness are based on the more flamboyant responses of the young and middle-aged. A toddler may have a rectal temperature of 103°F in response to the common cold; an 85-year-old may be unable to develop a respectable fever in response to a fatal pneumonia.

The quantity as well as the quality of symptoms is modified in the very old. Any number of disease states may be heralded by one or several of a limited number of symptoms, i.e., fatigue, anorexia, confusion or dementia, incontinence, changes in ambulation such as falls or a shuffling gait, weight loss, or a failure to thrive. Any of these requires investigation, as does any symptom which the aged person mentions. Often the elderly hesitate to speak of changes in their bodies because they think that what they are experiencing is a normal part of aging or because they are concerned that no one will take their complaint seriously. Even minor changes need to be explained.

A slight rise in temperature may signal one of the two most common causes of fever in the elderly, pneumonia and urinary tract infections. When a white blood cell count is done to investigate fever or other symptoms, it must be remembered that the normal white blood cell count decreases with age secondary to a fall in the lymphocyte count. The upper limit of normal is 9000 cells per cubic millimeter of blood (Caird, 1973).

CARDIOVASCULAR CHANGES

This system is especially vulnerable to the combined effects of the aging process and disease. Aging produces a loss of elasticity of the heart and blood vessels. The heart becomes a less efficient pump. It has decreased ability to beat faster in response to stress. The arteries stiffen and dilate. Kohn (1977) notes that the system is not designed to promote longevity.

Hypertension and atherosclerosis are dependent on the basic aging process, but other factors are involved in their development. Neither disease is present in the same degree in all individuals, nor is it as prevalent in all countries as it is in the United States. Epidemiologic studies of myocardial ischemia show a positive correlation between that disease and diets that are habitually high in any one of the following: total calories, fat, unsaturated fat, saturated fat, salt, simple sugars (DiGirolamo and Schlant, 1978). All or any of those describe many American diets.

PULSE RATE

Studies of the effect of aging on the resting heartbeat have produced variable findings (Howell, 1970; Kohn, 1977). Harris (1978) suggests 60 to 100 beats per minute as within normal limits. Clinically, it is necessary to know each older person's *usual resting pulse,* as a rate of 100 in someone whose usual rate is 80 is a significant change. The older person's heart rate returns to its resting rate more slowly. Consequently, the resting rate must be measured before the arthritic person laboriously climbs up onto the examining table or before other exertion. The pulse rate should be regular, but occasional premature beats occur more often with increasing age and may have no clinical importance.

BLOOD PRESSURE

There should be no more than 20 mmHg blood pressure difference in the arms. The systolic pressure rises with age until the age of 75 to 79; the diastolic pressure rises slightly to age 64 and then declines. The increased pulse pressure is an outcome of the decrease in elasticity of the larger arteries plus the increased irritability of the vasoconstrictor center in the medulla. The former is a normal outcome of aging; the latter is secondary to arteriosclerotic lesions, ischemia, or neuron damage (Harris, 1977). He suggests 160/100 mmHg as the upper limits of normal. Dr. W. Kannel, medical director of the Framingham Heart Study, cites the increased risk of coronary artery disease, congestive heart failure, and brain infarcts that accompany hypertension (Kannel, Wolf, and Dawber, 1978). He and his associates urge us to view hypertension as true pathology and not as inevitable, desirable, or innocuous. Treatment of hypertension should keep the blood pressure at 150/90 mmHg or less (Castelli, 1978).

HEART SOUNDS

The intensity should be comparable with that of a younger heart. Distant sounds may be caused by poor cardiac function, chest wall abnormalities such as excessive fat, or hyperexpansion of the chest from chronic obstructive lung disease (Harris, 1978).

The normal aged heart may have no murmurs. About one-third to one-half of aortic systolic murmurs are functional sounds from changes in the aorta as it lengthens and becomes tortuous. The murmurs of organic aortic stenosis are often louder, radiate into the neck, and produce a thrill. Thickening and distortion of the mitral and aortic valves can also produce a murmur comparable with valvular disease. Diastolic murmurs are always pathological.

POINT OF MAXIMAL IMPULSE

There may be considerable narrowing of the chest size, especially in women. This may make the point of maximal impulse (PMI) palpable at the anterior axillary line even when there is no significant left ventricular hypertrophy.

SIGNS AND SYMPTOMS OF HEART DISEASE IN THE ELDERLY

Heart disease is the most common cause of death in the elderly, and congestive heart failure is a common complication. The textbook description is usually based on its appearance in the middle-aged or "young" elderly, but the very old may present without the reliable symptoms of orthopnea, paroxysmal nocturnal dyspnea, and rales. If a client always has some ankle edema from varicosities, nocturia from the normal change in diurnal urination, and shortness of breath from poor cardiac and pulmonary reserves, the recognition of true failure can be difficult.

Dr. Harris has the following observations about symptoms of heart disease in the elderly.

Acute dyspnea may be the cardinal sign of myocardial infarction. There may be no chest pain, but sudden, acute confusion may also occur. Cheyne-Stokes respirations from arteriosclerotic interference of blood flow to the medullary breathing center may cause insomnia in the aged; congestive heart failure will aggravate the process. If patients have increased insomnia, start looking for other manifestations of heart failure. Patients being treated with vasodilating drugs may be benefited by a bedtime dose. Cough and wheezing may be secondary to early congestive failure. Vertigo, fainting, and any mental change may be secondary to a cardiac condition. Digitalis delirium is a possibility. Hemoptysis may signal heart failure or pulmonary emboli (Harris, 1978).

The very old may have a smaller heart size; a normal-sized heart on x-ray does not necessarily preclude the absence of heart failure. X-ray may also show an increased cardiothoracic ratio secondary to the decreased width of the thorax; this can be mistaken for an enlarged heart. The normal electrocardiogram (ECG) in the elderly shows no major differences from that of a normal young person.

ENDOCRINE SYSTEM

THYROID GLAND

The gland of even the very old is able to function adequately and to respond to stress (Goldman, 1971). Palpating the thyroid may be more difficult if cervical spine disease has shortened the neck; the gland will be lower in relation to the clavicle, and the lower poles less accessible.

Hypo- and hyperthyroidism can begin in old age. Both are easily overlooked. Only one system may develop a symptom, i.e., there may be just weight loss, or just congestive heart failure, or just decreased mentation (Morrow, 1978).

Hyperthyroidism may be present with a heart rate of less than 100 beats per minute if that is the maximum rate the aged heart can produce. The thyroid may be normal in size (Morrow, 1978). Seventy percent of people with hyperthyroidism have mild to moderate muscle weakness, most noticeable in the muscles used in stair climbing. Lid lag is common and is often

an early sign (Grob, 1971a). The manifestations of nervousness, insomnia, anorexia, weight loss, and palpitations experienced by the young may also be present in the elderly (McGavick, 1971).

Sixty to eighty percent of old people with hypothyroidism have the same signs and symptoms of the young, but the signals are easily assumed to be the effect of aging or chronic disease, e.g., coarse, dry skin; constipation; decreased sensitivity to cold; enlarged heart; skin pallor (McGavick, 1971). Weakness is the most common symptom (Grob, 1971a). A constant sensation of weakness and fatigue is abnormal in the healthy aged.

Hypothyroidism in the elderly mimics "senility." Hypothyroidism often develops after treatment with radioactive iodine or thyroidectomy. A neck scar should alert the examiner to that possibility.

Serum T_4 levels should show no change in the elderly. A below-normal reading is abnormal, and a borderline high may be significant. Serum T_3 levels decline with acute illness; a high is significant (Morrow, 1978).

PARATHYROID GLAND

Hyper- and hypoparathyroidism may occur, but the normal gland is able to function adequately throughout life.

PANCREAS

It is known that the older person's ability to deal with orally administered glucose is decreased. About 50 percent are at a two-standard deviation above that used to measure young adults. Whether this is a physiological normal result of aging or a pathological change is not known, nor is it known whether the underlying mechanism is the same or different than that which causes diabetes (Andrus and Tobin, 1977).

EYE, EAR, NOSE, AND THROAT

EYE

Although visual acuity and peripheral field vision decrease with aging, the eye is designed to produce good vision throughout life. The majority of older people can wear glasses that provide fair to excellent vision (Gordon, 1971). Blindness is not a normal outcome of aging. Individuals who are at risk of blindness because of disease can be encouraged to learn braille while some sight still remains.

Normal changes of the lid include thinning, wrinkling, increased pigmentation, and stretching. Bags below the eyes are from herniation of orbital fat. Increased tearing occurs when the lids no longer fit snugly over the globe and when the lacrimal puncta do not drain the eye well (Gordon, 1971). Dry eyes are also common.

The conjunctiva is thinner and more friable, and becomes less white with aging. The milky white arcus senilis around the cornea is almost universal after aged 80. Some black people will have an arcus in their second decade. Its appearance early in life may correlate with hyperlipidemia, but arcus senilis is not synonymous with heart disease (Rossman, 1977).

The pupillary sphincter becomes sclerotic and the opening smaller. The response to light becomes sluggish, or the pupil may become fixed. The elderly need a night-light to compensate for their inability to adjust quickly to sudden brightness, and they are equally at risk for stumbling and falling when they come into a dim room from bright sunshine.

Examination of the extraocular movement may show a defective upward gaze and convergence, but there should not be a lid lag (Grob, 1978a).

The lens continues to grow throughout life. With aging, less of the lens remains flexible and accommodation decreases. Most people over aged 40 can describe that phenomenon with more precision than they might prefer.

Vitreous floaters are a frequent occurrence after the fifth decade. They are secondary to benign changes in the vitreous but must be differentiated from retinal hemorrhage, which presents with a shadow that is constant with eye movement (Gordon, 1971).

The aged fundus has less luster and a more yellow appearance. The retinal arteries become narrower, straighter, more opaque, and less regular in size (Gordon, 1971).

The elderly person should have a yearly eye examination that includes visual acuity, visual fields, and intraocular pressure.

EAR

Examination of the ear usually shows no significant changes of aging though there may be a wasted appearance to the tympanic membrane (Howell, 1970). Complaints of dizziness or vertigo should be investigated as neither is a normal part of aging. There is degeneration of the inner ear and a decreased sense of balance.

Some people will experience a fluctuating hearing loss secondary to the effect of an abnormally high serum glucose. A sudden hearing loss in one or both ears is a therapeutic emergency; it may be from occlusion of a vessel in the organ of Corti and may improve with prompt treatment (Senturia and Price, 1971).

Most people develop a hearing loss that interferes with the effortless communication of earlier years. *Presbycusis* is the common progressive, sensorineural hearing loss of aging. It can begin comparatively early but may stabilize for long periods (Senturia and Price, 1971). It affects 50 percent of people over age 85. Older people with a noticeable hearing loss need a diagnostic evaluation to detect any treatable disease. The incidence of presbycusis is decreasing as better differential diagnosis becomes possible (Meyerhoff and Paparella, 1978). Baseline audiometry should be a health maintenance measure of all middle-aged people, as this measurement can aid in the diagnosis of a later hearing loss.

Senturia and Price (1971) note a positive correlation among good hearing and physical and mental health. A hearing aid becomes appropriate when the loss is more obvious than the aid or when the person has difficulty with ordinary conversation. People should be referred to an otolaryngologist or audiologist conversant with prescribing hearing aids and who has an agreement with hearing aid dealers whereby the potential wearer can use the aid on a trial basis. Auditory training such as lip reading should be made available.

Hearing loss is often more troublesome when there is background noise from other voices. Institutions in which older people live need to provide quiet rooms for small gatherings.

A hearing loss can foster a concern of being talked about. This may be a well-founded concern, as families, friends, and health care givers often do talk about the hard of hearing in their presence. When this is necessary, it should be acknowledged to the person that he or she is, indeed, the subject of the conversation.

NOSE AND THROAT

Neither shows significant change on examination. The sense of smell decreases secondary to loss of olfactory fibers. This can interfere with the ability to taste food or to smell harmful odors. Encourage the elderly to have a smoke detector in their homes. Foods can be made more flavorful with spices; the heavy use of salt may be a poor idea at any age.

The elderly may be plagued by a benign postnasal drip that causes frequent clearing of the throat (Howell, 1970). Those who had nasal allergies in their youth may have fewer or no symptoms in later years.

Muscular atrophy of the pharynx and larynx may lead to soft speech, another reason the older person may not be able to communicate well in a noisy room. Actual hoarseness that persists for more than 3 weeks needs investigation.

GASTROINTESTINAL SYSTEM

The physiology of the aging gastrointestinal system is described in detail in Chapter 22.

Oral disease is common in the elderly, who often need, but cannot afford, dental care. A good examination of the mouth necessitates removal of false teeth. Any lesion of the mouth deserves diagnosis. Smokers are at high risk of developing oral cancers. Their mouths need careful inspection and palpation, especially the floor of the mouth.

The mucous membrane of the mouth will be drier, and veins may be visible through the thinned epithelial covering. Yellow sebaceous glands (Fordyce spots) are often visible on the thinned buccal mucosa. The healthy tongue will be well papillated. Veins under the tongue may be varicose; large varicosities may be from cardiac or pulmonary disease. Microscopic examination of the tongue would show a drastic re-

duction of taste buds; only the ability to taste salt remains normal. People who rely on sugar, salt, and pepper as their main sources of pleasurable taste may sharply increase their intake of table sugar. The gums become paler because of a reduced blood supply; actual pallor may signal anemia. The teeth become yellower with age and may show cracks that have become stained. The teeth may appear longer if the gingival border has retreated. The extent of the periodontal disease can best be seen on x-ray.

Findings on the abdominal examination of the healthy older person should be similar to those of younger people. A nonenlarged liver may be palpable if there is downward displacement from the fixed diaphragm of chronic obstructive pulmonary disease or when severe kyphosis is present. The thin abdominal wall and weak musculature may also make it possible to feel a normal liver.

SKIN

Many of the changes are obvious on inspection. Areas of epidermis exposed to the sun show the most pronounced changes, especially in whites who have blue or green eyes and/or red hair. Darker-pigmented whites have better protection; blacks show the least effect from the sun's radiation. Fair-skinned people would do well to avoid unnecessary exposure to the sun at any age and to wear a sun hat and a protective substance containing para-aminobenzoic acid when they must be out-of-doors. Young people will probably ignore such advice; those who have had one or more skin cancers are more amenable. Pointing out that the sun hastens the process of skin aging may give some leverage.

The normal loss of subcutaneous fat is a loss of insulation; when coupled with the loss of connective tissue of the extensor surface of hands and forearms, blood vessels have poor support and rupture easily. The resulting purpura is benign.

Decreased oil-gland output may cause dry, itching skin. The elderly do not need a total body bath every day and do need to oil their skin. The oil merely keeps the water from evaporating from the skin. Vegetable shortening is cheap and useful. Thin lotions often contain more water than oil. The skin cannot absorb water; drinking water is part of keeping the skin hydrated.

Skin lesions must be diagnosed and removed if malignant. The following lesions are benign and need no treatment. Cherry angiomas are bright red, discrete papules found on the thorax, arms, face, and abdomen. Venous stars are bluish superficial veins radiating from a central point. They may be normal or a result of venous obstruction. Venous lakes are thin-walled papules filled with venous blood. They are often seen on the ears, face, lips, and neck of elderly men. Pressure on the lesions will empty them. A costal fringe is a fringe of superficial veins under the anterior rib margins and xiphoid process. Facial telangiectasis is a dilation of groups of capillaries of the nose and face and may be associated with exposure to wind, cold weather, or many three-martini lunches.

MUSCULOSKELETAL SYSTEM

Normal aging produces a loss in muscle mass. Arm and leg muscles become thinner and less firm. The small muscles of the hands are especially prone to wasting, but good hand grips should be present. In general, the older person lacks strength and endurance but has enough stamina to carry out daily activities if in good health (Grob, 1978b). Regular exercising will not regenerate lost muscle cells, but it can decrease the muscle wasting secondary to disuse atrophy. Intact muscle cells can regain strength and tone in a 6- to 8-week period.

There is a posture of generalized flexion in the very old. The head and neck are flexed forward; the dorsal spine is kyphotic. The elbows, wrists, hips, and knees are slightly flexed. There is also some muscular rigidity with resistance to passive movement of the neck and extremities (Grob, 1978a).

COMMON NIGHTTIME PROBLEMS

Nighttime muscle cramps of the legs occur, often for unknown reasons. They may be secondary to more than usual muscle activity, to

peripheral vascular disease, to decreased serum calcium or sodium, or to hypoglycemia. If no pathology is found, passive stretching or a hot bath at bedtime may be helpful. Quinine sulfate or Benadryl may provide relief (Grob, 1978a).

Restless legs, an abnormal sensation relieved by movement, may be present without disease in young or old but is more common with aging. Diabetes, lumbar degenerative joint disease, hypocalcemia, or alkalosis from hyperventilation should be considered.

Tendonitis of the rotator cuff of the shoulder, present in nearly all after 60, may make it impossible for the person to sleep on that shoulder.

OSTEOARTHRITIS

Cell changes begin in the second decade and increase with age. X-ray changes are apparent after age 50; after the age of 60, 25 percent of women and 15 percent of men experience symptoms (Grob, 1978b). Thirty percent of women have Heberden's nodes of the distal interphalangeal joints of the hands after age 80. These are generally considered a sign of osteoarthritis, but Rossman cites a 1965 study by Stecher who believes the nodes are hereditary and unrelated to other types of osteoarthritis (Rossman, 1977).

Osteoarthritis of the neck is most common at spinal nerves at C5 and C6. About 75 percent of people with symptoms are helped by aspirin and education about positioning of the head. The neck is to be kept in a neutral position of rest at all times, that is, bent neither forward nor back nor rotated to either side. The person should sit, stand, read, watch television, and sleep in this position. Sleeping on the abdomen is contraindicated. When osteoarthritis of the neck is present, even a mild whiplash can cause permanent neurological loss; the use of car seatbelts and headrests will minimize that danger.

People with symptomatic osteoarthritis of the lumbar spine may get good relief from a planned schedule of aspirin and maintaining a W position of flexed hips and knees when sitting and sleeping. A reclining chair or footstool will keep tension off the lower back; sleeping on the side with knees bent or on the back with a pillow under the knees will do the same.

OSTEOPOROSIS

Osteoporosis is a common change associated with aging; whether it is a disease or a normal change is not understood. The long-term research studies needed do not exist. It is known that there is a gradual loss of bone mass with aging in both sexes and among all races, but all men and black women have less bone loss than do white women. Osteoporosis ensues if there is an abnormal amount of loss. The unaffected bone is normal in composition.

Clinically osteoporosis leads to skeletal fractures, kyphosis, and reduced height; hip fractures may occur spontaneously, and the fall may be from the fracture rather than the fracture from the fall. The dorsal kyphosis secondary to compression fractures of the thoracic vertebrae may continue until the lower costal margins rest on the iliac crests. Muscles trapped between these bony parts can cause pain; the client can be assured that the symptom is benign, though that does little to relieve the discomfort.

Calcium deficiency may contribute to osteoporosis either from too little intake or from the decreased absorption that is part of aging. It is suggested that older people take in 1 g of calcium a day (1 mL of milk provides 1 g of calcium). Milk also contains the vitamin D necessary for calcium metabolism. If a calcium supplement is used, the carbonate is more effectively absorbed than the gluconate or lactate, both of which are often excreted whole in the stool (Barzel, 1978). Other sources of calcium are other dairy products, kale, mustard greens, tofu, tortillas, and pinto beans.

Gonadal deficiency is often implicated as a cause of osteoporosis because the incidence rises dramatically in postmenopausal women. Estrogen is often given to prevent osteoporosis following oophorectomy, but osteoporosis is not always a sequela of nontreated women. The routine use of estrogen to treat postmenopausal women is controversial (Barzel, 1978). Estrogen cannot replace bone loss after symptoms occur, but it does decrease the rate of calcium loss. Glowacki (1978) suggests low doses begun within 3 years of the menopause; if greater than 6 years have elapsed, he suggests estrogen only for symptoms.

Other factors which hasten bone loss are immobilization and perhaps just lack of exercise. Hyperthyroidism and hyperparathyroidism are possible, treatable causes of osteoporosis.

Animals fed an acid ash diet develop the same bone changes as humans who have osteoporosis (Barzel, 1978). Acid ash diets are high in animal proteins and some cereals. As protein intake rises, so does urinary calcium excretion. An intake 50 percent above a diet of 65-g protein per day has been associated with an increase in urine calcium. A too-high protein diet produces significant negative effects on skeletal mass (Heaney, 1979).

Daniell (1976) reports on a study of hand x-rays showing a 50 percent more rapid loss of bone among smokers than nonsmokers. He noted that nonsmoking women who had oophorectomies and nonsmoking women with an early menopause did not have an increase in early osteoporotic fractures. He concludes that smokers' bones may be at greater risk. Previous studies have shown that there are more bone loss problems in slender women. Daniell's study did not show that correlation, but he did note that some slender women use cigarettes to keep their weight under control.

NERVOUS SYSTEM

Measurement of changes in the nervous system presents many difficulties, and recent research sometimes contradicts earlier works. It is known that aging brings an increased threshold of perception of sensory stimuli of vision, hearing, light touch, and pain. The pathology of pneumonia, myocardial infarcts, and peritonitis is more easily missed because the older person feels little or no pain.

Sensorimotor responses show a lengthened reaction time after age 60, especially when a choice between two actions is necessary. It is the motor component that is more delayed.

Deep tendon reflexes of the arms can be elicited but are usually diminished in intensity. Beginning in middle age there is a loss of abdominal reflexes, especially if obesity or multiple childbearing is a factor. The deep tendon reflexes of the knee are generally intact, but the ankle reflexes are often absent and plantar reflexes may be unobtainable because of foot problems (Grob, 1978a). There is often a loss of vibratory sensation in the lower limbs.

The temperature-regulating center is less reliable; 96.9°F may be the normal oral temperature of the person over 90. The aged tend to feel chilly if the room temperature falls below 64°F.

Extrapyramidal changes can produce impassive face, slow movements, and decreased blinking, all of which may be accidentally diagnosed as parkinsonism, especially if the person also has a tremor. The elderly may have fasciculations of the calves, eyelids, hands, and feet; if no undue weakness or muscle wasting is present, the muscle twitchings are insignificant. The movements should be more irregular in rate and size and of a shorter duration than those of central nervous system disease (Grob, 1978a).

Biologic and psychologic aspects of the nervous system are difficult to separate. Sleep changes may combine both. Older people experience a decreased intensity of sleep with more numerous nighttime wakenings. They may need to take a nap during the day or to stay in bed somewhat longer at night to get the sleep they need. They require the same or slightly less total hours of sleep than in other stages of adulthood (Kales and Kales, 1972). Something is amiss if the older person gives a history of going to bed at 8:00 P.M. and trying to sleep until 7:00 A.M. What is amiss may be boredom, depression, or the institution whose rules assume the elderly need more sleep than the young.

Insomnia is a frequent complaint of the elderly. A detailed history will reveal whether the person is experiencing the normal sleep pattern of aging or true insomnia. The latter is often due to depression just as it is in other age groups, but it can also be caused by hypothyroidism, renal insufficiency, congestive heart failure, physical discomfort, or any of the acute disorders which produce confusion and dementia, i.e., electrolyte imbalance, hypoglycemia, liver failure, alcohol intoxication, head trauma, infectious diseases, and drug reactions.

Recent longitudinal studies of intellectual functioning show that most dimensions do not decline and that crystallized intelligence, i.e., verbal comprehension and use of firmly established habits, shows an increase in scores. Visual-motor flexibility requiring coordination between vision and motor performance shows a definite decline (Baltes and Schaie, 1974).

Global mental decline is not a part of normal aging, though the intellectual failure of organic disease is a grim possibility. That subject is discussed in Chapter 14, "Organic Brain Syndrome."

Many older people worry about memory loss, and depressed people complain of that symptom even when objective observation does not demonstrate a loss. I have heard the term *meta-memory* used at several recent conferences. The term refers to the way people describe their own memory to themselves. The older person who mislays an object may say, "My memory is failing me." The young person may say, "I am very absentminded today." Preoccupation with the fear of memory loss can interfere with memory. Helping older people to put their normal lapse of memory in a nonpathological perspective can relieve that worry and leave them free to learn and retain. They can also learn to use visual imagery and data organization to make remembering easier.

THE REPRODUCTIVE SYSTEM

FEMALE

Changes apparent on physical examination are secondary to declining estrogen levels. The levels drop significantly between 35 and 40 years and reach a plateau at about 60, after which there is little change (Pincus, 1955). The climacteric begins in the forties and usually spans 20 to 30 years. Cessation of the menses occurs when there is no longer enough estrogen to cause the endometrium to grow and shed, but estrogen levels may remain to maintain secondary sex characteristics into the sixties. Data suggest that postmenopausal estrogen comes from nonovarian sources (Talbert, 1977).

The menopause occurs at age 48 to 51 in many populations (Talbert, 1977). Menopause before age 40 may or may not be normal. Pregnancy is considered possible until there has been no menses for 12 months. Women who do not wish to conceive must be urged to use contraception until that year is completed.

BREAST CHANGES

Glandular breast tissue is gradually replaced by fat after age 35. Atrophy of the fat and gland occurs during the sixth decade. Such atrophy makes tumors more palpable. Normal shrinkage and fibrotic change may produce apparent nipple retraction similar to that of cancer, but the nipples can be everted if no cancer is present. The terminal ducts may be felt as firm, linear strands (Rossman, 1971).

VULVA AND VAGINA

During the sixties, the vulva begins to show hair loss, flattening of the labia, and skin atrophy. Any unexplained skin lesion must be biopsied to rule out cancer. The clitoris decreases in size. Bartholin's glands should not be palpable. The vaginal epithelium eventually becomes thin, pale, smooth, and dry. The introitus may admit only one finger, and the vagina is shorter. However a sexually active woman is likely to have normal vaginal pliability (Notelovitz, 1978). Notelovitz also notes that the same pesky pathogens that cause vaginitis in the young should be considered postmenopausally, as there is evidence that the flora of the vagina changes less than was previously believed. Gonorrhea should be considered when vaginal or urinary symptoms are present. A sex history should be as much a part of the history as it is in the young. Older women may hesitate to mention painful intercourse because of the cultural expectation that old people are asexual.

CERVIX, UTERUS, AND OVARIES

The cervix becomes smaller and flush with the vault. More nabothian cysts may form as the epithelium atrophies and endocervical glands are sealed over. The os may become stenotic and obliterated. There is withdrawal of the squamocolumnar junction into the cervical canal. Both of these latter changes make collecting a useful Papanicolaou smear more difficult and sometimes impossible. Cervical cancers peak in the forties and remain essentially at that level into old age (Upton, 1977). Uterine cancers are more prevalent in the elderly woman, especially if obesity, hypertension, or diabetes is present. Papanicolaou smears and pelvic examinations should be part of the older woman's health maintenance care, though an examination every other year may replace the yearly one (Somers et al., 1979).

The uterus becomes smaller and will be only 1 cm in size in very old women (Talbert, 1977). The ovaries become smaller and eventually are no longer palpable. Suspect pathology if the ovaries of a woman long past menopause are palpable, especially if only one is large enough to be felt.

Sexually, the woman will have no decrease in sensation of the clitoris. Her orgasms may be less intense and sometimes cause pain. The latter and any painful intercourse from atrophic vaginal changes can be treated with topical estrogen therapy.

MALES

The decline in reproductive function is much more gradual, and less research has been done on the effect of age on gonadotropin secretion.

The prostate shows nodular hyperplasia in whites and American blacks after the age of 50, but this finding is less common in Chinese men. The enlargement begins in the wall of the urethra and then includes the medial and lateral lobes. The posterior lobe is only indirectly involved. Consequently there may be little correlation between the size of the prostate palpable on digital examination and the severity of symptoms from prostatism. Cancer of the prostate almost always originates in the posterior lobe.

The testes decrease in size. Spermatozoa are manufactured into old age, but the number and motility decrease. There is less seminal fluid, and, therefore, the ejaculatory force decreases.

The penis shows progressive sclerosis of the arteries and veins. There is an increase in erectile impotence, but the causes are poorly understood. The older man will take longer to get an erection and may need more stimulation to do so. There is a longer refractory period.

Psychic erections occur less often, but many men continue to have erections in the rapid eye movement (REM) stage of sleep.

SEXUAL FUNCTION OF MALES AND FEMALES

There are insufficient studies of sexual functioning in the elderly. Those that exist are often based on few subjects. There is general agreement that both sexes can be sexually responsive throughout life if they are in reasonably good health and if they have an interested, interesting partner. People with good sexual activity when young are more likely to have a satisfactory sex life as they age. Those who develop problems as they age can often be helped by counseling offered by their usual health care provider. Those of us who care for the aged should know how to take a sexual history and to explain physiology of aging, and we should offer counseling. Glover offers an excellent chapter on that subject (1978).

RESPIRATORY SYSTEM

The normal changes of aging produce a system still able to support the usual activities of an older person. The normal elderly should have shortness of breath only from episodes of activity such as stair climbing, but not from walking at a reasonable pace on flat ground. They should have no cough or sputum production unless they smoke (Balchum, 1971).

PHARYNX AND LARYNX

The muscles atrophy and the voice becomes softer and more difficult to understand. Talking may require more energy. A quiet room can facilitate both speech and hearing.

CHEST AND LUNGS

The chest shows an increase in anteroposterior diameter secondary to osteoporosis and kyphosis, calcification of costal cartilages, reduced rib mobility, and partial contraction of the muscles of inspiration.

The lungs become less elastic, leading to an increase in residual volume and a decrease in vital capacity (Goldman, 1971). This should not produce symptoms in the resting state, but the hyperinflation produces hyperresonance to percussion and decreased breath sounds. There may be decreased movements of the diaphragm. None of the above need be thought of as true emphysema if there is no obstructive pattern during forced expiration (Balchum, 1971). If an older person is unable to blow out a match 6 inches away with the mouth wide open, there is excessive loss of forced expiratory volume, and a cause other than aging should be sought (Goldman, 1971). Blood gases will show a decline in pO_2 with aging; 75 mmHg is the mean in the seventh decade (Kent, 1978). pCO_2 and bicarbonate levels should remain normal.

After age 50 there is underventilation of the lung bases at all times (Balchum, 1971). In young people the lung bases are ventilated best, but with aging the rigidity of the lung improves the apical ventilation. The increased expansion of the upper areas can cause some collapse of the basilar lobes (Goldman, 1971). This may account for the atelectatic rales sometimes heard during the first few respiratory cycles when the lungs are auscultated. The health care provider needs to know what breath sounds are usually present in a particular older person's lungs so that a new finding can be accurately assessed. It should be remembered that crepitant basilar rales in the elderly can occur after only a few hours in bed (Agate, 1971).

LUNG DISEASE

The cough loses force secondary to increased rigidity of the thoracic structure and decreased strength of the expiratory muscles. The cilia become less active (Goldman, 1971). All these normal changes leave the lung able to cope with nonstressful situations but at an obvious disadvantage in the face of disease, surgery, and bed rest. The pneumonia that is a temporary inconvenience to the 20-year-old may have grave consequences for the 90-year-old. Deaths from pneumonia have decreased in number, but the incidence of the disease is the same (Klocke, 1977). Older people who have serious chronic disease can be offered the vaccine that prevents the three most common types of pneumonia and a yearly dose of influenza vaccine.

The peak incidence of tuberculosis is now in the older age group, usually from reinfection. Lung cancer and chronic obstructive pulmonary disease are related to smoking.

URINARY SYSTEM

Nondiseased kidney function is reduced but sufficient in normal aging, but disease in other parts of the body may reduce the kidney's ability to maintain homeostasis and excrete drugs. Reduced tubular function interferes with the ability to concentrate urine even in the face of decreased fluid intake (Kahn and Snapper, 1971). The elderly who have ambulatory or cognitive difficulties which make drinking fluids difficult and/or who take diuretic drugs are at high risk of developing dehydration. Good nursing care of the institutionalized elderly could benefit from the same enthusiasm for getting water into the body as for washing water over the body.

Nocturia can be a normal aspect of aging because of the loss of the previous diurnal pattern.

INCONTINENCE

Urinary frequency and increased residual volume occur in both sexes. Urgency and precipitant voiding may occur without underlying bladder disease; but neither incontinence nor bladder infections are a normal part of aging. When incontinence occurs, the person needs a detailed history and examination, as incontinence may be amenable to nursing interventions or medical treatment (See Chapter 36 for an in-depth discussion of incontinence.)

LOWER URINARY TRACT INFECTION

Bladder infections are one of the most common problems of the elderly of both sexes. Women under 65 have a less than 6 percent incidence with an abrupt increase to greater than 20 percent after 65. The critical age is 70 for men (Goldman, 1977). Retention and stasis in men is often secondary to an enlarged prostate. There

is some degree of prostatism in 75 percent of males over 65 years of age (Jaffe, 1971). The postmenopausal changes in the female urethra and vaginal epithelium can lead to a distal outflow obstruction with the same results as an enlarged prostate in men, that is, increase in residual urine and infection. The syndrome can be modified by the use of estrogen cream (Notelovitz, 1978). Postcoital voiding and other patient education given to young women who have bladder infections apply also to older women.

A study by Brocklehurst, Bee, and Jones (1977) showed 35 percent of 217 geriatric hospitalized patients having infected urine. Forty-six percent of those who initially had clean urine became infected during the year's study. There was a higher incidence among those with poor intellectual function, but the most common cause was fecal impaction leading to a dirty perineum. Their study showed better long-term treatment of cystitis with urinary antiseptics than with antibiotics for each discovered infection.

SUMMARY

Such are the developments of our bodies as we age. In biological terms, development continues only until maturity. In a broader sense, to develop is to cause to unfold gradually along lines natural to its kind. I suspect that those of us who write about aging are working out our own need to put aging in the latter perspective, and so I thank the reader who has made it possible for me to do that work.

REFERENCES

Agate, J.: The natural history of disease in later life, in I. Rossman (ed.), *Clinical Geriatrics,* Lippincott, Philadelphia, 1971.

Andrus, R., and J. Tobin: Endocrine systems, in C. Finch and L. Hayflick (eds.), *Handbook of the Biology of Aging,* Van Nostrand Reinhold, New York, 1977.

Balchum, O.: The aging respiratory system, in A. Chinn (ed.), *Working with Older People,* vol. 4, *Clinical Aspects of Aging,* DHEW, Rockville, Md., 1971.

Baltes, P., and W. Schaie: The myth of the twilight years, *Psychology Today,* **7:**35–40, March 1974.

Barzel, U.: Common metabolic disorders of the skeleton in aging, in W. Reichel (ed.), *Clinical Aspects of Aging,* Williams & Wilkins, Baltimore, 1978.

Brocklehurst, J., P. Bee, and D. Jones: Bacteriuria in geriatric hospital patients: Its correlates and management, *Age and Aging,* **64:**240–245, 1977.

Caird, R.: Problems of interpretation of laboratory findings in the old, *British Medical Journal,* **4:**348–351, November 1973.

Castelli, W.: Cardiovascular heart disease risk factors, in W. Reichel (ed.), *The Geriatric Patient,* HP Publishing Co., New York, 1978.

Daniell, H.: Osteoporosis of the slender smoker, *Archives of Internal Medicine,* **136**(3):298–204, March 1976.

DiGirolamo, M., and R. Schlant: Etiology of coronary atherosclerosis, in J. Hurst (ed.), *The Heart,* McGraw-Hill, New York, 1978.

Glover, B.: Sex counseling, in W. Reichel (ed.), *The Geriatric Patient,* HP Publishing Co., New York, 1978.

Glowacki, G.: Postmenopausal gyn problems, in W. Reichel (ed.), *The Geriatric Patient,* HP Publishing Co., New York, 1978.

Goldman, R.: Aging of the excretory system: Kidney and bladder, in C. Finch and L. Hayflick (eds.), *Handbook of the Biology of Aging,* Van Nostrand Reinhold, New York, 1977.

————: Decline in organ function with aging, in I. Rossman (ed.), *Clinical Geriatrics,* Lippincott, Philadelphia, 1971.

Gordon, D.: Eye problems of the aged, in A. Chinn (ed.), *Working with Older People,* vol. 4, *Clinical Aspects of Aging,* DHEW, Rockville, Md., 1971.

Grob, D.: Common disorders of muscles in the aged, in W. Reichel (ed.), *Clinical Aspects of Aging,* Williams & Wilkins, Baltimore, 1978a.

————: Prevalent joint disease in older persons, in W. Reichel (ed.), *Clinical Aspects of Aging,* Williams & Wilkins, Baltimore, 1978b.

Harris, R.: Special problems of geriatric patients with heart disease, in W. Reichel (ed.), *Clinical Aspects of Aging,* Williams & Wilkins, Baltimore, 1978.

————: The aging heart: Insight into biologic change and their clinical significance, *Geriatrics,* **32:**49–54, February 1977.

Heaney, R.: Can an excessive dietary intake of phosphate or protein contribute to the development of osteoporosis? from *International Symposium on Osteoporosis,* Biomedical Information Corporation, New York, 1979, p. 28.

Howell, T.: *A Student's Guide to Geriatrics,* Charles C Thomas, Springfield, Ill., 1970.

Jaffe, J.: Common lower urinary tract problems in older people, in A. Chinn (ed.), *Working with Older People,* vol. 4, *Clinical Aspects of Aging,* DHEW, Rockville, Md., 1971.

Kahn, A., and I. Snapper: Medical renal disease in the elderly, in A. Chinn (ed.), *Working with Older People,* vol. 4, *Clinical Aspects of Aging,* DHEW, Rockville, Md., 1971.

Kales, A., and J. Kales: The relevance of sleep research to clinical practice, in G. Usdin (ed.), *Sleep Research and Clinical Practice,* Brunner/Mazel, New York, 1972.

Kannel, W., P. Wolfe, and T. Dawber: Hypertension and cardiac impairment increase stroke risk, *Geriatrics,* **33:**71–83, September 1978.

Kent, S.: The aging lung. I: Loss of elasticity, *Geriatrics,* **33:**124–132, February 1978.

Klocke, R.: Influence of aging on the lung, in C. Finch and L. Hayflick (eds.), *Handbook of the Biology of Aging,* Van Nostrand Reinhold, New York, 1977.

Kohn, R.: Heart and cardiovascular system, in C. Finch and L. Hayflick (eds.), *Handbook of the Biology of Aging,* Van Nostrand Reinhold, New York, 1977.

McGavick, T.: Endocrine changes with aging significant to clinical practice, in A. Chinn (ed.), *Working with Older People,* vol. 4, *Clinical Aspects of Aging,* DHEW, Rockville, Md., 1971.

Meyerhoff, W., and M. Paparella: Diagnosing the cause of hearing loss, *Geriatrics,* **33:**95–99, February 1978.

Morrow, L.: How thyroid disease presents in the elderly, *Geriatrics,* **33:**42–45, April 1978.

Notelovitz, M.: Gynecologic problems of postmenopausal women: Changes in extra-genital tissues and sexuality, *Geriatrics,* **33:**51–58, October 1978.

Pincus, G.: Steroid metabolism in aging women and men, *Recent Progress in Hormonal Research: The Proceedings of the 1954 Laurentian Hormone Conference,* **11:**397, 1955.

Rossman, I.: Anatomic and body composition changes with aging, in C. Finch and L. Hayflick (eds.), *Handbook of the Biology of Aging,* Van Nostrand Reinhold, New York, 1977.

———— : The anatomy of aging, in I. Rossman (ed.), *Clinical Geriatrics,* Lippincott, Philadelphia, 1971.

Senturia, B., and L. Price: Otolaryngological problems in the geriatric patient, in A. Chinn (ed.), *Working with Older People,* vol. 4, *Clinical Aspects of Aging,* DHEW, Rockville, Md., 1971.

Somers, A., et al.: A whole life plan for well patient care, *Patient Care,* **13**(11):83–153, June 15, 1979.

Stecher, R.: Heredity of osteoarthritis, *Archives of Physical Medicine and Rehabilitation,* **46:**178–186, January 1965.

Talbert, G.: Aging of the reproductive system, in C. Finch and L. Hayflick (eds.), *Handbook of the Biology of Aging,* Van Nostrand Reinhold, New York, 1977.

Upton, A.: Pathobiology, in C. Finch and L. Hayflick (eds.), *Handbook of the Biology of Aging,* Van Nostrand Reinhold, New York, 1977.

THIRTY

ASSESSMENT OF THE FRAIL ELDERLY

Billie J. Robison

. . . and time said, "I take away all things I've given, but no more than that."
Valmiki (Ramayana)

LEARNING OBJECTIVES

- Name two factors that decrease the ability of the frail aged to cope with illness.
- List three coping mechanisms sometimes utilized by stressed elders.
- Name three techniques for establishing a trusting relationship and eliciting cooperation when assessing a frail elder.
- Identify at least three sources of information in a patient's records that can provide clues to the frail elder's illness other than those listed as part of the diagnosis.
- List at least four problems that occur so often in the frail elder as to be considered endemic in that population.

I became interested in the problems and needs of elders early in my nursing education; the interest intensified as my awareness of the scope and depth of those needs developed. For the past 4 years, I have been a family nurse practitioner in joint practice with a family practice physician. As a team we provide health care to about 325 elderly persons who reside in the six skilled nursing facilities (SNF) in our community. We also see elders in the office and on home visits by the nurse practitioner.

The initial history and physical assessments of the elderly we care for in skilled nursing facilities are performed by me as the nurse practitioner (see Figures 30-1 and 30-2). A therapeutic plan is developed for each patient and reviewed with the physician member of the team. I also do the admitting assessment, the routine monthly visits, annual reevaluations, triage of acute problems, and adjustments in therapy regimens, in consultation with the physician. This team approach model has been described by Loeb and Robison (1977).

My experience with hundreds of frail elders has reinforced my conviction that the nurse's attitude and approach can profoundly affect the outcome of assessment, the therapeutic interventions, and the motivation of the elder to move toward a higher level of well-being. This chapter focuses on the assessment of the frail elderly client and is based primarily on my experience as a nurse practitioner.

DEFINITION

The definition of the frail elderly used in this chapter is a bit broad—elderly persons who have reached a great age, in excess of 75, and who have during their long life accumulated multiple disabilities and/or chronic illnesses. Those changes combined with aged physiology, that is, with decreased ability of all major organ systems to respond to stress and maintain homeostasis, put those persons at increased risk of physiological and psychological decompensation. The frail elderly person is under constant stress from within and without and attempts to maintain daily activities as the psychological functions and strengths decline. The descent

into illness can be rapid; return to wellness is often slow and fraught with difficulties.

SPECIAL PROBLEMS WITH THE FRAIL ELDERLY CLIENT

The aged, as a group, have more health problems than the young. Their problems often involve more than one major organ system. Their physical disabilities are more likely to be multiple and chronic. Because of changes that occur in the aging physiology, their response to illness may be dampened and their symptoms may be vague and unspecific; in some cases the usual symptoms may be absent as, for example, in a "silent" myocardial infarction (Harris, 1978). Since they have lived a long time, they have accumulated more health history and are also likely to be less concise historians. Records may be widely scattered, and the clients' understanding of past diagnoses, surgeries, and treatments may be quite inaccurate. So, at the very least, it takes longer to obtain clients' histories.

A severe illness is more likely to affect multiple organ systems, complicating assessment and management and prolonging the return to homeostasis. Anemia, respiratory and urinary tract infections, and/or malnutrition can precipitate heart failure in an elder with heart disease. The heart failure can result in confusion and lead to renal failure and to electrolyte and fluid imbalances in rapid sequence.

The aging physiology also presents problems with treatment regimens. Aged people's responses to medications show wide variations. Their response to treatment is likely to be idiosyncratic. For example, an antidepressant drug such as Elavil may cause sedation in one person but severe agitation, restlessness, and insomnia in another. The multiple problems of the elderly may require prescription of multiple drugs, and the incidence of drug reactions can be expected to increase as additional drugs are prescribed (Chapron and Lawson, 1978).

Decreased hearing, visual acuity, touch, sensation, and mental alertness may result in errors in self-administered medications and noncompliance with a medical regimen (Chapron and Lawson, 1978).

HISTORY

DATE_____ D.O.B. _____ NAME_____

History of present illness:

Source:

Past history:
- ☐ Medical

- ☐ Surgical

- ☐ Miscellaneous

Review of systems:
- ☐ HEENT

- ☐ Cardiorespiratory

- ☐ GI

- ☐ GU

- ☐ Musculoskeletal

- ☐ Neuropsychiatric

FIGURE 30-1   A sample of the history used conjointly by a family nurse practitioner and physician team.

CHRONIC PROBLEM LIST

No.		No.	
1		11	
2		12	
3		13	
4		14	
5		15	
6		16	
7		17	
8		18	
9		19	
10		20	

ADDITIONAL COMMENTS

```
┌─────────────────────────────────────────────────────────────────────┐
│                      PHYSICAL EXAMINATION                             │
│                                                                       │
│    DATE_____  ADMITTING____  REEVALUATION_____  B.P._____  P____  R____  T____  │
│                                                                       │
│    General                                                            │
│                                                                       │
│                                                                       │
│    Skin                                                               │
│                                                                       │
│                                                                       │
│    Head, eyes, ears                                                   │
│                                                                       │
│                                                                       │
│    Nose, mouth, throat                                                │
│                                                                       │
│                                                                       │
│    Neck                                                               │
│                                                                       │
│                                                                       │
│    Chest                                                              │
│                                                                       │
│                                                                       │
│    Breasts                                                            │
│                                                                       │
│                                                                       │
│    Cardiovascular                                                     │
│                                                                       │
│                                                                       │
│    Abdomen                                                            │
│                                                                       │
│                                                                       │
│    Genitalia                                                          │
│                                                                       │
│                                                                       │
│    Rectal                                                             │
│                                                                       │
│                                                                       │
│    Extremities                                                        │
│                                                                       │
│                                                                       │
│    Neuromuscular                                                      │
│                                                                       │
│                                                                       │
└─────────────────────────────────────────────────────────────────────┘
```

FIGURE 30-2   A sample of a physical examination form used by a family nurse practitioner and a physician team.

ONSET	ACUTE PROBLEM	RESOLVED	PLAN

LAB:

_____ _____

PRESENT MEDS:

SIGNATURE_____

NAME_____   DATE_____

In addition to the physical problems many aged endure, they may also be assaulted by major psychic, social, environmental, and economic problems which include loss of status, loss of significant others, loss of security, inadequate financial resources, poor housing, poor mobility, and the brutalizing effects of "ageism." These problems can adversely affect the aged person's self-image, stress physiological and psychological systems, and precipitate illness and depression.

ASSESSING THE FRAIL ELDER

As people age, they do become more individualized and their personalities more deeply etched. When a nurse approaches a frail elder, it is important to be flexible and individualize the approach as the elder's condition, environment, and personality dictate. The health professional's first contact with the frail elderly client is frequently during a crisis period. Nurses are called to the home, for example, when the elder can no longer function, and we frequently meet them first in an acute or long-term care setting. We rarely see them in community settings, since the number and severity of the frail elder's disabilities are very likely to keep them confined.

Nurses see them at a time when they are not only acutely ill, but also besieged by the stress of adjusting to a series of rapidly changing environments—the ambulance, the emergency room, one or more hospital rooms, trips to x-ray and other departments, possible surgical assault, and eventual transfer to the skilled nursing facilities. In addition, the elderly person is frequently struggling with hopelessness and fear about the present and future.

An older person who is ill and coping with a new environment is subject to high levels of stress. The way elderly persons defend themselves will depend on their particular coping mechanisms. Examples of common defense mechanisms are: (1) passivity and withdrawal; (2) suspicion, hostility, and defensiveness; (3) excessive complaints and demands on relatives or staff; (4) use of charm and effusive praise to enlist support; and (5) denial of illness. The methods of coping are as individual as the elders who employ them. The assessment of the frail elder must include recognition and identification of individual coping patterns and reactions to stress.

INITIAL APPROACH

The examiner's approach to assessment and subsequent interactions can cause the elder to feel even more dehumanized and threatened, or the assessment can be designed as a therapeutic process to reduce fear, restore hope, rebuild a positive self-image, and motivate mobilization of psychic and physiological resources to bring about as swift and complete a return to health as possible. *An abrupt, impatient manner is always contraindicated; it will have the negative effects listed above.*

The approach to assessment must be individualized to suit the elder's needs. The standard model for taking a history and physical assessment may be quite appropriate for the alert, oriented elder who is not acutely ill and does not have sensory deficiencies; however, if the elder is acutely ill and has a hearing or vision loss, or is confused and withdrawn, the approach must be modified, as described later in this chapter.

The examiner first must establish a climate of reassurance and trust. A warm greeting with an extended hand and good eye contact will almost always result in acceptance of that hand; maintain the hand contact so long as the elder shows an inclination to do so. If the elder clings to the offered hand, the examiner can show acceptance and additional warmth by covering his or her hand with the other hand for a moment. After contact has been established and the examiner has made the introduction, it is important to explain the purpose of the visit. One should explain that one is there to identify the elder's needs in order that those needs can be better met. Then one should briefly describe the procedure. Explain, for example, that questions will be asked (some of them personal) and that a comprehensive physical assessment will be performed. It may be necessary to give a simple description of the examination prior to starting it. For example, "I will be looking in your eyes and ears, listening to your heart and lungs, feeling your stomach, and checking your arms and legs." If the patient is blind, the explanations are particularly important. As the examination proceeds, each step should be prefaced with an explanation. For example, "Next I will be checking your reflexes; I will be tapping certain parts of your arm or leg with a reflex hammer and it may cause that part to jerk." Such simple explanations help to alleviate the shock, fear, anger, and resistance that might occur if the patient were tapped without explanation. For the deaf client who can see, the demonstration of the instruments on oneself before they are used on the elder serves the purpose of improving understanding and helps comprehension. It also might amuse the elder and result in cooperation.

For the person who is both deaf and blind, which is not uncommon in the very old, touch is one's only means of communication. Gently guide the person's hand to feel the examiner's face, shoulders, and hands. Have the elder feel the instruments before you employ them in the examination. The patient's touch will help him or her to identify the examiner when next approached, and touching the instruments will help to identify the purpose of the visit. The investment of time and encouragement of touch communicates good will and respect for the individual's identity.

VIGNETTE 1

One of the skilled nursing facility residents whom I visit is both blind and deaf. When our contact first began she could, by using a magnifying glass, read 2-inch-high print made with a broad-stroke pen. I attempted to answer her questions, explain her treatments, and give the reasons her blood pressure needed to be checked. However, as her blindness progressed, she began to misinterpret much of the care provided by the staff. As a result she was frequently hostile, shouted at the staff, and was occasionally combative, which made her care very difficult. A pattern had evolved during our relationship in which I touched her frequently, sometimes hugged her, and always followed the same routine when I examined her. This pattern has allowed me to make contact with her, even during times when she has been hostile and combative with the staff. I greet her by taking her hand and having her touch my hair and my watch. She has not yet failed to recognize me, and she becomes quiet and cooperative. She talks during the entire visit, pouring out everything that has happened to her since my last visit, as she interprets it. While she talks, I maintain close contact by sitting beside her on the bed, our bodies touching. Touch and communication are maintained by hand holding and sometimes a hug. As she talks, she provides a full history of her problems—both physiological and social. Although the account is marbled with her suspicions and accusations directed at the staff, the basic history is accurate and can be further checked and reviewed with the staff for a clear picture of both her physical and psychological status. She recently developed a means of getting answers to her questions by instructing me to move her hand vertically for yes and horizontally for no. I have shared this technique with the staff in an attempt to improve their communication with this very handicapped but mentally alert elder. Because of the strong trusting relationship between this patient and me, she has been able to provide information which, when shared with the staff, aids them in better understanding her behavior and makes them more thoughtful and caring in their approach to her. As a result, she has been able to maintain a fairly high level of independence within the confines of her room and the areas with which she is familiar. She has also remained oriented, despite her tendency to be somewhat suspicious and threatened by the staff and her environment. (Probably a normal tendency in view of the severe sensory handicaps that she experiences.)

APPROACHING THE CONFUSED ELDER

When the very confused or the very agitated patient is approached, the history may have to be postponed. The nurse doing the assessment must concentrate on establishing enough contact to allow the patient to be approached in order to be able to assess the vital organ system and determine what the person's acute health problems are at that point. It may be necessary to assess only those problems and develop a health management plan first. After those problems are stabilized, then a history may be obtained from the patient. Records, the family, and other interested persons are resources that should be utilized in an attempt to understand what has happened to the patient to precipitate the present crisis.

For very agitated and combative patients, having someone face them and act as a distraction while the examiner approaches usually helps. Talking to the patient and using reassuring touch during the examination also has a calming effect. Standing behind the combative elder allows the examiner to auscultate the heart, lungs, and abdomen; palpate the abdomen for distention, rigidity, organomegaly, and abnormal masses; check for fecal impaction; and look for edema or signs of dehydration. At that time, examining the eyes, ears, nose, and throat may not be possible because the patient is too combative or resistant. Examination of the head may also have to be postponed, but it should not be missed. Ear canals impacted with cerumen are common, cataracts are endemic, and poorly fitting dentures and resulting ulcers of the gums may be factors contributing to malnutrition. Important data can be derived from the limited type of examination described, such as symptoms of congestive heart failure, pneumonia, bowel obstruction or fecal impactions, and signs of severe dehydration or edema that might suggest a fluid and electrolyte imbalance or renal failure. Laboratory studies can support or disprove clinical symptoms.

Recommended laboratory studies for screening include (1) SMA 20; (2) T_4 for thyroid function; (3) CBC to look for anemia, abnormal white blood cell counts, and other types of blood disorders; (4) urinalysis; and (5) chest x-ray. The last three tests can often indicate occult infectious processes. If the patient has been on medication, such as digoxin, Dilantin, barbiturates, or lithium, blood levels should be ordered for those drugs.

CAREFUL REVIEW OF EXISTING HISTORY

When a patient is admitted to the skilled nursing facility under the care of our team, the staff notifies the nurse member of the team to report the resident's arrival. Base data are collected at that time, including (1) age, (2) prior residence, (3) admitting diagnosis, (4) present medications, (5) mental status, and (6) activity level. Information about the activity level includes ability to perform activities of daily living, continence of bowel and bladder, and mobility.

Before the patient is seen, the nurse practitioner talks to the staff in order to get their impressions of the patient and reviews the medical record, if one has accompanied the patient. This information is scrutinized carefully for:

1. Information which may be missing
2. Tests to confirm diagnosis
3. Failure to treat identified problems
4. Medication for which there is no diagnosis
5. Combinations of medications that might be contraindicated
6. Medications that might give a clue to a history of drug or alcohol abuse and polypharmacy

The information is then carefully analyzed in an attempt to form a coherent pattern of the patient's past problems and interventions. This review serves to alert the examiner to possible unidentified problems when interviewing the patient and the family. For example, when someone enters the skilled nursing facility from an acute hospital and is on a regimen of thiamine, folic acid, and possibly vitamin B_{12}, without a diagnosis of alcohol abuse, it stimulates curiosity about whether this patient did have a problem with alcohol or suffered from malnutrition for other reasons. If so, what were the reasons?

Many times a careful review of the laboratory reports will reveal evidence of a urinary tract infection, with no evidence that the infection has been treated. This probably means that the patient still has a urinary tract infection, which may account for some of the confusion and/or other symptoms exhibited by the patient.

If the history indicates the patient was living at home alone and taking care of his or her own needs prior to acute hospitalization, and the patient arrives with a diagnosis of chronic brain syndrome, that history should cause one to question whether the diagnosis is correct. It could reflect a failure to identify underlying pathology that caused the patient to exhibit some confusion and could indicate that the person was labeled with a diagnosis of chronic brain syndrome only because of being old and ill. Investigation and treatment of the acute problem might clear this patient's thinking processes and make it possible for the elder to return to a former level of living.

Pay particular attention to any medications, sedatives, and tranquilizers, both major and minor, that the patient might have been taking. Often a patient will be taking a variety of medications that may include antiepileptic drugs, barbiturates, hypnotics, and major or minor tranquilizers. These drugs may have been prescribed over a period of time for various problems without a review of the total medication regimen. The patient may have been taking all those medications, and as the elder became more confused, the dosage may have been increased in an attempt to control the confusion and agitation, which was really caused by overmedication or the combination of drugs. Many patients who are admitted to the skilled nursing facility have been "cured" simply by stopping all drugs and allowing them about 2 weeks to return to a nontoxic condition.

The point of a careful review of the accompanying history and problems, even before one sees the patient, is to always have some skepticism toward a diagnosis of chronic brain syndrome. It also provides a base from which to approach the patient with a feeling of optimism and a tentative plan to restore this person to an improved level of function.

TALK WITH THE FAMILY

An opportunity to talk with the family before seeing the patient aids in evaluating a family's attitude toward the ill member. How does the family view the elder? Do they view him or her as difficult, a burden, incapable of getting better? Did they notice that the patient was getting a little forgetful and classify the forgetfulness as "senility"? Is the family concerned and helpful? Will a support system be available if the elder improves, so the elder can return to former surroundings? All these questions are part of the history and affect the assessment and management plan. Conflict in the family system can be suspected as contributing to the elder's present condition. Assessment of the family and the staff attitudes toward and expectations of the elder provide the assessor with clues as to how the elder views himself or herself. Those attitudes and expectations are the mirror in which the elder sees himself or herself reflected, and they have a strong impact in forming self-image. Enlisting family and/or staff support is crucial in motivating an elder to invest in hope.

The professional should be acutely aware of his or her own attitudes and feelings toward the elderly patient. Whatever those are, they will be transmitted, no matter how confused the elder might be. Optimism or lack of interest will be transmitted nonverbally, much more clearly than by any spoken word.

MEETING THE PATIENT

As I enter the room and first meet the patient, I take a little time to move objects around, set my bag down, and arrange my instruments, and I use that time to observe the patient. How is she or he lying? Is the patient watching alertly and with interest, or lying with eyes closed and without responding to the activity? Is the elder's face turned toward the wall? Does the elder look depressed? Angry? Hostile? Tense? Taking the time for observation gives the elderly patient a chance to get used to my being in the room and become prepared. It gives him or her an opportunity to become a little curious.

I approach with hand outstretched and let the elder set the pace. His or her response may be to reach for my hand or ignore it, or tell me to go away. The response has a strong impact on how I will proceed with the history portion of the assessment. After introducing myself I describe my role and explain the purpose of my visit. I sit in a chair that puts me at eye level, because sitting indicates an unhurried visit with time to talk, and the position is not one that increases a sense of helplessness in the elderly patient.

Most elders who are not severely confused are usually happy to find someone who seems genuinely interested and willing to sit and talk with them. They will pour out information. The nurses' problem will be to gather all the pertinent information without preventing the disclosure of what they need to talk about. Sometimes these histories take quite a while, because they are thought of not only as a source of significant information, but also as a therapeutic catharsis for the patient. However, there are patients who are so threatened by finding themselves in a long-term care environment that their only protection is denial and hostility. Quite often an elderly person will be unwilling to tell one anything and will be suspicious, angry, and bitter about his or her status. The need to retain control will be demonstrated by refusal to participate.

VIGNETTE 2

A 94-year-old male, Mr. A., was an example of this type of patient. His elderly wife could no longer keep him at home because he was becoming more and more confused, had urinary urgency and frequency, and was unable to get to the bathroom without assistance. Because of her frail health, she had reached a point where she was no longer able to care for him. In the nursing facility, he was aware enough to realize where he was and was extremely frightened by this situation and also very angry. I approached him on three occasions in an attempt to do a history and physical. Each time he absolutely refused to talk to me or to allow me to do more than a cursory examination. He was so threatened by his situation that to have forced my services on him would have been both a physical and psychic assault. The only solution was to telephone the family, share the problem with them, and ask them to try to persuade him to allow me to do the assessment and share the necessary information. The family interceded, and Mr. A. did become willing to share his feelings, his symptoms, and his goals with me.

This gentleman was very clear about his goals. There was only one place he wanted to be and that was home. Based on his goal, a plan was developed and Mr. A. was motivated to participate. We began bladder training, and we discovered a urinary tract infection which was treated. He began a physical therapy program designed to teach him to transfer from his bed to wheelchair and from his wheelchair to the toilet. Strengthening and gait-training exercises for walking were added as he progressed. Eventually, because of his obstructive uropathy with residual retention, a urinary catheter had to be inserted. The catheter provided a side benefit, eliminating the urinary frequency that had caused loss of sleep at night. As a result, he was more able to put his energy into participating in his physical therapy during the day. He was discharged home within 1 month, ambulatory, with assistance from a home care health agency. I believe very strongly that if Mr. A.'s feelings, fears, and desires had not been considered in his assessment, he would not have obtained the level of independence that he developed. A history should include identification of the patient's goals. When those goals are determined, they should become a priority item in the care plan. Accomplishing those goals may become the foundation which restores the hope and motivation that allows an elderly person to return to independent living. If there is no possibility for independent living, accomplishing those goals can be what makes life *worth* living to that elder.

PRIORITIES

When one is doing a history, it is important to make a fairly quick assessment of the patient's strengths, attention span, and level of fatigue. If the patient looks very tired or weak, the examiner will want to concentrate on obtaining the information that is important to the patient's immediate well-being. Health problems of the elder's parents and other relatives may be irrelevant to the present needs of an elder who has already lived to a great age. More information can be obtained after the patient has stabilized.

After completing the history, always thank the patient for sharing. Then ask if there is anything that he or she would like to talk about that might help in understanding him or her better. Often this question will cause an outpouring of grief and anger, tales of disappointment and sorrow over events and relationships in life. The nurse should be prepared to accept the weeping that frequently occurs in response to the question and recognize that the healing process has already begun as the elder unloads the burden of emotion long carried within.

MENTAL STATUS EXAMINATION

Assessment of mental status begins early, based on information gathered from records and family as well as on observation of the level of consciousness and the elder's behavior. Usual simple tests include questions which test the elder's recent and remote memory, orientation to person, place, and time, calculations and current information about the social or political structure of the society (i.e., What is your name? Name of the president? Where are we now?) (Caird and Judge, 1977).

Care must be exercised in asking mental status questions to avoid the impression of an interrogation. Such an impression may cause the elder to feel threatened and result in withdrawal or hostility. It is best to start with questions the elder is most likely to be able to answer without a great deal of thought, such as birth date, birthplace, and information about close family members which most elders retain even when confused. Questions should be asked in a conversational tone with a show of interest. If those questions are answered successfully, then gradually more complex questions are introduced.

Old people are usually very concerned about their mental status. They fear becoming confused and "senile." When they are unable to call up memories quickly, they often assume that

they are showing signs of the dreaded "senility." Since this is a subject that already causes a great deal of anxiety, being unable to recall quickly increases their stress level and makes it less likely that they will be able to provide the information asked of them. One goal during a mental status examination is to help the patient be as comfortable and relaxed about the questions asked as is possible. By going from the simple, easily answered questions to the gradually more complex, the patient experiences success and is more relaxed about answering complex questions. If the patient is very confused and rambling, take time to listen carefully. Often significant clues about the patient's history can be picked out of the flow.

The conclusions of the mental status examination should not be written in stone. That status may show a dramatic improvement after the patient's physical and emotional problems have been identified and resolved.

PHYSICAL EXAMINATION: SPECIAL PROBLEMS

Certain problems which cause both mental confusion and debilitation should be expected and looked for in the elderly. They are so common as to be endemic in that population, and they may be missed because their onset is insidious and the symptoms are vague. These problems include:

- Dehydration: Look for poor skin turgor, peaking of the skin when it is gently pinched, dull sunken eyes, dry mouth mucosa, increased pulse, low fever, concentrated strong-smelling urine, and an elevated blood urea nitrogen in the laboratory reports. Kee (1973) reports that in a dehydrated patient, the hemoglobin and red blood cell count may be above normal limits; however, in anemia because of hemoglobin concentration those tests may appear within normal limits.
- Fecal impactions: Check the abdomen for distention and left lower quadrant tenderness and masses. Always do a rectal examination. Do not be trapped by a recorded history of a recent bowel movement. It is easier for an

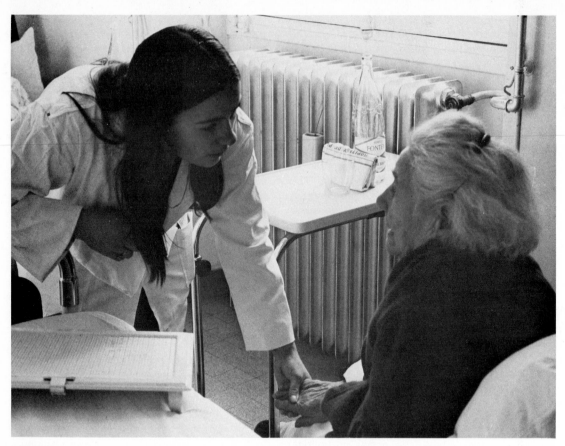

FIGURE 30-3 Examiners must first establish a climate of reassurance and trust in the interaction. A warm greeting with an extended hand and good eye contact will almost always result in acceptance of that hand; maintain the hand contact as long as the elderly person shows an inclination to it. If the client clings to the offered hand, examiners can show acceptance and additional warmth by covering the client's hand with their other hand for a moment. (*World Health Organization, photo by E. Schwab.*)

overworked employee to record a bowel movement than to give an enema.

- *Anemia:* Pale mucosa and pallor are clues, but a CBC is essential. If anemia is present, consider occult gastrointestinal bleeding as a possible causative factor. Investigate for a history of aspirin or other anticoagulant intake. Look for signs of undernutrition, both clinically (loose skin folds and emaciation) and in laboratory reports, such as anemia, decreased protein, and albumin.

- *Urinary tract infections:* These may be present in males because of hypertrophied prostates causing obstructive uropathy and in females because of atrophic mucosa and improper hygiene. Both sexes are at risk because of in-adequate fluid intake and incomplete emptying of the bladder (Jennings, Nordstrom, and Schumake, 1973).

- *Pneumonia and/or congestive heart failure:* Both often appear together, one precipitating the other. The frail elder is often generally debilitated, and suffers from arteriosclerotic heart disease and valvular insufficiencies. They rarely fully expand the lungs and are likely to have been immobile; hence they are at risk for cardiac decompensation and pneumonia (Coni, Williamson, and Webster, 1977).

- *Depression, both endogenous and exogenous:* The frail elder has usually experienced over-whelming physiological and psychological stress prior to entry into the health care system.

- *Drug toxicity and oversedation:* Many elders are on cardiac drugs, digoxin being one. Many of them will be on dosages of 0.25 mg per day. As elders age, kidney function decreases. Digoxin is eliminated through the kidney, and, if renal impairment is present, the patient may quickly build up toxic dosages (Kayne, 1976). Also patients with cardiac problems are usually on a diuretic which can cause electrolyte and fluid imbalances. Even potassium-sparing diuretics can cause hypokalemia. Because of changes in the aging physiology, drug dosages that would be therapeutic in a younger patient may be toxic in an older patient. The drugs may be poorly eliminated or more slowly metabolized. Drugs that have a long half-life such as certain sedatives, hypnotics, and antipsychotics can build up to toxic proportions (Chapron and Lawson, 1978). We frequently encounter patients who are on hypnotics such as flurazepam, 30 mg at bedtime with an order for a repeat. There are very few aging physiologies that can tolerate that dosage for very long, and flurazepam has a long half-life (Soloman et al., 1978). The end result of such a regimen may be a patient who is agitated all night, lethargic and drowsy all day, and frequently very, very confused. Other drug regimens that should alert one to a possibility of overdosage or toxicities include barbiturates, lithium, major and minor tranquilizers, and hypoglycemics.
- *Foot problems:* Thickened hypertrophied mycotic toenails may hide ulcerations. Hammertoes and thick, painful plantar calluses may have caused instability of gait leading to a fractured hip or cessation of ambulation (see Chapter 21).

NEED AND BENEFITS

The proportion of the very old, those over 75 years of age, is increasing. Califano (1976) reports that in 1940 only 7 percent of the total population was 65 and over. Today that proportion is 11 percent, and estimates are that by the year 2030, 18 percent of the population will be 65 or over. There is also a change in the pattern of the aged. In 1940, 30 percent of older people were 75 or over; by the year 2000 they will compose 45 percent of the elderly. Faye Abdellah (1977; 1978) reports that persons currently reaching their sixty-fifth birthday will on the average live 16 more years, or to age 81.

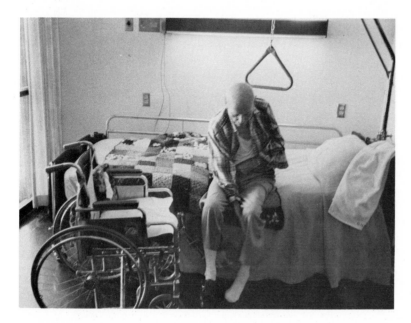

FIGURE 30-4 This man is 90 years old. When one is taking a history it is important to make a fairly quick assessment of the patient's strengths, attention span, and level of fatigue. If the elderly person looks very tired or weak, the examiner will want to concentrate on obtaining the information that is important to the patient's immediate well-being. (*Courtesy of Anthony J. Skirlick, Jr.*)

As those numbers of elders increase, so will the need for nurses who are knowledgeable in common threats to elder's health, who are able to develop programs to prevent illness, support wellness, and assist frail elders to attain and maintain their maximum potential for health.

The development of knowledge of the special needs and common threats to the health of frail elders and skills in meeting those needs by nurses, combined with sensitivity and appreciation of the uniqueness of each elder, will allow the nurse to function as a therapeutic agent and as a potent client advocate. The interventions of the nurse can result in increased successful outcomes and greatly improve the quality of life for the elders so served. The frequency of successful interventions is a powerful antidote to the hopelessness and helplessness frequently experienced by health care providers when confronted with the complexities of the multiple problems of the frail elder and results in enrichment of the provider's professional life.

REFERENCES

Abdellah, Faye G.: Long Term Care Policy Issues: Alternatives to Institutional Care, Annals AAPSS, 438, July 1978, Department of Health, Education, and Welfare, Health: United States 1976–1977, PHS, HRA (NCHS, NCHSR), DHEW Publication no. HRA 77-1232, Hyattsville, Md., 1977, pp. 3–26.

Caird, F. I., and T. G. Judge: Assessment of the Elderly Patient, 3d ed., Pitman Press, Bath, England, 1977, p. 94.

Califano, Joseph A., Jr.: The aging of America, Questions for a Four Generation Society, Annals AAPSS, 438, July 1978, pp. 97–98, Bureau of the Census, Demographic Aspects of Aging and the Older Populations of the United States, Current Population Reports no. 59, January, 1976, pp. 9–26.

Chapron, Dennis, and Jon Lawson: Drug prescribing and the elderly, in William Reichel (ed.), Clinical Aspects of Aging, Williams & Wilkins, Baltimore, 1978, pp. 20–26.

Coni, N., D. Williamson, and S. Webster: Lecture Notes on Geriatrics, Blackwell Scientific Publications, distributed by Lippincott, Philadelphia, 1977, pp. 205–206.

Harris, Raymond: Special problems of geriatric patients with heart disease, in William Reichel (ed.), Clinical Aspects of Aging, Williams & Wilkins, Baltimore, 1978, p. 45.

Jennings, M., M. Nordstrom, and N. Schumake: Physiologic functioning in the elderly, Nursing Clinics of North America, 7(2):242, June 1973.

Kayne, Ronald C.: Drugs and the aged, in Irene M. Burnside (ed.), Nursing and the Aged, McGraw-Hill, New York, 1976.

Kee, Joyce L.: Fluid imbalance in elderly patients, Nursing 73, April 1973, pp. 40–43.

Loeb, Phillip, and Billie J. Robison: Experience of a physician-nurse practitioner team in care of patients in skilled nursing facilities, Journal of Family Practice, 4(4):727–730, April 1977.

Soloman, F., et al.: Sleeping pills, insomnia and medical practice, New England Journal of Medicine, 300(14):803–808, April 5, 1978.

THIRTY-ONE

THE HOME ASSESSMENT

Valerie L. Remnet

I make the most of all that comes,
The least of all that goes.
Sara Teasdale

LEARNING OBJECTIVES

- Discuss the three factors that need to be determined at the outset of an interview of the aged.
- Discuss four areas to assess in the physical environment of the aged for safety.
- Discuss four factors in assessment of interpersonal relationships.
- List the major factors in the assessment of physical and psychological dynamics.
- Describe the mental status questionnaire (MSQ).[1]
- Describe the three major types of service plan the elderly might need.

---

[1] The MSQ can be found in Chapter 14.

The home visit is a valuable therapeutic tool in two ways. First, one can make an individualized assessment of the needs of the elderly person. Second, one can make an optimum "fit" between these needs and the available services in the community. A crucial aspect of the assessment of elderly clients is that they are likely to have a conglomerate of social, physical, and psychological problems (Gaitz and Baer, 1970). These problems may serve to further accentuate individual differences, which are already more pronounced because of senescence. Old people are not a homogeneous group. They vary widely in health, personality, behavior, and socioeconomic background. The processes of aging vary from one individual to another, within each individual's organs, parts, and body systems, and progress at different rates. The span of years of the aging phase of life can be longer than that of any other phase (Spark and Brody, 1972).

Thus, the aged, because of their life experiences and current problems, need individual assessments of: (1) the physical environment, (2) interpersonal relationships, and (3) personal dynamics, both physical and psychological, which are influencing present functioning. Such assessments can be done most effectively in the elderly person's home milieu by a trained professional.

INTERVIEWING THE AGED

In his writings on situational assessment and intervention, Siporin (1972) states that a basic principle of the assessment process is that of client participation, that evaluation can properly be done only with the active engagement and collaboration of the client in a joint worker-client enterprise. *To help the client through a diagnostic experience is a basic helping intervention.* Situational assessments, moreover, involve judgments about discrepancies between the actual life situation of the client and what is considered normative or appropriate for a well-functioning individual (or group) at certain stages of life. This calls for self-awareness on the part of the professional and consideration of cultural, class, and other values and criteria being used. Such discriminations and judgments

need to be validated in direct discussions with the client.

In order to have an effective discussion with the elderly person, Burnside (1980) relates three factors which need to be determined at the outset. These are (1) assessment of distance, both physical and psychological, (2) assessment of hearing and vision, and (3) assessment of comprehension. She states that $1\frac{1}{2}$ to $2\frac{1}{2}$ feet is usually an effective and comfortable distance between the interviewer and interviewee and that they should be facing each other. Older persons seem to respond more readily when they can look directly at the interviewer. Also, psychological distance, which involves the interaction between the interviewer and the elderly person, must be sensitively evaluated. Burnside found that when there was a reciprocity in the interview, in which the aged are allowed the ego-enhancing role of an authority on the subject of survival and aging, the interview was more effective and, more importantly, therapeutic for the elderly person. Also, some persons may react readily to warmth and closeness and others may be suspicious and guarded, and the interviewer will need to go slowly and schedule several interviews in order to build up trust and rapport.

Burnside relates that hearing can be assessed by asking interviewees if they can hear what is said. They may say that their hearing in one ear is better than the other and would prefer interviewers to sit on that side. Also, if the elderly have a diagnosis of cataracts or glaucoma, it will be necessary to sit closer. Comprehension ability will be maximized if interviewers will (1) consider interviewees' cultural and educational background, (2) pace themselves to the slower responses of the aged, (3) use short sentences, (4) speak slowly, and (5) limit the number of questions.

ASSESSMENT OF THE PHYSICAL ENVIRONMENT

The assessment of the physical environment of the home involves both its safety for the client and its potential information about the person's past and present life-style. The influence of en-

TABLE 31-1

ASSESSMENT OF HOME SAFETY

1. Throughout the interior there are several common features which should be checked for safety. For example:
   a. Are scatter rugs firmly anchored with rubber backing?
   b. Are electrical cords in good repair, especially a heating pad?
   c. Light, heat, and ventilation
      (1) Is there adequate night lighting?
      (2) Are stairways continually illuminated?
      (3) Is temperature within comfortable range (70–75°F)?
      (4) Is the heater vented properly?
      (5) Is there cross ventilation?
   d. Is furniture sturdy enough to give support?
   e. Is there a minimum of clutter, allowing enough room for easy mobility as well as less fire hazard?
   f. Are emergency telephone numbers posted in a handy place and easily read, such as doctor, fire department, ambulance, paramedics, nearest relative?
   g. If the client has limited vision, does phone have enlarged dial?
2. The kitchen can be evaluated for the following:
   a. Stove, refrigerator, and sink
      (1) Is the stove free of grease and flammable objects?
      (2) Is baking soda available in case of fire?
      (3) Are matches used or is there a pilot light?
      (4) Is the refrigerator working properly?
      (5) Is the sink draining well?
   b. Is food being stored properly?
   c. Is trash taken out daily?
   d. Is there a sturdy stepping stool in evidence?
   e. Are there skid-proof mats on the floor?
3. In the bathroom, are safety measures observed?
   a. Are handrails beside the tub and toilet?
   b. Are skid-proof mats in the bathtub and/or shower?
   c. Are electrical outlets a safe distance from the tub?
4. Outside the home, points to consider include:
   a. Walks and stairs
      (1) Are there raised or uneven places on the sidewalks?
      (2) Are stairs in good repair?
      (3) Are the top and bottom stairs painted white or a bright contrasting color to improve visibility?
      (4) Are handrails securely fastened?
   b. Are screens on doors and windows in good repair?
   c. Is there an alternate exit for the house?

vironment on behavior varies with the individual's capabilities. Newcomer (1973) has found that the environment may have little effect on the capable person who may be able to change the environment or leave it. However, as capabilities decrease, the individual may have less of a possibility to manipulate the situation. According to DeLong (1970) underlying all perceptions of space are a person's senses, and in the aged there is a decreased sensitivity in the sensory apparatus. Thus, the sensory contact of the elderly with their social and spatial environment is diminished, and they must negotiate with that environment with reduced information.

Functioning with such reduced information can increase the accident potential in the environment. A home which was safe and in good condition when the person was in the middle years now might need some changes and repairs to compensate for the elderly person's declining abilities. However, the suggestion of any changes must be made with the appropriate timing and emotional support. As Roberts (1980) states, "Man's sense of space is closely related to his sense of self, it is an intimate transaction with his environment." Thus, in order to give recognition to the supportive changes needed in the home, the aging person must also give recognition to a declining ability to function.

The assessment can be made on a brief tour of the residence. Such a tour is done only at the invitation of the person. Experience has demonstrated that most people are proud to act as host or hostess and show the interviewer through the house. Areas which should receive special attention in an assessment for home safety include (1) the outside of the house, (2) the kitchen, and (3) the bathroom. Table 31-1 could serve as a checklist for a nurse on a home visit.

In addition to assessing the home for safety, the tour can provide information about the person's past experiences, hobbies, life-style, and interpersonal relationships. Many elderly have objects which they value because of a long association. Smith (1956) describes these objects as windows which look into the person's past.

These objects acquire even greater value in their owner's eyes as he ages, and as he feels more and more the need for reassuring glimpses into that past wherein he sees triumphs and affection which he cannot glimpse in the bleak future. Moreover, inanimate objects have a reassuring constancy, a quality which the aging person often needs to encounter in a world of rapid change. . . . The expected sameness, when encountered, brings reassurance. . . . An aged hand cradles the bowl of a pipe and derives as much comfort from the touch as from the fragrant smoke. For sameness, dependable sameness, means that a person need not readjust as he must to change. And it is very pleasant for the old person to use an adjustment long perfected. Here is the effortless peace of habit.

Items for consideration in this assessment could include: (1) the colors used in decorating the house, (2) the presence of flowers, pictures, photographs of relatives and friends, (3) the presence and types of books, records, magazines and newspapers, (4) the presence of mementoes, hobbies, or craft work, and (5) the presence of clocks, calendars, and mirrors.

ASSESSMENT OF INTERPERSONAL RELATIONSHIPS

Interpersonal relationships may include the family, friends, neighbors, clubs, and religious affiliations. Family dynamics are usually brought out early by the elderly client. Weiner et al. (1967) found that frequently clients present a distorted picture of their families. Clients may state that relatives are all against them or that they are treating them with indifference. The relatives, in turn, feel misunderstood and are angry about clients' accusations. "Just as a child expects that his parents can relieve his pain, undo all harm, so does the senescent parent unconsciously expect his children to remove the burdens of his age." While they are dissatisfied with themselves, senescent persons demand from their children the impossible, that they make them unaware of their weakness (Anthony and Benedek, 1970). Thus, care should be taken to distinguish between the objective circumstances and the subjective states.

Such factors as the proximity of the children and frequency of contact need to be assessed. It is important to evaluate (1) the family's understanding of the situation, (2) what they are doing about the situation, (3) what they can realistically continue to do, and (4) what they are unable to do. "Filial maturity requires the adult child's capacity to accept and resolve what he cannot do, as well as mature acceptance of the can-and-should do filial role" (Spark and Brody, 1972). Also, it is relevant to explore previous relationship patterns between the elderly person and the family. The family's current attitudes and behavior will be in continuity with previous experiences.

Friends and neighbors are important sources of primary relationships. Atchley (1972) writes that the demands of the friend role are flexible and can be adjusted to fit the individual's capability in terms of health and energy. It is the greatest source of companionship next to that of spouse. In areas where the older population dominates, group neighborliness is in evidence. Sheldon (1956) traces this group spirit back to the time when women had their babies together, and they got used to helping one another right from the start. Thus, it is important to assess the presence of friends and neighbors, their proximity, frequency of contact, and services exchanged.

However, there is no uniformity among the aged about what they want for themselves. An example of such differences is given by Field (1968) in a story of two elderly ladies who lived in the same house. One of the ladies wrote day after day, "Nobody came to see me today." The other lady's diary contained the same sentence over and over again, "Nobody came to see me today, thank God." The loneliness of the first lady would not be understood by the second lady, just as the contentment of being alone, expressed by her, would not be understood by her neighbor. Thus, one can be alone without being lonely, just as one can be with family, friends, clubs, activity groups, and religious activities and still feel isolated and lonely. In assessing social activities outside the home, past and present attendance patterns and the degree of involvement of the person are significant. It is essential to discover what the meaning of personal relationships and activities has for the individual. There is no reason to expect that the elderly will change their whole life-style just because they are growing old.

Also, it is important to observe pets in the home. Many older people who have no close fulfilling personal relationships lavish their affection and attention on pets. Vickery (1972) writes that this investment of strong emotional feelings and attachments on animals becomes a sublimation or redirection of normal feelings whose expression may have been thwarted because of lack of close human relationships.

In addition to recognizing the continuity of life-style and present relationships, the interviewer also needs to assess recent changes in the life-style and relationship patterns. Burnside (1970) writes of loss as a constant theme with the aged. By far the most painful loss and the most difficult is the loss of a loved spouse. Death of friends through the years is another significant loss. Kaplan (1957) states that losing relatives and friends makes an older person feel insecure and without protection. Financial and role losses may prevent elderly persons from attending clubs and religious activities which might have become significant parts of their previous socialization pattern. Burnside (1969) writes that one needs to remember always that any loss experienced by the aged person in the past couple of years would be considered a potential reason for grieving. Also, anniversary dates of any significant loss need to be noted. These dates may be particularly stressful, especially if there is unresolved grief work.

ASSESSMENT OF PHYSICAL AND PSYCHOLOGICAL DYNAMICS

Many aged will try to maintain their life-style, even when their failing capacities make it a practical impossibility. Thus, the aging person's physical capabilities and psychological state need to be assessed in relation to the capacity for self-care. Factors to help assess physical capabilities include (1) general health, (2) personal care and safety, (3) mobility, (4) dietary needs, (5) housekeeping and maintenance, and (6) management of finances (see Table 31-2).

In conjunction with the assessment of an elderly person's physical capabilities, an evaluation of mental state in relation to ability to perform the necessary activities of daily living is relevant. This evaluation may include (1) a mental status questionnaire, (2) assessment of self-esteem, (3) changes in body image, (4) use of defense mechanisms, and (5) presence of depression.

Kahn et al.'s (1960) mental status questionnaire can be used to assess the presence of chronic brain syndrome (see the table in Chapter 14). Chronic brain syndrome develops gradually. Symptoms may include (1) lack of affect, (2) impairment of memory, and (3) confusion and lack of orientation. Generally, chronic brain syndrome is considered to be irreversible. Depression may resemble chronic brain syndrome. However, a person with chronic brain syndrome is disoriented, whereas a person who is depressed remains oriented. Acute brain syn-

TABLE 31-2
ASSESSMENT OF PHYSICAL CAPABILITIES

General Health

1. Has the elderly person had a recent physical examination?
2. Is there a regular family doctor?
3. Are hearing, eyesight, teeth adequate or corrected?
4. Is the corrective device in good working order (hearing aid working, glasses prescribed in recent years and for the client, lens in good condition)?
5. Can the person move or sit without feeling dizzy and falling?
6. Can the person control the passing of urine and bowel movements?
7. Can the person manage a special disability without help (an amputation, severe arthritis, colostomy, insulin injections)?

Personal Care and Safety

1. Can the person accomplish the following activities of daily living
   a. Attend to daily grooming (shaving, combing hair, brushing teeth, cutting fingernails, and toenails)?
   b. Get in and out of bed?
   c. Get on and off the toilet, in and out of the bathtub?
   d. Dress and undress?
2. If the person is capable of personal care, is he or she well groomed?
3. Do slippers and shoes fit securely, have nonskid soles?
4. Are sleeves to robes and/or dresses close-fitting, to minimize fire hazard?
5. Are devices, such as canes, walkers, wheelchairs or other prostheses, in good repair?
6. Are medicines in a special place, well-labeled, prescribed for the person, and within expiration date?

Mobility

1. Can the following be accomplished with competence
   a. Walk around a room?
   b. Leave the building?
   c. Walk up and down stairs?
   d. Walk around the block?
   e. Drive a car?
   f. Use public transportation?
2. Is the person doing the exercises of which he or she is physically capable?

Dietary Needs

1. In maintaining nutritional needs, can the person shop, prepare meals?
2. Is the person eating properly balanced meals, drinking enough fluids?
3. If on a special diet, is the person both knowledgeable and capable of preparing it?

Housekeeping and Maintenance

1. Can the person perform housekeeping tasks as follows
   a. Wash and dry dishes?
   b. Dust and maintain household order?
   c. Do the laundry and ironing?
   d. Vacuum and/or mop the floors?
   e. Clean the bathroom?
   f. Keep the stove and refrigerator clean?
2. Is the person able to do yard work?
3. Can the person perform seasonal tasks, such as washing walls, repairing screens, washing windows, moving furniture, pruning the garden?

TABLE 31-2
ASSESSMENT OF PHYSICAL CAPABILITIES (*Continued*)

Management of Finances

1. With financial matters, can the person manage daily purchases, write checks, and pay bills on time?
2. Does the person have a knowledge of budgeting and wise shopping practices?
3. Does the person feel he or she has adequate finances to meet his or her needs?

drome has a rapid onset, and mental functioning may be less uniformly affected. Generally, acute brain syndrome is reversible.

The level of self-esteem can be a significant factor in both the elderly person's motivation to function and willingness to accept needed help. Changes in self-esteem may be initiated by retirement. Field (1968) noted,

> With retirement, an older person is suddenly faced with the realization of a reduced income, or no income, and the urgent need to adjust to it; with time on his hands and not having learned what to do with it; with a loss of companionship as mutual interest in work recedes into the background; and a loss of status because he is no longer productive.

(See Chapter 41 for more information on retirement.)

Further role constriction can negatively·influence the elderly's self-esteem. Loss of spouse and friends, restricted mobility due to ill health, and withdrawal from community organizations due to economic limitations can add to the aged person's problem of rolelessness. Rolelessness can lead to loneliness, social isolation, or alienation. Wood (1953) wrote,

> Loneliness, with its related problems, is the result of frustration of man's biosocial needs by the processes of desocialization in modern society, that is, by the reduction of modes and opportunities for spontaneous and unreserved social participation.

And Schacht (1970) wrote,

> Social isolation can be construed in the sense of the absence of positive interpersonal relationships . . . the individual who

tried to establish meaningful contact with another and is not successful. Alienation is an awareness of non-belonging or non-sharing.

While according to Mead (1934),

> It is in the form of the generalized other that the social process influences the behavior of the individuals involved in it and carrying it on . . . in abstract thought, the individual takes the attitude of the generalized other.

Thus, the aged person's loss of self-esteem, as reflected by society, may be a factor in the withdrawal from, rather than a reaching out for, needed services.

The concept of the generalized other also applies to the younger members of society. Society reflects positively on them, not only because they are productive, but also because they possess youth, vigor, and physical beauty. Such qualities are valued highly by our society. As the normal aging process gradually reduces the possession of these qualities, thus changing one's body image, the individual can become quite threatened. "There is reason to believe that the status losses such changes imply and the consequent threat to self are much more significant psychologically than any diminution of actual functional capacity" (Kuhlen, 1956). Thus, considering our societal values, relatively insignificant changes such as graying hair and increasing weight can be a threat to the individual. However, body image changes in chronic illness can be significantly more threatening. Leonard (1972) believes,

> Any alteration in the body is a disturbance of one's integrity, a threat to one's self. . . . There are frequently feelings of shame

when a person loses control of such bodily functions as bowel and bladder function and speech. . . . Shame is the personal, private judgment of failure passed on one's self by himself. . . . A disabled individual often has fears of death, incapacitation, pain, abandonment, loss of self-esteem, and disturbance of interpersonal relationships. For the most part these fears are based on fact and reality; they are not delusions.

Thus, it is important to assess not only elderly persons' perceptions and feelings about their body changes and capacity to function but also to assess the perceptions and feelings of their families and significant others in their lives.

DEFENSE MECHANISMS

Vickery (1972) writes that in order to cope with the many uncomfortable changes that life brings, an individual utilizes unconscious though healthy psychic reactions known as defense mechanisms. She cites some of the more common ones used by older adults.

1. *Denial* is a familiar defense mechanism by which people treat situations in the outer environment that make them feel uncomfortable as though they did not exist.
2. *Exclusion of unwanted stimuli* is a mechanism closely related to denial but of quite different dynamics. In this defense, people experience lowered psychic energy and an inability to deal with all stimuli coming to the consciousness from the outside. To protect their waning capacities, they begin to exclude some, hearing what they want to hear and seeing what they want to see.
3. *Rationalization* is the avoidance of the discomfort of acknowledging the truth by formulating more acceptable explanations. A parent who longs for more attention from an adult child may say, "My son would like to come to see me more often, but, after all, he is such an important and busy man."
4. *Projection* is the ego ascribing to another person what are in reality its own traits and unconscious wishes. Jealous mothers-in-law will say, "What more could you expect

from such a thoughtless, demanding, self-centered person as my son's wife!"
5. *Regression* is the utilization of ways of control that brought emotional satisfactions in earlier stages of life. The man who blows his top is using the adult version of the child's temper tantrum.
6. *Manipulation* is a healthy ego defense used by many older people to secure the protection and the help of a stronger individual when their egos are feeling weak and threatened. It takes the form of flattery, flirting or seductive conduct, complaints of helplessness, or displays of pain and stress. In these ways the older person strives to elicit the sympathy and attention of the authority figure.
7. *Reminiscing* is the use of past experiences as the frame of reference for a large portion of the individual's thought content and much of his or her conversation. Through reminiscing the person strives to maintain self-esteem, work through personal losses, and reaffirm his or her sense of identity. Any sense of depression that may accompany reminiscing is neither deep nor chronic.

Defense mechanisms are overlapping and interrelated. They are the ego's attempt to deal with reality and the stresses the aging person is facing. According to Moses (1972), in working with the elderly, "one does not try to tamper with their defenses unless modification of the life situation is feasible. . . . It is necessary to assess the degree of ego strength and to avoid depth insight because of the danger of rekindling old, unresolved conflicts." Thus, it is important to be aware of and assess both the defenses utilized by the elderly person and the degree of ego strength.

DEPRESSION IN THE ELDERLY

Depression in the elderly can be associated with environmental changes, loss of self-esteem, and/or changes in body image. Goldfarb (1967) states that the most common disorder, syndrome, or illness in the geriatric patient is depression. He writes that the components of depression, which are multiple, can include (1) early and late causes, (2) loss of resources, (3) decreased mastery, (4) feelings of helplessness with resulting fear and anger. He states that the depressed patient longs for assistance, which has come to be equated with or supplanted by a desire for understanding, for evidence of regard, and obligation regarded as "love." Thus, by being aware of the components of depression, one can more effectively assess the aging person's overt behavior. (See Chapter 10.)

ASSISTANCE PLAN FOR THE ELDERLY

The individualized assessment of the aging person and his or her needs may take several home visits. A relationship which will be therapeutic to the individual takes time to develop; thus, as previously mentioned, pacing one's self to the responses and needs of the elderly person is essential. The types of services that must be considered in the assistance plan are shown in Table 31-3.

In working out an accepted plan of assistance with elderly persons, it is important to be aware of their values, life-style, and habits. Frequent visits to the home will enhance this awareness. The plan should minimize the need for changing lifelong habits and patterns.

It is difficult to change patterns established throughout a lifetime, particularly when there is little need to keep pace. The habitual ways do not suit the changing conditions. The old person becomes anxious about new untried methods and grows increasingly conservative, wishing to use the ways that have proven adaptive but which now make him less capable of mastering new tasks. The need to do things differently grows burdensome. (Lidz, 1968)

In addition to recognizing the need to integrate needed assistance into the life-style of the aging individual, Milloy (1964) gives two criteria for recommending services (with the exception of protective services): (1) Will using the service increase or maintain the person's capacity for mastery? (2) Will it tend to lessen the client's sense of isolation and increase feelings of being needed? If the services being considered for the elderly person satisfy these criteria, they will both assist in maintaining the person's residence in the community and increase socialization. In order to establish an optimum "fit" between the elderly's needs and services, it is important to be aware of community resources in the four categories shown in Table 31-3.

In summary, the home visit can (1) serve as the basis for a therapeutic relationship between

TABLE 31-3
TYPES OF SERVICES REQUIRED

Basic services: Those services needed by all persons in the community.

1. Emergency financial assistance
2. Comprehensive outpatient medical care
3. Mental health services

Adjustment and integrative services: Those services that help older persons participate in community life, adjust to new social roles, and retain and utilize their capacities.

1. Counseling services
2. Legal aid
3. Retirement counseling
4. Adult day center
5. Senior citizen group activities
6. Information and referral service

Supportive services: Those services that help older persons retain their established living arrangements when they no longer can do so through their own efforts.

1. Homemaker services
2. Home health aides
3. Visiting nurse service
4. Home counseling service
5. Friendly visitor
6. Telephone reassurance service
7. Meals-on-Wheels
8. Transportation

Protective services: Those services that protect the civil rights and personal welfare of older persons who are subject to neglect and/or exploitation by relatives, friends, the community, or the aged persons themselves.

1. Public guardianship
2. Conservatorship

the older person and the interviewer, (2) provide the milieu in which necessary information can be obtained to work with the client in formulating a plan which will best meet individualized needs, and (3) serve as a base for follow-up visits as the interviewer acts as a liaison between the aging person and the community's resources. A vignette follows which exemplifies the salient points made in this chapter.

VIGNETTE: THE HOME VISIT

I visited Mrs. M. at the request of her daughter, Mrs. B. Mrs. B. said that her mother was "driving me to the end of my rope."

"No matter what I do for Mother, it is not enough!" "I visit Mother every day, and sometimes on my lunch hour, but she still calls me at least five times a day insisting that I come and see her right away. When I say I cannot, she tells me she just might die before I see her again. I cannot do my work well anymore because I cannot concentrate. I keep thinking, 'Suppose she did die, I would never forgive myself.'"

Mrs. B. went on to say that her mother was much worse since her hospitalization for a stroke 3 months ago. "I guess she has made a good recovery for her age, but she gets confused more often. I do the best I can to help her keep her home up, but I just cannot do anymore. I have my own family to look after, too."

I scheduled a home visit with Mrs. M. for later in the week. Mrs. B. said she would join me there if she could. As I approached the house, I noticed it was in good repair. There were no stairs involved. I rang the doorbell and had to wait several minutes for Mrs. M. to come to the door. I introduced myself and she welcomed me into her home. Mrs. M. walked slowly. "I get up around nine every morning, but it takes me until noon to be able to move around the house much."

I commented on her colorful dress and how pretty it was. Mrs. M. smiled and said she and her daughter had made it. "I do not feel ready for the day until I wash myself *completely* [she emphasized this point]. Even on days when I cannot get into the

tub, I take a sponge bath. Then I get dressed and I'm ready for the day." Mrs. M.'s attire was complete with hose, shoes, jewelry, and makeup.

Mrs. M. stated that she was hard-of-hearing. "I have a hearing aid but I do not wear it much, I have had a lot of trouble with it." I sat close to her and I noticed that she watched my lips intensely. As long as I spoke slowly, we had no difficulty in communicating.

Mrs. M. introduced me to "Mr. Cat" who had been living in the house for about 3 weeks. "I usually do not like animals, but he scratched on my door one night and looked so hungry, and he was so thin. He found me! Look at how fat and healthy he is now!" Mr. Cat snuggled and purred on Mrs. M.'s lap as she stroked him. Both looked contented.

With pride, Mrs. M. invited me on a tour of her home. Her eyes twinkled as she showed me her bedroom. "Not bad for an old lady, is it?" I complimented her on her taste and said the room reflected a person who enjoyed pretty things. She replied, "I have always loved pretty things. When I used to go dancing I wore frilly dresses. How I loved to dance!" In the bathroom I noticed there were no handrails or nonskid mats in the tub. Mrs. M. commented that she was taking more sponge baths recently and missed getting into the bathtub.

In the living room Mrs. M. pointed with pride to her daughter's painting which hung on the wall. Family photographs were on the TV. Handmade flower arrangements were on display throughout the room. In the kitchen I noticed that Mrs. M. had had a breakfast consisting of a boiled egg, toast, and cereal. "I like to start the day with a good meal, but I am getting forgetful and cannot cook dinners like I used to do." I interjected the idea that perhaps she and her homemaker could prepare some dinners together. Mrs. M. replied, "That might be helpful. I just do not want someone coming in my home and trying to take over like the last girl did!"

We went out onto the patio and Mrs. M. showed me her little garden. "A man comes once a week to look after it. I am not able to do much in the yard anymore, but I could not do without my garden." I commented that her neighbors must enjoy looking at such a lovely yard. Mrs. M. looked wistful. "I do not know my neighbors now; they are mostly young folk. My old neighbors have either died or moved away. I have been here 17 years so there has been a lot of change. I used to walk up and down the blocks and know so many people, now they are all gone. I cannot even walk a half a block now, I get so weak." As we came back into the living room, Mrs. M. paused and looked into a mirror. "I am getting so wrinkled, of course I am 84 years old!" I replied that I had noticed her smile more than her wrinkles. Mrs. M. looked at me closely as if evaluating what I had said, then accepting it, looked pleased.

Mrs. M. told me of her gentleman-friend who had lived with her for 7 years. He moved back to Chicago when she was hospitalized 3 months ago. "I miss him so, we shared so many good times. I have written to him several times telling him that I am okay now and invited him to come back. He has not answered. Maybe he is sick now. I guess I will just have to advertise for another man. It is a shame to have a spare room empty!" I felt that this demonstrated a positive adaptation to loss.

"I have raised four children and they have all turned out good, so I have done my bit! I am not afraid to die, it is the waiting that is hard. My daughter is so good to me, but I am just a burden to her now. I am not much use anymore." Mrs. M. looked dejected. Her fingers reached up to touch her cameo brooch. As I looked at it admiringly, she said softly, "It was my mother's."

At this point in the interview, Mrs. M.'s daughter arrived. Mrs. M.'s mood changed. "I need surgery, you know, but my daughter will not take me to the doctor." Mrs. B. reminded her mother that they had been to the doctor the week before and that he had said he did not want to operate on her hernia right now. Mrs. M. did not acknowledge her daughter's reply but went on to say that her daughter hides her hearing aid. Mrs. B. went and got her mother's hearing aid,

checked it to see that it was working. She gave it to her mother saying, "It was on the shelf in your bedroom where you always keep it, Mother." Again, Mrs. M. did not respond.

Throughout the interview I had interjected questions from the mental status questionnaire. Mrs. M. had missed three. Her anxiety was visible when she could not answer a question. She quickly rationalized her inability to name the present president by saying, "I have not had the time to read the paper everyday."

Mrs. M. spoke with irritation when she could not hear the conversation between her daughter and me. "I know you are talking but I cannot hear you!" Her dark eyes blazed! Immediately I realized that I had unintentionally changed my position and Mrs. M. could no longer read my lips. I apologized and corrected my position. Mrs. M. looked pleased with herself. I was pleased at this demonstration of ego-strength.

We discussed the number of hours a homemaker would be needed. Mrs. M. accepted the plan that the homemaker would work *with* her. Also, she liked the idea of going out for a walk. Her daughter looked relieved when I stated that I had just the right homemaker in mind. As I prepared to leave, Mrs. M. said, "You will come back and see me?" I assured her that I would look forward to visiting with her again and thanked her for her hospitality.

FOLLOW-UP VISITS TO IMPLEMENT ASSISTANCE PLAN

Based on my home visit with Mrs. M., several of her needs became apparent. An assistance plan was formulated to meet these needs as follows:

1. *Home safety:* I suggested to the daughter that handrails on the tub and a nonskid mat in the tub would help Mrs. M. to be able to take baths.
2. *Integrative services:* I investigated a senior day center in the area. The center provided activities on Tuesdays and Thursdays from

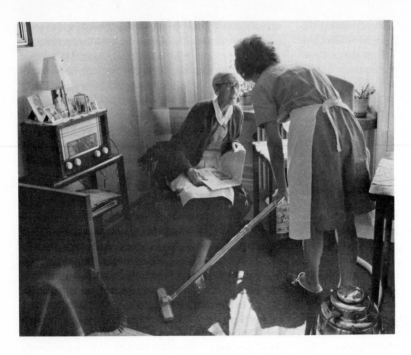

FIGURE 31-1 Regular domestic help is one of the most needed services for the elderly. (*Reprinted with permission of the World Health Organization, photo by E. Mandelmann.*)

10:00 A.M. to 2:00 P.M., as well as transportation and a free lunch. Also, I found out that the men outnumbered the women three to one. When I discussed the center with Mrs. M. she was ready to go to the next session. This socialization should increase Mrs. M.'s self-esteem, as well as help to fill her need for male companionship.

3. *Supportive services:* Since the day center met on Tuesdays and Thursdays, a homemaker was placed in the home on Monday, Wednesday, and Friday from 1:00 to 5:00 P.M. In this way, Mrs. M. would have someone with her every afternoon when she was up and about. The homemaker was a middle-aged, positive, cheerful woman who could "work with" Mrs. M., letting her maintain her role as lady of the house, while reducing her frustrations at not being able to do all the tasks alone. Part of the homemaker's time was to be spent taking Mrs. M. out for walks in order to gradually build up her strength. Drives to a nearby park and shopping center were included for short-range goals. The long-range goal was to maximize Mrs. M.'s abilities to cope in all areas of functioning.

4. *Counseling in the home:* Goals included providing Mrs. M. with positive reinforcement in all her new activities and promoting her acceptance of her physical limitations. Supportive counseling was provided for her daughter, Mrs. B. She was encouraged to ventilate her feelings of frustration toward her mother. Long-range goals included helping the daughter to understand the dynamics of her mother's behavior and being able to separate her objective performances to help her mother from her mother's subjective evaluations.

REFERENCES

Anthony, E. J., and T. Benedek: *Parenthood,* Little, Brown, Boston, 1970, p. 205.

Atchley, R. C.: *The Social Forces in Later Life,* Wadsworth, Belmont, Calif., 1972, p. 316.

Burnside, I.: Grief work in the aged patient, *Nursing Forum,* 8(4):416–427, 1969.

————: Interviewing the aged, in I. Burnside (ed.), *Psychosocial Nursing Care of the Aged,* McGraw-Hill, New York, 2d ed., 1980, pp. 3–14.

————: Loss: A constant theme in group work with the aged, *Hospital and Community Psychiatry,* **21**(6):173–177, June 1970.

DeLong, A. J.: The micro-spatial structure of the older person: Some implications of planning the social and spatial environment, in L. Pastalan and D. Carson (eds.), *Spatial Behavior of Older People,* University of Michigan Press, Ann Arbor, 1970, p. 83.

Field, N.: *Aging with Honor and Dignity,* Charles C Thomas, Springfield, Ill., 1968, pp. 14, 22.

Gaitz, C. M., and P. E. Baer: Diagnostic assessment of the elderly: A multifunctional model, *Gerontologist,* **10**:47–52, 1970.

Goldfarb, A. I.: Psychiatry in geriatrics, *Medical Clinics of North America,* **51**(6):1515–1527, November 1967.

Kahn, R. L. et al.: Brief objective measure for the determination of mental status in the aged, *American Journal of Psychiatry,* **117**:326, 1960.

Kaplan, J.: The day center and the day care center, *Geriatrics,* **12**:247–251, April 1957.

Kuhlen, R. G.: Changing personal adjustment during the adult years, in J. E. Anderson (ed.), *Psychological Aspects of Aging,* American Psychological Association, Washington, 1956, pp. 21–29.

Leonard, B. J.: Body image changes in chronic illness, *Nursing Clinics of North America,* **7**(4):684–695, December 1972.

Lidz, T.: *The Person,* Basic Books, New York, 1968, p. 484.

Mead, G.: *Mind, Self, and Society,* University of Chicago Press, 1934, p. 155.

Milloy, M.: Casework with the older person and his family, *Social Casework,* **45**(8):450–456, 1964.

Moses, D. F.: Assessing behavior in the elderly, *Nurs-ing Clinics of North America,* **7**(2):225–233, June 1972.

Newcomer, R.: Environmental influences on the older person, *Aging: Prospects and Issues,* Andrus Gerontology Center, University of Southern California, Los Angeles, 1973, pp. 79–89.

Roberts, S. L.: Territoriality: Space and the aged patient in intensive care units, in I. Burnside (ed.), *Psychosocial Nursing Care of the Aged,* McGraw-Hill, New York, 2d ed., 1980, pp. 72–83.

Schacht, R.: *Alienation,* Doubleday, Garden City, N.Y., 1970, pp. 157–158.

Sheldon, J. F.: Some problems of older people, in J. E. Anderson (ed.), *Psychological Aspects of Aging,* American Psychological Association, Washington, 1956, pp. 3–11.

Siporin, M.: Situational assessment and intervention, *Social Casework,* **53**:91–109, February 1972.

Smith, E. S.: *The Dynamic of Aging,* Norton, New York, 1956, pp. 176–177.

Spark, G. M., and E. M. Brody: The aged are family members, in C. J. Sager and H. S. Kaplan (eds.), *Progress in Group and Family Therapy,* Brunner/Mazel, New York, 1972, pp. 712–725.

Teasdale, Sara: The philosopher (poem), in A. L. Alexander (ed.), *Poems That Touch the Heart,* Doubleday, Garden City, N.Y., 1963, pp. 236–237.

Vickery, F. E.: *Creative Programming for Older Adults,* Association Press, New York, 1972, pp. 107–109.

Weiner, L., A. Becker, and T. Friedman: *Home Treatment,* University of Pittsburgh Press, 1967, p. 121.

Wood, M.: *Pathos of Loneliness,* Columbia University Press, New York, 1953, p. 9.

THIRTY-TWO

ASSESSMENT OF SAFETY FACTORS

Bernita M. Steffl

He who has health has hope, and he who has hope has everything.
Arabian Proverb

LEARNING OBJECTIVES

- List at least five areas or specific dimensions of prevention for older adults and describe one preventive measure for each.
- Identify in teaching or work with clients a comprehensive list of safety measures for accident prevention.
- Identify the rationale for implementation of safety measures in above objective.
- Identify for their own application (by clients, family, or friends) at least one preventive precaution or intervention against stroke.
- Defend and document the statement that "nutrition, exercise, smoking are the three most important aspects of preventive health maintenance for older adults."

Some years ago Dunn (1958) wrote about the role of older people in the future economy of the United States, proclaiming (1) that the greatest reservoir of experience and maturity was among older people, and that there was opportunity to transform upper years of life from a social liability into a social asset; (2) that we must change society to accept the concept that old age is a period of great value to society; and (3) that the nation could no longer afford to waste its principal unused resource. The implication was the need for a change of ideas, practices, and laws concerning the aged.

It has taken us more than 20 years and the impact of the increase in the elderly population to awaken to Dr. Dunn's predictions! Now, in 1980 we are looking more at preventive health in old age. It has become an economic necessity, and perhaps we are realizing that sooner or later the elderly are us! We are becoming more definitive in health maintenance for the elderly, and we have done away with mandatory retirement.

A THEORETICAL FRAMEWORK FOR PREVENTION

The World Health Organization's definition of health says, "Health is a state of complete physical, mental and social well being and not merely the absence of disease." To provide this kind of health is an overwhelming task and requires commitment from health professionals.

The task may be better accomplished if we use an organized approach or scheme of prevention—a theoretical framework—a model which helps us to maximize physical, psychological, and sociological potential.

A very workable theoretical framework based on philosophy and principles of public health includes these three interfacing concepts:

1. *Levels of prevention.* Leavell and Clark (1965) developed a model of primary, secondary, and tertiary prevention which has become classic in the delivery of health care (see Figure 32-1). The goal, of course, is to apply primary prevention wherever possible. For example, prevention of dental cavities or obesity is much more productive than treatment; however in our work with the aged we will be focusing more on secondary and tertiary prevention or early diagnosis and rehabilitation. *Prevention* as used in this chapter means "anticipating; making impossible or hindering advancement." Such prevention requires anticipatory action based on knowledge of the natural history of a disease or disorder. This leads us to the epidemiologic concept.

2. *Epidemiology.* This is defined as the mass phenomenon of a disease, the study of the state of health (or dis-ease), and distribution of individuals, groups, and masses by evaluating agent-host-environment relationships (Wilner, Walkley, and O'Neill, 1978). An unsophisticated definition would be "learning about the who, what, when, and where of events that affect health in its broadest sense." The word itself comes from the Greek *epi,* meaning "upon," *demos,* meaning "people," and *logus,* meaning "reasons," and so literally it means "study of what falls upon the people." The epidemiologic approach is especially helpful to the nursing process because it demands orderly thinking and precise expression of one's observations and deductions and also specificity in defining the problem. Not only the facts themselves, but the process of defining and arranging them

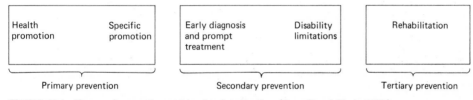

FIGURE 32-1 Phases of prevention and levels of application. (*Leavell and Clark, 1965.*)

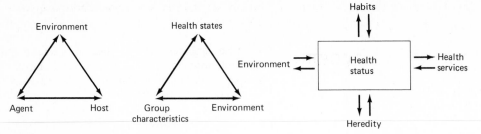

FIGURE 32-2 Examples of epidemiologic models. Most models emphasize the interrelationship of the host-agent-environment triad in the same way.

into organized sequences, have real meaning for the nurse. Epidemiology, though, is more than a total of accepted facts; it includes arrangement into chains of inference events which extend more or less beyond the bounds of direct observation. Facts are related to one another in order to construct explanatory hypotheses concerning the natural history of a disorder and its eventual prevention or control (Corrigan and Corcoran, 1966). These epidemiologic facts and the nature of the problem then dictate the most productive and feasible level of prevention (see Figure 32-2 for diagrammatic examples of models).

3. *High-level wellness.* We use levels of prevention and the epidemiologic approach for the ultimate goal of high-level wellness, that is, maximizing the potential of each individual's capability for balance and purposeful direction within the environment where he or she is functioning (Dunn, 1971; see Figure 32-3). Just as the World Health Organization's definition of health includes more than the absence of disease or infirmity, high-level wellness means more than just being free from sickness; yet most of us think we are well when we are not sick. High-level wellness fits the study and care of aging so well because most old people are not "all sick" or "all well" simultaneously or all the time. There are changes from day to day. This requires ongoing observation and assessment to monitor for indicators of change toward health or illness. This kind of preventive and restorative nursing requires a great deal of skill and a high level of ability in decision

making. Such nursing can change the progress of a patient in a way that long-term care can be shortened or lengthened. In essence, the concept of high-level wellness might help us to always consider and maximize the wellness and focus upon health potential rather than the sickness of individuals. In a nutshell, when we work with the elderly, it is much more encouraging and productive to concentrate on what is left than what is gone. Will Rogers might have said, "It's like looking at the doughnut instead of the size of the hole in the middle." Doctors, nurses, and health workers frequently forget to do this, perhaps because their training has been oriented toward disease rather than maintaining wellness. Disease may be more interesting, and it is easier to fight sickness

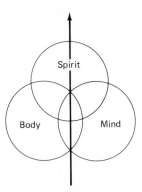

FIGURE 32-3 High-level wellness symbol. The three interlocking orbits represent the human body, mind, and spirit as an interrelated and interdependent whole. The arrow symbolizes the life cycle of the individual striving to achieve purpose in living and growing in wholeness toward the maturity of self-fulfillment. (*Dunn, 1971.*)

than to struggle for a condition of greater wellness.

NUTRITION, EXERCISE, SMOKING

When one examines research and information related to preventive longevity, that is, what can be done to maximize the quality of life into old age, three elements keep surfacing over and over—nutrition, exercise, and smoking. They are the key or the crux and are very difficult to change and control because they depend on human behavior.

NUTRITION

It is clear that nutrition is one of the major environmental factors in resistance to disease and tolerance to stress, and it is possibly a variable in the extension of current life expectancy (Weg, 1978).

Both overnutrition and undernutrition increase the probability of death. Both can be prevented to a considerable extent by simple addition or subtraction of nutrients; but changing the motivation of individuals to eat more or less makes preventive nutrition very difficult. Much of the problem is putting to work information that we already have, but securing new information is generally easier than applying old. The elderly are vulnerable to poor diets, food fads, and advertising. Health education tends to be in the hands of merchants. We eat what we are sold, rather than demand what is good for us.

The main problems in preventive nutrition education in older adults are: (1) caloric intake (too little is most common); (2) constipation; (3) dentures, chewing, and periodontal disease; (4) medications related to diet; (5) changes in ability to taste and smell; and (6) hydration (Cadigan, 1979).

Confusion, malaise, listlessness, and iron-deficiency anemia result from prolonged nutritional deficits and are not uncommon among the elderly ill who live alone. Dehydration is probably the most devastating nutritional deficit which happens all too often and has such serious consequences as fostering breakdown of skin and tissue. A lack of fluid and bulk in diets of the elderly causes and aggravates colitis, di-

verticulitis, constipation, and hemorrhoids. Adequate nutrition and hydration can alleviate all these.

Some still controversial but very significant research findings in preventive nutrition have to do with calcium and vitamin intake. Some researchers are of the opinion that increased calcium intake for older women in addition to estrogen therapy is needed to overcome bone loss associated with menopause. Osteoporosis is the most common disability in later life, and with it comes increased probability of bone fracture. It has been suggested that people be screened for loss of density of the alveolar (tooth-supporting) bone, because studies show that loss of calcium and phosphorus appear early in the jaw (Albanese, 1974).

The results of intake of supplementary vitamin A, niacin, ascorbic acid (vitamin C), and thiamine (vitamin B) have been studied in humans as well as animals. The researchers and subjects have reported improved health from such treatments. For example, Exton-Smith (1968) says that variations in these vitamins may have only minor significance in young people, but in older persons the homeostatic mechanisms may be impaired and that, therefore, the environmental or pathological stresses to which the elderly are particularly prone may upset this precarious physiological balance.

Speculation about supplementary vitamin E and lecithin will be left to the reader. More research is indicated. Few medical practitioners order these, yet many elderly profess to "feel better" when taking them in daily supplements.

The amount of food eaten and amount of fat intake are two more topics of controversial studies. Though no one has yet produced a sufficiently effective method of reducing obesity, we can practice all levels of prevention here. The relationship between obesity and degenerative disease is enough to suggest that obesity prevention is a major means of preparing for a healthy old age. We also have good evidence that the higher the intake of fat, the shorter the life-span (Schlenker et al., 1973; Weg, 1978).

Evaluation of past nutrition education activities has shown that classroom lectures are ineffective in teaching older persons. Poor hearing and eyesight, lack of sustained concentration, and lack of skill and experience among those who are teaching the aged are some reasons for the ineffectiveness of this method. Informal group discussions are more effective, even though more time-consuming. An individual approach is necessary. We must remember that individual differences increase with age and that physiological changes and rate of aging are uniquely individual. In this manner one can involve the consumer-participants in identifying their needs, involve them in demonstrations, and provide for special dietary counseling and promote socialization.

According to Mann (1973), the following are some specific facts to consider in preventive nutrition education and practice:

1. Cultural sets, attitudes toward food, are established early in life and are almost unchangeable in the aged.
2. Physical mobility and vigor of food-seeking ability diminish with age.
3. Though micronutrient requirements are not changed, calorie requirement is lessened with age.
4. Malabsorption is increased as teeth are lost and gastric mucosa and enteric enzymes diminish, so the need for therapeutic diets increases.
5. Economic buying power diminishes, and so availability of food is lessened.

Nutrition cannot be overemphasized for the elderly. It certainly affects the recovery from illness, and the ability to eat is a symbol of hope for older persons and their families (Cadigan, 1979). (See Chapter 23.)

EXERCISE

Why exercise? Heart disease was a relatively minor affliction in the United States until we changed from an agricultural to an industrial society. Lack of exercise is now a key factor in this and many other diseases of the mature years. The major benefits of a planned exercise program are:

1. Developing an efficient cardiovascular system
2. Lowering blood pressure
3. Relieving stress and tension
4. Controlling body fats efficiently
5. Decelerating the deterioration of bones with age
6. Providing a day-to-day feeling of well-being

The sad and simple fact is that there are no shortcuts to a consistent, effective exercise program. It cannot be squeezed into the daily routine now and then or accomplished only on weekends. An effective exercise program must be routine, at least three times a week, and aerobic. Aerobic means "with oxygen"; that is, the body must be exercised enough to use additional oxygen and use it efferently (Hunt, 1978).

However, aerobic exercises should be avoided until at least 2 hours after eating. The best time for all exercise is before a meal; otherwise we confuse the cardiovascular system, which is busy digesting. Shock (1972) says that, in order for physical activity to benefit the body physiology, one has to "exercise till it hurts." That is, the physical exertion must persist to extend circulation to the very smallest capillary!

Exercise is good for all systems. It enhances not only biological but psychological and sociologic functioning. Last but not least, "sexercises," simple fundamental pelvic exercises for a full, happy, and vital sex life, have been advocated for years (Prudden, 1961).

SMOKING

Smoking is a killer that even exercise cannot disarm. It has repeatedly been identified as one of the most powerful negative predictors of longevity. There are well-designed studies on disease-free aging which show the significance of cigarette smoking. There is no doubt that if we (professionals as well as the general public) apply present knowledge about smoking, we could improve the health of the middle-aged and aged in our population (Public Health Service, Office on Smoking and Health, 1979).

Nurses have many opportunities to practice primary and secondary prevention in their health teaching about smoking. Even for people who have smoked for many years, quitting affects future health, and risk of developing fatal diseases attributable to smoking drops sharply.

The Surgeon General's Advisory Committee on Smoking and Health reveals the following conclusive statements which are helpful to initiate prevention (Brown, 1973):

1. Cigarette smoking initiates disease process by causing progressive damage.
2. Cigarette smoking initiates disease process with continual repair and recovery to a critical and irreversible point.
3. Cigarette smoking promotes disease by positively supporting pathology or interfering with the organism's normal capacity to cope.
4. Cigarette smoking increases probability of a critical event in temporary situations such as myocardial damage when there is increased demand for oxygen and the supply is diminished (by smoking).
5. The effect of one disease upon another may be greater in smokers than nonsmokers.

SPECIFIC DIMENSIONS OF PREVENTION FOR OLDER ADULTS

The thrust of current prevention is on health education for self-health maintenance. All of us, including the elderly, need to take more responsibility for our own health for obvious socioeconomic reasons.

Older people are very interested in and receptive to education, and the medical profession is becoming more and more involved in preventive education. Contrary to the opinion and attitudes of many, old people are able to learn and, in fact, are eager to learn, especially about themselves. Researchers have demonstrated and proved that old people learn as well as young people, given adequate time (Birren and Schaie, 1977).

Newer health education programs such as the one at Georgetown University's Department of Community Medicine advocate teaching lay people more than signs and symptoms for early detection of disease. Physicians there say the "medical mystery must go." Some people like being passive patients, but people who wish to be more active will have increased opportunity to learn how to stabilize and maintain health. Dr. Keith W. Sehnert has been a pioneer in this trend. He has written a current best seller *How to Be Your Own Doctor (Sometimes)*. He says, "You already are acting as your own doctor most of the time. The trouble is you haven't been trained for the job . . . and I am far more concerned about dangerous ignorance than dangerous knowledge."

The health-activated older person needs to learn to use (on a less sophisticated level) many of the same skills employed by health professionals, including (1) keeping health records, (2) measuring vital signs, including blood pressure, (3) examining the body for abnormal signs of illness, coping with injuries and emergencies, and (4) learning to deal conservatively with common self-limiting illnesses that do not require a visit to the physician's office. Physicians will be paid for prevention instead of cure, and that will be most fitting, especially since the word *doctor* comes from the Latin word *docere*, meaning "to teach" (Sehnert and Eisenberg, 1978).

MENTAL HEALTH

What can we do to prevent mental deterioration of the elderly? We can begin promoting positive mental health by believing and expecting that not all old people are "senile." It simply is not so. In addition, we must learn to differentiate organic conditions, such as chronic brain syndrome, from withdrawal and depression. A great deal of isolation, alienation, and disengagement comes from mutual withdrawal of patient and nurse. For example, Mr. C., who has been in the nursing home for 2 months, communicated less and less. The student nurse, who chose him as her patient for the semester, reported after 4 weeks, "I'm going to terminate with Mr. C. He says he doesn't feel like talking and just sits there. I don't think he even cares if I come and I'm not getting anything out of it." The student was encouraged to examine her own feelings and behavior and recognized her own withdrawal. She continued to see Mr. C., and a meaningful relationship developed and persisted for more than a year.

It is easy to withdraw and disengage from a client if the client refuses to cooperate or seems "out of it." Personnel working with the elderly first of all need preparation in mental health concepts. If we know what to look for and are *careful* in our psychosocial assessment, we can, in a short time, learn a great deal about a person, which might help to maximize his or her potential.

Whether an elderly person is physically ill or well, we can promote positive mental health with meaningful activity—and also productive, if possible—meaningful in relation to the person's cohort group and cultural background, and productive because most of the present generation of old people relate usefulness to productivity.

Preventive mental health occurs by helping elderly individuals with loss and grief work, providing a "lifeline," that is, communication and/or interaction with a significant other. And, according to Oberleder (1969), we should encourage those in middle age to work out and let out anger to prevent "senility."

Biofeedback may also serve a preventive role in aging. Biofeedback consists of producing positive feelings through control of brain waves. Relaxing is the common denominator. Brain-wave activity is recorded as a continuous flow of changing frequencies of electrical waves, the most frequent being alpha waves. When we are in a state of rest, relaxed and inattentive with eyes closed, alpha waves appear on the graph. Zen priests during meditation produce almost continuous alpha waves. So it would seem that one way to relax would be to produce alpha waves at will. Though the subject is still in a relatively developmental state and still controversial, there is a possibility here of a real contribution in preventive psychiatry by "self-regulation" (Riss, 1973).

By nature of their contact with the aged, nurses are often in a key position to prevent three common tragedies in the aged. They are:

1. Failure to differentiate between acute and chronic organic brain syndrome. The transitory confusion from an acute illness, electrolyte imbalance, or medication may cause the patient to be too quickly labeled as "senile."
2. Failure to differentiate organic mental disorders from depression which has resulted in withdrawal.
3. Suicide. It is on the increase in the United States, and the highest rate is in males over age 65. Our role in prevention is to recognize and work with anxiety and depression. Men-

tal health is covered in more detail in Chapters 5, 10, 12, 13, and 14.

MULTIPHASIC HEALTH SCREENING FOR SENIOR POPULATIONS

Multiphasic screening for detection and prevention of chronic illness is a modern development in public health. A number of these programs are now in existence in the United States and abroad, at national and local levels by voluntary and official agencies. Screening efforts are generally guided by vital statistics (see Table 32-1). In the United States, chronic disease conditions most often screened for in the elderly are cancer, diabetes, hypertension, respiratory diseases, and glaucoma.

Though screening programs can be very valuable in preventive education and in providing a certain amount of medical care to individuals who cannot afford such examinations, there are pitfalls. A health screening program must be well planned and coordinated to include follow-up care for the findings. Otherwise we create or compound problems. In addition, we must be aware that passing a simple screening test sometimes gives a person a feeling of false security and not passing creates undue anxiety. Good preplanning and nursing follow-up counseling with clients and their families are essential.

Strokes: The Fear of the Elderly Advanced diagnostic tools, monitoring of blood pressure and microcirculation (Duling, 1979) are creating increased optimism about staving off strokes (Drake, 1973). Research indicates that strokes can be prevented or greatly minimized.

About one-half million persons become victims of stroke each year, and no other disease is more costly in terms of the care needed by those who survive. Prevention is infinitely preferable to treatment of stroke, not only in terms of the individual, but also in substantial benefits to the community.

Prevention, of course, entails identifying persons at risk of developing embolisms, thrombotic or stenotic occlusion of vessels supplying

TABLE 32-1

DEATHS AND DEATH RATES FOR THE 10 LEADING CAUSES OF DEATH IN SPECIFIED AGE GROUPS: UNITED STATES, 1977*

Rank Order in 1977	Cause of Death and Age†	1977	
		Number	Rate
	45–64 Years, All Causes	437,795	1,000.0
1	Diseases of heart	153,652	351.0
2	Malignant neoplasms, including neoplasms of lymphatic and hematopoietic tissues	132,514	302.7
3	Cerebrovascular diseases	22,926	52.4
4	Accidents:	19,167	43.8
	Motor vehicle accidents	8,000	18.3
	All other accidents	11,167	25.5
5	Cirrhosis of liver	17,166	39.2
6	Suicide	8,368	19.1
7	Diabetes mellitus	7,798	17.8
8	Influenza and pneumonia	6,691	15.3
9	Bronchitis, emphysema, and asthma	5,357	12.2
10	Homicide	3,783	8.6
	All other causes	60,373	137.9
	65 Years and Over, All Causes	1,242,344	5,288.1
1	Diseases of heart	548,352	2,334.1
2	Malignant neoplasms, including neoplasms of lymphatic and hematopoietic tissues	232,226	988.5
3	Cerebrovascular diseases	154,623	658.2
4	Influenza and pneumonia	39,871	169.7
5	Arteriosclerosis	27,371	116.5
6	Accidents:	24,092	102.5
	Motor vehicle accidents	5,750	24.5
	All other accidents	18,342	78.1
7	Diabetes mellitus	23,599	100.5
8	Bronchitis, emphysema, and asthma	16,288	69.3
9	Cirrhosis of liver	8,622	36.7
10	Nephritis and nephrosis	5,834	24.8
	All other causes	161,466	687.3

* Refers only to resident deaths occurring within the United States. Rates per 100,000 population.
† Eighth Revision International Classification of Diseases, adapted 1965.
SOURCE: *Monthly Vital Statistics Report,* Department of Health, Education, and Welfare, National Center for Health Statistics, Publication no. (PHS 79-1120), vol. 28, no. 1, May 11, 1979, p. 22.

the brain or in the brain, as well as those susceptible to intracranial hemorrhage.

Considerable research is now being devoted to identification of patients with cerebral transient ischemic attacks (TIA). It is estimated 85 percent of TIA patients develop strokes. Researchers, such as Leonberg (1974), contend that, through a prophylactic program, stroke may be reduced from 15 to 50 percent in these patients. Leonberg's prophylactic treatment includes a thorough evaluation of patients for high-risk factors at the time of TIA and the continued monitoring and follow-up treatment of the high-risk factors, such as hypertension, hyperlipidemia, and polycythemia. One of the most useful, safe, simple, and rapid means of assessing microcirculation in monitoring patients is examination of the conjunctival microcirculation in relation to both morphologic and dynamic features. Nurse awareness and ability to assess for TIA, or "little strokes," may help shape the future of potential stroke victims (Keller and Truscott, 1973).

Vascular reconstructive surgery following TIA, aimed at improving the brain's blood supply, also offers concrete hope of staving off a stroke. Such surgery is performed under an operating microscope, which allows the surgeon to anastomose arteries smaller than a millimeter in diameter. The procedure was developed in the mid-1960s simultaneously by two surgeons, Dr. Raymond M. P. Donezky, of the University of Vermont, and Dr. M. Gazi Yasargil, of the University of Zurich.

As an alternative to surgery in TIA patients, many physicians have used anticoagulant drugs. Though these drugs have tended to reduce frequency and severity of ischemic attacks, the incidence of strokes seems to have been the same. Fields and Hass (1971) have done studies using aspirin to alter platelet stickiness, with the possibility of preventing coagulation in its earliest stage. Rodvien and Mielke (1978) also report on work with drugs which inhibit platelet participation in thrombus or atheroma formation that might help prevent strokes under certain circumstances.

Identifying the patient at risk is a difficult and costly task. Because procedures such as angiography require hospitalization, are expensive, and entail some risk, efforts are being made to develop simpler, noninvasive screening methods. Two of these, thermometry and opacity pulse propagation measurements, are currently being evaluated. The basis for using thermometry lies in differing origins of blood supply. With a highly sensitive instrument, blood flow across the forehead is measured by light reflections. Thus far this procedure correlates well with arteriographic findings. Further innovations in instruments, to replace or enhance the usefulness of the trained observer and present clinical tests, are still relatively unexplored potentials of computerized soft-tissue tomography, ultrasonic tools, and intracranial pressure monitoring (*Medical World News*, 1974). Exercise testing for tolerance is still one of the most valuable noninvasive tools of modern medicine (Merrill and Froelicher, 1977).

Numerous studies are being conducted in this whole area of follow-up of patients with TIA, but a leading neurologist says,

> The traditional dictum that there is nothing that can be or should be done for a stroke still holds good in too many hospitals. House officers in some institutions are still being trained not to admit people with strokes unless they are in a coma.

As noted in *Medical World News* (1974), if follow-up for prevention becomes a reality,

> Everyone with an acute stroke, big or little, needs to be admitted to the hospital for reestablishment of blood flow to an ischemic area before it becomes an infarct and for evaluation, assessment, and a plan for preventive monitoring.

We should also be aware of the fact that over the past 15 years techniques have been developed and introduced which make it possible to treat vertebrobasilar aneurysms surgically, with reasonable safety. Improved diagnostic measures and techniques have disclosed more of these aneurysms, and technical surgical advancements are changing the view that these lesions are for the most part inoperable (Drake, 1973).

One cannot leave this topic without a few words about the hazards of electronic equipment in critical care areas. A study of cardiac electronic monitoring and therapeutic devices in 11 major hospitals in Detroit revealed that equipment was being carelessly used, was poorly designed, and was seldom tested or properly repaired (Green, 1973). This has very definite preventive implications for nurses.

Preventive Dental and Mouth Care Preventive dental health should also start early in life to be truly effective. Dental problems of old age have often reached a state of irreversibility. Nevertheless, emphasis must be placed on maximizing dental function for nutritional as well as aesthetic reasons. Loss of teeth and periodontal disease increase with age, as do a number of nutritionally related clinical and oral problems, such as loss of taste, dry mouth, burning and sore tongue, oral mucous membrane disease, temporary mandibular joint discomfort, and bone atrophy. Preventive measures include a well-balanced diet, elimination of sugar, reduction of snacks, adequate water intake, chewing of firm foods, and avoidance of soft, retentive foods. Fluoridation of water is very helpful in preventing caries. If fluoridated water is not available, topical applications of fluoride should be considered.

Many dentists now have hygienists instruct all their patients in preventive techniques, such as proper brushing with soft, fine bristles and using dental floss to prevent deleterious buildup of plaque and excessive dental erosion. Many older people have stained teeth and use harsh toothpastes with whiteners; some of these whiteners may contain formaldehyde, which is unsafe (Nizel, 1972).

Ill-fitting dentures not only affect dietary intake and thus nutritional status, but they cause irritability and frustrations which also affect the psychosocial behavior, emotional climate, and total well-being.

Public health workers have long been aware of the lack of dental care available to the elderly. Medicare has not helped much either; however, we can promote programs to assist the elderly in this by pointing out to health professionals, as well as the elderly, how much dental health affects total health. Dental assessment should be part of every physical examination.

Dental care has not had high priority in the value systems of many elderly individuals or among nurses; however, the nurse is in a unique position to assess and teach oral hygiene to save teeth and maximize function when dentures are necessary. It is encouraging to note the increased attention to the problem by dentists such as the Geriatric Dental Group of Portland, Oregon, who have developed programs on preventive education and control of oral disease in the elderly (Gerhards, 1978).

Vision and hearing losses are covered in Chapters 33 and 34, respectively, and so they will not be covered in this chapter.

Drugs The number of prescribed drugs increases with age, and many elderly are taking from 10 to 15 prescribed drugs and even more over-the-counter drugs daily. As the spectrum of disorder increases in the aged, so does the pharmaceutical answer to the problem. With so many drugs available, it is not surprising that drug interactions in the elderly are increasing and have reached epidemic proportions.

The danger with drugs has also increased because more patients are treated on an outpatient basis and manage their own medications, and because of failure of patients to tell physicians of what they believe to be trivial self-treatment.

Jessup (1974) lists the following nursing responsibilities in drug administration:

1. The nurse must be a coordinator of the efforts of other health professionals.
2. The nurse needs to detect, describe, and assess accurately the symptoms of clients.
3. The nurse must be a professional doubting Thomas, a real devil's advocate, in questioning the advisability of an order if in doubt.
4. The nurse must be a teacher; clients' compliance to a drug regimen in the home is better when they receive sufficient education.
5. The nurse has a responsibility to be a monitor of the older person's response to a drug regimen.

Alcoholism It is estimated that 10 percent of the drinking population in the age group 55 to 64 are alcoholics. That means there are about 2 million elderly alcoholics in the United States. The aging alcoholic-addict is the least visible, too often protected by family and well-meaning friends, and often out of reach of conventional modes of treatment. However, many older alcoholics are "new alcoholics," and prospects for reversing the problem are good (*Aging and Addiction in Arizona,* 1979).

At St. Luke's Alcohol and Drug Abuse Program in Phoenix, Arizona, a peer group treatment plan for older persons implemented by Don Goddard (a senior citizen) has been so successful that the advisory committee has published a position paper to arouse public awareness to the problem and to propose recommendations for rehabilitating older alcoholics (*Aging and Addiction in Arizona,* 1979).

Accident Prevention   Accidents are the third-ranking cause of death and a leading cause of injury to the aged and cut across all levels of prevention (Butler and Lewis, 1977). It is important to keep in mind that the most common debilitating accidents among the aged are falls. Current research indicates that these accidents due to falls show a greater involvement of host-linked factors than environmental factors and that there is a higher rate of accidents among the aged with impaired functional capacity (Margulec et al., 1970). We also know that most falls and accidents happen in the home and in the bedroom. These facts justify time, money, and energy to educate both the professional and the client about accident prevention.

Education for accident prevention cannot be isolated or packaged into a handy program. The persistence of the problem, in spite of many attempts to educate the public and change behavior, has demonstrated that the approach must be comprehensive, consistent, and integrated into daily activities of living. It requires sophisticated assessment skills. For example, assessment skills used when walking an older client include (1) noting how his or her shoes fit (ill-fitting and improperly fastened shoes, clothing, or mechanical devices can cause pain and falls), (2) assessing functional capacity of the limbs and the respiratory tract, and (3) assessing for sensory deprivation. If their sight is failing, the elderly may be reluctant to acknowledge this loss and may attempt to compensate. In doing so, they may take more risks and increase the possibility and probability of accidents. Though compensatory behavior is desirable, the nurse must be aware that there are dangers, such as inability to hear warning signals and smell smoke.

Older people can be counseled about preventive measures, such as not rising from a horizontal position too rapidly after rest, especially in the dark. Blood pressure changes take a few minutes. They should also be cautioned to beware of sharp moves of the head because of changes in the balancing mechanisms of the inner ear (Butler and Lewis, 1977). More specific safety precautions are listed at the end of this chapter.

Fires   Accidental death and injury from fire are most frightening, and in many cases easily prevented were it not for the frailties of human behavior. We have all heard and read about tragic nursing home fires killing helpless people; each year many elderly die from fires caused by smoking in bed in their own homes.

There is no question about the necessity of a multidisciplinary approach to prevent fires. This shared responsibility makes it easier to shift the day-to-day surveillance (and pass the buck) for fire drills and in-service education. Usually the nurse-administrator is accountable for the in-service education of staff and clients in fire prevention and control. Fire drills may seem mundane and silly. We make jokes about them; however, with the turnover of personnel in nursing homes for the aged, it would seem that we should be very rigid about prevention education and persist in routine practice drills for safety in these settings. Local fire departments and the Red Cross are valuable and helpful resources for teaching fire prevention and rescue techniques. These services are usually free in every community.

The persistence of nursing home fires raises the question of how good the regulatory systems are for licensing and obtaining government support. Elias Cohen, a former State Aging Commissioner and now professor in the Department of Community Medicine, University of Pennsylvania, has repeatedly and emphatically stated the need for standards which can be enforced to adequately protect the dependent elderly in extended care facilities (*Hospital Practice*, 1972).

PREVENTIVE PROTECTIVE SERVICES FOR THE AGED

A large number of elderly people are swindled and deceived every year by consumer fraud, land and property swindles, and medical quackery. Many of our present-day older population have not had much opportunity for any legal education, even most necessary protective legal education, and may not have needed much legal service earlier in their lifetimes. Add those with illness in various stages and a large number of foreign-born who may not read or write English well, and we have a group very vulnerable and susceptible to fraud. Every community ought to have an information and referral service and directories for its elderly.

Nurses are often quite ignorant about the scope and realm of legal protection and legal aid for the elderly. The following are common legal protections of person and property for which elderly persons and their families should be familiar with (Davis et al., 1974).

Power of attorney is the legal means of giving someone the power to act in one's behalf in financial matters. Authority can be limited to particular or extended to all matters; it can be temporary or permanent. This involves signing a document that is witnessed and notarized. A copy is filed with the County Recorder's office. Note that this does not require a lawyer, but it would seem desirable to have a lawyer handle it.

A *guardian* is a person, appointed by a court, who is given legal jurisdiction over another. A guardian has essentially the same powers and duties as a parent with respect to a child. A guardian has limited power, however, over the property of the older person. An appointment is accomplished by filing a petition to the Superior Court, and the guardian is then accountable to the court. The law offers some safeguards for the person over whom a guardian is to be appointed.

A *conservator* is a person, appointed by a court, who is given legal jurisdiction to protect and manage property of another person. This is accomplished in the same manner as guardianship.

Helping older people make plans to protect their money and property is a recognized preventive measure. It seems simple, yet most nurses are ignorant about common legal protective procedures that all elderly should carry out.

Making a will is at the top of the list of ways to protect money and property. Most people avoid this and hate to do it, particularly those elderly who have never learned about the increasing cost and the complications when a person dies without a will. For example, in the absence of a will, the court usually decides who will inherit the estate of the deceased. In making a will, the person must decide on an executor. Residence requirements may be necessary for the executor. A handwritten will is valid, but a lawyer's help is advisable.

Joint ownership of bank accounts and trusts is a method of legal protection to manage property and income. Most banks and trust companies are equipped to provide help and advice in the area of joint ownership.

Making *burial plans* and arrangements may seem morbid to some, but it serves a real preventive function in regard to the family. It is helpful when one can bury a parent or spouse according to his or her wishes. The elderly often feel less of a burden if they are able to state their wishes and participate in plans for their demise.

The American Association of Retired Persons has instituted many programs and services to help older people protect themselves where legal counsel and procedures are indicated and where unscrupulous entrepreneurs are a threat.

DISCHARGE PLANNING—HOME CARE—DAY CARE

Discharge planning is planning for and providing comprehensive, coordinated continuity of care. Patients have the right to expect planning and referral to comprehensive care after leaving an acute care setting, and all health care professionals have the responsibility to provide them. The concept is receiving increasing recognition at health care facilities because of requirements for quality assurance utilization review. Ideally, and to be most effective, discharge planning begins before admission to the facility, and the process includes prevention, intervention, and postvention (Steffl and Eide, 1978).

Home care in its broadest sense is the provision of health care and supportive services to a sick or disabled person in his or her place of residence. A home care patient is one whose needs and home and family situation are such that the required care can be more appropriately provided at home. Visits to a physician's office, clinic, or hospital out-patient department are not feasible or cannot meet his or her needs, but professional observation and treatment are not required 24 hours a day, and the nursing and other therapeutic services the physician prescribes may be brought on an intermittent basis, with good results.

Day-care centers, as the name implies, provide supervision and care for older people who cannot function entirely on their own. Most adult centers are designed primarily for recreation and socialization, but day-care centers also offer more therapeutic resocialization and daily activity for individuals who are more physically dependent. The goal is to provide daytime therapeutic protective service. This may also make it possible for family members to continue to work. For example, if a day-care center is available, Ms. Doe, a successful professional middle-aged woman, may not have to institutionalize her mother or give up her job because the mother is too disoriented to be left alone.

CONSIDERATIONS IN HEALTH PROMOTION IN THE AGED

The following specific preventive health measures for older individuals are taken from a guideline by Elsie A. Giorgi, M.D. (1971). Dr. Giorgi emphasizes multidisciplinary responsibility by identifying (in parentheses) who might be responsible for each measure.

1. Prevention of injury (primary prevention)
   a. Install good lighting, especially on landings and stairwells (general; health educator; builders).
   b. Install handrails on both sides of staircases and halls or at least on one side, designed to show when top and bottom steps have been reached (general; health educator; builders).
   c. Paint top and bottom steps and risers in easily seen colors; use nonskid treads (general; health educator, builders).
   d. Eliminate loose extension cords, small mats, sliding rugs, slippery linoleum (general; health educator; builders).
   e. Use rubber-backed nonskid rugs and nonskid floor waxes (general; health educator).
   f. Tack down edges of rugs or use wall-to-wall carpeting (general, health educator).
   g. Advise use of corrugated soles on shoes (aged; health educator).
   h. Provide adequate lighting from the bedside tables to the bathroom with baseboard light and easily available switches and flashlight at bedside (general; health educator; builders).

   i. Use levers rather than doorknobs (aged; health educator).
   j. Provide telephone at bedside (aged; health educator; telephone company; builders).
   k. Eliminate casters on chairs, rickety tables, sharp-cornered furniture, and high beds (aged; health educator; furniture manufacturers).
   l. Advise against looking up when climbing stairs or moving the head suddenly to the side, since this may interfere with the blood supply to the brain and cause fainting (aged; health educator).
   m. Avoid sedation (aged; physician).
   n. Label medications distinctly and completely and indicate whether they are for internal or external use. Provide good illumination at the medicine cabinet to avoid errors in self-administered medicine (general; pharmacist; health educator).
   o. Avoid smoking in bed (general; health educator).
   p. Make certain that markings of dials on stoves are distinct (general; stove builders).
   q. Use controls outside the tubs and showers (general; bathtub manufacturers).
   r. Give complete instructions on accident prevention to all personnel in hospitals and other institutions (general; health educator; nurses).
   s. Install grab rails and nonskid mats or emory strips in bathtubs (general; bathtub manufacturers).
   t. Use high sinks, high toilet seats, and high refrigerators to prevent undue bending of the head, which may cause dizziness and falls (aged; fixture manufacturers).
   u. Train all concerned in use of wheelchairs carefully (general; health educator; nurses; wheelchair manufacturers).
   v. Use care in the feeding of aged people to prevent aspiration and asphyxiation in presence of poor gag reflex (aged; nurse; health educator).
   w. Frequently reevaluate capability for driving motor vehicle (aged; physicians; Bureau of Motor Vehicles).
   x. Provide pedestrian escort in bad weather and sometimes even in good weather, de-

pending on the person's physical and mental capabilities (aged; physician).

   y. Test vision and hearing frequently and treat eye, ear, and foot abnormalities immediately to prevent stumbling, etc. (aged; physician).

2. Specific prevention of disease and early disease detection (secondary prevention)

   a. Instruct (if possible) concerning familial incidence (genetically and unknown genetically induced) of disease (general; physician; health educator).

   b. Have periodic checkups to discover and effectively treat the conditions which may lead to chronic illness (general; physician; health educator).

   c. Schedule more frequent periodic health examinations in the aging person because of constant breakdown of tissue. Give close attention to all symptoms and signs. Avoid "not expecting to feel well" when one becomes older (aged; physician).

   d. Be aware that aging persons can mask usual signs and manifestations of severe illness, such as fever, and acute abdominal disease. Be suspicious.

   e. Treat defects immediately while motivation is still present, e.g., foot, eye, and hearing trouble, arthritic changes, sustained and intermittent high blood pressure, and early congestive heart failure, rather than procrastinate because of chronological age (aged; physician).

   f. Continue immunizations required for particular age groups (e.g., tetanus, influenza, smallpox) (aged; physician).

   g. Avoid exposure to communicable disease insofar as possible (general; health educator; physician).

   h. Have periodic screening tests for early detection of occult disease to arrest it before damage is severe or irreversible (annually in young and mature, biannually in aging or chronically ill). These should include the following: hemogram, sedimentation rate, urinalysis, electroencephalogram, stool specimen after being meat-free for 4 days, 2-hour postprandial blood sugar, x-ray of heart and lungs, cancer detection tests such as sigmoidoscopy, Papanicolaou vaginal smear, acid phosphorous; sputum if a smoker of cigarettes (general and aged; physician; health educator).

   i. Thoroughly and completely evaluate specific body system if any tests show deviation from normal, no matter how slight (general; physician).

   j. Replace hormones as indicated (early) rather than attributing fatigue, etc., to "old age" (aged; physician).

   k. Prevent pressure point erosion and ulceration (especially in bed-bound or partially bed-bound patients) by frequently turning patient and padding crucial areas.

3. Personal health habits (primary prevention)

   a. Stress the need for maintenance of optimal weight (general; physician).

   b. Instruct in the value of good nutrition and the harmful effects of certain foods such as polyunsaturated fats and high calorie foods.

   c. Motivate toward optimum body care (cleanliness, good dental repair, adequate attention to feet, etc.) (general; health educator).

   d. Stress the need for initiation and continuation of an adequate exercise program (general; physician; health educator).

4. Social habits and mental health (tertiary prevention)

   a. Constantly motivate toward optimal fulfillment in all spheres of living rather than just work and family (general; physician; health educator).

   b. Prepare for period of loss of family and work roles by discussing these possibilities frequently in the mature years (general; physician).

   c. Motivate for substitution for work, community, and family roles by specific and general interest along other lines, such as hobbies, volunteer work, clubs, and trips (preaging group and aged; physician; health educator).

   d. Provide easy availability of proper substitute interests (aged; physician; social service). [The Mount Sinai Hospital–based Geriatric Day Center is an example of this. Here a small group (20 persons) is engaged in recreation and discussion sessions which closely resemble group psychosocial therapy. The basic plan is to keep the groups small so that they are given closer, more individual attention which motivates them to resuming their lost community role.]

e. Family instruction on the adverse effects of overprotectiveness of senior citizens. It is just as important to know how to intervene as it is to know when to intervene. They should be allowed and encouraged to do as much as possible for themselves. The latter applies in institutional settings, also. Families should be instructed about poor communication or misunderstanding based on guilt feelings which ultimately lead to irreversible disruption of families (aged; physician; social worker).

5. Obtaining health care and prepayment for health care (primary prevention)

a. Free selection of physician should without question remain the prerogative of each person. It is fair, however, to acquaint everyone with the criteria which usually (though not always) apply to the selection of a well-trained, well-motivated physician including type of hospital associated with and type of training necessary for specialization (general; health educator; social worker).

b. All, especially the aging, should be made aware of the resources available to them in their particular community to serve their health needs. If they are medically or socially indigent, they should be informed as to how they may secure the proper assistance (general and aged; public health; health educator; social welfare department).

c. Prepaid health insurance should be encouraged. However, it is good to secure authoritative advice as to which plan best covers the individual needs of the person (general; physician; social worker; health educator).

SUMMARY

The greatest stresses on health in late adulthood are anxiety, poor nutrition, smoking, and lack of physical activity. Prevention is difficult because alleviation requires a change in behavior; therefore, a scheme of prevention by design for nurses seems desirable. The theoretical framework discussed at the beginning of this chapter suggests a design for prevention based on levels of prevention using an epidemiologic approach to promote high-level wellness. These concepts should be applicable and helpful in developing nursing care plans, continuity of care, and comprehensive health services for elderly individuals and groups.

REFERENCES

Aging and Addiction in Arizona: Community Advisory Committee, St. Luke's Hospital, Phoenix, Ariz., 1979.

Albanese, Anthony A.: Nutrition problems of the elderly, speech delivered at National Dairy Council Conference, Chicago, June 1974; reported in *Phoenix Gazette,* June 12, 1974, p. K-2.

Birren, James E., and Warner K. Schaie: *Handbook on the Psychology of Aging,* Van Nostrand Reinhold, New York, 1977, pp. 421–447.

Brown, Merilyn: Health maintenance and aging: role of cigarette smoking, unpublished paper, College of Nursing, Arizona State University, Tempe, March 1973.

Butler, Robert N., and Myrna I. Lewis: *Aging and Mental Health,* 2d ed., Mosby, St. Louis, 1977, pp. 224–225.

Cadigan, Marianna R. D. (Chief Nutritionist, Maricopa County Health Department, Phoenix, Ariz.): Interview, June 24, 1979.

Corrigan, Marjorie J., and Lucille E. Corcoran (eds.): *Epidemiology in Nursing,* Catholic University Press, Washington, 1966, pp. 241–242.

Davis, Harold C., and Committee on Legal and Protective Services: *Legal and Protective Services for the Aging,* Community Council, Phoenix, Ariz., 1974, pp. 12–17.

Drake, Charles G.: Surgical treatment of vertebral-basial aneurysms, *Current Concepts of Cardiovascular Disease,* **8**(6):27, November/December 1973.

Duling, Brian: Duling's fantastic voyage, *American Heart Quarterly,* **2**(2):1–4, Spring 1979.

Dunn, Halbert L.: *High Level Wellness,* Beatty Publishing Company, Arlington, Va., 1971, pp. vi, 1–7, 56–63.

——: *Role of the Older Person in Tomorrow's Economy,* reprinted from *Problems of U.S. Economic Development,* vol. 1, Department of Health, Education, and Welfare, 1958.

Exton-Smith, A. N.: The problems of subclinical malnutrition in the elderly, in A. N. Exton-Smith and

D. L. Scott (eds.), *Vitamins in the Elderly,* John Wright and Sons, Ltd., Bristol, England, 1968.

Fields, W. S., and W. K. Hass (eds.): Aspirin, platelets, and stroke: Background for a clinical trial, in *International Symposium on Neurohematology,* Houston, Tex., 1970, Warren H. Green, St. Louis, 1971.

Gerhards, Michael: Issues in dental services for the elderly, presentation at Western Gerontological Society, April 12, 1978, Tucson, Ariz.

Giorgi, Elsie A.: *Aging and Mental Health,* leaflet used at workshop, Los Angeles, Feb. 6, 1971.

Green, H. L.: Hazards of electronic equipment in critical care areas: A research approach, *Cardiovascular Nursing,* **9**(2):7–12, March/April 1973.

Hospital Practice: Nursing-home fire: The anatomy of a tragedy, government impact on hospital practice, May 1972, pp. 139–153.

Hunt, Howard F.: *How Much Exercise Do We Need?, Blue Print for Health,* XXVII(1), Blue Cross Association, 840 North Lakeshore Drive, Chicago, IL 60611, 1978, pp. 41–49.

Jessup, Linda E.: Nursing responsibilities in drug administration, in R. Davis (ed.), *Drugs and the Elderly,* Andrus Gerontology Center, University of Southern California, Los Angeles, 1974, pp. 59–62.

Keller, Margaret R., and B. Lionel Truscott: Transient ischemic attacks, *American Journal of Nursing,* **73**(8):1330–1331, August 1973.

Leavell, Hugh Rodman, and E. Gurney Clark: *Preventive Medicine for the Doctor and His Community,* McGraw-Hill, New York, 1965, pp. 14–37.

Leonberg, S. C.: Stroke prevention program may aid high-risk patient, *Internist Observer,* January/February 1974.

Mann, George V.: Relationship of age to nutrient requirements, *American Journal of Clinical Nutrition,* 26:1096–1097, October 1973.

Margulec, Itzhak, Gershon Librack, and Meir Schadel: Epidemiological study of accidents among residents of homes for the aged, *Journal of Gerontology,* **25**(4):342–346, 1970.

Medical World News: Staving off strokes, Feb. 8, 1974, pp. 47–53.

Merrill, Sylvia A., and Victor F. Froelicher: Exercise testing, *Cardiovascular Nursing,* **13**(6):23–28, November/December 1977.

Nizel, Abraham E.: *Nutrition in Preventive Dentistry: Science and Practice,* Saunders, Philadelphia, 1972, chap. 27.

Oberleder, Muriel: Emotional breakdowns in elderly people, *Hospital and Community Psychiatry,* **20**(7):21–26, July 1969.

Prudden, Bonnie: *How to Keep Slender and Fit after Thirty,* Random House, New York, 1961, pp. 144–160.

Public Health Service, Office on Smoking and Health: *Smoking and Health Bulletin,* March/April 1979, pp. 43–81, Rockville, MD 20857.

Riss, Jean F.: Health control through bio-feedback, *Modern Maturity,* **14**(6):67–68, December/January 1972–1973.

Rodvien, R., and C. H. Mielke: Platelet and antiplatelet agents in strokes, current concepts of cerebrovascular disease, *Stroke,* **XIII**(2):5–8, 1978.

Schlenker, E. D., et al.: Nutrition and health of older people, in *Symposium of Nutrition,* San Juan, Puerto Rico, reprinted from *American Journal of Clinical Nutrition,* **26**(10):1111–1119, Department of Health, Education, and Welfare, 1973.

Sehnert, Keith W.: *How to Be Your Own Doctor: (Sometimes),* Parade, Los Angeles, Feb. 24, 1974, pp. 11–12.

———— **and Howard Eisenberg:** *A Doctor in Every Home, Blue Print for Health,* Blue Cross Association, 840 North Lakeshore Drive, Chicago, IL 60611, 1978, pp. 56–66.

Shock, Nathan W.: Lecture in *Seminar on Biology of Aging,* Andrus Gerontology Center, University of Southern California, Summer 1972, unpublished.

Steffl, Bernita M., and Imogene Eide: *Discharge Planning Handbook,* C. B. Slack, Thorofare, N.J., 1978, pp. 1–6.

U.S. Department of Health, Education, and Welfare: *Coordinated Home Care Programs,* USDHEW Publication no. 1579, Washington, 1966, pp. 1–3.

Weg, Ruth B.: *Nutrition and the Later Years,* Andrus Gerontology Center, University of Southern California Press, Los Angeles, 1978, 78–124, 132.

Wilner, Daniel M., Rosabelle Price Walkley, and Edward J. O'Neill: *Introduction to Public Health,* 7th ed., Macmillan, New York, 1978, pp. 334–346.

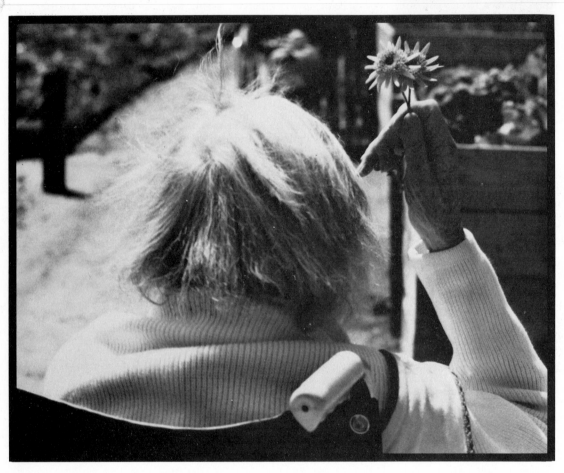

SEVEN

Anthony J. Skirlick, Jr.

IMPORTANT CONSIDERATIONS OF THE ELDERLY ADULT

The person who has never started anything is the one who
has never wondered when, or how, or if it would ever
end.
The rest of us have visions of being thrown out, carried
out, or just left standing inside, not ever realizing the job
was done.

William E. Bradshaw

THIRTY-THREE

THE SENSES

Irene Mortenson Burnside

. . . Last scene of all,
That ends this strange eventful history,
Is second childishness, and mere oblivion,
Sans teeth, sans eyes, sans taste, sans everything.
William Shakespeare
As You Like It

LEARNING OBJECTIVES

- Identify the four most common eye diseases associated with the elderly and list five guide-lines for care in each disease.
- Define presbyopia.
- Describe abnormal changes in the eye.
- Describe effective ways of working with the blind and visually handicapped.
- Define illusions.
- Describe common illusions which occur in aged clients.
- Define presbycusis.
- Define phonemic regression.
- Describe 10 nursing interventions for the deaf or hard of hearing.
- Describe four nursing interventions important in the loss of appetite or taste in aged clients.

This chapter is about the senses of vision, hearing, touch, taste, and smell; pain is also included. Blindness will be covered in depth in the next chapter, and touch is covered in detail in Chapter 35; neither of these subjects will be handled in this chapter.

Problems involving visual and hearing deficiences are rampant in the elderly. It is well to remember that serious problems in vision and hearing will also have psychological repercussions in the older person. For instance, an important research finding indicates that vision and its correction may indeed precipitate some of the very mental problems that workers are trying to eradicate (Snyder et al., 1976). It is well-known that being hard-of-hearing correlates with paranoid ideas and suspicious and guarded behavior (Eisdorfer, 1965; Cooper et al., 1974).

In the first part of this chapter, the four most common eye diseases in the elderly and implications for care will be discussed. A section on illusions follows; this is an area often overlooked. An excellent, research-oriented essay on visual perception and communication is recommended because of the pragmatic stance it takes (Shields, 1977). Figure 33-2 shows fields of normal vision. Hearing and guidelines for working with the hard-of-hearing are discussed, then taste, smell, and pain.

NORMAL CHANGES

The word *presbyopia* comes from the Greek *presby* meaning "old," and *opys,* meaning "eye." Presbyopia is impaired vision as a result of loss of elasticity in the crystalline lens of the eye. Presbyopia begins at about age 40 and usually is correctable with eyeglasses.

EYE DISEASES

Trachoma, a chronic contagious form of conjunctivitis, is a worldwide affliction causing much visual disability. It is now almost entirely limited to underdeveloped countries. In the United States, trachoma is limited to the Indian reservations in the Southwest; nurses working with Indian populations need to be well-informed about trachoma.

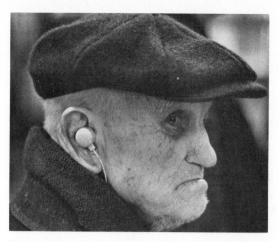

FIGURE 33-1 We do need to reward and reinforce positively the aged who wear their hearing aids. Many get discouraged and disgruntled with them and will not use them, or use them only sporadically. (*Courtesy of Harvey Finkle.*)

In the United States, four major eye diseases are associated with the elderly: (1) cataract, (2) glaucoma, (3) macular degeneration, and (4) diabetic retinopathy. These eye diseases, while prevalent in the elderly, are not peculiar to the aging eye; in fact, all except diabetic retinopathy can be present at birth. Good general health, diet, and living conditions are important for a high level of resistance to eye diseases, as well as other diseases which may occur in late life (Faye, 1971). Nurses working in prevention programs, screening clinics, and health maintenance programs will be applying those aspects of health care with their older clients.

CATARACTS

Susruta performed the operation of couching a cataract in India as early as 2000 years before Christ. The term *couching* means the treatment of a cataract by displacing the lens of the eye into the vitreous humor. Cataracts are a universal eye condition, and today the medical removal of cataract is successful in over 95 percent of the cases due to newer instruments, techniques, anesthetics, and drugs. *There still remains, however, the problem of detection and prevention of cataracts, because cataracts are the most common disability in the aged eye* (Kornzweig, 1971) (see Figure 33-3).

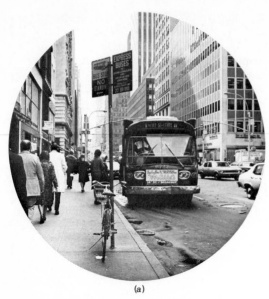

(a)

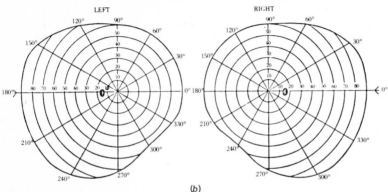

(b)

FIGURE 33-2 (a) Normal vision. A person with normal or 20/20 vision sees this street scene. (b) The field of vision (peripheral vision) with both eyes is 180°, recorded on these charts. (*Photo courtesy of The Lighthouse, New York Association for the Blind.*)

Cataracts and Visual Function A cataract is an opacity, or clouding, of the lens of the eye which blocks or changes the amount of light for vision. The lens is located behind the pupil and the colored iris. Normally the lens is transparent, and it helps to focus images onto the retina at the back of the eye which transmits them to the brain.

The underlying cause of cataracts is not determined, although it is known that a cataract is associated with chemical changes which occur in the lens (National Society for Prevention of Blindness, 1975).

The visual function of the person who has

cataracts will depend on the location of the opacity in the lens. If the opacity is generalized over the eye, haze over the vision will occur both indoors and out, but the haze may be worse in bright light. If the opacity is in the front layers of the lens, then there will be complaints of glare when outdoors or in an intense light; the intense light brings the pupil down over the opacity and, therefore, cuts down on the vision.

If the center of the lens is opaque, there will be a constant haziness to the vision. Even when the light is average or a bit dim, the old person may be able to function well although he or she will complain that it is like "looking through

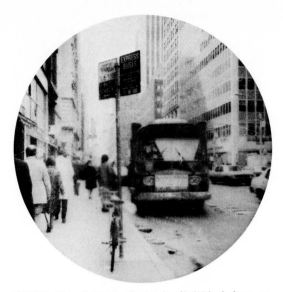

FIGURE 33-3 Cataract. Acuity is diminished from an opacity of the lens. The field of vision is unaffected. There is no scotoma, but the person has an overall haziness of view, particularly in glaring light. (*Courtesy of The Lighthouse, New York Association for the Blind.*)

Christman (1970) found that old people who were incapable of self-care, even those who were thought to be hopelessly "senile" and helpless, showed remarkable improvement following cataract surgery; the improvement was probably due to the reversal of sensory deprivation. After the surgery nearly all the patients fed themselves, stopped bedwetting, navigated without assistance, and became more interested in personal grooming, socialization, television, and reading.

Surgery is the ultimate goal in cataract treatment, but it need not be done if the person has mobility and can still do close work. It is encouraging to old persons if you tell them that cataract surgery is successful in more than 95 percent of the cases (Kornzweig, 1971). The modern techniques used are wound incision, advanced types of surgery, the removal of the lens with a cryo (freezing) probe or by emulsification and suction. Surgery is usually advised when there is a point of "life interference"—that is, the visual difficulty interferes with everyday activities.

dirty windows," or "having a skin" over the eyes. An interviewer can see the "skin" or milkiness in such eyes.

When the pathology of the lens is on the back layers of the lens, there will be good distance vision but inability to read well, because the focal point for reading will coincide with that of the opacity.

One must remember that cataracts which occur as a secondary complication require other dimensions also in their management, e.g., when there is macular degeneration present as well as a cataract. I once interviewed a 90-year-old woman who had macular degeneration in one eye and a cataract in the other.

Cataract Surgery Ophthalmologists have repeatedly observed that after cataract operations, elder patients may develop psychotic reactions characterized by delirium (Linn, 1965). Nurses should be alert to such mental changes. Linn's classic article describes mental problems following surgery and warns against an incapacitating depressive reaction. *Reducing mental confusion and disorientation is a primary responsibility in gerontological nursing.*

Complaints to Listen For

- Blurred vision is one of the first complaints. The client may complain that the light is not bright enough to read by. Objects have to be held closer to the eye to be seen.
- Double vision or spots may become noticeable as the cataract develops. Lights may not be clearly outlined but seen as if there were two or more. In some instances the client may see spots and experience loss of detail.
- A frequent change of eyeglasses may indicate the presence of a cataract near the center of the lens.
- The person may express being "dazzled" by intense light, an occurrence which is noticeable to others as a milky or yellowish spot in a normally black pupil.
- Having any one or all of these signs or symptoms does not necessarily mean that a person has cataracts. Their presence does indicate the need for a thorough eye examination.

The following is one example of a nursing home resident who managed to solve a vision problem by altering the lighting and of the drastic results that ensued.

VIGNETTE 1

Mr. G. was an 86-year-old man who spent 10 years in hospitals and/or nursing homes. He lived in a 187-bed nursing home and was struggling with his diminishing sight caused by cataracts. He was often extremely depressed about his failing vision, yet he had done some remarkable things on his own to help compensate for the vision loss. For example, he removed the glass from his radio clock and could "feel the time" with his fingertips. He used a felt-tip pen to mark off the days on his calendar so he could see what the current date was. He had always enjoyed reading, a privilege that was slowly being denied him, and he particularly liked to read at bedtime. He had a friend buy a high-wattage bulb to replace his overhead light bulb. However, to direct the light down on his reading material more, he dropped a large bath towel over the small metal fixture. He fell asleep one night while reading, and the intense heat from the bulb caused the towel to catch fire. The three patients were evacuated from the room and were uninjured.

This is one example of how elderly persons attempt to solve problems on their own. It is also a good example of "exciting" stimuli for nursing-home residents who admitted they detested the ennui of institutional life. Boredom will be discussed in the next chapter. Group discussion the day after the fire focused not on the danger but on giving me a vivid account of the fire scene and praises for the firemen, who jolted the usual placid night scene of the nursing home when "they roared into the parking lot with three big trucks, and firemen in helmets and bunkers, carrying axes, swarmed in here" (Burnside, 1976).

Implications for Care

1. Older persons can adjust to wearing contact lenses, but much time, patience, and encouragement may be required.
2. If there is a preexisting retinal damage, then close-vision reading aids, large print, or telescopic lenses are recommended.
3. Often case finding for low-vision correction is not done in homes for the aging. The result of such neglect may be that the old person tends to accept the loss of vision as an inevitable part of aging.
4. In fact, it seems to be a major task just to keep glasses from getting lost (and after loss of several pairs, some people use none).
5. It is important to tell those with cataracts that *"you need more light on your work, but less light near your eyes"* (National Society for Prevention of Blindness, 1975).
6. Cataract patients may also need tinted lenses to help them handle the glare even when indoors or while watching television. A pair of clip-on flip-up polarized plastic lenses may help (gray tints of 50 to 60 percent absorption are the most acceptable). These can be used whether down or over regular glass, or they can be placed in flipped-up position and be used as a sun shade. Some old people wear green visor caps to help reduce glare (Burnside, 1979).
7. Observe for signs and symptoms of depression following communication of the diagnosis; having to relinquish a driver's license and driving; and giving up pleasurable activities such as reading or sewing.

ACUTE GLAUCOMA

See Fernsebner's (1975) article on the early diagnosis of acute angle-closure glaucoma. She describes the onset of acute glaucoma as often developing within hours and occurring with such severe symptoms that it may suggest neurological, gastrointestinal, sinus, or dental disorder. A simple finger tension test can be done by the nurse for gross screening of acute-closure glaucoma. (A tonometer test is preferred and should be done.) The fingers are placed on the client's eyelids to feel the tension—the eye in such an instance might "feel as hard as a golf ball" (Fernsebner, 1975).

Wide-angle glaucoma is responsible for the chronic form of the disease and is more difficult to locate. Campaigns and screening efforts must continue so that glaucoma can be detected before it reaches the critical stages and becomes manifest; this is generally thought to be over 40 years of age (see Figure 33-4).

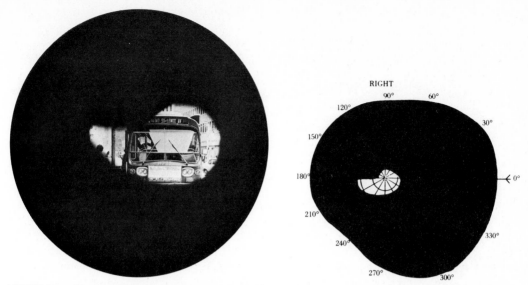

FIGURE 33-4 Glaucoma. Advanced glaucoma involves loss of peripheral vision, but the individual still retains most central vision. Early detection and cooperation with good medical care can prevent this drastic loss of vision. (*Courtesy of The Lighthouse, New York Association for the Blind.*)

An Elusive Disease Of the four major eye diseases, glaucoma still eludes detection in community health programs, especially in the early population. It is sometimes called "the silent disease" because it has no really definite symptoms; by the time it is reported, much irreversible damage has occurred. The late symptoms are field loss, blurring, and halos. A combination of tests, measurement of eye pressure with a tonometer (or by a new method called *applanation tonometry*), a careful examination of the optic nerve with an ophthalmoscope, and measurement of the central field of vision with a screening device, help diagnose glaucoma in its early stages. Eye pressure can appear to be normal, but the disease may still be progressing. Cases can be easily missed in mass screening programs. Even in the later stages of this eye disease, the visual function may seem to be normal and may remain at 20/20 even when there has already been an extensive amount of damage to peripheral vision. When clients begin to collide with things or to lose words on the printed page, they suspect trouble.

Treatment Plan When glaucoma is identified, it can be treated with drops or pills or a combination of the two. The treatment is aimed at trying to prevent the flow of aqueous humor which causes pressure against the optic nerve and subsequent atrophy of it.

Unfortunately old people may find the treatment disagreeable. The pills are diuretics and may keep the person going to the bathroom at night. Urinary frequency disrupts sleep.

The drops which do constrict the pupil may also darken the vision; this is especially true if there is a cataract present. If adequate instructions and explanations are not given by the nurse, the old person may not adhere to the treatment plan. The important thing to always remember regarding glaucoma is that early detection and a religious adherence to the medical treatment are crucial.

Glaucoma Susceptibility It is known that members of the family of a person with glaucoma are more susceptible to the disease than other persons in the same age group. The combination of local eye drops and drugs has been so effective controlling the increased intraocular pressure that eye surgery for glaucoma is less needed than it used to be. The person has to be under constant surveillance, however, and tested at regular intervals to make sure that the therapeutic regimen is effective.

Kornzweig (1971) states that the removal of a cataract in a person who has both cataracts and glaucoma will cure both conditions in a large number of cases, and it is particularly true for the aged in whom the combined diseases are frequently found. That phenomenon had been suspected for a long time.

Signs and Symptoms of Chronic Glaucoma Having any of the symptoms listed below does not necessarily mean a person has glaucoma; they could be caused by some other less serious eye trouble. But it is well to remember that these symptoms might not even be present, and yet one could have early glaucoma.

1. Frequent changes of glasses, none of which is satisfactory
2. Inability to adjust the eyes to darkened rooms, such as theaters
3. Loss of side vision
4. Blurred or foggy vision
5. Rainbow-colored rings around lights
6. Difficulty in focusing on close work

Instructions for Persons with Glaucoma The following are suggestions recommended by the National Society for the Prevention of Blindness (1975):

1. Follow the ophthalmologist's instructions carefully.
2. Use only the prescribed drops every day and at the time of day advised.
3. Do not use any other eye drops or washes without consulting the health care person.
4. Do not take any other drugs or medications, no matter how harmless they seem, without checking with the ophthalmologist.
5. If consulting another physician, be sure to mention that you are being treated for glaucoma.
6. Situations which make you nervous or worried can raise the pressure in the eyeball. Try to avoid such situations.
7. Although coffee and tea are stimulants which may raise the pressure when taken in large quantities in a short period of time, they need not be harmful when used moderately.
8. Alcoholic beverages, including beer, may actually lower the pressure in the eyeball.
9. Tobacco may cause constrictions of the blood vessels supplying the optic nerve (which connects the retinal cells to the brain) and adversely affect the glaucoma.
10. Always keep a light on in the room when watching television.
11. Have a complete physical examination yearly. Good health means more satisfactory results in the treatment of the glaucoma.
12. Proper diet, good dental care, plenty of sleep, fresh air, and exercise are all necessary.
13. If you have a cold, infection, or other illness, seek prompt medical treatment and avoid self-treatment.

As stated previously, the nurse should watch and listen for signs and symptoms indicating depression.

Important points to remember about glaucoma are as follows: (1) it usually strikes after age 35, (2) it is difficult to detect in the early stages, and (3) it can usually be controlled if caught early.

MACULAR DEGENERATION

The causes of macular degeneration in the aged are not known. It may be an inherited or a familial condition. Some persons think that the condition in the aged may have a genetic basis. Others think that the circulation to the macular area may diminish because of arteriosclerosis.

The macula lutea is a small area in the retina that is hardly more than $\frac{1}{16}$ inch in diameter. In spite of its tiny size, it is the area for central vision or daylight vision (as opposed to side vision or night vision), the vision for great distances, for reading fine print, sewing fine stitches, and perceiving color the most clearly. It is also the area in which one can identify other people's features at a distance (see Figure 33-5).

A survey of over 1000 residents in a Jewish home and hospital for the aged revealed that one-third of those over age 65 had some degree of macular degeneration. *The condition does increase with age and affects 24 percent of persons*

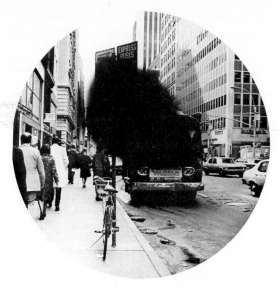
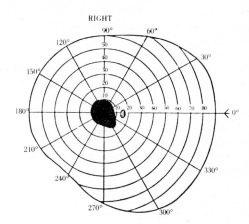

RIGHT

FIGURE 33-5 Macular degeneration is also a prevalent eye disease. The area of decreased central vision, called a *central scotoma*, is shown. The peripheral or traveling vision remains unaffected. (*Courtesy of The Lighthouse, New York Association for the Blind.*)

between age 65 and 80 and 38 percent of those over 80 years of age (Kornzweig, 1971). Vision is reduced to 20/70 in the moderately advanced cases. In the advanced cases vision can be 20/200 or less. The side vision is usually maintained, and affected persons can get around and take care of themselves. They do complain bitterly, though, when forced to give up reading, writing, and sewing, and, of course, it is also sad when there is difficulty in identifying their neighbors. Low-vision aids are very helpful to these persons (Kornzweig, 1971). In macular degeneration the adjustment in daily living may be less difficult if the degeneration is gradual.

Implications for Care

1. Low-vision lenses are particularly helpful for cases of macular degeneration.
2. Early detection is important for medical treatment and to prescribe low-vision glasses (over 50 percent of all visually handicapped persons over 65 years of age have macular degeneration).
3. Old people can use hand magnifiers quite well.

4. Suggest use of stand magnifiers if there is tremor or severe arthritis.
5. Telescopic lenses should be tried.
6. High-vitamin diet to combat insufficiency of vitamins A and B complex is important (Kornzweig, 1971).
7. Reassure older persons that they will not become totally blind.
8. Watch for signs and symptoms of depression.

DIABETIC RETINOPATHY

In past years the number of older persons who have lost vision and sometimes become totally blind as a result of sustained diabetes mellitus has grown considerably. Diabetic retinopathy is now the most common cause of blindness which results from a metabolic disease, and especially among the aged. This increase has occurred because there are now more diabetic patients who are living longer because of early diagnosis and better control of the diabetic state.

Diabetic retinopathy is nearly always bilateral and does not usually appear until the person has had diabetes for 15 to 25 years. The degree of retinopathy is not well correlated to the severity and the degree of control of the diabetic condition (Kasper, 1978).

Diabetic retinopathy starts with the forming of a small dilatation of a capillary, called a *microaneurysm.* Both blood and serum seep out of these involved capillaries, exudates form, and hemorrhages occur. The hemorrhages may be so severe that the vitreous cavity is completely filled, and then vision is totally blocked.

The argon laser beam is used to treat cases of diabetic retinopathy. The beam obliterates the blood vessels responsible for the bleeding. Early cases are helped, but late cases only rarely improve. The basic causative factors are still unknown except, of course, the diabetes itself (Kornzweig, 1971).

It is not so difficult to find the retinal pathology which occurs in diabetes because most of the clients are under medical care and are, therefore, referred for eye care promptly when and if there are any changes in vision. Early case finding is needed to prevent the recurrence of hemorrhages. Treatment is not satisfactory, although laser photocoagulation is used with aged patients (Kasper, 1978).

Cataracts are also a frequent companion of diabetes mellitus and usually are formed in the back layers of the lens.

Although the emphasis is on low-vision center and the use of what vision there is even though it may be slight, it is well to remember that the diabetic who is also visually handicapped must be prepared to function sometimes as a blind person; this could happen when a vitreous hemorrhage has affected vision.

Special Problems With the aging process comes an increase in special problems. If old persons live alone, they may not seek medical help. A community without an outreach program may be unaware that such individuals exist.

Implications for Care

1. Good medical care and correct medication to control the diabetes
2. Diet
3. Exercise routine
4. Control of weight
5. Visual aids as needed

6. Orientation and mobility training classes for clients in a state of temporary blindness

HEMIANOPSIA

Hemianopsia (also spelled *hemianopia*) is a vision loss in half of the visual field and can be readily discovered by a confrontation field test. One eye of the aged person is closed by placing the palm of the hand over it; the other eye is fixed on the examiner's finger. The examiner's finger is brought around from behind the seated client and on the side of the eye which is being tested and is moved until the person is aware of the finger. It is done on each eye separately. The check is also done from above and downward and then below and upward. Homonymous hemianopsia can be seen in Figure 33-6. It is usually caused by a vascular accident.

Hemianopsia, which may occur in either the lower or the upper fields, can occur in one or both eyes. It may be due to pressure on the optic tract (Kornzweig, 1971) (see Figure 33-7).

EYEGLASSES AND PROPER LIGHTING

Clients should be advised about the importance of correctly prescribed glasses, that they should have them made individually, and that they should not buy ready-made ones in department stores or by mail order. It is recommended that safety lenses of shatter-resistant glass or plastic be used in all glasses.

Wearing glasses may create problems for some of the elderly. Some of the problems indicated on a questionnaire I sent to nurses included (1) loss, (2) identification, (3) breakage, (4) cleanliness, and (5) ensuring wearing (Burnside, 1972). The glasses become especially problematic for the confused aged person who is ever losing them and for others who love to read but cut down on reading because of these problems. Some old people continue to wear glasses they have had for many years, and some wear other people's glasses. Some elderly buy dime-store bifocals to use, and some carry a magnifying glass with them. Whether a person wears glasses, whose they are, and how effective they are should be recorded in the initial assessment

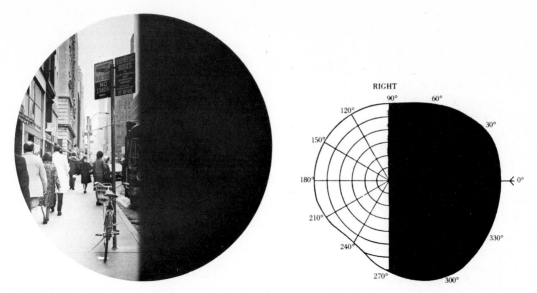

FIGURE 33-6 Hemianopsia is a defect in the optic pathways between the eye and brain. Vision is lost in half of a field. The most common defect occurs in corresponding halves of the right field of vision and causes reading impairment, right homonymous hemianopsia. It can also occur on both left halves of the field of vision. (*Courtesy of The Lighthouse, New York Association for the Blind.*)

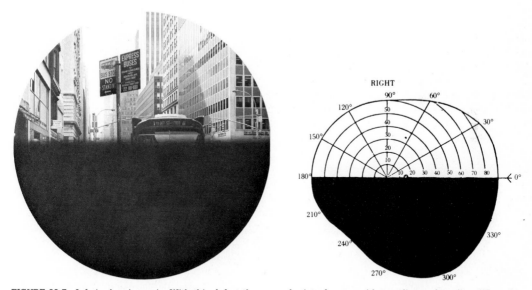

FIGURE 33-7 Inferior hemianopsia. With this defect there may be interference with traveling and reading. When the visual defect is in the upper half, it is called *superior hemianopsia*. (*Courtesy of The Lighthouse, New York Association for the Blind.*)

made by the nurse. However, it is well to remember that time, energy, and money can often be wasted if the solutions are not acceptable to the aged client. Our suggestions may simply be rejected.

Ways to Improve   It is a goal to improve the ability to read, to see television, or even to dial the phone. The phone does add to the pleasurable moments of an elderly person. There is available on the market an enlarged telephone dial to place beneath the ordinary phone dial. The numbers and letters are magnified five times and glow in the dark. The gadget is inexpensive and easy to attach.

While doing close work, the elderly should be instructed to take a position that is comfortable for doing the work. *Always remind the aged person that there should be sufficient illumination* (see Figure 33-8). The light should be diffused evenly in the work area to eliminate glare. A glare can be either from a light shining into the eyes, for example, a bare light bulb, or it can be a reflection from a nearby object. It is advisable to leave a second lamp burning so that when the client looks up from the work the eyes will not need to adjust from the brightly lit surface to the darkness of the surrounding room.

Shadows should be avoided by the reader's sitting in such a position that the light comes over the left shoulder, if the reader is right-handed, or over the right shoulder if left-handed (see Figure 33-8). Advise the client to take a rest at times, to shift position, and look off into the distance or close the eyes momentarily (Southern California Society for the Prevention of Blindness, 1972). This is important advice for older women who still do much fine needlework, for instance, crocheting, tatting, needlepoint, or embroidery.

SUNGLASSES

While sunglasses do provide relief from the glare of the sun, it goes without saying that they must not be worn while driving at night or in the fog. The glasses should fit well enough that light and glare do not enter the eye over and around the

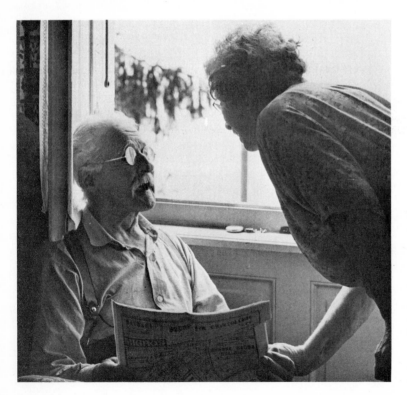

FIGURE 33-8   Reading affords many older persons great pleasure; we should do all we can to encourage it by preserving the sight. Note how the elderly man in this photograph has placed himself to receive the best possible light. Older persons' vision can be improved greatly by simply improving the lighting. *Nurses must incorporate such information in nursing care plans.* Attention to lighting is extremely important. One woman in a facility explained her lack of interest in reading. "There's only a 25-watt bulb in the middle of our four-bed room. How can I read?" (*World Health Organization, photo by C. Huber.*)

lens. For a client who wears glasses regularly, there is a need for corrective prescriptions ground into sunglasses.

It is well to have all glasses, aids, and prostheses labeled with the person's name, as losing and misplacing glasses can become a pervasive problem in late years.

GLARE: A PROBLEM FOR THE AGED

Increased susceptibility to visual glare is one problem in the aged population that nurses should be aware of and then pose interventions for the glare. Attending to the glare problem in the elderly helps nurses function better with these clients in a variety of settings. For example, there are glares in the acute hospital or long-term care setting—the glare through windows or from light-colored and brightly polished corridors when the sun hits them. In the interview room, if the aged person is seated facing a window with bright light, the glare can be very bothersome and distracting. I am reminded of a student who came into my office. We had had a lecture on being sensitive to the problems of old people, and glare was one problem discussed. In a few moments the student said, "I am really aware now how much the bright sunshine coming in that window does bother me; would you pull the drapery, please?" Glare is "a harsh, uncomfortably brilliant light, specifically bright sunlight" (Webster's, 1973). Hatton (1977) points out in her excellent article about glare that the visual efficiency is lowered and this may cause a disabling effect; there can be discomfort which can range all the way from slight irritation to actual pain.

Hatton classifies glare into two types: simultaneous and successive. The simultaneous glare happens when the peripheral field is of much lower luminance than the source which is more powerful. The successive glare is defined as one in which the eyes pass from a field of a lower level of illumination, and one to which the eye has adapted, to a field with much higher illumination.

Three factors interact with age to determine the minimum amount of light to which the eye can respond: (1) the region of the retina which is stimulated; (2) the stimulus size, duration, and wavelength of both the light used to preadapt the eye and the test light itself; and (3) the amount of time spent in the dark or dark adaptation (Fozard et al., 1977).

We are familiar with the temporary loss of vision that we experience when we enter a darkened restaurant or theater in the daylight. But we tend to not be as cognizant of the effects of too much illumination and the effects of glare. It has been suggested that increased opacity in the lens of the eye is the primary cause of an increasing sensitivity to glare.

IMPLICATIONS OF VISUAL CARE OF THE ELDERLY

The following list was adapted from Hatton (1977).

1. Fine-detail work should be done under localized light.
2. Background light should not be brighter than the central field.
3. Printed matter should not be on glossy paper and should be printed with ink with low reflection factors.
4. Avoid all glossy and polished surfaces, glass-covered items and chrome, for example.
5. Remember that persons over 60 require twice the illumination as a 20-year-old person for given tasks.
6. Diffuse lighting rather than light from one direction is best for most environments.
7. Light in an inside room should be almost equal to the light in rooms connected to it.
8. Room-darkening shades are important when there is too much light from windows. (These shades are a great deal more expensive than ordinary shades, and the client should be alerted to that.)
9. Light-colored walls and ceilings should have matte finish, not high gloss.
10. Desk lamps and table lamps or pull-down fixtures are needed for close work.
11. Very high levels of illumination should be used only when needed because as the brightness of light increases, the permissible ratio of light to dark increases.

12. Stairways should not be between or at the edge of differing levels of lighting.
13. Steps should be color coded at the edges.
14. Adequate lighting is necessary at all stairs.
15. Night-lights are essential.
16. Light switches must be close to the bedside within reach.
17. Turn one's head aside when switching on a bright light.
18. Sunglasses are helpful for glares outside as are hats with brims or bills.
19. Suggest an umbrella on cloudless bright days to protect field of vision.
20. Evaluate the susceptibility to glare in all placements and environments.
21. Patients in rooms should be placed away from glaring lights, for example, in critical care units.
22. Night driving suggestions to prevent scotomatic glare (night blindness) are:
    a. Never look directly at the oncoming headlight.
    b. Travel on divided highways to reduce the distance of approaching glares.
    c. Travel on routes that are lighted to decrease the contrast of lights.
    d. Glare tolerance tests should be given to old drivers to sort out those who might be a hazard.
23. Teach the older individual about glare.
24. Check lighting when complaints arise of tired eyes or feelings of tension.
25. Appropriate lighting intervention must be carried out by the health care individual.
26. The nurse can serve as a consultant for input into building, remodeling and decorating projects which involve the older client.

ILLUSIONS

There are two definitions of illusions which apply to this section: (1) "a misleading image presented to the vision," and (2) "perception of something objectively existing in such a way as to cause misinterpretation of its actual nature" (Webster's, 1973).

I have listened to so many descriptions of illusions by old people that I am now convinced it is an area in which clinicians will have to intervene. Instructors will also need to alert students and assist them to become skillful in real-ity testing during illusional states. Elsewhere I have documented information of illusions described by colleagues; the reader is referred to that listing (Burnside, 1979).

Research Needed   The visual world and the visual field, especially that of visual illusions, could be a fascinating area for nurses to explore. Gibson (1966) deals with the subject. The perception of people, surfaces, objects, space, all depend on the elderly person's past experiences. Those perceptions based on the past, if coupled with visual changes in the aging process, may account for some of the unusual and interesting illusions described by the aged.

Segall (1966) reported on the use of visual illusions, and a detailed account of many illusions and the feelings engendered after people experience drug-induced illusions is well described by Castaneda (1972).

Misleading cues to an environment can cause accidents for both young and old if they make incorrect assumptions about objects, space, distance, and obstacles which are of a hazardous nature.

Prevalence of Illusions   Among the aged illusions are common, and they are not by any means restricted to mentally ill individuals. Are illusions due to failing eyesight in the aged, poor lighting, misperceived environment, or other causes? Several excellent samples of hallucinations and illusions are given by Jaeger and Simmons (1970).

One elderly person admitted to a hospital reacted to bed rails by requesting to be "let out of jail." Finally a nurse realized how the aged person might be viewing the rails from her prone position in bed. As the aged lady looked to each side of her, the rails on her bed did indeed appear to be jail window bars. Another instance occurred in an acute psychiatric ward on a 4:00 P.M. to midnight shift. A frightened elderly patient kept telling me about "the huge white ghosts outside." I walked to the window of her room, and outside the ward were several large laundry carts piled high with dirty linen, but carts and linen both were white even in the darkness (Burnside, 1979). It is important to actually look in the direction the patient is looking when he or she describes such illusions so that one can better test their grasp of reality.

Misperceptions in Environment Speaking of illusions can immediately label an old person as confused and disoriented, which may well be true. However, all of us have experienced illusions of our own. I have mistaken a radar screen for a large Ferris wheel; in moments of fear, I have thought of bushes and trees as shaped like sinister humans, and so on. In foreign countries, I perpetually mistake something for some other object in my effort to identify it and/or find something familiar. I suspect it is much the same for old people who are placed in the foreign places we design for them.

But illusions are funny things, too. They often relieve boredom and monotony. I recall hearing of one lady of more than 90 years who put her toaster cover on her radio and then wandered around the kitchen looking for her radio (Miller, 1978).

Old people misperceiving their environment can upset and/or enliven wards in both acute hospitals and nursing homes. One hot midnight in a large county hospital, an old woman threw a pitcher of ice water on her roommate and began screaming, "Fire, fire, fire!" She saw a large red neon light down the street from the hospital and thought there was a fire. Hospital personnel responded with alacrity and then dismay, as the drenched woman had to be pacified and changed (Burnside, 1976).

In old people, hallucinations, or illusions, may not be symptoms of mental illness so much as misperceived incoming data. One group leader listened as an elderly woman in the group muttered about "feathers" and looked at the leader's long skirt. The pattern in the fabric did somewhat in fact resemble feathers (Burnside, 1976). It requires patience and time for the nurse to pursue reality in the face of persistent delusions or illusions, but it is a nursing responsibility to describe and reinforce reality for the older confused client. The task is tedious and time-consuming and requires patience, and perhaps that is why it is not pursued often enough.

VIGNETTE 2

A colleague shared the story of an elderly woman newly admitted to a nursing home. The schedule of the nursing home was not explained to her; she was not aware of the changes of shifts that occur in nursing homes and hospitals. At 11:30 every night

the woman heard much noise and commotion from the employee's parking lot. She fantasized that the personnel waited until that time of the night to remove the dead bodies from the facility. As her fantasies grew, so did her insomnia, and she spent restless, sleepless nights fearing her own demise. She verbalized her fears to a nurse, who then intervened. A reality-oriented nurse took the woman out to the parking lot one night at shift change to show her exactly what occurred there at 11:30 P.M. From then on the patient was reassured.

This vignette includes several important points for nurses to remember: (1) awareness that the fear of dying may exist; (2) sensitivity to how difficult nights can be for some institutionalized aged persons; and (3) realization of how elderly people may readily misperceive their environment. This is especially true because *many aged are written off as confused when actually they are misperceiving the milieu.* Since this happens so commonly, student nurses should be taught to be on the alert for such occurrences and immediately intervene to correct misperceptions. We must help the elderly person come as close to reality as possible.

VIGNETTE 3

In Sarasota, Florida, two elderly couples drove into the bay and drowned. They were out for an evening of chamber music. They mistakenly drove down a boat ramp into Sarasota Bay during a driving rainstorm. The police said that two long wooden docks lead out into the water. They drove right between the docks. The ramp goes downhill gradually. The couples were in two cars. The lead vehicle probably thought they knew where they were going, and the other simply followed it down the ramp, according to the police (*San Jose Mercury,* 1979).

COLORS

Sicurella (1977) feels that even when glare is completely absent and lighting is appropriate, there may be little to help a visually impaired person see an object unless there is sufficient color contrast between the object and the background. If the color of an object is sharply contrasted against the background, then very high levels of illumination and the proper positioning of the object will become less critical.

All objects have three visual characteristics: opacity, transparency, and reflectivity. The one specific rule that seems to be general is the finding that white lettering on a black background is better seen than black lettering on a white background (Sicurella, 1977).

IMPLICATIONS FOR CARE REGARDING COLOR

The following list is adapted from Sicurella (1977).

1. *Kitchen:* There are problems in measuring quantities, proportioning foods into amounts, reading gauges, judging cooked food (whether done or not), and physical hazards. Because there is a lack of contrast in most kitchens, attach sheet of black contact paper to wall above counter to have light foods show up better. Use white contact paper for measuring, pouring dark liquid. Provide two cutting boards, one light colored and one dark colored for cutting foods of various colors.

2. *Dining areas:* Use contrasting colors so that food can be better seen. Use cups and saucers with colored edge bands to help determine the edges. Smoked-glass tumblers can be seen on cloth better than clear-glass ones. Use caution in selecting tablecloths; overhead light above may bring out the worst in a bright tablecloth. Avoid warm to hot colors and also patterned tablecloths which tend to confuse the eye. Newcomer (1974) described the difficulty in eating if one places white dishes on a light table and the aged cannot see the edge of the plate. I once served white angel food cake on a white plate on a white table and wondered why the oldsters did not immediately reach for it.

3. *Living area:* Subdued lighting in the living area makes it a problem area. Watch for low freestanding objects in the living room. Horizontal planes with edges beyond the base on furniture may cause collisions. The lower the object, the greater the possibility of tripping over it. Avoid sharp edges and corners. Select low tables with tops which contrast with the floor and are more easily seen. Electrical and telephone cords traversing the old person's path can be real hazards.

4. *Bathroom:* Lighting in bathroom is critical because usually the person wants it directed on the face. Consider a mirrored medicine cabinet with built-in fluorescent light fixtures on each side to reduce the brightness, illuminate the face more uniformly, and reduce shadows. Often bathrooms are painted high-gloss white; suggest other paint.

5. *Bedroom:* The safest and the most practical beds are those without head- and footboards. The lighting in closets is very important. Install a pull-chain, porcelain, wall light socket inside closet above the door. It is called "display lighting" and is ideal because it illuminates but the light source is out of sight above the head and behind. Pale blue colors in room decor, bedding, patients' clothing, staff uniforms are not recommended as color choice for the aged. Bright blue is one of the colors poorly seen by the elderly due to changes in the eye.

6. *Work and/or desk area:* Use a dark blotter for stationery to provide line of demarcation. Use black felt-tip pens. Use a black telephone with white symbols and clocks with dark background and white symbols. Base of Rolodex should be dark. Check that dividers are legible. Arrange files to side of the drawer rather than front to back so that light sheds directly on the title tabs in the side-to-side arrangement. In a front-to-back grouping, the titles face away from the light.

OUTDOORS

The outdoor environment can be treacherous for old people who have vision problems. Curbs and cracks in the sidewalks may create problems in navigation because they may not be visible to the aged with failing eyesight. Many old people who drive cannot see the exits of parking lots as the curb blends with the street; consequently, they often drive off the curbs, much to the surprise and consternation of their passengers. Bright sunny days can hamper people's movement because of intense sunlight, or sun shining on snow, or foggy weather where signs, cues, environmental landmarks normally observed are changed or appear distorted.

Visually Impaired The following suggestions are offered for working with visually impaired old people (Burnside, 1974):

1. Make sure the individual has adequate lighting at all times, especially for reading, sewing, writing, and similar activities.
2. Avoid bright glare, e.g., highly polished floors, enamel walls, windows without curtains or shades.
3. There should be a soft light on at night, especially in the bathroom, kitchen, or other areas where the individual is likely to go.
4. Old people should be discouraged from taking long drives at night because of night blindness.
5. Large-print books, newspapers, calendars, and magazines should be made available (Burnside, 1970).
6. Many useful aids can be procured, e.g., ordinary-size playing cards with enlarged figures and oversized cards.
7. Talking-book records and machines can be obtained free from the Library of Congress.
8. Face the individual when speaking.
9. Wear bright red lipstick to facilitate lip-reading.
10. Do not cover your mouth when speaking; keep mustaches and beards trimmed so lips are visible.
11. Do not smoke or chew gum when speaking to such a person.
12. All elderly persons should have pockets in their clothing for carrying treasured things.
13. It is important for them to have a transistor radio.
14. Special dials for phones are available which enlarge the numbers and glow in the dark.
15. Do not move furniture or belongings without explaining what you are doing and why.
16. Give detailed instructions for anything you plan to do. Wheelchair patients, in particular, need to be told about obstacles, warned when they will be pulled backwards, etc., to diminish their fear.
17. Large clocks and large calendars are a must for orientation.
18. Do not use colors which merge, e.g., white dishes on a white table, beige light switches on beige walls.
19. Eyeglasses must be cleaned often and the prescription checked to see if vision is corrected properly.

HEARING

"She had no teeth and was partly deaf. One wondered whether new spectacles, dentures and a hearing aid would have transformed her appearance and enhanced her ability to communicate with others" (Townsend, 1962, p. 274). This quotation describes the plight of many older persons whom nurses will be working with. Shanck (1980) has written about communication problems one can expect to encounter in an elderly population. An excellent article on auditory perception and communication by Corso (1978, p. 531) reminds us that "the problems of speech and hearing cannot be isolated from the individual's total pattern of behavior."

NORMAL HEARING CHANGES

Presbycusis is normal hearing loss which is attributable to age alone. It is used as a diagnosis only if no other cause for hearing loss can be found (Goodhill, 1979). These persons have great trouble in hearing sibilants such as *s, sh,* and *ch.*

PREVALENCE OF HEARING LOSS

Hearing loss is more prevalent in elderly men than in elderly women. The aged gradually lose the ability to hear high-pitched sounds. The reader is referred to Ruben's chapter in *Clinical Geriatrics* for further details (Ruben, 1979). Noises also often can be mistaken for sounds other than what they really are. Again, a nurse's sensitivity and patience in exploring and following through with feedback on such comments is important. Nighttime can be a difficult period for the aged, as was previously noted in the example of the newly admitted woman who could not correctly identify noises in a parking lot.

Some oldsters can be encouraged to take up

lipreading; this is a neglected field, and we need more persons to teach it. Hearing aids also require more attention (Burnside, 1972). When working with aged individuals who tend to be suspicious and guarded, it is best to move slowly until they trust you.

Cooper et al. (1974) studied 132 mental hospital patients who averaged 68 years of age. None had had mental illness before the age of 50; at the time the study was done, it was found that 65 were paranoid. Over 46 percent of those with paranoid ideation had a hearing loss, compared with 38 percent of the control group. The deafness of the paranoid subjects had been of long standing.

Wells (1976) reminds us that three eminently treatable causes of deafness, cranial arteritis, syphilis, and sarcoid, are often overlooked. In one article he writes about early diagnosis and proper therapy with disorders occurring in the five senses and stresses the importance of staving off the dimming of the senses. Hearing problems create havoc in one-to-one relationship therapy, in group work, and in any interview. Screening out extraneous noise, keeping instructions simple, facing the person, and not covering one's mouth while speaking are but a few of the things to remember when conversing with the aged hard-of-hearing.

HEARING PHONE-A-TEST

The Chicago Hearing Society has devised a free and simple telephone hearing test which is used to reach elderly citizens who might not be aware they have a hearing loss.

The Phone-A-Test Center often receives more than 100 calls per day. The taped screening has four warbled tones. They are of different pitches and intensities. If the caller cannot hear all four tones, it is recommended the caller contact the family physician, an audiologist, or the Hearing Society.

COURTESY AND THE HARD-OF-HEARING

One hardship suffered by persons with a hearing loss is the isolation, real or fancied, that their handicap imposes upon them. This is increased by the embarrassment people with normal hearing sometimes show in their presence. To help both groups, the National Association of Hearing and Speech Agencies and other organizations devoted to aiding the communicatively handicapped offer these suggestions:

1. Remember that there are all degrees and several kinds of hearing loss. People may have anything from a slight to a profound loss. They may have trouble hearing only high-pitched or low-pitched sounds. They may hear you but not be able to understand you. They may hear well in some situations and not at all in others. They may hear poorly at one time and almost normally at others. Do not group all persons with hearing loss into one category. They are individuals and their hearing problems are individual. Take time with them. You may be pleasantly surprised and rewarded.

2. When you meet a person who seems inattentive or slow to understand you, consider the possibility that hearing, rather than manners or intellect, may be at fault. Some hard-of-hearing persons refuse to wear hearing aids. Others wear aids so inconspicuously or cleverly camouflaged that you may not spot them at first glance.

3. Remember that the hard-of-hearing may depend to a considerable extent on reading your lips to understand what you are saying. They do this even though they may be wearing a hearing aid, for no hearing aid can completely restore hearing. You can help them by trying always to speak to them in a good light and by facing them and the light as you speak. However, do speak to them; most of them benefit from sound.

4. Speak distinctly but naturally. Shouting does not clarify speech sounds, and mouthing or exaggerating your words, or speaking at a snail's pace, makes you harder to understand. On the other hand, try not to speak too rapidly. Normal, well-articulated, well-modulated speech is best.

5. When you are in a group that includes a hard-of-hearing person, try to carry on your conversation with others in such a way that he or she can watch your lips. Never take advantage of this handicap by carrying on

private conversations in low tones the person cannot hear.

6. Do not start to speak to the hard-of-hearing abruptly. Attract their attention first by facing them and looking straight into their eyes. If necessary, touch their hand or shoulder lightly. Help them grasp what you are talking about right away by starting with a key word or phrase, e.g., "Let's plan our weekend now," "Speaking of teen-agers. . . ." If they do not understand you, do not repeat the same words. Substitute synonyms: "It's time to make plans for Saturday" (National Association of Hearing and Speech Agencies, n.d.).

VIGNETTE 4

Mr. B., a 74-year-old man living in his own home, gradually became hard-of-hearing. His spouse patiently repeated sentences for him because he detested wearing his hearing aid. (He had spent $500 for a hearing aid and felt he had been bilked.) He felt very self-conscious about the hearing aid even though it was really not very conspicuously attached to his glasses. He said he resented having to put on reading glasses so he could hear! The spouse became very annoyed because she had to repeat so much of what she said. Often it did appear that he did not listen attentively to the person speaking and then would vex them with "What?" His teen-age grandchildren, however, did not tolerate such behavior. They refused to talk loudly and repeat what they said; instead, they quietly and steadily insisted he wear his hearing aid and rewarded him with long conversations when he did.

The lesson to be learned here is that we need to reward and reinforce the aged positively when they do accept and use prosthetics and also give them feedback. The hard-of-hearing aged need to realize how exhausting and what a strain it can be to have to raise one's voice, continually repeat things, or have an inattentive listener. When the effort expended to converse becomes very great, many persons will avoid the interaction if possible, which only increases the isolation and alienation felt by the hard-of-hearing aged person.

HEARING AIDS

Hearing aids create many problems for the aged users and their caretakers. The parts of a hearing aid are small and intricate and clients with palsy, severe arthritis, or partial paralysis may not have the manual dexterity needed to handle them. Some hearing aids are so noisy and so difficult to adjust that the individual will not wear them. Batteries get lost, wear out, and/or are difficult to obtain. See Shanck's practical suggestions for improving care in this area (Shanck, 1980).

There are aged people who have been duped into buying an aid and may have been bilked; they simply will not spend more money on repairs or a new aid. The cost of hearing aids prevents many poor elderly persons from obtaining them, and yet they are such a vital prosthetic.

"SENTRIES OF SOUND"

Lately the media have presented articles on training dogs to do the hearing for deaf persons, and about the work of the American Humane Society program. Dogs are trained to carry messages between deaf couples living in the same house, to help a deaf mother find a crying child, and to guard against burglars and prowlers at night.

The San Francisco Society for the Prevention of Cruelty to Animals has a "hearing dog" program where lost or abandoned dogs are trained to hear and then live with deaf people. The Hearing Dog Center trains dogs to respond to sounds ranging from the usual ones, such as a knock at the door or the ring of a telephone, to unusual noises, such as a prowler. The program developed from a study by the Minnesota Society of the Prevention of Cruelty to Animals in 1975 based on the idea from the deaf who observed their dogs for clues to sounds. Training takes about $2500 and 4 months; the dog learns to respond to voice commands, hand signals, and a variety of household sounds and is trained to lick its master's face in bed when a smoke alarm sounds. Dogs are given free to the deaf and made available to those with severe or profound deafness, especially deaf people over age 18 with infants and who do not have hearing people living with them. More of these hearing dog centers are needed to provide deaf persons, especially the elderly deaf, with a loving useful companion and a home for a lost or abandoned dog (Stix, 1979).

GUIDELINES FOR COMMUNICATING WITH THE HARD-OF-HEARING[1]

When talking to the hard-of-hearing, you will be able to help them understand you more clearly by following these simple suggestions:

1. Talk at a moderate rate.
2. Keep your voice at about the same volume throughout each sentence, without dropping it at the end of each sentence.
3. Always speak as clearly and accurately as possible. Consonants should be articulated with special care.
4. Do not overarticulate; mouthing or overdoing articulation is just as bad as mumbling.
5. Pronounce every name with care. Make a reference to the name for easier understanding, e.g., "Joan, the girl from the office," or "Penney's, the downtown store."
6. Change to a new subject at a slower rate, making sure that the person follows the change to the new subject. A key word or two at the beginning of a new topic is a good indicator.
7. Do not attempt to converse while you have something in your mouth, such as a pipe, cigar, cigarette, or chewing gum. Do not cover your mouth with your hand.
8. Talk in a normal tone of voice. Shouting does not make your voice more distinct, although many seem to think it does. In some instances shouting makes it more difficult for a hard-of-hearing person to understand.
9. Address the listener directly. Do not turn away in the middle of a remark or story. Make sure that the listener can see your face easily and that a good light is on it.

---

[1] Sacramento Hearing Society, Inc., 1717 Morse Avenue, Sacramento, CA 95825.

10. Use longer phrases which tend to be easier to understand than short ones. For example, "Will you get me a drink of water?" presents much less difficulty than, "Will you get me a drink?" Word choice is important here. "Fifteen cents" and "Fifty cents" may be confused, but "a half-dollar" is clearer.

A regulation on hearing aids to protect individuals with hearing impairments was established by the FDA in 1977 (*Federal Regulations,* 1977). It requires persons with a hearing loss to have obtained a medical evaluation of the impairment by a physician, preferably a specialist in ear diseases, within 6 months prior to purchasing a hearing aid. The physician must provide a written statement of the medical evaluation indicating that the individual is eligible for a hearing device. The primary concern underlying this requirement is that an unnecessary or partially effective hearing aid might be substituted for primary medical or surgical treatment (*FDA Drug Bulletin,* 1977).

Nurses could explore the possibilities of training for those hard-of-hearing and deaf old people.

TASTE

Taste may be one of the special senses in the aged that nursing really has ignored; at the risk of sounding defensive, I must say it is easy to overlook some facts of care in the aged because the problems are so multiple, so complex, and so consistent. Added to this may be a lack of resources—both financial and community. Taste buds diminish with the advancing years; studies show various results. Nurses are confronted most frequently with the adamant aged (or family of peers) who request items not on the regular diet. The need for more spices as well as more seasoning and texture is often expressed. One old man enjoyed having "extras" at his bedside—a bottle of hot sauce, a jar of peanut butter, strawberry jam, etc. "Minipantries" are discouraged in many institutions, however.

Food has tremendous psychological importance for the aged individual. Many old persons find comfort in eating food they were accustomed to early in life. We should remember this in planning care. In the face of so many losses, nurses should make a real effort to see that the food served is palatable and enjoyable. Eating alone, ill-fitting dentures, special diets, and poorly prepared food (hot food served cold, cold food served warm) only increase the reasons why an old person does not enjoy eating, or will not eat, or both. I found that eating is one of the pleasurable things for aged group members. Food can be a surprise and, therefore, a stimulus. It can have psychological importance, and often food is an excellent way to reach the more regressed aged.

Engen (1977) states that although a number of researchers have observed that taste sensitivity decreases with age, one must consider the conclusion with caution because not all experiments have been able to verify that finding. He also points out that when an increased aversion for bitterness is found in taste tests, it could be more characteristic of the modalities than of detection.

SMELL

Susan Schiffman and Marc Pasternak (1979, p. 73) studied discrimination of food odors in the elderly and suggest that "the ability of subjects to judge qualitative odor differences between food flavors may decrease with age." Interestingly, elderly subjects were the best at discriminating fruits from the other stimuli presented; they also preferred fruits to the rest of the stimuli. The researchers felt the inability to discriminate might be due to primary sensory loss. The decrease noted with age could be due to other factors such as disease, sex differences, and smoking (Engen, 1977).

However, regressed patients do respond to colognes, shaving lotions, and pleasant odors. On a couple of occasions I handed an elderly woman a bottle of cologne, and she practically took a sponge bath with it. How many old men in institutions can enjoy the aroma of a pipe or a cigar? Or splash shaving lotion on themselves? Or how many old people can smell food cooking, in itself a pleasurable sensation?

To overcome the sterile atmosphere of in-

stitutions, one nursing home was built so that vents from the bakery led into the hallway to the dining room.

TOUCH

Touch as a therapeutic strategy is covered in Chapter 35, and so it will not be covered in detail here.

In an outstanding rehabilitation hospital in Lidingo, Sweden, the occupational therapist showed me a sandbox on legs that the carpenter had made so that wheelchairs could get close to it. The sand was warmed, and hidden in it were a variety of surprises (rocks, shells, marbles — objects with a variety of textures). The patients were encouraged to run the warm sand through their hands and fingers and the heat of the sand on sore stiff hands, the tactile sensations, and the surprise of the objects when found all combined to be a therapeutic effort.

The reader is referred to Kenshalo (1977) for a survey of research about aging and somesthesis. (Somesthesis, body sensibility, includes those sensations which arise from normal and intensive stimulation of the skin.)

PAIN AS A DANGER SIGNAL

> ADAPTATION
> *Pain sits within me.*
> *Unmoveable.*
> *I now move around it.*
>
> Irene Mortenson Burnside

Pain as a danger signal is an important facet of any discussion of the senses. The aged often accept much unnecessary pain because they think it is concomitant with growing old. According to Savitz (1968), aged persons will deny that pain exists in order to avoid examination. I recall a friend's mother who refused to have a physical examination; when she finally did consent, she was discovered to have an inoperable cancer. Old people in pain often cannot endure the long waits in clinics and physicians' offices when they go to be examined. They have to go to the

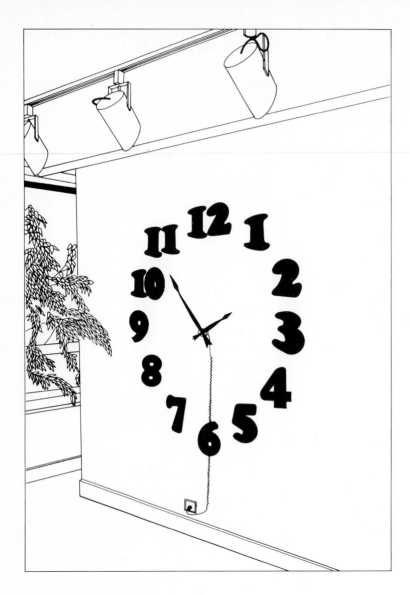

FIGURE 33-9 The importance of clocks and calendars is often ignored in planning residences for the aged. In an article I explained the importance of clocks and calendars for the orientation of the older person (Burnside, 1970). This drawing indicates that an entire wall could accommodate a clock with lighting from above so that it is easily seen.

bathroom; they get weary sitting on uncomfortable chairs; they get annoyed with the chaos that may exist; and they resent being hurried and jostled about. No wonder they talk about "the good old days when the doctor made home visits."

Pain, as it relates to specific disease entities and nursing care problems of the aged, is discussed in other chapters of this book. Lipowski (1970) has written a most interesting article on this subject, and the reader is also referred to Mitchell (1973) and the article "Pain and Suffering" in the *American Journal of Nursing* (March 1974). Szafran and Birren (1970) state that the available data do not permit a general statement about changes in pain sensitivity with age.

Pain and the associated behaviors may be reinforced in the client's environment and have been of such long-standing duration that these behaviors have become a way of life for the client. Also if the pain problem is difficult to diagnose, that is, if it is strangely distributed or has a peculiar onset or time pattern, the examiner must consider that the real problem is depression. It is most difficult to differentiate between pain and depression in the elderly person (Fordyce, 1978).

Another problem with pain among elderly clients is that they may prefer to rationalize functional impairments as pain. The client may actually have short-term memory loss or problems in sensory perception (cataracts, hearing loss, etc.). The client claims pain and/or associated functional impairment, and then can rationalize for not doing previous social activities or tasks. If one went ahead and did the activities or the tasks as usual, one would risk revealing the loss or the disability and its severity. This phenomenon has been observed enough that it should always be considered when there is a puzzling pain problem in the elderly client (Fordyce, 1978).

SUMMARY

There has been heavy emphasis in this chapter on the senses of vision and hearing, interventions by nurses, and prevention of sensory deprivation. Assessment of vision and hearing is an important part of any physical examination and should be done carefully. Nurses have the responsibility to assess an aged person's environment to increase the person's function and potential. Clocks and calendars will improve orientation (see Figure 33-9). As nurses increase their knowledge and research about normal aging and the senses, and study, assess, and manipulate environments, they will more effectively assist older people who are coping poorly in their surroundings. A code to indicate special problems in nursing home residents was designed by Miriam Breyer (see Figure 33-10).

Because elderly patients, unlike other age groups, often do not complain of pain in dis-

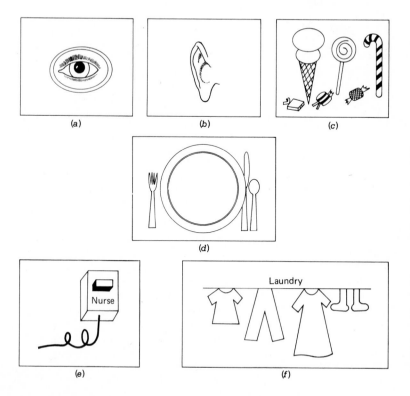

FIGURE 33-10 The drawings on this communications aid are intended to alert bedside staff members to various problems of residents. The drawings are done on a card which is then covered with clear contact paper. Drawings are placed at the foot of the bed. The problems or special needs indicated are (a) vision; (b) hearing; (c) no sweets—diabetic; (d) where food is to be placed on tray (for blind residents and those with hemianopsia); (e) inability to use call light; (f) who does the resident's laundry (the latter can be a real problem in some facilities). (*This communication aid was designed by Miriam Singer Breyer, Dr. Kelly Canelo, and Sylvia Muzzio, Mission Hills Convalescent Hospital, San Jose, Calif., in their work on "The Sensory Project."*)

eases, the nurse must really examine closely not only for pain but for conditions usually painful in other clients. The reader is referred to Chapter 27 for assessment of pain in the older client.

REFERENCES

Burnside, Irene Mortenson: Accoutrements of aging, in Lois B. Knowles (ed.), *Nursing Clinics of North America,* June 1972, pp. 291–301.

————: Clocks and calendars, *American Journal of Nursing,* **70**(1):117–119, January 1970.

————: The special senses and sensory deprivation, in Irene Mortenson Burnside (ed.), *Nursing and the Aged,* McGraw-Hill, New York, 1976.

————: A nurse's perspective: Blindness in long-term care facilities, *The New Outlook for the Blind,* **68**(4): 145–150, April 1974.

————: Psychosocial caring: Reality testing, relocation, and reminiscing, in Irene Mortenson Burnside, Priscilla Ebersole, and Helen Elena Monea (eds.), *Psychosocial Caring Throughout the Life Span,* McGraw-Hill, New York, 1979.

Castaneda, C.: *Journey to Ixtlan,* Simon & Schuster, New York, 1972.

Christman, E. H.: Cataract operation on the institutionalized elderly, *Eye, Ear, Nose and Throat Monthly,* **49**(8):31–35, August 1970.

Cooper, A. F., et al.: Hearing loss in paranoid and affective psychosis of the elderly, *Lancet,* **2**(7885): 851–854, 1974.

Corso, John F.: Auditory perception and communication, in James E. Birren and K. Warner Schaie (eds.), *The Handbook of the Psychology of Aging,* Van Nostrand Reinhold, New York, 1978.

Eisdorfer, Carl: Developmental level and sensory impairment in the aged, *Journal of Projective Techniques,* **24**(2):129–132, 1965.

Engen, Trygg: Taste and smell, in James E. Birren and K. Warner Schaie (eds.), *Handbook of the Psychology of Aging,* Van Nostrand Reinhold, New York, 1977, pp. 554–561.

Faye, Eleanor E.: Visual function in geriatric eye disease, *The New Outlook for the Blind,* **65**(7):204–208, September 1971.

FDA Drug Bulletin: New hearing and health care practices, **7**(2):8, May/July 1977.

Federal Regulations: Hearing aid devices: Professional and patient labeling and conditions for sale, **42**:9286–9296, Feb. 15, 1977.

Fernsebner, Wilhelmina: Early diagnosis of acute angle-closure glaucoma, *American Journal of Nursing,* **75**(7):1154–1158, July 1975.

Fordyce, Wilbert E.: Evaluating and managing chronic pain, *Geriatrics,* **33**(1):59–62, January 1978.

Fozard, James L., et al.: Visual perception and communication, in James E. Birren and K. Warner Schaie (eds.), *Handbook of the Psychology of Aging,* Van Nostrand Reinhold, New York, 1977.

Gibson, J. J.: *The Senses Considered as Perceptual Systems,* Houghton Mifflin, Boston, 1950, 1966.

Goodhill, Victor: Deafness, tinnitus and dizziness in the aged, in Isadore Rossman (ed.), *Clinical Geriatrics,* Lippincott, Philadelphia, 1979.

Hatton, Jean: Aging and the glare problem, *Journal of Gerontological Nursing,* **3**(5):38–44, September/October 1977.

Jaeger, Dorothea, and Leo W. Simmons: *The Aged Ill,* Appleton Century Crofts, New York, 1970.

Kasper, Robert L.: Eye problems of the aged, in William Reichel (ed.), *Clinical Aspects of Aging,* Williams & Wilkins, Baltimore, 1978, pp. 393–401.

Kenshalo, Dan R.: Age changes in touch, vibration, temperature, kinesthesis, and pain sensitivity, in James E. Birren and K. Warner Schaie (eds.), *Handbook of the Psychology of Aging,* Van Nostrand Reinhold, New York, 1977.

Kornzweig, Abraham L.: The eye in old age, in Isadore Rossman (ed.), *Clinical Geriatrics,* Lippincott, Philadelphia, 1971.

Linn, Louis: Psychiatric reactions complicating cataract surgery, *International Ophthalmology Clinics,* **5**(1):143–154, March 1965.

Lipowski, Z. J.: Physical illness: The individual and the coping process, *Psychiatry in Medicine,* **1**:91–103, April 1970.

Miller, Diane: Personal communication, 1978.

Mitchell, Pamela H.: *Concepts Basic to Nursing,* McGraw-Hill, New York, 1973.

Mobile Life-Line: Sentries of sound, **1**(9):May 1978.

National Association of Hearing and Speech Agencies: 919 18th Street, N.W., Washington, n.d.

National Society for the Prevention of Blindness, Inc., and Affiliates: *Cataract: What It Is and How It Is Treated,* New York, February 1975.

Newcomer, Robert: Personal communication, 1974.

Pain and suffering, *American Journal of Nursing,* **74**(3): 489–519, March 1974.

Ruben, Robert: Aging and hearing, in Isadore Rossman (ed.), *Clinical Geriatrics,* 2d ed., Lippincott, Philadelphia, 1979.

Sacramento Hearing Society, Inc.: 1717 Morse Avenue, Sacramento, CA 95825, n.d.

San Jose Mercury, January 14, 1979, p. 14a.

Savitz, Harry A.: Geriatric axioms, aphorisms, and proverbs, *Journal of the American Geriatrics Society,* **16**(4):758, April 1968.

Schiffman, Susan, and Marc Pasternak: Decreased

discrimination of food odors in the elderly, *Journal of Gerontology,* **34**(1):73–79, January 1979.

Segall, Marchall H.: *Influence of Culture on Visual Perception,* Bobbs-Merrill, Indianapolis, 1966.

Shanck, Ann: Communication disorders: A problem in rehabilitation of the aged, in Irene Mortenson Burnside (ed.), *Psychosocial Nursing Care of the Aged,* 2d ed., McGraw-Hill, New York, 1980.

Shields, Eldonna: Aging changes that affect the older person's ability to maintain neural control, *The Registered Nurse Consultant to the Immediate Care Facility,* American Nurses' Association, Kansas City, 1977, pp. 64–73.

Sicurella, Vincent J.: Color contrast as an aid for visually impaired persons, *Visual Impairment and Blindness,* **1**(6):252–257, June 1977.

Snyder, Loraine H., et al.: Vision and mental function of the elderly, *Gerontologist,* **16**(6):491–495, 1976.

Southern California Society for the Prevention of Blindness, Inc.: *Glaucoma . . . Sneak Thief of Sight,* Los Angeles, May 1970.

———: *Your Eyes . . . for a Lifetime of Sight,* Los Angeles, July 1972.

Stix, Harriet: Hearing dogs fill gap for deaf parents, *San Jose Mercury News,* San Jose, Calif., March 2, 1979, p. 3.

Szafran, J., and James E. Birren: Perception, in James E. Birren (ed.), *Contemporary Gerontology: Issues and Concepts,* Andrus Gerontology Center, University of Southern California, 1970.

Townsend, Peter: *The Last Refuge,* Routledge, London, 1962, p. 274.

Webster's New Collegiate Dictionary, Merriam, Springfield, Mass., 1973.

Wells, Charles E. C.: Helping stave off a dimming of the five senses, *Medical Opinion,* **51**(2):20–25, February 1976.

OTHER RESOURCES

FILMS

Age-related Sensory Losses—An Empathic Approach, 15 min/color, Institute of Gerontology, University of Michigan, Wayne State University, Detroit.

Cataracts, 13½ min/color, National Society for the Prevention of Blindness, Inc., Public Relations Dept., 79 Madison Avenue, New York, 10016.

See No Evil, Seth Pinsker, 16 mm/15 min/b&w, discussion guide available.

RECORDED SELECTIONS

"Choice Magazine Listening Service" offers subscribers who are visually impaired 8 hours of recorded selections each month. Articles, fiction, and poetry from publications such as *The New York Times, Esquire,* and *The Wall Street Journal* are included. Choice, 14 Maple St., Port Washington, NY 11050.

MISCELLANEOUS

Insulgage gauge, a visual aid for diabetics with low vision who self-inject insulin, Char-Mag Company of Glendale, Inc., Milwaukee, WI 53217.

Once Again—with Feeling, pamphlet designed by Miriam Singer Brewer about sensory losses and communication with nursing home residents for the aged resident, families, and nurse's aides. Miriam Singer Brewer, Gerontology Center, San Jose State University, San Jose, Calif.

"Touchables," a gadget that can be attached to a push-button type telephone and uses double-faced tape to enlarge the size of the buttons. Designed for persons who have poor vision. Buddy Company, 1350 S. Leavitt St., Chicago, IL 60608.

THIRTY-FOUR

SENSORY DEPRIVATION AND BLINDNESS

Irene Mortenson Burnside

And there she stood, as strange as something loaned,
slowly growing old and blind,
and was not prized. . . .
Rainer Maria Rilke

LEARNING OBJECTIVES

- Define sensory deprivation.
- Define perceptual deprivation.
- Define perceptual monotony.
- List six needs the older blind person may have.
- Describe 10 nursing interventions which were recommended by blind individuals.

This chapter is divided into two sections; the first is about sensory deprivation and the second is about blindness in elderly persons. Several nurses have described blind elderly persons who suffered from severe sensory deprivation (Abarca, 1980; Burnside, 1974; Mummah, 1975, 1976). Since the two conditions are closely related, it seemed natural to place them in the same chapter. The prevalence of blindness among the elderly is such a difficult problem that I felt it was important to include a special section with detailed suggestions for nursing interventions with blind elderly persons.

In the years since Hebbs (1937) studied perception in human beings by studying sensory deprivation, there has been increased interest in the area (Lilly, 1956; Solomon et al., 1965). Bower (1967) studied sensory stimulation in the treatment of senile dementia. Sensory deprivation has increasingly become a subject of scientific concern; the area is a fertile field for study by gerontological nurses.

Nurses have written about the importance of space and place for patients (Minckley, 1968). DeMeyer (1967) discussed the environment of the intensive care unit (ICU). More recently, the impact of the environment on the acutely ill patient in the ICU has been considered (Roberts, 1976, 1980). The reader is referred to Mitchell's excellent chapter, "Sensory Status," in *Concepts Basic to Nursing* (1973) and to the chapter on sensory deprivation by Roberts (1976).

As nurses better understand the specific aging process of the senses, the consequences of extreme isolation, and sensory deprivation for the aged, they are able to intervene more effectively. The sensory deprivation of institutionalized individuals is receiving much publicity because of nursing home scandals and exposure and also because residents in these homes often provide captive audiences for researchers. Public health nurses and visiting nurses are frequently in a position to study the sensory problems of community-based aged persons, since they often discover or are referred to such aged individuals.

Nurses should be able to lead sensory retraining groups with ease. The goal in such groups is to provide stimuli to improve recognition of the environment and adult-to-adult interaction, albeit with elementary techniques.

TERMS USED

SENSORY DEPRIVATION

Several terms may be used to describe the state of sensory impoverishment. *Sensory deprivation* is a common one; others are *perceptual deprivation, sensory restriction, confinement, touch-hunger,* and *stimulus-hunger.* The term *sensory restriction* may be used, and because of the actual loss incurred by some aged individuals, *sensory loss* may be used to indicate that lessened sensory input has its roots in impaired or decreased vision and/or hearing. These changes may be the result of normal aging changes or of pathological conditions.

PERCEPTUAL DEPRIVATION AND RESTRICTION

The terms *perceptual deprivation* and *perceptual restriction* signify an absence or lessening of meaningful patterning of sensory stimuli. Perceptual monotony indicates that the patterns of sensory stimuli are normal, but there is no variety. Social isolation may be one form of perceptual monotony which is due to a static environment and little social contact (Boore, 1977).

Sensory-perceptual restriction means that there is reduction of the normal amount and the pattern and variety of the sensory input. A *sensory-perceptual overload* means there is an increase in sensory stimulation which results in a loss of the normal ability to discriminate patterns.

Schultz (1965) made these predictions regarding sensory deprivation:

1. Conditions of diminished sensory input will result in measurable changes in activity level.
2. Restricted variation of sensory input will activate the sensoristatic drive state, which will become increasingly intense as a function of time and amount of deprivation.
3. When conditions of sensory restrictions disturb the sensoristatic balance, gross disturbances of functioning will occur in perception, cognition, and learning.
4. When stimulus variations are restricted, the organism will lower its sensory thresholds

and thus become increasingly sensitized to stimulation in an attempt to restore the balance.

5. Organisms will exhibit evidence of learning in situations where the only apparent reinforcement is a change in sensory variation.
6. There are individual differences in the need for sensory variation.
7. Reduction of the patterning or meaning of the stimulus input will result in greater behavioral effects than simple reduction of the level of stimulation.

SENSORY ACUITY AND PERCEPTION

If we refer to the ability to be aware of simple stimuli, such as light and dark, noise, touch, taste, odor, or vibrations, the terms *sensory acuity, sensation,* or *sensory processes* are used. If the stimuli are more complex, then the term used is *perception.* Perception signifies that there is a meaning or interpretation of the stimuli, rather than just the awareness of the sensation itself.

BOREDOM AND ENNUI

Although boredom is not peculiar to old age, it may become intolerable during the retirement years. The bored old people I have known were in three types of institutions: Veterans' Administration hospitals, state hospitals, and nursing homes. The antidote, of course, is to educate staff and patients to engage in more creative activities and to provide stimulus and opportunities for more purposeful living. That is much easier written than done.

In a classic old article, "The Pathology of Boredom," Woodburn Heron (1957) states that "monotony is an important and enduring human problem." The study was done to find out how humans would behave where nothing at all was happening.

As the subjects lay in isolation, cut off from stimulation, the content of their thought gradually changes. At first they tended to think about their studies, about the experi-

ment, about their personal problem. After awhile they began to reminisce about past incidents, their families, their friends, and so on. To pass the time, some tried to remember in detail a motion picture they had seen; others thought about travelling . . . some counted numbers into the thousands.

Irritability increased as time went on, and there were times when they were easily amused. At times they lost their sense of perspective, and after long isolation, some began to see "images."

The findings of Heron have application for long-term institutionalized individuals. Perhaps reminiscence is one way they handle their boredom. If this is true, then the need for reminiscing takes on even greater significance (see Chapter 8).

One poet has eloquently described boredom:

> INERTIA[1]
> *Nothing wild —*
> *and wooly fog*
> *enfolds this game, clogged*
> *with a lull and yawn*
> *and a lukewarm luck*
> *that warms no bones.*
>
> *The dirty*
> *dog-eared back*
> *of the day, like a card*
> *cast from the deck,*
> *lies on the lake,*
> *and its two-spot eyes*
> *stare at the sky*
> *but take in no trick.*
>
> *The doldrums*
> *have dealt this deuce*
> *of a dull day . . .*

Richman and Richman (1978) developed a technique known as *sensory training,* a structured program of both sensory and social stimulation for the mentally impaired, regressing aged

---

[1] A. M. McGaffin, in R. Humphries (ed.), *New Poems,* Ballantine Books, New York, p. 97. Reprinted with permission.

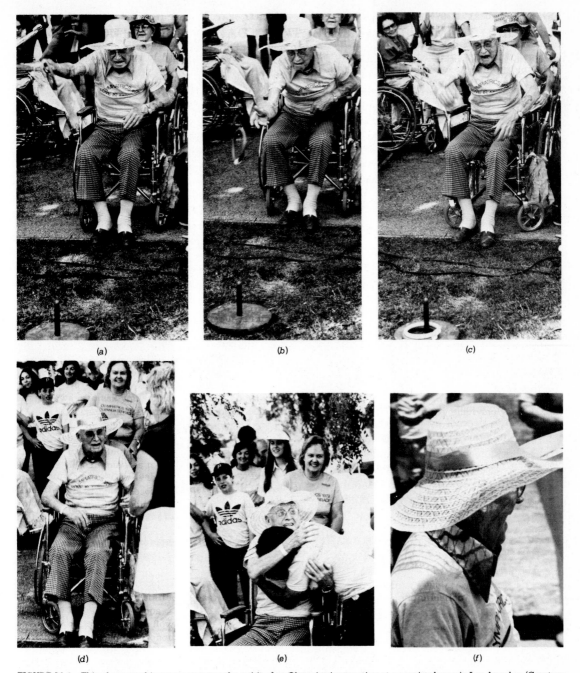

(a)   (b)   (c)

(d)   (e)   (f)

FIGURE 34-1   This photographic essay captures the spirit of an Olympiatrics meeting at a nursing home in Los Angeles. (*Courtesy of Anthony J. Skirlick, Jr.*)

person. The sensory training combines repetition, reinforcement, and immediate reward, and there are a series of graded exercises. "It is not a question of which is the best treatment for everybody, but what is the best treatment for which person at this particular time and in this particular physical and mental condition?" They point out that the technique is intended to be called sensory *training* and not sensory *stimulation,* because a population may need a reduction in sensory input or a more gradual increase of stimuli. The authors suggest that there are schizophrenic patients who strenuously resist and do not respond to sensory training because they need less stimulation, not an increase, at that time.

The application of sensory training to those with sensory handicaps, such as the blind, has also been recognized. These persons often feel quite isolated, and the sensory techniques do provide a socially supportive accepting milieu.

SENSORY-PERCEPTUAL OVERLOAD

The most common sensory-perceptual overload occurs in the aged person hospitalized in an acute facility, particularly an intensive care unit. While it is true that overstimulation and a bombardment of the senses could overload the aged person and also be a problem, it will not be covered more fully in this chapter because of lack of space.

ASSESSMENT

During the assessment, the aged person's behavior and mental state need to be evaluated, especially emotional state and cognitive functioning. The function of each sense organ is examined, and the use or nonuse of prostheses must be noted.

Limited mobility may be an important factor causing sensory-perceptual restriction, especially for persons confined to a wheelchair. Aged persons who have arthritis, cardiovascular or respiratory disease, Parkinson's disease, amputations of limbs—all who have decreased mo-

bility—are at high risk for sensory-perceptual restriction.

SENSITIVITY TO SENSORY STIMULATION

"The individual's sensitivity to such [sensory stimulation], his ability to integrate it and to attend selectively to it is a continuing dynamic process" (Birren, 1964, pp. 81, 83). The aging individual needs to develop effective perceptual habits for processing sensory information to be able to cope with the environment and make as few errors as possible. Some aged do this poorly, particularly those persons with organic brain syndrome. Aged people often respond slowly and, of course, make many mistakes. It is easy for caretakers to become impatient with them, because even the smallest environment changes can upset the aged person. One example of an error in response was observed in a group of chronic brain syndrome patients. An aged lady stirred her coffee with an orange crayon I had given her when I asked her to draw the proverbial October pumpkin. I had unwittingly given her two tasks simultaneously, which had complicated the matter for her. It is important not to overload such individuals with instructions and/or stimuli. Crowded information given to the aged person causes the first message to be erased (Birren, 1974). Nurses should be cautioned not to crowd information if they do not want to mask previously given information.

RECEPTION AND INTEGRATION OF INFORMATION

Birren (1964) states that a human's ability to do complex skills, and even that person's survival, depends upon the reception and the integration of information from such specialized nerve endings as those in the eye, ear, skin, and muscles. But there is not necessarily a direct relationship between the sensitivity of the sensory receptors and the individual's behavior. There can be some loss of acuity without noticeable behavior impairment, since usually there is a wide safety margin and people have more sensory output than is needed for detection and discrimination of signals. And it is possible for the individual to adapt to sensory loss by using the information which is available from other sense organs. It is important to note that Birren's findings suggest that nurses should try to further such adaptation by increasing the information available from other sense organs. If vision is poor, can "hearing the environment" be maximized? If blindness is a problem, can auditory stimuli and cues be increased? If there is a hearing loss, can visual aids in the environment be increased to help the individual process information more easily and readily? Signs, textures, posters, arrows, bright color-coding, written messages are but a few of the possibilities.

Because there may not be a direct relationship between the sensitivity of the sensory receptors and the adequacy of behavior (or its "appropriateness," as psychiatric jargon would have it), some of the sensory losses of the elderly may escape the eyes of caretakers. But when the behavior becomes inadequate, the oldster is in trouble whether in a facility or in the community. It would be utopian if we could prevent the occurrence of such behavior, but since there are behavioral problems, nurses have the responsibility to observe and discover what may be awry.

Group workers may uncover problems with the senses; these are important findings. A patient might not read anymore because glasses need correction. It is not uncommon for aged people to be wearing someone else's glasses. One ophthalmologist giving eye examinations in a long-term care facility was careful to make sure each person had on his or her own glasses before he began the eye examination. An old man I knew gave his best friend his hearing aid because it helped his friend more than it did him! One should always keep in mind that old people who seem to be dull and not very sharp may actually have hearing problems. Communication and socialization may decrease with increased hearing loss.

SOCIAL ISOLATION

Difficulty in communication can greatly increase social isolation, especially in those with cerebrovascular accidents and Parkinson's disease, and those who cannot manage the language.

The level of stimulation the person is used to will need to be ascertained—by asking the aged person, relatives, or friends. Energy levels can be particularly low for an aged person at certain times; for example, lack of sleep, overexertion, a long trip, or a recent hospitalization can deplete an aged person's energy reserve. These are a few reasons why stimulation level will need to be carefully monitored. Since some aged, especially the frail, cannot verbally express their needs (or admit to their low energy level, etc.), the caretaker will have to be astute about observing nonverbal cues which indicate weariness, exhaustion, lack of sleep.

It is not uncommon to find non-English-speaking elderly persons, and one needs to make a special effort to teach them. Often they are isolated and alone for long periods of time in institutions, except perhaps for mealtime interactions, medications, baths, etc. The blind elderly person who speaks little or no English can become very isolated.

Abarca (1980) observed the results of isolation and sensory deprivation in a one-to-one relationship with a 65-year-old. Blind persons in particular need sensory input; absence of stimulation can lead to hallucinations, and in some instances the severity of their hallucinations can be reason for a transfer to a mental institution or to a less desirable section of a nursing home.

PHYSICAL ISOLATION

Many elderly persons are isolated because of the barriers or fences which are placed around them. The sight of a person surrounded by rails on a bed, the arms of a wheelchair, or the frame of a walker should immediately alert the nurse to the fact that the person probably has less touching, less physical contact, simply because of these enclosures.

It is not uncommon, when one is in an area where there are elderly persons in wheelchairs, to see one of them reach out to touch another person, especially a child. Such a gesture often indicates that some individuals who must use wheelchairs, crutches, canes, and walkers have a great need for the comfort and stimulation of touch.

Caring for the brain-syndrome patient is difficult, but it becomes an even more complex problem when that patient is also blind. Constant testing of reality, through touching, is an all-important means of decreasing sensory deprivation (Burnside, 1973). Staff members sometimes have to realize that the prevention of regression is an important goal in the care of these persons. Mummah (1975, 1976) pioneered in group work with frail, blind Japanese residents.

BLINDNESS

In the United States it was not until the late 1960s that attention was paid to the aged who are functionally blind (Smith, 1971). In the past several years increased attention has been paid to the aging visually impaired population because of the changes which are occurring in our society. Of all blind persons, 50 percent are over age 65, and 60 percent are age 55 and over. If one uses the estimate that 50 percent of blind persons fall into the category of aging, there will be approximately 299,250 geriatric blind persons by the end of the century (Worden, 1976). The diseases which may cause blindness are discussed in the preceding chapter.

Depression is a common problem among the aged. Often they are depressed because of a loss, and it is not uncommon for elderly persons who are losing their vision to have spells of varying degrees of depression. In-service educators in programs for visually impaired and blind persons will need to take this into account and intervene appropriately. Loss of a driver's license due to vision deficits is a common cause of depression in both men and women.

NEEDS OF THE OLDER BLIND PERSON

Worden (1976) delineates the needs of the older blind person in the following categories:

1. Health care. Availability/accessibility of adequate health services must be considered.
2. Housing. A change in housing becomes a problem for many.
3. Income maintenance. The aging blind population often are at the low income level.
4. Employment opportunities are limited.
5. Socialization. This is the most serious gap in the services to older blind people.
6. Self-care and learning of self-care skills.
7. Supportive services.
8. Mobility. Improved by use of such human guide techniques as the long cane.

SUGGESTIONS BY BLIND PATIENTS FOR APPROPRIATE ASSISTANCE

Two hospitalized blind persons gave explicit instructions for nurses to make adaptation easier for them, as reported by Perks (1975) and Simmons (1975). The following implications for helpers were drawn from the two articles:

1. Approach slowly, introduce yourself, and do not startle the patient with sudden movements and/or noises.
2. Ask questions of the blind person, not the accompanying person.
3. Try to place the person as near to the bathroom as possible so a normal degree of independence can be maintained.[2]
4. Show the person the bed and allow him or her to feel around the edges.
5. Indicate where the locker or closet is and what shelves are inside, but try to permit the patient to sort out belongings. (So the patient will know later on where they are.)
6. Show the patient around the ward several times slowly to permit familiarity with the territory.
7. Instruct about radio, telephones, how to get talking books, etc.
8. Do not talk down to blind persons.
9. Introduce the patient to other patients on either side and give them an opportunity to shake hands. Have the patient take your arm as you move about.
10. Always pin the bell to the bed and indicate where it is, how it works.

---

[2] This is particularly true for the elderly who may have a high frequency of urination.

11. At mealtime, tell patient where the food is placed.
12. Instruct "feeders" to say when the next mouthful is coming and what it is.
13. Be meticulous about removal and cleaning of artificial eyes and dentures. Eye sockets can become very uncomfortable if artificial eyes are not cared for properly.
14. If a urine test is required, put an identifying mark on the container so that it can be found easily by the blind person.
15. Take the time to read their correspondence for them if they wish.
16. Be sure to speak to blind patients, since often no one speaks to them.
17. Always return pitchers of water and other objects to their rightful and expected place, so blind patients will not knock them over.
18. Keep flowers away from the edge of the table since they are easily knocked over, but place them close enough so the patient can enjoy the fragrant smell.
19. When sending to x-ray or other departments, indicate on chart that the person is blind.

WHAT TO DO WHEN YOU MEET A BLIND PERSON

All too often, people feel unnecessarily awkward when they meet a blind person. To help you and the blind person feel more at ease in various situations, consider the following pointers (*What to Do When You Meet a Blind Person*, 1977):

1. When you walk with blind people or guide them across streets, let them take your arm. Blind people who go about by themselves have usually come to know the width of certain streets. Unless there is an unusual obstacle, you need not say when the curb is approaching except when asked.
2. When giving directions to blind people, be absolutely sure to use the terms *right* and *left* accurately. They depend upon directions far more than sighted people.
3. If a blind person is using a guide dog, remember that the dog is working—do not distract it by petting, etc.
4. When you meet a blind person escorted by a guide, speak to the person directly, not through the guide. Do not shout; the person is blind, not deaf!
5. It is not necessary to avoid the subject of blindness. You may use the word *see* as much and as often as you would with a sighted person.
6. In making introductions to a blind person, you may help by saying, unobtrusively, "To your right is Mr. Jones, and next to him is Mr. Smith. . . ." This helps the blind person to associate the right voice with the right person. It also helps if the person introduced comes forward directly after you speak his or her name and says something to the blind person or shakes hands.
7. In shaking hands, a blind person will generally hold out his or her hand for you to shake. If not, do not insist on grabbing for it.
8. If you take a blind person to a party, tell him or her quietly where things are and make introductions normally. But do not force people on the blind person or try to introduce everyone at once.
9. When showing blind persons to a chair, merely put their hand on the arm or back of it. They will seat themselves.
10. When you enter a room where a blind person is, say something at once to make your presence known.
11. If you live or work with a blind person, keep doors either fully opened or closed. The arrangement should be understood. Any furniture moving should be discussed.
12. In a restaurant, read the menu to your blind friend. Explain how the food is arranged on the plate by the clock technique.
13. Always ask whether a blind person wants help. Many blind people can do things for themselves and resent indiscriminate help.
14. Think twice before giving to blind beggars.
15. Remember that the blind person has lost no individuality with the loss of sight.

IMPLICATIONS FOR INTERACTION WITH BLIND INDIVIDUALS

The following suggestions are taken from a previously published article (Burnside, 1974).

1. Directly face the person when speaking.
2. Touch the person; a handshake helps the person place where you are.
3. Pockets on clothing are a must.
4. A transistor radio is important for each blind person.
5. A rope or cord to the bathroom to guide them may be useful; be careful not to make it a hazard, however, or the blind person may trip over it.
6. Do not move things around, either personal belongings or furniture.
7. Remove the glass face of a clock so the person can tell time by touch.
8. Devise a calendar with raised letters.
9. Arrange for talking books, available free from the Library of Congress.
10. Speak clearly, slowly, and distinctly, while facing the blind people. If their attention span is short or if they are confused, it is helpful to touch them while you speak. For elderly patients who hallucinate, it is especially important to touch them while you are speaking to them.
11. Speak before you touch, however, or you may startle the person.
12. Check the person's hearing; if it is impaired, you may have to move in closer or talk directly into the ear.
13. Face them (do not talk from behind them) to improve hearing.
14. Give detailed instructions about all things you plan to do; there are no nonverbal or visual cues to assist them. In group meetings, especially, explain to the blind person what is occurring.
15. Do not leave aged blind people alone in their rooms for long periods of time; they may begin to hallucinate.
16. Do not change daily schedules—blind people often judge the time of day by the day's regular events. They do not have dawn and dusk for reminders.
17. Use as many external cues as possible, e.g., clocks that chime, noon whistle, intercom, radios.
18. Constantly use sensory stimulation through touch, sounds, and smell, since visual stimulation is absent. Increase such stimulation if there are signs of apathy or withdrawal, or a diagnosis of brain syndrome.
19. The newly blinded individual should be told about this disability in a straightforward manner in order to decrease its impact (Cull, 1973).

Freedman and Inkster (1977, p. 1) make the following recommendations: (1) a serious outreach effort must be made to bridge the gap between medical and blindness systems; (2) physical restoration services must be made available to the aging blind; (3) rehabilitation services should be made freely available to the elderly blind and their families, and should be tailored to their individual needs; (4) self-help and self-study for the elderly should be encouraged through programmed study, on cassettes, and step-by-step guides.

SUMMARY

This chapter stresses the need for nurses to be sensitive to sensory deprivation in aged individuals and to increase their facility in working with the blind. Kornzweig (1971, p. 209) suggests that efforts must always be directed toward prevention of blindness and that "in a certain sense, blindness is an indication of failure, and it would act as a spur to greater efforts toward prevention."

The poet Muriel Spark (1968) has beautifully described the void and sense of loss often associated with blindness:

> Capacity, I understand
> Is limited to fixed perfection,
> Being a measure of displacement;
> The void exists as the bulk defined it,
> The cat subsiding down a basement
> Leaves a catlessness about it.

REFERENCES

Abarca, Maria E.: One-to-one relationship therapy: A case study, in Irene M. Burnside (ed.), *Psychosocial Nursing Care of the Aged,* 2d ed., McGraw-Hill, New York, 1980.

Birren, James E.: Psychology of aging, paper presented at *Aging: Issues and Concepts* (workshop), Las Vegas, Nev., April 18, 1974.

_____: *The Psychology of Aging,* Prentice-Hall, Englewood Cliffs, N.J., 1964, pp. 81, 83.

Boore, Jennifer: Old people and sensory deprivation, *Nursing Times,* **73**(45):1754–1755, Nov. 10, 1977.

Bower, H. M.: Sensory stimulation and the treatment of senile dementia, *Medical Journal of Australia,* **1**:1113–1119, June 1967.

Burnside, Irene M.: A nurse's perspective: Blindness in long-term care facilities, *The New Outlook for the Blind,* **68**:145–150, April 1974.

_____: Touching is talking, *American Journal of Nursing,* **73**(12):2060–63, December 1973.

Cull, J. G.: Psychological adjustment to blindness, in A. Beatrix Cobb (ed.), *Medical and Psychological Aspects of Disability,* Charles C Thomas, Springfield, Ill., 1973.

DeMeyer, J.: The environment of the intensive care unit, *Nursing Forum,* **6**:262–272, Summer 1967.

Freedman, S. Saul, and Douglas E. Inkster: The impact of blindness in the aging process, *Mary E. Sweitzer Memorial Seminar Report,* Washington, 1977, chap. 1, p. 1.

Hebbs, D. O.: The innate organization of visual acuity: Perception of figures by rats reared in total darkness, *Journal of Genetic Psychology,* **51**:101, 1937.

Heron, Woodburn: The pathology of boredom, *Scientific American,* **196**(1):52–56, January 1957.

Kornzweig, Abraham L.: The eye in old age, in Isadore Rossman (ed.), *Clinical Geriatrics,* Lippincott, Philadelphia, 1971.

Lilly, John C.: Mental effects of reduction of ordinary levels of physical stimuli on intact healthy persons, *Psychological Research Reports,* **5**:1–9, 1956.

Minckley, Barbara: Space and place in patient care, *American Journal of Nursing,* **68**(3):511–516, March 1968.

Mitchell, Pamela H.: *Concepts Basic to Nursing,* McGraw-Hill, New York, 1973.

Mummah, Hazel: Fingers to see, *American Journal of Nursing,* **76**(10):1608–1610, October 1976.

_____: Group work with aged blind Japanese in the nursing home and in the community, *New Outlook for the Blind,* **69**(4):160–167, April 1975.

Perks, Jennifer: Nursing a blind patient, *Nursing Times,* **71**(44):1728–1729, October 30, 1975.

Richman, Leora, and Joseph Richman: Sensory training, ten years after, paper presented at *Eleventh Congress of Gerontology,* Tokyo, August 1978.

Rilke, R. M.: *Selected poems,* in C. F. McIntyre (trans.), University of California, Berkeley, Calif., 1971, p. 73.

Roberts, Sharon: *Behavioral Concepts and the Critically Ill Patient,* Prentice Hall, Englewood Cliffs, N.J., 1976.

_____: Territoriality: Space and the aged patient in intensive care units, in Irene M. Burnside (ed.), *Psychosocial Nursing Care of the Aged,* 2d ed., McGraw-Hill, 1980.

Schultz, Duane: *Sensory Restriction: Effects on Behavior,* Academic, New York, 1965, p. 32.

Simmons, Julie: The personal touch, *Nursing Times,* **71**(44):1729–1730, October 30, 1975.

Smith, Patricia Scherf: Aging and blindness: A public symposium, *The New Outlook for the Blind,* (9):201–219, September 1971.

Solomon, Phillip, et al.: *Sensory Deprivation,* Harvard, Cambridge, Mass., 1965.

Spark, Muriel: Selected lines from "Elementary," from *Collected Poems: I,* Knopf, New York, 1968.

What to Do When You Meet a Blind Person, Allied Health Education, Harrisburg, Pa., 1977.

Worden, Helen W.: Aging and blindness, *The New Outlook,* (12):433–437, December 1976.

OTHER RESOURCES

PUBLICATIONS AND PAMPHLETS

American Foundation for the Blind, Inc., 15 W. 16th St., New York, 10011
Blindness and Diabetes
Dog Guides for the Blind
Facts about Aging and Blindness
Facts about Blindness
How Does a Blind Person Get Around? (JoAnne Murphy, 1974)
I'm Blind Let Me Help You (Irving R. Dickman)
Recreation and Hobbies for the Blind, June 1977 (selected references compiled in the M. C. Migel Memorial Library)
Travel in Adverse Weather Conditions (Richard L. Welsh and William Wiener, 1976)
Travel Concessions for Blind Persons
Understanding Braille
What Do You Do When You See a Blind Person?

Dickman, Irving R.: *Living with Blindness,* Public Affairs Pamphlets (no. 473), 381 Park Avenue South, New York 10016, May 1977.

Division for the Blind and Physically Handicapped, Library of Congress, Washington
Braille alphabet and numerals
Free library service for the blind and physically handicapped
Request for free talking book library service, September 1968.
Commercial Sources for Spoken Word Cassettes
Reference Circular, May 1973, 15 pp.
Regional and subregional libraries for the blind and physically handicapped.

Compensating for Sensory Loss. Kathy Carrol (ed.), Human Development Series, Ebenezer Center for Aging and Human Development, Minneapolis, MN 55408.

Minneapolis Society for the Blind, Inc. *Caring for the Visually Impaired Older Person,* Minnesota Society for the Blind, Inc., 1936 Lyndale Ave. South, Minneapolis, MN 55403.

MULTISENSORY KITS

Bi-Folkal kits are multisensory kits that have been prepared for use in programming for older adults. Each kit includes slides, tapes, and articles to taste, smell, and feel and is centered on an event of time in the older person's life-span such as "Remembering Train Rides." Bi-Folkal Productions, Inc., 440 South Perkins Blvd., Burlington, WI 53105.

FILMS ABOUT BLINDNESS

American Foundation for the Blind, 15 West 16th St., New York, NY 10011: *Not without Sight,* 19½ min/16 mm/color. Rental, $25 per screening; purchase, $150. 1973.

Communicating with Deaf-Blind People, 18 min/16 mm/color. Rental, $8 per screening; purchase, $150. 1964.

Helen Keller in Her Story, 50 min/16 mm/b&w/two reels. Rental, $35 per screening. 1954.

Sykes, 13 min/16 mm/color. Sykes Williams, elderly blind musician. Filmakers Library, Inc., 290 West End Ave., New York, 10023.

ORGANIZATIONS

Division for the Blind and Physically Handicapped, Library of Congress, 1291 Taylor St., N.W., Washington, 20542.

Bureau of Education for the Handicapped, Office of Education, 7th and D Streets, S.W., Washington, 20202.

Office for the Blind and Visually Handicapped, Department of Health, Education, and Welfare, 330 C St., S.W., Washington, 20201.

American Foundation for the Blind, 15 West 16th St., New York, 10011.

National Society for the Prevention of Blindness, 79 Madison Avenue, New York, 10016.

The Seeing Eye, P. O. Box 375, Morristown, NJ 07960.

American Printing House for the Blind, 1838 Frankfort Ave., Louisville, KY 40206.

Recording for the Blind, Inc., 215 East 58th St., New York, 10022.

THIRTY-FIVE

THE THERAPEUTIC USE OF TOUCH

Irene Mortenson Burnside

The art of touch is an integral part of nursing intervention.
Kathyrn Barnett

LEARNING OBJECTIVES

- Compare and contrast task-oriented touch vs. affective touch.
- Discuss the effects of cultural patterns on using touch.
- Compare and contrast therapeutic vs. nontherapeutic touch used with the elderly.
- List several different types of therapeutic touch appropriate with elderly clients.
- Identify the barriers which interfere with touching aged persons.
- List 10 reasons for the use of touch with an elderly patient.

Some of the ideas in this chapter were originally presented as a speech to the Norwegian Nurses' Association, Kristiansand, Norway, May 11, 1978.

Touch can be a powerful therapeutic way of communicating with the aged client. Yet, it is not well covered in current nursing literature, and only recently have nurses begun to research the impact of touch on patients or clients. Touch is a powerful, inexpensive therapeutic nursing intervention, and it is interesting that the nursing profession has not studied or researched touch more, since touch is such an important component of all nursing. This chapter is divided into three sections. The first is an overview of the nursing literature. The second is an overview of articles written by members of other disciplines. The third explains implications for practice.

DEFINITIONS OF TERMS

The sense of touch may also be known by more technical terms such as the *tactile system* or the *haptic system*. The word *haptics* was coined by Geza Revesz (1950) when he pointed out in his study of blind persons that they must depend on their information about the world through touch. *Haptic* refers to the sensations which are received through the organs of touch, through tensions, and through movement of muscles, bones, and tendons (Roger et al., 1953).

Articles on touch can be found under all three of the above terms. Problems in vision and hearing still receive the most attention of all the sensory processes in publications like the *Journal of Gerontology*. Most of the articles indexed were on the subject of vision; a few were on the sense of balance or on hearing.

The terms used in this chapter will include *toucher,* the person initiating the touching, and *touchee,* the person receiving the touch. When I use the word *touch,* I will always mean physical contact. Physical touching may convey powerful psychological messages which are also necessary in effective caring of the elderly. Two other terms are *task-oriented touching* and *affective touching* (Burnside, 1977).[1] As nurses we must touch patients or clients in task-oriented ways, taking a blood pressure, giving a back rub, pro-

---

[1] The term *affective touch* was used by DeWever in her study (1977).

viding support during ambulation or transfer, etc. *Affective touch* is that form of touch which expresses caring, concern, affection, or control. It occurs when the helper wants to touch or feels moved to touch the aged person. If there is a purpose involved, it is not the performance of some physical nursing task. Rather it is a psychological purpose, as when a nurse quietly and calmly touches an apprehensive client to allay anxiety.

REVIEW OF THE NURSING LITERATURE

THERAPEUTIC EFFECTS OF TOUCH

Kathyrn Barnett (1972a, 1972b), a nurse researcher, wrote two excellent, helpful articles about the use of touch in nursing. Even though she did not focus on touch as used with the elderly person, her research includes important data on the older toucher and touchee. Barnett observed 516 instances of touch in a proprietary and nonproprietary hospital in Dallas, Texas. The occurrence of touch by age groups (as recorded for both the touchers and touchees) provides some data in relation to use of touch. The hand, forehead, and arm were the most frequently touched. No health team member touched a patient's finger, toes, ankle, or genitalia.

McCorkle (1974) studied the positive effects of a nurse's touch on seriously ill patients. In 1973, DeWever completed a dissertation on the relationship of baccalaureate nursing students' personalities and their perceived discomfort in touching patients.

Greenberg (1972) studied therapeutic effects of touch on a sample of 10 elderly psychotic state hospital patients. She concluded that touch did have a positive effect on her interactions with these individuals. All the patients were females 65 and older who exhibited overt psychotic symptoms. The study needs to be replicated, and it should include men in the sample, or a sample entirely of men should be studied to discover any possible sex-related differences in response to touch, an important consideration in touching. [Greenberg's study was done for her

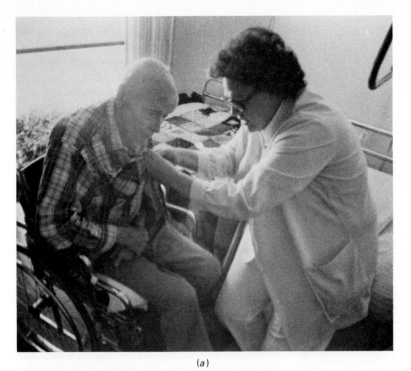

(a)

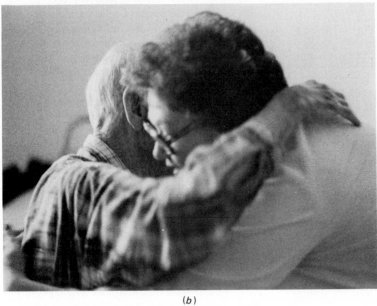

(b)

FIGURE 35-1 Task-oriented touching occurs frequently in the care of bed patients who are transferred daily from bed to wheelchair and back to bed. (*Courtesy of Anthony J. Skirlick, Jr.*)

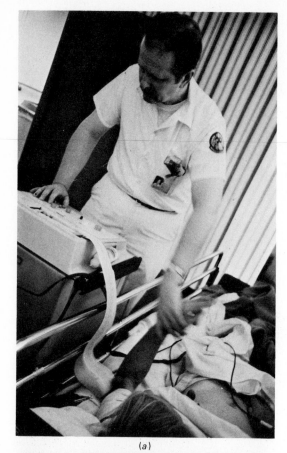

(a)

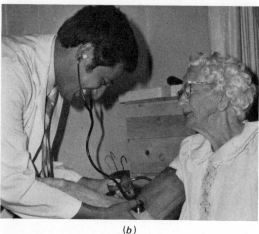

(b)

FIGURE 35-2 Task-oriented touching occurs in relation to many disciplines, as in administration of an electrocardiogram or in taking of a blood pressure reading by a pharmacist/researcher monitoring drugs in a nursing home. [(a) *Courtesy of Anthony J. Skirlick, Jr.;* (b) *courtesy of Will Patton.*]

master's thesis, and although there are undoubtedly many other master's theses on the subject, I have located only these: Trowbridge (1967), McCorkle (1972), Baldwin (1970).]

The reader is urged to study "The Language of Touch" by Sandra Weiss (1979).

CAUTION ADVISED

Several authors suggested that touch be used circumspectly (Barnett, 1972a; Boore, 1977), and of course psychiatrists also tend to be so inclined. Some geropsychiatrists, however, often stress the importance and need of touching the elderly client (Weinberg, 1969).

Mercer (1965) felt that touch could facilitate the healing process greatly or it could be detrimental, and that the results depended on the individual case. Margaret DeWever (1977) studied nursing home patients' perception of nurses' affective touching. The definition of affective touching was physical contact outside that needed for procedural duties. Results suggested that some subjects would experience discomfort if an older male nurse affectively touched the subject, if a male nurse touched or held the subject's hand, or if a nurse, male or female, placed his or her arm around the shoulders of the subject. This particular form of touch was perceived as uncomfortable by the greatest number of subjects (see Figure 35-4). However, DeWever found that most of her subjects were comfortable when nurses touched them in most circumstances, and so she concluded that touch should be used, but used judiciously.

According to Betty Sue Johnson (1965), there is great potential for hope when touch is introduced as part of the interaction regardless of how the nurse structures a verbal relationship. The nature of that change will depend partly on how each individual interprets the touch according to his or her background. The culture one grew up in and also one's present level of social maturity will be important. Johnson suggests that changes which occur will depend on the conscious effort of the nurse to use touch as part of a goal-directed plan and as a communication tool.

Jean Hardy (1975) feels that touch is central to nursing and is a primary way to establish empathy and to express care to the patient. Her

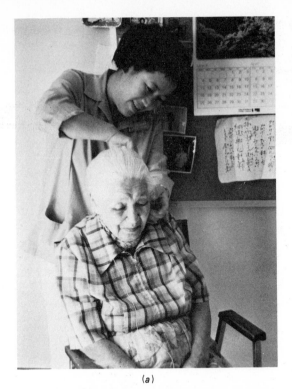

(a)

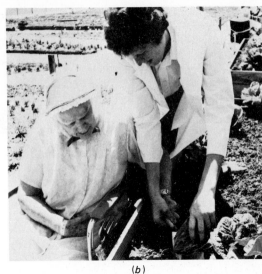

(b)

FIGURE 35-3 (a) The importance of touch during grooming can be noted; (b) A young hospital administrator assists a hemiplegic resident to harvest the plants grown in the elevated garden beds. [(a) and (b) *Courtesy of Anthony J. Skirlick, Jr.*]

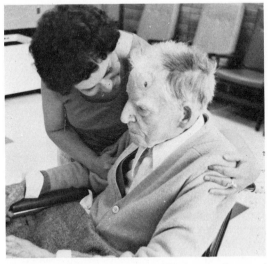

FIGURE 35-4 DeWever's study in 1977 of nursing home residents revealed that placing arms around the shoulders of a subject (whether toucher was a male or female) was perceived as uncomfortable by the greatest number of subjects. (*Courtesy of Anthony J. Skirlick, Jr.*)

article focuses on the back rub and describes how it should be given. It is an excellent article for instruction of home health aides and geriatric nurses' aides.

Leah Cashar and Barbara Dixson, nursing instructors, analyzed instances of personnel touching patients in a state psychiatric hospital setting. They concluded that there are three broad categories of touch: (1) reality orienting, (2) support, and (3) physical protection. They encourage more conscious consideration to be given the use of touch. These authors also remind us that nonverbal communication more accurately reflects emotions than the verbal, but that the nonverbal is very often less accurate because of its interpretations by others (Cashar and Dixson, 1967).

Shirley Farrah (1971) suggests that the use of touch is necessary in sensory loss and it will help the patient by providing much needed additional stimulation.

Jennifer Boore (1977) points out that the

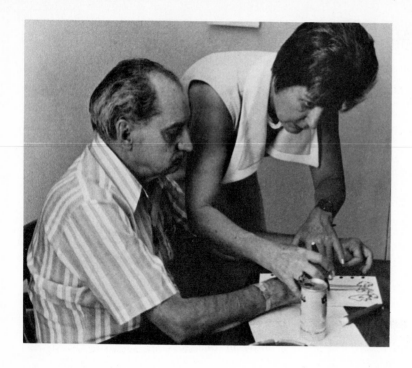

FIGURE 35-5 In Chapter 17 I described group work with the cognitively impaired elderly. Touching as you teach them is effective, as seen in this photograph which shows one individual of the group drawing (after his beer was finished). (*Courtesy of Will Patton.*)

sense of touch seems to be lost only as a result of a pathological condition, e.g., in diabetic neuropathy. She feels that the most common condition in which a person loses the sense of touch is the cerebrovascular accident. The paralysis of one side of the body is accompanied by the loss of the person's kinesthetic sense.

Irene Burnside (1973) wrote about the use of touch in group work with six elderly residents diagnosed as having chronic brain syndrome and observed that gradually members were comfortable touching not only the leader but the other group members as well. She used touch profusely and emphasized its use in the opening and closing of group meetings. Touch can also be a reward.

NONNURSING LITERATURE

GENERAL INVESTIGATIONS OF TOUCH

Lawrence Frank (1957) provided an extensive comprehensive review of literature on touch as a communication, but unfortunately that review is now over 20 years old and needs updating.

Esther Brown (1961) wrote that an important aspect of the healing process was to be able to communicate both verbally and nonverbally with the client and that to be able to use both of them communicating therapeutically was a skill of high order.

Masters and Johnson (1972) state that touch often carries its own message and that it can be asexual. It can represent a personal attitude or emotion. It can give comfort and reassurance. It also can be a sensual touch which has no further goal than the sheer enjoyment of tactile perception.

J. Dominian (1971) writes about the importance of touch in one's ability to communicate and also points out that it is an aspect of human behavior which various disciplines are interested in. Psychologists are concerned with the role of touch in development and maintenance of such characteristics as human perception, learning, memory, thinking, and intelligence. Dynamic psychologists are interested in the significance of touch in the personal and interpersonal life of the client. Psychiatrists, says Dominian, should share the interests of both groups and be concerned about clinical disturbances of touch—the pathology involved in self-mutilation, abnormal sensation, haptic, pain, etc. Writing from the viewpoint of a psychiatrist, Dominian suggests that all physicians and nurses learn to use their hands for touch in the way they would perform a delicate medical, surgical, or nursing procedure.

Neurologists J. Dyck, Paul Schultz, and Peter O'Brien (1972) were concerned with touch in regard to disturbances which arise in the ascending, descending, and central pathways, sensations of pain and temperature which may lead to neurological syndromes. At the Mayo Clinic in Rochester, Minn., they studied quantitation of touch-pressure sensations in persons age 6 to 83 and tested sensation in the index finger and great toe. They found that the threshold of touch-pressure was higher in the toe than in the finger of the old compared with the same measurements for the young, and for the subjects over the age of 40 years the threshold was higher in men than women. The goal of their study was to obtain normative values to use in comparison with patients who had disorders of primary sensory neurons. They also wanted to determine the differences in site, age, and sex.

Joy Huss, an occupational therapist, wrote a most sensitive article, which was the 1976 Eleanor Clark Slagle Lecture for the American Occupational Therapist Association (Huss, 1977). She describes her experiences in the use of touch over her 18 years as an occupational therapist. She advised her profession to begin to use touch in a caring manner and felt that in time it could make a difference in our culture. Her advice applies to the nursing of the elderly, as well.

Arthur Burton (1967) presented a psychiatrist's view that "touch is the fundament of being-in-the-world for it is the vehicle par excellence by which the person locates himself in space-time." He goes on to say,

If one enters a ward of regressed schizophrenic patients who have been hospitalized for long periods, the "noisy" silence of the ward is startling until one realizes the arms which flail out to touch are a substituted form of communication. They want again to make tactual contact to reassure themselves of their continuity and existence. The same is true of a geriatric ward.

The need to touch supersedes the need to verbalize, and offers reinforcement on a level more congruent with deficit status. The anticipation of decline and death in such patients forces them to cling tactually, not only to the world, but to the unconscious residual of the mother symbiosis. (p. 97)

The same author feels that the problem of touching is more a problem of the psychotherapist than the client. "It is because the psychotherapist does have a need to touch his patient that the taboo comes into play" (Burton, p. 1967, p. 98).

Burton and Heller (1964) in an earlier publication wondered whether medicine had dichotomized itself into those who touch the body and those who do not; nurses might ponder the same question. In their article they describe the origins of the taboo of touching the body and discuss the taboo in psychotherapy in relation to the schizophrenic patient.

Helen Colton, in the *Los Angeles Times,* described a study at Purdue University (Colton, 1977). Researchers had library clerks alternately touch and not touch the hands of students returning books. Almost uniformly, students who had been touched reported happier and most positive feelings about themselves, the library, and the clerks than those who were not touched. The touch lasted half a second, and many students did not even remember having been touched.

Ernst Beier (1974) has pointed out that nonverbal cues can be measured and are expressions of an individual's unconscious motivations. He suggests a cautionary note that "we often create our own problems by stimulating the world around us without knowing what we're doing. Our nonverbal behavior often serves ends that are obscure to nearly everyone, especially to ourselves" (p. 56).

Duncan Holbert, 62, a polio victim, had been in an iron lung for many years. He said, "Tactile contact is vitally important. People are so unconscious about touching. They touch something or someone every day, wherever they go. I finally realized why I had felt so lonely. It was because of my need to touch. I used to burst into tears [over this]. When someone touches me, it's like

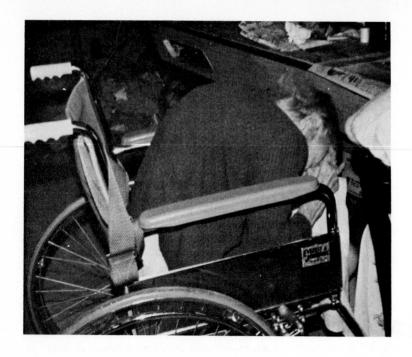

FIGURE 35-6 "The need to touch supersedes the need to verbalize, and offers reinforcement on a level more congruent with deficit status" (Burton, 1967, p. 97). (*Courtesy of Susan Bryant.*)

an electric shock that brings me out of that unusual lonely state" (Holbert, 1977).

CULTURAL ASPECTS OF TOUCHING

Researchers have discovered significant differences in the attitudes of different cultures toward touching. Nurses should keep these cultural attitudes in mind as they consider the therapeutic use of touch.

Edward Hall, an architect long interested in proxemics, carefully studied the cultural influence in use of space and touch in interactions (Hall, 1966). He examined the Japanese bow which forces physical distance and requires other persons to stand away. As a health precaution, Japanese do not use handshakes because of a fear of spreading germs.

Regarding Chinese culture, I was adamantly told by an elderly gentleman, "Touch belongs in the bedroom." Colton described a filming of Americans in China. When the film was shown to the Chinese authorities, they disapproved of a scene where an American woman was touching the feet of an elderly Chinese woman while she described how her feet had been bound as a child. The Chinese were offended. It is difficult, however, to say whether it was the touch itself or rather their wish not to record that particular treatment of Chinese women for others to see. She reminds us that churches also are encouraging touching, shaking hands, etc. And she ends with Bob Hope's flip and simultaneously wise statement, "If people aren't cuddled, they curdle" (Colton, 1977, p. 6).

As we approach a particular individual, it is wise to proceed slowly if we do not know his or her life-style, background, or cultural beliefs. At the same time we should avoid making hasty or simplistic judgments based only on a general knowledge of a person's culture.

At a professional meeting held in Japan, I met a Japanese psychiatrist who had studied in the United States. As I walked up to him, I thought I should bow, but instead I shook his hand to present myself. I was totally unprepared for what happened. I did not even have a chance to extend my hand because when he recognized me, he put his arms around me and hugged me. I had planned to approach him in his homeland with formality, but he greeted me as Americans might greet one another. And it shattered what I thought I had learned from Edward

Hall and my Japanese friends and clients! For another example see Figure 35-7b.

IMPLICATIONS FOR NURSING CARE

A sharp man in his eighties was in one of my groups. He was blind and confined to a wheelchair. Once he stated in the group meeting that the owner of the nursing home was in the building. I wondered how he knew since none of the rest of us did. When the owner passed the doorway, I checked with Mr. T. "How did you know?" He replied, "Easy. We never get hugged by the nurse's aides unless the owner is here. This morning I was hugged." Touching does not always relay messages of sincere caring! But this story does reveal that insincerity in gestures is quickly picked up by many aged persons.

Nurses should keep in mind, however, that nonaffectionate persons may be threatened by affectionate persons. This is especially evident in a health care environment. Sometimes elderly institutionalized clients are wary of overly affectionate staff members. They can be observed to move away or even to put up their hands or arms as if in self-defense. It is possible that such immediate nonverbal reactions to touching result from previous harsh treatment.

It is important for the toucher to consider the life-style and the background of the aged person. The frail centenarian who is almost blind and deaf and has no close relatives needs to be touched in a different manner than a 69-year-old dowager who is living in the community quite self-sufficiently with many friends, relatives, and community activities. Watch for and listen to cues given by the older person who is interacting with you because you will most surely be rejected in one way or another if you trespass beyond the line of private space or what is acceptable touching for that individual. Be careful about touching "loners." We learn what is acceptable and/or therapeutic by astute observation, sensitivity, and sometimes trial and error.

VIGNETTE 1

I was working with an internist in a nursing home one day. He approached a shabby, isolated old man in the corner of the day room. The internist quickly asked me for a quarter and then reached out and shook hands with the old man. He responded only slightly to the internist until he felt the coin in his hand, placed there when the internist shook his hand. He brightened up and said to the internist, "Thank you, old man." The internist explained to me later that the man had been a loner, a hobo who had been sleeping under one of the bridges. He had apparently been a panhandler prior to his admission to the nursing home. The internist used touch but also included something out of the man's life-style to begin a relationship with him.

TASK-ORIENTED VERSUS AFFECTIVE TOUCH

In a rather simplistic way I have divided touch into two categories, task-oriented and affective touching. However, there are times when both might occur during nursing interventions when, for example, a gerontological nurse practitioner checks the vital signs of a client who is apprehensive. The nurse might hold the aged person's arm or hand for awhile at the end of the interview and physical examination. In one article the nurse practitioner said she was greeted as often with a hug as she was with a handshake (Loeb and Robison, 1977). Her use of touch with the frail elderly is described in Chapter 30.

Handshakes are one safe and easy way to begin the use of touch with a new client. During an initial interview, much can be learned from a handshake, e.g., you can feel palsy, warmth, coldness, perspiration, arthritis, clamminess, and very thin hands. At times you can also feel whether the aged person is clinging to your hand or wants to let go quickly. This can give you some clues to the degree of dependency you will be encountering in the oldster (Weinberg, 1969).

Frequently one observes staff members patting the head of an elderly patient who is sitting down, especially if the older person is in a wheelchair. Such behavior should be vigorously discouraged; it is a gesture often used with small children and can be seen as patronizing.

However, wheelchair patients are often inaccessible to easy forms of touching. It is difficult to put an arm around the shoulder or waist of a person in a wheelchair. Wheelchairs are one of the "fences" we use. Others include geriatric chairs (commonly called "geri" chairs), and bed rails are the worst fences of all. How difficult it is to touch old people we have so carefully and sometimes carelessly fenced in. Getting them beyond the fences means also that touching is important in the daily transfer of individuals (see Figure 35-7a).

We do need to be cautious about how we use touch. Touching could knock the older person off balance—particularly a person who is using a cane, crutches, or walker. Walking down the hall with your arm around an aged person's waist, or arm in arm, is relatively easy. But nurses should always be aware of the problems that a gesture can cause to a frail or handicapped older person, since the fear of being thrown into disequilibrium can overcome the intended therapeutic effect of touching.

THERAPEUTIC TOUCH AND THE ELDERLY

Nurses have always been in close contact with patients and often touch them, sometimes in "untouchable places." Early in one's career one must develop an individual philosophy or attitude about the use of touch. Few nurses seem to study their own art of touching and how effective or ineffective they are. Yet many nurses have described to me the effects of their touching. They know its therapeutic power. They remark on how comfortable they are in using touch. Yet, when I press for their rationale, they say, "It was intuition," or "I just knew that I should." Nurses have learned to process behavioral cues rapidly—so rapidly in sorrow, or discomfort. They do not identify that step which is, "I did it because . . . ."

DIFFERENT APPROACHES

There are differences between the use of touch with the younger client and with the older. For one thing, you do not have to be so cautious and so overly professional about your use of touch

with the older person; perhaps touch has fewer sexual overtones for some elderly people. If it does have sexual overtones, it can still be therapeutic for the older person, for example, a buxom nurse's aide who fluffs pillows leaning over her patients might rekindle the excitement in life by giving them something in the daily routine to look forward to.

It seems to me that old people have lived in their bodies a long time; they seem to know the contours of their bodies, the dimensions and the boundaries. Some of the confused aged I have worked with seem to know their own bodies in a way that adolescents and/or young adults do not. I see this even in the very demented. Shall I call it "body ease?" I do not know another term to describe it. But one exception to this general truth about older people is the poststroke patient who very often gets very confused and does not know which leg is which, or says strange things about his or her limbs. Such behavior is the result of the stroke. We have constantly to remember the interplay between physical illness and mental illness. For instance, depression in an older poststroke patient is very common. A lowered self-esteem and change in body image are a result of a severe blow to the body, such as a stroke or the trauma of a colostomy or a mastectomy. These people often feel that they are "untouchable," and the warm touch of a caretaker may help restore their sense of self-esteem.

Touch is therapeutic for old people because of the loss of significant others. For example, I nearly always touch centenarians, because most of them have outlived everybody who has been significant in their lives. We also need to touch old people who seem to have given up and are apathetic and listless. Touching old people also helps compensate for sensory deficits—failing eyesight, blindness. One should be more cautious with the deaf and the hard-of-hearing, because research shows they tend to be more guarded and more suspicious than people who hear well.

You can interact better with confused old if you will hold their hand or touch their arm or shoulder during the time you are conversing with them. That has tremendous significance for working with the confused, disoriented elderly. Touch, powerful as it is with the demented

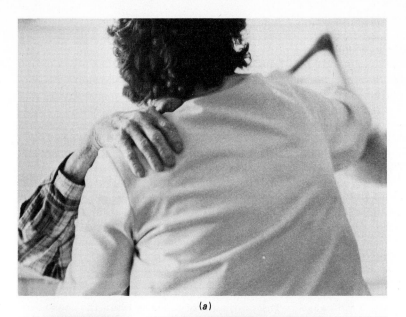

(a)

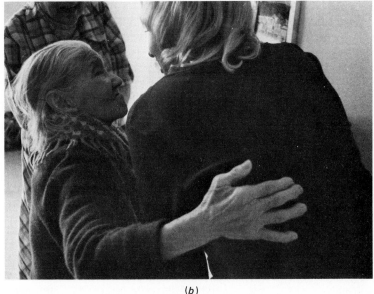

(b)

FIGURE 35-7 Health personnel must deal with their own feelings of being touched by the elderly. (a) For example, the dependency needs of the frail elderly may require touching that seems excessive to some personnel. I recall once being told by an uptight director of nurses when an elderly man in a wheelchair reached for my hand, "Don't let him touch you; he once had syphilis." (b) Contrary to customs I described elsewhere in this chapter, this tiny Japanese lady was delighted to see her former nurse and touched her profusely when she visited. (*Courtesy of Anthony J. Skirlick, Jr.*)

aged, was mentioned only about four times in 60 articles or chapters I reviewed on dementia.

Regarding the use of therapeutic touch, remember:

1. There are differences in approaches to the younger and the older person, e.g., a young schizophrenic and an 80-year-old burned-out schizophrenic.

2. Do not be overly professional and "uptight" about the use of touch.

3. Some old people are more comfortable with their bodies than teen-agers or middle-agers.

4. Use touch for sound reasons, e.g., loss of sig-

nificant others, to compensate for sensory deficits, or because confused clients are in touch longer when you touch them during interactions.

5. The helper must be aware of the elderly client touching the helper.

SPONTANEITY

The spontaneity of the touch may be one of the powerful factors in its use. Spontaneity exists, I suppose, for the very reason that the toucher does not stop to analyze what is happening and why and what will be done about it. It is safe to say that such nurses have had enough successes with spontaneous touching, that they are not afraid of any risks that might be lurking in wait. The seduction rate of nurses by elderly patients, I think, is probably quite low.

Perhaps we as instructors are overly cautious in our teaching about the use of touch with the older person—for whatever reason. We may even discourage newcomers to the field of gerontological nursing about using touch. However, it has been my experience that the touch of the elderly, especially the frail elderly, is of great therapeutic value in interactions.

NONTHERAPEUTIC TOUCH

What needs to be researched carefully is *nontherapeutic touching*. From such studies we could discover the observed cues that reveal when the aged person does not wish to be touched or the situations when the use of touch is not helpful. Only our elderly clients can tell us when our touch is nontherapeutic. Two common problems occur which I shall call *off-place* and *off-time.*

OFF-PLACE

Often the place of interaction indicates that one should proceed with caution. For example, if a female nurse is on the night shift and sits on a male patient's bed, that might set up an intimate scene which could cause unexpected or unhelpful results. The behavior elicited from the aged person may surprise the nurse, although when the scene is replayed and analyzed, the behavior usually is not so surprising.

VIGNETTE 2

A nurse working the afternoon to midnight shift went into the room of a very ill old man in his eighties. She gave him evening care which apparently seemed sensuous to the confused disoriented old man. He had admitted to the nurse on previous occasions when he was lucid that he had been a habitué of bordellos. As the nurse approached the door and snapped out the overhead lights, he cheerfully called out to her, "Good night and your money is there on the dresser, Myrtle."

OFF-TIME

The off-timing of touch is often the reason for the poor acceptance or outright rejection of the act of touch by the touchee. Yet, timing is such an individual matter for both toucher and touchee that it is most difficult to analyze. It should be acknowledged that there are days and times when the nurse is withdrawn and cannot comfortably be touched or feel comfortable touching a client. Discussing the discomforts of touch is one important aspect of beginning to understand why one does or does not touch certain individuals, or why a patient is not amenable to being touched.

PERSONAL AWARENESS

Nurses need to analyze the impact of touch on themselves. How one uses touch depends on one's family background, cultural patterns, comfort with touch, and professional admonitions. The available role models are also influential, especially for nurse's aides who learn often by mimicry. Experiential exercises in the classroom or with peers can facilitate personal awareness.

TOUCH AS PART OF A CARE PLAN

Touch with the elderly may be initiated as part of the nursing care plan in one or more of the following situations or states:

1. During loneliness expressed by an aged person.
2. During pain, expressed or observed.
3. During the dying state (whether the patient is aware of approaching death or not).
4. During the translocation shock.
5. During reality-testing.
6. During diminished states of awareness (e.g., following anesthesia sleep to wakefulness).
7. During sensory deprivation.
8. During interviews to reduce anxiety.
9. During confusional states.
10. To indicate caring quality of the helper.
11. To increase self-esteem.
12. To increase information and input for the blind.
13. To instruct in rehabilitation (e.g., in post-stroke persons).
14. To support aged grieving or sad relatives.

QUESTIONS

We need to answer, mainly through experience, many questions about the use of touch. The amount of pressure to use is critical—how much pressure? Why do we use firmer pressure at some times than others? When an elderly patient becomes very angry, it may help to hold him or her firmly to help him or her gain control. In contrast, a dying person may request the gentlest of touching for several reasons: pain, isolation, fear, need for tenderness, and reassurance. A dying person may need long periods of touching.

Whom do we touch and whom do we not touch? Why do we touch them at all? What form of touch do we use? It is a long way from a handshake to a hug, and there are many variations in between. Is the touch skin-to-skin, or is it through rubber gloves, or through clothing or bedclothes? How much of your skin or body actually does touch the body of the older person? What objects can we introduce to increase tactile experiences for our clients?

SUMMARY

The review of the literature offers encouragement in the use of touch, but several authors caution us not to be overzealous in its use. The current literature reveals one study regarding the use of touch with the elderly person (DeWever, 1977). There are no specific studies of articles which describe or analyze nontherapeutic touch. I think that the best resource still available to nursing is the research done by Barnett (1972a, 1972b). Her guidelines are excellent and timeless. They are included here as a summary for the reader, since they apply perfectly to the care of the aged (Barnett, 1972b).[2]

- The greater the patient's sense of isolation and sensory deprivation, the greater the need for relatedness to others through touch.
- The greater the patient's altered body image, the greater the need for acceptance through touch.
- The greater the patient's feeling of depersonalization, the greater the need for identity through touch.
- The greater the patient's regression, the greater the need for communication through touch.
- The greater the patient's anxiety, the greater the nurse's responsibility regarding the appropriateness of the use of touch.
- The greater the patient's dependency, the greater the nurse's responsibility regarding the appropriateness of the use of touch.
- The greater the patient's self-concealment, the greater the need for communication through touch.
- The greater the patient's need for privacy, the lesser the need for touch.
- The greater the patient's need for territorial imperative, the lesser the need for touch.
- The lesser the patient's self-esteem, the greater the need for confirmation through touch.
- The greater the patient's sense of rejection, the greater the need for acceptance through touch.
- The greater the patient's fear of death, the greater the need for relatedness to others through touch.

---

[2] Adapted from *Nursing Research,* vol. 21, no. 2, March/April 1972, with permission. Copyright American Journal of Nursing.

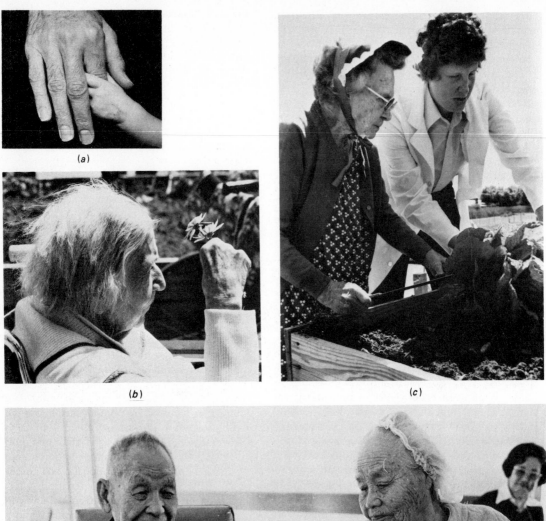

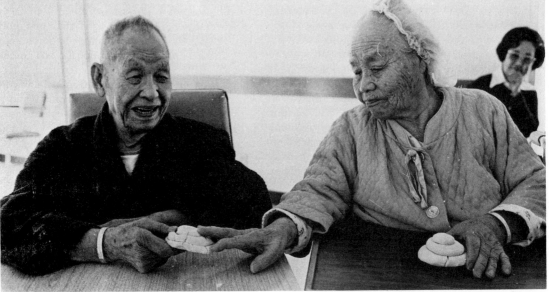

FIGURE 35-8 Touching involves more than physical contact with other adults. The aged should be able to touch pets, children, flowers and plants, and craft materials, as seen in these photographs. [(a) *Courtesy of Dorothy Larimer, Children's Hospital, Medical Center, Oakland, Calif.;* (b) *and* (c) *courtesy of Anthony J. Skirlick, Jr.;* (d) *courtesy of Chiari Endo.*]

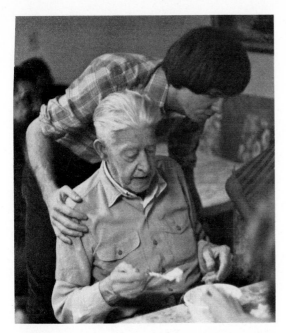

FIGURE 35-9 "The greater the patient's feeling of depersonalization, the greater his need for identity through touch" (Barnett). This tenet is especially applicable to those newly admitted residents who feel stripped and bereft and who experience translocation shock. (*Courtesy of Anthony J. Skirlick, Jr.*)

REFERENCES

Baldwin, Beverly: A study of the reaction of patients to the intrusive behavior of nurses, master's thesis, University of Iowa, 1970.

Barnett, Kathryn: A survey of the current utilization of touch by health team personnel with hospitalized patients, *International Journal of Nursing Studies,* **9:**(4):195–209, November 1972a.

———: A theoretical construct of the concepts of touch as they relate to nursing, *Nursing Research,* **21**(2):102–110, March/April 1972b.

Beier, Ernst G.: Nonverbal communications: How we sent emotional messages, *Psychology Today,* **7:**53–56, October 1974.

Boore, Jennifer: Old people and sensory deprivation, *Nursing Times,* **73:**1754–1755, Nov. 10, 1977.

Brown, Esther L.: *Newer Dimensions of Patient Care,* pt. I, Russell Sage Foundation, New York, 1961.

Burnside, Irene M.: The therapeutic use of touch with the elderly, in Herbert Shore and Marvin Ernst (eds.), *Sensory Processes and Aging,* Dallas Geriatric Research Institute, Dallas, 1977.

———: Touching is talking, *American Journal of Nursing,* **73**(12):2060–2063, December 1973.

Burton, Arthur: *Modern Humanistic Psychotherapy,* Jossey-Bass, San Francisco, 1967.

——— **and Louis Heller:** The touching of the body, *Psychoanalytic Review,* **51**(1):122–134, Spring 1964.

Cashar, L., and B. K. Dixson: The therapeutic use of touch, *Journal of Psychiatric Nursing,* **5**(5):424–451, May 1967.

Colton, Helen: The touchstone of togetherness, *Los Angeles Times,* pt. V, Nov. 27, 1977, p. 4.

DeWever, M.: An investigation of the relationship of baccalaureate nursing students' personality and their perceived discomfort in touching patients, doctoral dissertation, University of Houston, 1973.

———: Nursing home patients' perception of nurses' affective touching. *The Journal of Psychology,* **96:**163–171, July 1977.

Dominian, J.: The psychological significance of touch, *Nursing Times,* **67:**86–89, July 22, 1971.

Dyck, J., Paul W. Schultz, and Peter C. O'Brien: Quantitation of touch-pressure sensation, *Archives of Neurology,* **26**(5):461–471, May 1972.

Farrah, Shirley: The nurse/the patient—and touch, in Margery Duffey (ed.), *Current Concepts in Clinical Nursing,* vol. II, Mosby, St. Louis, 1971.

Frank, Lawrence K.: Tactile communication, *Genetic Psychology Monographs,* **56:**211–251, November 1957.

Greenberg, Barbara M.: Therapeutic effects of touch on alteration of psychotic behavior in institutionalized elderly patients, unpublished master's thesis, Duke University, Durham, N.C., 1972.

Hall, Edward T.: *The Hidden Dimension,* Doubleday, Garden City, N.Y., 1966.

Hardy, Jean: The importance of touch for patient and nurse, *Journal of Practical Nursing,* **25:**26–27, June 1975.

Holbert, Duncan: *Hospital Tribune,* Dec. 5, 1977, p. 17.

Huss, Joy: Touch with care or a caring touch, *American Journal of Occupational Therapy,* **31**(8):11–18, January 1977.

Johnson, Betty Sue: The meaning of touch in nursing, *Nursing Outlook,* **13**(2):59–60, February 1965.

Loeb, Philip M., and Billie Joy Robison: Experience in physician-nurse practitioner team in care of patients in skilled nursing facilities, *Journal of Family Practice,* **4**(4):727–730, 1977.

McCorkle, Ruth: Effects of touch on seriously ill patients, *Nursing Research,* **23**(2):125–132, March/April 1974.

————: The effect of touch on seriously ill patients, master's thesis, University of Iowa, 1972.

Masters, William H., and Virginia Johnson: Touching—and being touched, *Reader's Digest,* December 1972, pp. 66–69.

Mercer, Lianne S.: Touch: Comfort or threat? *Perspectives in Psychiatric Care,* **4**:20–25, May/June 1965.

Revesz, Geza: *Psychology and Art of the Blind,* translated by M. A. Wolf, Longmans, New York, 1950.

Roger, G. Barker, et al.: *Adjustment to Physical Handicap and Illness,* Bulletin 55, revised, *Social Science Research Council,* New York, 1953, p. 275.

Trowbridge, Judith: Nurse-patient interpretations of the nurse's touch, master's thesis, Loma Linda University, Loma Linda, Calif., 1967.

Weinberg, Jack: Lecture, summer institute, Andrus Gerontology Center, University of Southern California, Los Angeles, July 1969.

Weiss, Sandra: The language of touch, *Nursing Research,* **28**(2):76–79, March/April 1979.

OTHER RESOURCES

SLIDES/CASSETTE

The Meaning of Touch, a slide/cassette program designed to be used as a teaching-learning tool to sensitize students, professionals, and paraprofessionals to sensory needs of the aged. The package includes 80 colored slides, a list of the slides, a narrative script with theory on touch, and a bibliography. For further information write: Professor Bernita M. Steffl, College of Nursing, Arizona State University, Tempe, 85281.

FILMS

Cries and Whispers, commercial film, Ingmar Bergman.

Minnie Remembers, 5 min/16 mm/color. Mass Media Ministries, Inc., 2116 N. Charles St., Baltimore, Md 21218.

The Mortal Body, 12 min/16 mm/b&w. Filmakers Library, Inc., 290 West End Ave., NY 10023.

THIRTY-SIX

URINARY CONTINENCE: ASSESSMENT AND MANAGEMENT

Thelma J. Wells
Carol A. Brink

Hail fellow, well met,
All dirty and wet:
Find out if you can,
Who's master, who's man.
Jonathan Swift

LEARNING OBJECTIVES

- Recognize attitudes held by people in general and the health professions in particular.
- Describe the normal process.
- Describe age changes.
- Assess key physical, psychosocial, and environmental factors.
- Explain common interventions.
- Explain specific interventions.
- Describe management of urine control and soiling.

Urinary continence management is a complex skill which derives from physiological ability through a process of social learning. The interweaving of physical and psychosocial aspects of urinary continence management will be discussed throughout this chapter. To understand such interweaving, it is essential to recognize some of the social and professional attitudes about excretory functions. These attitudes may be a source of vague anxiety, a cause of interpersonal communication difficulties, and act as barriers to effective nursing practice.

LAY TERMINOLOGY

Common terminology for personal urinary continence management reveals an interesting lack of directness. An individual may feel uncomfortable talking about excretory needs or dysfunction; some individuals may find it almost impossible to discuss such problems because of a constraint against offensive words and/or an ignorance of health professional terminology. This may be especially true when an older individual is trying to communicate with a young care provider. Health care providers need to be sensitive to excretory needs, alert to possible communication barriers, and nonjudgmental of other's terminology. They must strive to be more comfortable in using common lay terms with their clients. If an elder has increasing difficulty with urine control, wet pants and garments are an inevitable outcome. Yet this symptom of difficulty, wetness, may be so embarrassing and so detrimental to self-esteem that the elderly person living in the community fails to seek help. Such a person may try a variety of actions with limited success; e.g., covering up the wetness with multiple padding and strong scent, restricting fluids to an inadequate level, or excessive toileting to the point of virtual self-imprisonment. But perhaps the oddest situation occurs when an elderly person with urine control difficulty does seek professional help and is told that "wetting is normal in aging; get used to it." Such a comment is demeaning and not true. In the institutionalized elderly it is not uncommon to hear a rather desperate denial in response to questions of urine control ability while observing (both visually and olfactorily) a confirmation of difficulty. The comment, "I don't know where that [urine on the bed, chair, or floor] came from" may indicate several things. It could be denial, reflect a significant recent memory loss, or attest to sensory failure. Or it could be a combination of all these and other factors. More creative, but equally desperate, patient responses to proximal wet environments include, "The roof leaks," "It rained in," or "Someone put it there." These responses may be greeted with hilarity by the staff and serve as an encouragement for the patient to perform the "comic" routine for others. A laughing response might be interpreted by some as acceptance and/or camaraderie, but is more likely to be seen as disparaging and callous. Certainly it does not seem to be a helpful exchange for the beginning of a trusting and confiding client-nurse communication process.

PROFESSIONAL TERMINOLOGY

Care providers are wont to use their own terminology with clients. Hence, they are apt to ask an older person, "Are you incontinent?" or refer to someone as such. [It might be well to note that the common lay meaning for this word has nothing to do with lack of urine control. *Webster's New Twentieth Century Dictionary* (1978) gives the first definitions for *incontinent* as "not restraining the passions or appetites, particularly the sexual appetite; indulging lust without restraint; unchaste; lewd."] Asking about or referring to someone in that context may be even more sensitive than asking about their personal urination ability. *It would seem wiser not to use the word* incontinent *with clients.*

How does one discuss this subject with older people? Care providers typically tend to avoid using explicit lay terms such as *pee* and resort to the professional euphemism for urine, *water*. Thus, one hears the older person asked, "Do you have trouble controlling your water?" or, in a more jovial manner, "Any trouble with the water works?" The rationale for these professional euphemisms is much weaker than that used for lay terms. Such usage may confuse some older people who might well wonder why the care provider is concerned about the plumbing in their homes. Or the client might wonder about the subterfuge, since the substance in question is known by all to definitely not be water. It seems both sensible and logical to use the word *urine* with older clients. Health professionals do need to be alert, of course, to the possibility that the word may not be understood. In those cases, explore further to find and use the client's term.

Lay terminology for excretion is a critical and sensitive area, but so is the professional vocabulary. Medical-nursing dictionaries typically define incontinence as "the inability to control excretory functions" (Miller and Keane, 1978, p. 512). Such a broad definition merely denotes the general contextual domain. It is remarkable that such a nonspecific word is accepted with such credence. Care providers blithely write or check "incontinent" on client information forms and sincerely believe they are conveying valuable data. Knowing that someone is "incontinent" of urine is equivalent to knowing virtually nothing about them. The term does not, for instance, inform as to frequency of the urine difficulty: night, day, both? It does not indicate severity of the problem: occasionally, often, always? It does not denote the magnitude of the urine control loss, e.g., 5 or 500 mL? It does not convey the duration of the problem: for the last 2 years or since admission to a care facility? It does not relate whether the client is aware of this difficulty. And it does not report any of the significant circumstances impinging on urinary continence control, e.g., access to the toilet, adequate fluid intake, medications. *In short, the term incontinent is a nonspecific word which does not impart any relevant, descriptive information about a client's urine control problem.*

It would appear that the popularity of the term *incontinent* is related to its implications in nursing; that is, the word is not meant to convey client information but is a task message among nurses. Wells (1975, p. 1908) notes that "it usually means 'Bring more sheets and pads when you get to that one!'" If this is true, then the greater danger in the term's usage is not so much a lack of specificity as its connotation: unquestioning acceptance of loss of urine control with increased age combined with routinized, passive, soiling-focused nurse behaviors. The underlying professional issue is a philosophical "What is nursing?" concern. *Is nursing the elderly a process of pathetic endorsement of devastating loss or a dynamic force to maximize the older individual who is experiencing loss?* If gerontological nursing is the latter, then it should be action-directed, not passive-responding. The nurse caring for the elderly should be nonaccepting of the label *incontinent* for clients and bombard the users of such terminology with a host of vital questions. Helpful objective data would become the descriptive base, ensuring the greater likelihood of success in resolving urine control difficulties.

SOCIETAL REFLECTIONS

Problems with terminology, both lay and professional, stem from pervasive social attitudes about excretion. Perhaps the most annoying documentation of social aversion to accept excretory behavior is the dearth of public toilets and their placement in out-of-the-way corners. Whatever one's vocabulary awareness and abstract discrimination, great determination and excellent physiological ability are needed to successfully find a public toilet. Such facilities tend to be distant from main activity areas with poor directional routing, often through hazardous areas. Toilets in high-use businesses are not always available to the public. For example, grocery stores and laundromats frequently bar all but employees from toilet use, and often establishments with toilets for the public require a key-release procedure. This lack of accessible and suitable public toilets is a major restraint for many older peoples' socialization opportunities and even their acquisition of essential goods and services.

While "hide the toilet" appears to be a social game, "hide the knowledge" is its counterpart in the health profession. Basic textbooks seldom include more than a page for urinary continence discussion. Nursing textbooks characteristically focus that discussion on catheter management. Although clinical research into urine control difficulties can be traced to the ancient Egyptians (Glen, 1979), it is only within the last 30 or so years that the literature reflects significant progress in understanding the problem. Nurses, often the care givers to those suffering from lack of urine control, rarely have published more than general commentaries on this significant clinical problem. Clearly, good clinical nursing research studies are needed.

SIGNIFICANCE OF URINE CONTROL DIFFICULTY

Normal aging, per se, has not been found to be a deterrent to continence; physical and mental health seem to be the key factors (Isaacs and Walkey, 1964). However, the frequency of urinary incontinence does increase as age increases, particularly for those over 85, and is most often associated with immobility and intellectual failure (Coni et al., 1977).

Surveys in European hospitals of older people with urinary incontinence show prevalence figures ranging from 13 to 48 percent, with Willington (1975d) estimating that about 30 percent of unselected elderly admissions are incontinent. In the United States, the Department of Health, Education, and Welfare (1975) Long-Term Care Facility Improvement Study reported that 55 percent of patients in the skilled nursing homes surveyed had some problem with urine control and an additional 5 percent had a catheter or other collecting device. It is difficult to obtain information about urine control problems for elderly people living in the community. Two British surveys revealed incontinence incidence figures of 20 to 31 percent for noninstitutionalized older persons (Brocklehurst et al., 1968; Milne et al., 1972). Other European community studies report incidence ranges of 1.6 to 42 percent in samples of elderly populations (Milne, 1976).

The data clearly suggest that lack of urinary control is a significant problem, particularly in nursing the ill and frail old. Therefore, nurses must be knowledgeable about the principles of urine continence management, preventive measures aimed at continence control, and alternative therapeutic interventions for resolving or reducing difficulties with urine control.

DYNAMICS OF URINARY CONTINENCE

PHYSIOLOGICAL BASIS

The physiological basis of urinary continence, maintenance of urine-holding and expulsion processes, is complex and not well understood. Organ-oriented specialists, i.e., urologists, neurologists, and gynecologists, tend to view the functional process of urinary control from the confines of system-specific territory. The literature thus reflects variation in terminology for similar concepts, dependent on the author's primary affiliation. Further, there are divergent views and varying levels of consensus for each field's findings and theoretical stance in the urine control process. In 1971, the International Continence Society (ICS) was founded to act as a forum for multidisciplinary clinicians and scientists working in the continence maintenance domain (Glen, 1979). Recognizing the significance of communication barriers, the ICS has a standardizing committee to define terminology and investigative techniques. The future holds a promise of both increased knowledge and greater communication clarity. At present, most useful for this chapter's purposes is a broad overview of normal urinary continence ability. Specific physiological debate within this overview is best found in the current literature or the texts cited.

It is helpful to consider the development of urinary continence during childhood. Willington (1975c) notes three stages: automatic bladder action, conditioned reflex training, and conscious inhibition. In the first, the infant's bladder fills and empties as a simple spinal reflex. Mothers may become conditioned to associate infant intake and output with diaper changing times, but the infant lacks central nervous system development for such awareness. The second stage, conditioned reflex training, builds on normal neurological growth in the child. It requires the awareness of a sensory stimulus (full bladder) with motor response (voiding) in a suitable place (potty chair or toilet). The last stage, conscious inhibition, is the discriminating ability to delay and requires full cerebral cortical development, attained at about 2 years of age. A subtle and intricate process of sensory awareness, motor ability, appropriate environmental associations, and time-body regulation all must function together for voluntary control of urine excretion in a socially acceptable manner. This high-level ability is achieved for day hours by most normal 2- to 2½-year-olds and for nighttime as well for the majority of children by 5 years (Cook et al., 1978).

Figure 36-1 illustrates the physiological processes for urine storage and expulsion. The bladder has been aptly described as "a balloon with three holes, two for the ingress of urine and one for its egress" (Robertson, 1978, p. 20). This remarkable internal urine reservoir is essentially one muscle, the detrusor. It is smooth muscle which displays unique characteristics, most of which are still in a stage of exploration. Among its attributes is tone, the bladder's resistance to stretch (Miller and Keane, 1978); this is a "plasticity" property demonstrated in cystometrograms which display the relationship between bladder pressure and volume (Ganong, 1975). It might seem reasonable that as fluid volume increases in a container, pressure in the container

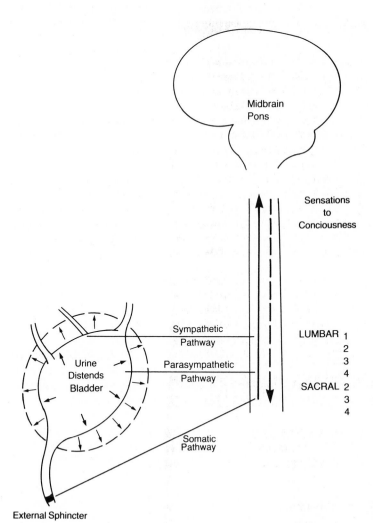

FIGURE 36-1 Storage and expulsion of urine.

would increase at a similar rate. But this is not true for the bladder. As urine enters via the ureters, there is an initial slight rise in pressure, but as filling continues, the pressure levels off; i.e., the bladder significantly increases its holding capacity while maintaining a low-pressure profile.

The opening of the bladder into the urethra is called the *bladder neck* or *outlet.* Considerable debate revolves around the nature of its continence control mechanisms. A striated muscle in the anterior urethral wall serves as the external urinary sphincter. To maintain continence, the pressure in the bladder must be lower than that in the urethra. This higher intraurethral pressure is achieved by bladder neck mechanisms, posterior urethra factors such as tonus, elasticity, and length, and the external sphincter under voluntary control (Bissada and Finkbeiner, 1978).

Neurological aspects of urine continence are involved and sometimes obscure. As smooth muscle, the bladder is innervated by both parasympathetic and sympathetic fibers. However, the role of the latter is not well understood, and only the parasympathetic pelvic nerves seem to be essential. Somatic innervation evolves from the striated muscles of the pelvic floor and external urinary sphincter via the pudendal nerve. Basically, bladder activity is a spinal reflex which ensures urine storage and expulsion even if cerebral connections are not intact, as in infants owing to developmental level and in any individual with spinal cord trauma above the reflex center. However, as solely a spinal reflex, bladder function is not only involuntary but also less effective. Cerebral involvement is essential for urination control, normal bladder storage efficiency, and a coordinated voiding sequence. Thus, spinal cord pathways must be intact and a number of supraspinal centers functioning for proper urine continence. No one brain center has been identified as primary; rather, various central nervous system regions appear to function either for inhibition or facilitation in urine continence management (Bissada and Finkbeiner, 1978).

The general process of urine storage and expulsion can be understood as follows. Sensory receptors in the bladder wall are activated as the bladder distends, sending impulses along parasympathetic pathways to the spinal cord re-flex center at the level of sacral nerves 2 to 4. Bladder status input travels up the spinal cord to a variety of areas in the brain. The individual's first desire to pass urine occurs when the bladder holds approximately 150 mL (Ganong, 1975). If the individual thinks that it is an inappropriate or inconvenient time to void, inhibitory impulses arise from several cerebral sites and travel back to the bladder to prevent the voiding sequence. The bladder can continue to fill, doubling its volume, without the individual experiencing discomfort because of its smooth muscle plasticity. It is not until about 400 mL of urine is in the bladder that the individual experiences "a marked sense of fullness" (Ganong, 1975). Neurologically, increasing numbers of bladder volume receptors have been stimulated by wall distention and are bombarding the sacral cord center where impulses are increasingly sent off to the brain. Through experience, the individual knows that soon it will be necessary to seek an appropriate place to void. As the bladder continues to fill toward its maximum capacity, an average 500 mL in the adult, the pressure in the bladder significantly rises, approaching urethral pressure. The individual experiences noticeable discomfort and may display such signs as increased perspiration and various motor activities, e.g., leg crossing and hand wringing. It becomes a matter of time before voluntary inhibition is overridden by changes in the bladder-urethra pressure gradient. The individual learns to avoid this discomfort, stress, and possible embarrassment by heeding bladder-fullness sensations.

A series of facilitating mechanical and neurological events assist the individual who desires to void and has found the appropriate place. Males typically stand to urinate, a posture which utilizes gravitational effects while allowing a comfortable and free-flowing position for the longer male urethra. Females usually sit to void, facilitated by an upright trunk which can bend forward to increase abdominal pressure, thus aiding bladder emptying. Toilet seats are specially contoured primarily for comfort, but the uniqueness of the seat also serves as a positive stimulus to voiding. Once in position, the individual voluntarily initiates the voiding sequence. The muscles of the perineum relax, the bladder contracts, the diaphragm is lowered, and there is some contraction of the abdominal muscles. Contraction of the bladder increases the pressure within it, bladder outlet resistance is decreased, and urine flows into the urethra and out past the relaxed external sphincter. Cerebral centers continue to facilitate bladder emptying by keeping the bladder contracted until empty when the muscles relax and the external sphincter contracts.

AGE CHANGES AFFECTING MANAGEMENT

Three separate but interrelated aspects of aging impinge on or are specific to urinary continence in the elderly. These are (1) age decrement in functional abilities associated with continence, (2) age changes within the bladder and continence mechanisms, and (3) consequences of chronic illness, the frequency of which increases with age. However, loss of urine control is not a normal outcome of aging. Older people can experience many age changes which might but do not affect their ability to control urine. Many older people have significant functional loss and chronic illness but maintain urine continence. Increased age is a risk factor in control of urination. The age aspects noted may work separately or in concert, requiring elderly individuals to spend considerable attention and energy to maintain continence. When combined with a wide variety of situational factors, age aspects may result in a temporary loss of urine control. And sometimes the effects of increased age yield a permanent failure in continence ability.

FUNCTIONS ASSOCIATED WITH CONTINENCE

Weg (1975) states that while physiological function declines with time, the changes are gradual and remaining capacity is more than enough for independent living. Nonetheless these changes may require alteration and adaptation which affect urine continence management. Since urine is produced in the kidney, age decrement in that organ is critical. Most significant to urine control is the fact that the kidney's ability to concentrate urine declines with age (McLachlan, 1978). The normal cycle of more urine formation during day than night hours may reverse, resulting in a larger nocturnal urine production (Goldman, 1977). Goldman (1977) attributed the common finding of nocturia in old age to a basic disturbance in the diurnal rhythm of urine excretion. Brod (1971) proposed an additional night effect for individuals with cardiac failure which would also add to increased urine production. Such a person's kidneys may receive an increased blood flow when the individual is quiet and recumbent as at night and bodily requirements for cardiac output are less. Further, functional decrements in aging may affect the individual's continence plan through increasing the time needed to find and get to the toilet, requiring modification of urination behaviors.

The Bladder and Continence Mechanisms It is probably most accurate to state that little is known about bladder function in normal elderly people. However, a study by Brocklehurst and Dillane (1966) provides interesting data. Utilizing cystometrograms, they studied 40 continent women over age 65, of whom 16 had diagnosed neurological disorders. Selected bladder function findings can be summarized as follows:

1. Forty-three percent had a capacity of 250 mL or less.
2. About 50 percent had incomplete bladder emptying with residual urine quantities of 50 mL or more.
3. Bladder contractions during filling suggested some loss of cerebral inhibition.
4. Late onset of desire to void was found with the majority requesting desire to void only at full bladder capacity.

The authors note that such bladders could be called *neurogenic;* that is, the cause for the dysfunction is most likely to be found at the cerebral rather than bladder level. Concluding that only 6 of the 40 cystometrograms could be considered normal, they remark, "Thus, abnormal cystometrograms would appear to be the rule in old age" (Brocklehurst and Dillane, 1966, p. 301).

The female urethra may be described as hormone-dependent and is affected in menopause by a loss of vascularity and a flattening of its walls (Robertson, 1978). Brocklehurst and Brocklehurst (1978) report an unpublished study by Dymock who examined 100 female geriatric patients and found that 69 had marked to minimal protrusion of the urethral mucosa (urethrocele). It was not determined whether the urethrocele was a result of urethral prolapse or edema, but it was significantly correlated with inflammation and incontinence. The literature does not reflect significant male urethra changes with aging. However, a gland which surrounds the urethra at the base of the penis, the prostate, enlarges as the male grows older (benign prostatic hypertrophy) and can act to cause bladder outflow obstruction, presenting as urine retention and/or dribbling (Jaffe, 1978).

In females, pelvic floor musculature may alter during aging. Significant causes are gravitational effects over time, postmenopausal tissue atrophy, and a multiparous obstetrical history (Zacharin, 1979). The result may be vaginal wall relaxation which allows the bladder or rectum to bulge into the vagina (cystocele and rectocele, respectively), or the uterus may lose some or all of its suspensory position and fall into the vagina (prolapse), creating pressure changes within the bladder by organ displacement and/or outlet incompetence (Glowacki, 1978). Atrophic (senile) vaginitis, the consequence of hormone depletion postmenses, may be found in elderly women and is characterized by a fragile, dry vagina with superficial erosions and a thin, whitish discharge which may be blood-tinged (Bates, 1979). Probably because of common embryologic origins, this condition is associated with atrophic urethritis and urine control difficulties (Robertson, 1978).

Chronic Illness The prevalence of chronic disorders is generally higher in older people (Harris, 1978). Three such conditions have been found to be commonly associated with bladder dysfunction: cerebrovascular accidents, parkinsonism, and diabetes mellitus (Tarabuley, 1974). Brocklehurst (1951) stated that in addition to cerebrovascular accidents, increasing mental confusion and confinement to bed were the most important precipitating factors in loss of urine control. Indeed, dementia (organic brain failure) is thought to cause disorganization of higher brain function to the extent that voluntary control of urine is permanently lost (Agate, 1970). The associated loss of intellectual ability to plan ahead for prophylactic bladder emptying also contributes to spontaneous voiding commonly observed in the dementia patient (Coni et al., 1977). Any condition which limits mobility and/or causes chronic pain would impinge on urine control, and arthritis is found to affect 38 percent of older people (Harris, 1978). Thus, many chronic illnesses, common and uncommon, affect continence management. Sometimes the relationship seems obvious, but in other instances it is not entirely understood. However, in all cases either an insult to the brain or spinal cord has occurred and/or body movement has been restricted.

NURSING ASSESSMENT

Noting that assessment is the first step in the nursing process, Marriner (1975) states that a nurse must gather data to help identify and define the client's problem before a logical plan of care can be developed. While this basic point may seem obvious, it is often not done for clients' urine control problems. A combination of social and professional attitudes about excretory behavior, discussed earlier, contributes to avoidance of urination behavior analysis. The care provider may not know how to assess urine control difficulty or what to do with the data collected. And, busy with the press of many demands, nurses may not feel they have time to accumulate the information needed, especially when communication with the patient may be hampered by deafness, dysphasia, or intellectual impairment.

Social and professional repugnance for excretory activity is silly, injurious, and obstructive. Nurses, as advocates of health, should lead the way toward more enlightened and frank discussion of basic human excretory behaviors. Since urine continence is complex, an assessment guide can be a useful tool. Such a guide has been developed to accompany this chapter and can be found in Table 36-1. However, the time issue should be addressed. Very simply, how do you want to spend your time: mopping up urine and changing wet beds or trying to prevent those situations from happening? If you prefer the latter, then you are an active, thinking nurse, and you *must* take the time to gather a data base from which to act. Consider the issue from a patient's view. As a patient, how would

TABLE 36-1

URINARY CONTINENCE MANAGEMENT: NURSING ASSESSMENT GUIDE

Date of review:
Name
Birthdate   Age
Sex: M   F
Marital status: S   M   WID   DIV

I. Current continence profile—patient interview (for all patients)
   A. Tell me about your typical pattern of passing urine.
      1. How many times would you say you usually pass urine from morning waking to bedtime?
         1 2 3 4 5 6 7 8 9 10   10 (describe):
      2. Do you have *regular* times when you pass urine during the day?
         No   Yes   (describe)
      3. What is the usual amount of urine you pass *each time* during the day?
         <half a cup   A cup   A pint   A quart
      4. Do you usually wake during the night to pass urine?
         No   Yes
         a. If yes, how many times would you say?
            1 2 3 4 5   5 (describe):
         b. If yes, do you usually wake at *regular* times to pass urine during the night?
            No   Yes   (describe)
         c. If yes, what is the usual amount of urine you pass *each time* during the night?
            <half a cup   A cup   A pint   A quart
      5. Have you noticed a change in your typical pattern of passing urine?
         No   Yes   (describe)
      6. Do you have any problem or concern about passing urine?
         No   Yes   (describe)
   B. I want to ask you some specific questions about passing urine.
      1. Once you are aware that your bladder is full, how long can you usually delay emptying your bladder?
         a. No ability to delay
         b. 1 to 5 minutes
         c. >5 minutes to 15 minutes
         d. >15 minutes to 30 minutes
         e. >30 minutes to 1 hour
         f. >1 hour (describe)
      2. Do you have any difficulty starting to urinate?
         a. Strain to start   No   Yes
         b. Slowness   No   Yes
         c. Burning   No   Yes
         d. Itching   No   Yes
         e. Pain   No   Yes
         f. Other (describe)
      3. Once you have started to pass urine, do you have any difficulty during urination?
         a. Starts and stops   No   Yes
         b. Strain to keep flow going No   Yes
         c. Burning throughout   No   Yes
         d. Other (describe)
      4. Do you feel that you completely empty your bladder?
         No   Yes
      5. If sexually active, do you notice any difficulty with urination after intercourse?
         Not active   No   Yes   (describe)
      6. Does urine ever come away from you when you don't want it to?
         a. During coughing/sneezing/laughing   No   Yes
         b. Changing position such as standing up   No   Yes

    c. Constantly leaking   No   Yes

    d. Other (describe)

    e. If yes, how much?

         A few drops   A tablespoon   Half a cup   >half a cup   (describe)

    f. If yes, how long has this been going on?

         (1) A week or less

         (2) >a week to a month

         (3) >a month to 6 months

         (4) >6 months to 1 year

         (5) >1 year (describe)

7. Have you had any urine problems in the past? (Probe: urinary tract infections).

     No   Yes   (describe)

    a. If yes, how was this treated?

    b. If yes, was the problem resolved?

         Yes   No   (comment):

8. How often do you usually have a bowel movement?

    a. >than once a day (describe)

    b. Once a day

    c. Every other day

    d. Other (describe)

9. Do you regularly take a laxative?

     No   Yes   (describe)

II. Continence problem analysis—care provider summation (for those with continence problems)

  A. Statement of the patient's urine continence problem

  B. Patient response to the problem (circle those that apply)

     Does not appear aware   Denying

     Indifferent   Feels hopeless

     Motivated to resolve   Other (describe)

     Embarrassed

  C. Functional ability (circle as apply, comment as appropriate)

1. Communication:	good	fair	poor
2. Mentally oriented:	always	usually	never
3. Mobility:	unlimited	limited	none
4. Self-drinking:	independent	needs some help	totally dependent
5. Self-toileting:	independent	needs some help	totally dependent

  D. Pertinent physical assessment, patient data

    1. Abdomen

      a. Any scars from prior surgery?

         No   Yes   (describe)

      b. Any sign of bladder distention?

         No   Yes   (describe)

    2. Genitalia (both sexes)

      a. Any sign of redness?

         No   Yes   (describe)

      b. Is there a rash?

         No   Yes   (describe)

      c. Are there any lesions or nodules?

         No   Yes   (describe)

      d. Is there a discharge?

         No   Yes   (describe)

3. Female
    a. Is the urethra bulging?
        No   Yes   (describe)
    b. Is anything protruding from the vagina?
        No   Yes   (describe)
        (1) If no, can you see a bulge(s) in the opening of the vagina?
           No   Yes
        (2) If there is/are a bulge(s) in the vaginal opening,
           (a) Is it from the upper part (anterior wall)?
           (b) Is it from the lower part (posterior wall)?
    c. Can you feel any object in the vagina?
        No   Yes   (describe)
    d. Can the patient feel your finger in the vagina?
        No   Yes
        (1) If yes, can she squeeze her vagina around it?
        (2) If yes, is this squeeze strong or weak? (circle which)
4. Male
    a. Is the penis circumcised?
        No   Yes
        (1) If no, is the foreskin freely movable?
           No   Yes
    b. Is the relaxed penis small and withdrawn into itself?
        No   Yes
    c. Is the scrotum enlarged?
        No   Yes   (describe)
    d. Is the scrotum tender?
        No   Yes   (describe)
5. Rectum
    a. Are there hemorrhoids?
        No   Yes   (describe)
    b. Is there a discharge?
        No   Yes   (describe)
    c. Do you feel stool in the rectum?
        No   Yes
        (1) If yes, is it soft or hard? (circle which)
6. Urine data
    a. What is the color?
    b. What is the odor?
    c. Is there anything abnormal from the urinalysis report?
    d. Is a clean-catch specimen indicated?
E. Fluid intake and urine output status
    1. Average 24-hour fluid intake per __ days:
    2. Average 24-hour urine output per __ days:
    3. Average frequency of wetting in 24 hours per __ days:
        0 1 2 3 4 5 6 7 8 9 10 11 12 13 14 15 or indicate
    4. Typical times of wetting in 24 hours per __ days:
        A.M. 12 1 2 3 4 5 6 7 8 9 10 11
        P.M. 12 1 2 3 4 5 6 7 8 9 10 11
F. Current relevant medical diagnoses (circle those that apply)
    1. Neurological: stroke   parkinsonism   dementia   other   (describe)
    2. Urological: UTI   prostatic enlargement   urethritis   other   (describe)
    3. Gynecological: Prolapse rectocele   cystocele   vaginitis   other   (describe)

    4. Musculoskeletal: arthritis   rheumatism   fracture   other   (describe)

    5. Other medical conditions: diabetes mellitus   heart failure   other   (describe)

G. Relevant medications taken regularly (circle those that apply)

    1. Drugs which alter the senses: hypnotic sedative   tranquilizer   analgesic narcotic

    2. Drugs which alter urination: diuretics   bladder relaxants   bladder stimulants

    3. Other (describe):

H. Significant past health

    1. Any abdominal or pelvic operations?

        No   Yes   (describe)

    2. Female

        a. Number of pregnancies:

        b. Number of deliveries:

        c. Menopause: No   Yes   If yes, age __

 I. Significant environmental factors

    1. Distance of toilet from patient: __ feet

        Comment:

    2. Are toilet/bathroom modifications needed?

        No   Yes   (describe)

    3. Are toilet alternatives needed?

        No   Yes   (describe)

    4. Is a signal/call device available?

        No   Yes   (describe)

    5. How do care providers assist the patient in continence management?

NOTE: UTI = urinary tract infection.

you want to spend your time: sitting pantless in a pool of urine, sitting pantless on a dry paper, smelling, itching, and being socially avoided? If you do not find these attributes of incontinence appealing, then you are an empathetic, sensitive nurse.

PHYSICAL ASSESSMENT

Skills pertinent to a thorough physical appraisal include inspection, palpation, percussion, and auscultation. The first two are certainly familiar to nursing since observation and touch have long been used as instruments of assessment. Percussion and auscultation may be less familiar and have been well described in other texts (Bates, 1979; Crane, 1975). Obviously a complete physical assessment is essential for adequate base-line data and full analysis of clinical problems. However, it seems most appropriate to focus this discussion on basic, preliminary observations which can and should be made by all nurses. Greater knowledge can be obtained in

assessment texts or the helpful programmed instruction series in the *American Journal of Nursing,* especially the sections on the female pelvis and the male genitalia (Cohen, 1978a, 1978b, 1979). Preliminary analysis of loss of urine control in an individual requires that the nurse examine the abdomen, external genitalia, rectum, and, in the female, the vagina. Items essential to the examination include (1) a good light source, (2) gloves and lubricant for the rectal and vaginal inspection, and (3) privacy. If an institutionalized patient shares a room, either the roommate can be asked to leave during the brief examination or the patient can be brought to an examining area. During internal examination, rectum or vagina, the patient should be as comfortable as possible. Stiff, fixed, or flaccid limbs may require careful positioning and pillow propping.

Abdomen Normally a bladder cannot be seen or felt unless it is distended and needs emptying. However, an overdistended bladder, one that retains urine to the point of overflow, may be revealed in examining the abdomen. The urine overflow presents as continual wetness or intermittent dribbling, caused by excessive bladder pressure which overcomes outflow resistance. When assessing the abdomen for signs of urine retention, one should first look at the contour. In a thin individual a distended bladder may appear as a slight suprapubic bulge which usually extends no more than 4 to 5 cm above the symphysis pubis. Such a bladder feels smooth and tense, but pliable. Note, though, that in an obese person's abdomen, the bladder would be neither visible nor palpable. In such individuals gentle palpation of the "bulge" or suprapubic area should produce tenderness if bladder distention is present and sensation is intact. Remember that in the diabetic patient with peripheral neuropathy bladder sensation may be absent and no discomfort elicited on palpation. Percussion of a urine-filled bladder produces a dull sound and helps identify its outline.

Urinary retention causing bladder distention is associated with many common treatable disorders in old people including fecal impaction. An assessment of the abdomen should include superficial and deep palpation generally as well as auscultation of bowel sounds. Increased bowel sounds may be heard with diarrhea or early intestinal obstruction, both conditions associated with fecal impaction (Bates, 1979).

External Genitalia Inspection of the elderly female should include the labia, urethral orifice, and vaginal opening; of the male, the foreskin, glans, urethral opening, and scrotum. Any unusual redness, swelling, lesions, nodules, or discharge should be noted and described. It is not uncommon to find chafing in skin folds from heat and moisture or a urine rash, both of which are susceptible to infection. Lesions or nodules need to be felt for tenderness, consistency, and mobility, i.e., soft or firm, freely movable or fixed, and thus reported. Such information is helpful in distinguishing between possible benign cysts and carcinoma.

In elderly males a retracted penis is not uncommon and becomes a problem primarily in situations where the use of a urinal in bed is required or an external urinary device for soiling management becomes necessary. Cystocele, rectocele, and uterine prolapse are not uncommon in elderly women and may be easily visualized (Bates, 1979). Urine leakage may be observed in such individuals by asking them to strain or bear down during inspection; positive findings should be noted. If any unusual discharge is present, a culture could be helpful.

Vagina Many elderly women are reluctant to have a pelvic examination even if it is offered. Anticipated discomfort and fear of abnormal findings as well as embarrassment or apathy may be factors involved in such a response. Cooperation in mentally disoriented patients may be impossible to achieve. Thus, the examination advocated in this preliminary assessment requires merely the introduction of one lubricated, gloved finger into the vagina. This simple inspection is highly informative, easily done, and well tolerated by older women. Any firm object palpated should be further evaluated. Such an object might be the cervix which is usually small in older women. However, a cervix might be missing in some older females who have had prior gynecological surgery. A pessary, inserted for uterine support, might be discovered, and, if so, its history and effect elucidated through patient interview, record review, and gynecological consultation.

An important neuromuscular evaluation, pelvic floor tone, can be made with the one-finger vaginal inspection. The examiner asks the patient whether she feels the finger within the vagina and asks her to squeeze it by tightening the muscles around it. Avoid having the patient hold her breath, squeeze her thighs, or simply bear down; such movements utilize muscles other than those being evaluated. Greenhill (1979, p. 198) notes, "A weak muscle offers little resistance to pressure; even if the patient succeeds in tightening the muscle, the contractions are weak and confined to a narrow area."

Rectum A rectal examination is done primarily to rule out a fecal impaction or chronic constipation. A gloved, lubricated finger is gently inserted into the rectum, stool is felt for and, if present, consistency noted. Any unusual mass should certainly be reported immediately.

INTERVENTIONS

Brocklehurst and Brocklehurst (1978) have presented a helpful distinction in which loss of urine control is considered to be transient or established, i.e., temporary or permanent. Elderly people will be most helped if the care provider considers it the former, exploring for cause and resolution, until proved otherwise, in which case major effort is made to deal satisfactorily with the loss of urine control. The Nursing Assessment Guide (Table 36-1) yields information that can be used to prevent, reduce, resolve, and manage loss of urine control. Discussion will proceed from general continence interventions directed toward common situations affecting the individual and the environment, to specific interventions which serve as explicit continence treatments, and finally to interventions aimed at more effective management of urine control loss and soiling.

GENERAL

Hydration Adequate fluid intake is probably the single most significant factor in urine continence management. There is consensus in the nursing literature that the elderly person with urine control problems needs between 2000 and 3000 mL of fluid per day unless contraindicated by medical conditions such as cardiac or kidney failure (Maney, 1976; Wells, 1975; Kick, 1973). The stress on adequate fluid is essential for several critical reasons. Primary is the obvious requirement for sufficient urine in the bladder to stretch wall receptors, signaling the spinal reflex and higher centers of the need to pass urine. Isaacs (1976) writes of a need to amplify this signal for continence management and warns that restricted fluid intake may lower awareness of bladder sensations with resultant incontinence.

No reputable literature could be found which advocated general fluid restriction for the elderly with urine control difficulty. However, several sources recommended encouragement of fluid intake during day hours with restriction after an evening time: 5 P.M. (Agate, 1970), 6 P.M. (Adams, 1977), and 8 P.M. (Maney, 1976). This practice addresses a nighttime wetting issue

and rests on two key assumptions about the elderly: first, that adequate fluid can be consumed before the restriction period and, second, that lack of fluid intake for 10 to 12 hours should be directly related to lack of urine output during that time. Both assumptions may be false. Achieving an adequate fluid intake in an elderly oriented person with urine control loss is difficult. Such an individual's innate desire is to restrict fluid. To reverse this trend, considerable discussion needs to be pursued with a focus on "flushing out the system" and maintaining general health as essential aspects of assisting continence. Achieving an adequate fluid intake in the disoriented elderly is a consuming process of staff perseverance and ingenuity. In either case it is not always possible to achieve an adequate intake before a fixed time. Earlier discussion of kidney changes with age suggest that urine output at night may be on a different rhythm for the old. Apart from threats to comfort which fluid restriction suggest, the procedure may be unsuccessful because of its resultant understimulation of the bladder. Schaefer and Martin (1975) write of enuretic behavior therapy treatments for children and note that the bladder needs relevant stimuli (fullness) before one can expect an appropriate response (waking to void). Because of these factors and a lack of research, nighttime fluid restriction for the old should be carefully considered and pursued only with great caution.

The importance of adequate fluid intake in the elderly person with urine control loss is critical to other aspects of successful functioning. There is a known direct effect of dehydration on mental processes in the old (Adams, 1977; Brocklehurst and Hanley, 1976); inadequate fluid intake and attendant electrolyte deficiencies cause a drop in blood pressure (Guyton, 1977). Thus, old people with low fluid intake may become confused and disoriented; subsequent lack of mental attending to continence may increase loss of control. Secondly, inadequate fluid intake is associated with constipation which is associated with urinary incontinence (Brocklehurst and Hanley, 1976; Willington, 1975c). When the body receives insufficient oral fluids, the stool, which is made up in part of water, becomes dry and hard. Large amounts of such stool in the rectum can press on the bladder outlet, forming an obstruction to urine flow.

One of the first interventions for urinary continence is a fluid intake of 2000 to 3000 mL per day. This can be achieved through careful planning and family/staff cooperation. In the home it is essential to measure the commonly used drinking vessels in order to plan and monitor intake. Whether in home or hospital, a client directly involved in the fluid intake plan and record is more apt to be successful. Fluid need not be thought of as uninspiring and dull. Although individual diet, health history, and economics may set some specific limitations, a wide variety of substances count as fluid, e.g., ice cream, popsicles, jello, beer. It is helpful to attach family or staff routines to fluid intake, e.g., drink a cup of coffee while watching a favorite morning TV show or have a glass of juice while waiting for a physiotherapy session. Consultation with a dietician may yield greater fluid selection and presentation variety; consultation with an occupational therapist may help with individuals who cannot manage ordinary drinking glasses and cups. Sufficient fluid intake in the institutionalized, disoriented elderly may require the intense focus of one staff member. A successful approach, observed in some English geriatric units, is to assign one staff person to mouth care and fluid intake responsibilities. Since poor oral hygiene deters fluid intake which, in turn, compounds poor oral hygiene, there is logic in combining the two tasks. While personalized nursing is always preferred, a task assignment for critical and high-need areas such as fluid intake seems justified.

Bowel Regulation Another early and significant intervention for urinary continence management is bowel regularity. Constipation and fecal impaction may impede urine outflow, causing urinary retention and overflow. Fecal impaction may also present as mucous, watery diarrhea, the result of hard stool irritating the bowel's mucous membrane. The role of dehydration in constipation has been noted; obviously an adequate fluid intake is a helpful preventive approach. Other factors associated with constipation include a lack of dietary roughage, inactivity, inattention to the call to defecate, and laxative dependence (Adams, 1977). Nursing ac-

tions can reduce or resolve these difficulties. High-fiber diets are considered highly effective in constipation management (Burkitt and Meisner, 1979); nurses need to work with dieticians and the client's family to provide tasty, desirable high-fiber foods. An activity program would not only facilitate bowel regularity but provide motivation for urinary continence. Frequently, staff note that patients with urine control difficulties maintain continence when taking part in interesting activities.

The urge to move the bowels occurs as feces enter and distend the rectum, stimulating stretch receptors which send impulses to the spinal cord. Fecal movement toward the rectum occurs commonly after meals and is, perhaps, most urgent during the first hour after breakfast (Guyton, 1977). Quick attention to bowel movement urges, privacy, and toilet comfort will facilitate regularity. Laxative abuse is not only a public response to advertising and cultural norms, but may be also a well-meant but overenthusiastic nursing intervention for the elderly. Bowel-regulating programs with laxative, enema, and suppository may be too vigorous for many old people. There is a tendency to standardize such programs so that the 300-pound stroke patient gets the same treatment as the 80-pound individual with parkinsonism, the common result being diarrhea and fecal incontinence in the latter. Bowel programs tend to become routinized and may continue for someone who no longer needs one or for someone who does need one but needs less assistance than provided. Bowel regularity programs are helpful but should be individualized, kept to the minimum assistance needed, and be reevaluated periodically. Note, too, that constipation can be a symptom in many diseases including cancer of the colon; a thorough evaluation is needed for individuals newly experiencing constipation and for those not responding to simple interventions (Brocklehurst, 1977).

Urinary Tract Infections Urine, normally sterile, is also an excellent culture medium for bacteria which, if present, are cleared from the bladder by the process of urination (Robertson, 1978). Infection is likely to occur in situations where the bladder cannot empty completely, leaving residual urine in which organisms can multiply. Urine concentrated with sugar is even more conducive to bacterial growth; thus, the uncontrolled elderly diabetic is particularly prone to bladder infection (Lye, 1978). Infrequent voiding results in bladder distention and has been cited as a cause of urinary infection (Lapides et al., 1971). It is thought that persistent distention leads to ischemia of the bladder wall with subsequent reduction in its ability to resist infection. Brocklehurst and Hanley (1976) believe that the common cause of bladder infection in females is through fecal contamination of the urethral orifice. Since *Escherichia coli,* an organism normally existing in the gastrointestinal tract, is most frequently cultured from older women's urine, proper wiping and good hygiene after defecation are critical for women (Walkey et al., 1967). Males are also especially susceptible to urinary infection after a prostatectomy (Brocklehurst and Hanley, 1976). Secretion from the prostate gland is thought to contain an antibacterial substance which is lost after resection.

Urinary infection in an older person can be either acute or chronic. Symptoms of acute cystitis such as burning, urgency, and increased frequency may occur and are similar to those found in younger people. Fever, however, is often missing, whereas mental confusion and/or loss of urine control may not only be present, but serve as the first sign(s) of the infectious process. Standard treatment with appropriate antibiotics should resolve the symptoms (Brocklehurst and Hanley, 1976). Chronic infection is sometimes associated with loss of urine control, nocturnal frequency, or precipitancy, but at other times it is completely asymptomatic, and in any case is secondary to underlying bladder disease. Successful treatment is limited since reinfection usually occurs within 3 to 4 months. A therapeutic trial of an antibiotic helps determine the relationship of infection to symptoms (Lye, 1978). If symptoms are unrelieved and relapse of infection occurs, further treatment is not usually pursued (Brocklehurst and Hanley, 1976). Wear (1975) believes that urinary tract infections in the elderly require urologic evaluation including both intravenous pyelography and cystoscopy.

The diagnosis of urinary infection, acute or chronic, is made on the basis of a count of bacteria found in the urine (Walkey et al., 1967). A count of greater than 100,000 organisms per milliliter is thought to represent true infection rather than specimen contamination. Also, the presence of two or more different organisms in the urine is indication of contamination (Lye, 1978).

The collection of a proper urine specimen is often difficult, especially in the elderly female patient where skin and vulvar organisms are frequent contaminants. The midstream clean-catch method attempts to reduce contamination of urine but is difficult to acquire from frail, ill elderly who are often confused and/or immobile. Two people may be needed to assist the patient in obtaining the specimen. Careful cleansing of the external genitalia is required with particular attention to the female labia minora, male foreskin if present, and for both the urethral orifice. Sterile saline, sterile water, or plain soap and water are suggested as cleansing agents (Walkey et al., 1967; Lye, 1978; Beyers and Dudas, 1977). Walkey et al. (1967) recommend that antiseptics not be used for cleansing since they have been shown to reduce actual bacterial count. Collection of urine in a sterile container is advised. Specimens from patients being diuresed should be collected in the morning. Remember that urine bacterial colony counts depend on fluid intake and urine flow rate (Robertson, 1978). A urine specimen can be stored in domestic refrigerators for up to 48 hours (Lye, 1978). Suprapubic aspiration, a medical procedure, provides an alternative way of collecting uncontaminated urine (Brocklehurst and Hanley, 1976). However, this procedure in old people is equally beset with difficulties. Clearly, clinical investigation is needed to explore ways to secure clean urine for analysis.

Drug Effects Drugs commonly prescribed for old people that precipitate loss of urine control and disrupt continence management efforts are diuretics and the relaxants or central nervous system depressants. A diuretic is given chiefly to rid the body of excess fluid and, therefore, increases urinary output. One should consider the time of administration and realize, for example, that a diuretic pill prescribed twice a day (bid) may well be given or taken at 9 A.M. and 9 P.M., thus increasing the probability of involuntary wetting during the night. It may be possible to facilitate nighttime continence by giving both tablets at the same time in the morning without reducing their overall diuresing effectiveness. Drowsiness is only one side effect of the major tranquilizers such as Thorazine, Haldol, and Mellaril (Pfeiffer, 1978). Minor tranquilizers, including Librium and meprobamate, are all capable of producing delirium in an old person since they affect the cerebral cortex. Hypnotics like chloral hydrate and Dalmane, as well as sedatives, including the barbiturates and Valium, diminish awareness, create confused states, and severely alter the conscious ability to remain continent. More creative, less drug-dependent, interventions for sleep, restlessness, and anxiety are needed. When relaxants or central nervous system depressants are absolutely essential, they should be given in doses as low as possible and with the realization that urinary continence may be compromised.

There are other drugs that directly affect bladder muscle function incidental to their original purpose (Bissada and Finkbeiner, 1978). For example, drugs such as levodopa, the antihistamines, phenothiazines, and tricyclic antidepressants have been shown to produce voiding difficulties or urinary retention. Conversely, Dilantin, digitalis, methyldopa, reserpine, Valium, and Librium have been associated with symptoms of stress incontinence, nocturnal enuresis, and/or urgency.

Gynecological/Genitourinary Consultation Because so many gynecological/genitourinary conditions can cause or contribute to loss of urinary continence, every older person with complex urine control difficulty deserves a consultation with a specialist in the relevant field. Careful observation by the nurse can serve as an impetus for fuller evaluation by a physician or nurse practitioner who should seek specialist consultation for complex or difficult diagnoses. The nurse should act not only as a competent observer to facilitate communication with other professionals but should be an advocate that such communication take place. Rampant ageism is evident in the denial of or apathetic response to appropriate gynecological/genitourinary consultation for urine control problems in the older person. Comments such as "too

expensive" and "wouldn't do any good" are shortsighted and ignorant reactions which need to be addressed with vigor and facts. Male continence problems are commonly associated with benign prostatic hypertrophy. Jaffe (1978) notes that approximately 70 percent of such prostatic obstructions can be removed by a relatively simple operation (transurethral resection). Common female continence problems with a gynecological origin are atrophic vaginitis and urethritis which respond well to estrogen therapy, and conditions of vaginal and pelvic floor relaxation such as cystocele, rectocele, and prolapse which can be treated with vaginal pessaries or surgical intervention (Glowacki, 1978).

ENVIRONMENTAL FACTORS

Toilet Distance and Discrimination The best place to pass urine is in the toilet where environmental cues, privacy, and typical voiding behaviors combine to assist satisfactory bladder emptying. A good toilet is sufficiently close, large, and comfortable to be an appropriate haven for those in need. How close a toilet needs to be is determined by the individual's mobility rate and urine holding capacity. An unpublished study in Scotland evaluated oriented, continent, ambulant elderly patients and toilet distance (Scottish Home and Health Department, 1970). The study recommended that toilets be no more than 30 to 40 feet from such patients during day use. Coni et al. (1977) thought that relatively immobile patients should be no further than 49 feet (15 meters) from a toilet. Clearly, each patient is different, and the nurse is well advised to actually measure bed and chair distances to the toilet and to time mobility rates on an individual basis. A change in room or bed assignment, or relocation of a favorite chair closer to the toilet, could give some older people a slight time advantage, all they might need to keep urine control. A plea, too, should be made for clarity in toilet labeling in institutions. If corridor toilets must have modern international symbol designation, could they also have the more familiar toilet notation? Institutions might also consider distinctive color coding as a further aid to toilet location. How helpful it would be if the individual could rely on the certainty that all red doors, for example, concealed a toilet.

Clothing Manipulation of clothing can add a significant time factor to some older people's toilet venture. There are many useful suggestions for easy clothing management and toileting such as elastic waist bands for trouser and lapover backs for skirts (Elphick, 1970; Lowman and Klinger, 1969; May et al., 1974). Occupational therapists can be especially helpful in clothing modification which might aid toilet use. It ought to be stressed that lack of clothing, i.e., underpants, may be a handicap in continence control. Underpants may serve as a reminder to preserve dryness, a self-monitor of urine leakage, and a stimulus to toilet use when wet.

Chairs Consideration needs to be given, too, to chair design and bed height; both should facilitate mobility. Jordan (1978) recommends chairs for the well elderly with seat height of 17 inches and depth of 16 inches with no more than a slight backward slope. Norton et al. (1962, 1976) studied the institutionalized elderly and recommended a variety of chair heights from 15 to 19 inches but noted that most would find a 17-inch chair height suitable. The latter study includes other useful information for chair selection. In addition, physiotherapists can be helpful in chair choice as well as acquiring special assisted-rise chairs, e.g., spring or hydraulic lift devices.

Toilet Size and Design Toilet size is critical, especially when mobility devices are used. Wheelchairs require a turning space of 5 by 5 feet (Jordan, 1978), and walking frame "turning circles" require even more room: 5 by 6 feet (Scottish Home and Health Department, 1970). Toilet stall door design can be a hindrance to both privacy and access. Inward-opening door closure is impeded by wheelchairs or walking frames in all but very large toilets. Thus, Jordan (1978) urges stall doors 32 inches wide which swing out to a space at least 4 feet wide. Grab bar placement is critical, with physiotherapy advice most helpful. One suggestion is that grab bars be placed on both walls of a stall and run parallel to the floor at a height of 33 inches (Jordan, 1978). Home toilets can be adapted with grab bars through community services; a toilet support frame available at hospital supply agencies may be useful. The standard toilet seat is 16 inches from the floor, too low for many individuals with stiff hips. Plastic or metal toilet seat inserts can be obtained from supply companies to raise seat height to 20 inches, or home adaptations can be made (Lowman and Klinger, 1969). Obviously toilets need to be well illuminated, with comfortable warmth and humidity.

Toilet Alternatives: Commodes, Bedpans, and Urinals When toilets are too distant, too small, or otherwise unsuitable, alternatives are needed. A good commode has all the essentials of a good chair, e.g., suitable height and stability. All commodes are not good commodes, and even a good commode is not right for all patients. Commodes for home use tend to be fixed chairs and are generally stable. Commodes for institutional use tend to be lightweight and sometimes have wheels which, even with locking mechanisms, still have mobility. Commode purchase requires consideration of all available models and advice from physiotherapists. An institution is best served with a variety of evaluated commodes and clear criteria for appropriate use with specific types of patients.

Bedpans, receptacles for urine and feces, are of ancient origin and serve as toilet use for individuals confined to bed. The term *bedpan* is a broad generality for a number of varying vessel designs. Figure 36-2 displays five common bedpans, each of which offers different advantages. The standard bedpan is of a large oval shape with rounded sides. It is quite stable but is cool to touch if made of stainless steel. A cutaway style plastic bedpan is available which, while perhaps less stable, provides easier handling for attendants and may have some further advantage in rim design. Pediatric bedpans are modeled on the standard adult form but are smaller; they may be easier to use and more comfortable for small, frail elderly individuals. Fracture bedpans are of a shovel design and come in a large and small version. Both have a projecting handle at the front and a tapered back to facilitate placement with minimal pelvic movement. All these bedpans are easily obtained through local health supply dealers or catalog mailings. It is most useful to have a variety of bedpans available for those elderly requiring one. The nurse and the patient may need to try several models before the most helpful one is found. At best

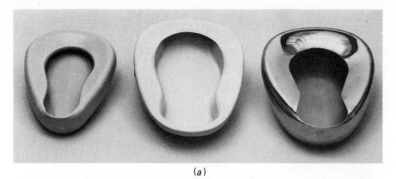

(a)

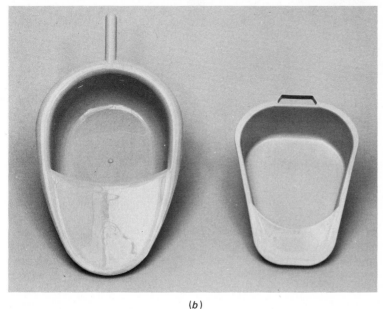

(b)

FIGURE 36-2 Five common bedpans. Standard one has a large oval
shape and is usually of stainless
steel. A plastic bedpan, though less
stable, is easier to handle. Fracture
bedpans are a shovel design; a large
and small version are shown. (Courtesy of Carol A. Brink.)

bedpans are a poor toilet alternative as supine voiding reduces or negates muscle involvement which aids in bladder emptying.

The male urinal is of a fairly standard bottle shape which varies by degree of neck curvature and handle design, factors which relate to ease of placement and handling. The quest for an equally satisfactory female urinal is probably as ancient as the success of the male version. Noting that female urinal criteria are more complex than those for males, Norton (1970, p. 29) discovered that "every conceivable variant of the bottle-shaped container has been explored over the past 50 years." The two female urinals pictured are typical of the more common designs (see Figure 36-3). The wide-mouthed version is

sometimes called "duckbilled." Its opening is larger and more recessed than the narrow-mouthed model whose advantage is in the smaller area needed for placement. Both designs offer advantages to patients with different body shapes and functional needs. Urinals for both sexes can be of great assistance but need to be carefully selected. A number of homemade versions have been suggested. For frail males who need to stand to void, a pint-size plastic bowl fixed on a stick at penis height has been proposed (Elphick, 1970). Lowman and Klinger (1969) note that women might void into a funnel connected with wide-bore tubing to a container. Certainly some elderly men and women have devised their own homemade urinal systems;

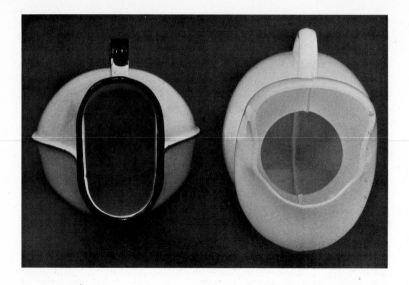

FIGURE 36-3 Female urinals. The wide-mouthed version is sometimes called "duckbilled." (*Courtesy of Carol A. Brink.*)

they ought to be made comfortable to share their advice and continue using home aids if desired.

Signal Devices If one needs assistance to get to the toilet or alternative, a signal device is essential. All institutions have some sort of device at each bed for signaling nurses, but it is not uncommon to find it unattached for individuals who need it. Exploration sometimes reveals a purposeful intent to stop patients from calling the nurse with a variety of reasons given: "calls too much," "wets anyway," and "doesn't really have to go." All such responses indicate a desperate need for nursing action, none of which includes signal device withdrawal. Patients may seek attention by calling the nurse and, if so, need a supportive care plan to establish trust. Patients' loss of urine in the bed and feelings of having to pass urine without doing so are important observations which need to be noted and evaluated more fully. Safety of patients and continence management require signal device attachment for all patients within reach of bed unit call systems. Home clients needing assistance or such institutional patients away from bed units or unable to work such a device might use a small handbell to call for attention. Clients at home can arrange for light, bell, or voice call systems through relatively simple handyman home alternatives.

SPECIFIC CONTINENCE INTERVENTIONS

Exercise Two types of exercise may be useful in urinary continence management for the elderly. One is known generally as *pelvic floor exercises;* the other is a newer and less-developed technique known as *bladder tolerance training.*

Pelvic Floor The development of pelvic floor exercises is generally attributed to Kegel's work with postpartum females in the late 1940s (Kegel, 1949). He developed a series of exercises to reduce or resolve urinary stress incontinence; the success rate in clients without surgical or obstetric injuries and without neurogenic or other systemic disease is reported to be better than 86 percent (Greenhill, 1979). Although many elderly women might have one or more of the conditions known to negatively influence this therapy, they still should be taught and encouraged to use pelvic floor exercises (Willington, 1975a). Clients with mental dysfunction and those who lack motivation will be slow or unsuccessful learners, but most older women will benefit from an exercise program. At the very least this conscious attention and positive action for continence management will enhance psychological states, and some older women may significantly increase muscle strength to achieve better continence control. Before the exercises are taught, pelvic floor strength needs to be evaluated and should be periodically re-evaluated during the course of the program (Nursing Assessment Guide). The elderly woman needs a full explanation of the techniques; illustrations and printed guides may be helpful. Mandelstam (1977) cautions that improvement is gradual and most effective if done regularly for at least 3 months. Pelvic floor exercises are probably most successful as part of a regular and continual continence management program.

It is useful to start the exercise sessions during client toileting when sight, sound, and feeling enhance learning the muscle control techniques. Remember that voiding exercises are dependent on adequate fluid intake. While sitting on the toilet or commode with her legs apart, the client is asked to begin urination and then to stop midstream by tightening the muscles around the urine outlet and vagina. "Squeeze the urine off" may be a helpful directive. Try to have the client avoid increasing abdominal pressure by grunting or breath-holding responses as the pressure increase will press on the bladder and work against stopping the urine flow. Ask the client to keep the urine "shut off" for 3 or 4 seconds and then "let it go." This on/off exercise may be practiced several times during a voiding.

A nonvoiding exercise should then be learned and regularly practiced. Instruct the client to sit on a firm-seated chair with an upright back support. Have her place her feet flat on the floor and put her knees apart; this technique reduces exercising extraneous muscle groups. She should then squeeze tight the muscles around the urine outlet and vagina. Pretending to be shutting off urine flow might help. If the client has pelvic floor sensation, she should feel the vagina close and lift up. Again, try to have her avoid increasing abdominal pressure. Ask her to hold the tightness for 3 seconds, relax for 3 seconds, and repeat. If the client has difficulty with the exercise focusing on the urethral and vaginal areas, encourage her to squeeze her rectum shut as if to stop diarrhea. After she has become familiar with the sensation of anal tightening, encourage the process of learning more specific urethral and vaginal tightening

sensations. Various suggestions for practice periods throughout the day have been given, from 15 to 30 tightenings every half-hour (Greenhill, 1979) to 10 tightenings four times a day (Nursing Update, 1976). Individual client energy, ability, motivation, and need are relevant factors in arranging an exercise schedule.

Pelvic floor exercises are also relevant for older men with dribbling incontinence related to prostatic surgery. In such cases, the exercise focuses on squeezing the rectal sphincter shut. Practice may be helped initially if the nurse inserts a finger into the rectum and asks the client to tighten the muscles around it. Remember to encourage relaxation of other muscle groups and have the client avoid increasing abdominal pressure. During proper muscle tightening the penis retracts, a useful monitor of a successful exercise. Krauss et al. (1975), who report reduction or resolution of postprostatectomy incontinence with this technique, suggest that the exercise be practiced 20 to 30 times every waking hour starting 2 days preoperatively and continuing postoperatively as necessary. Again, individual assessment, teaching, and planning are necessary for a satisfactory exercise program.

Bladder Wilson (1976) writes of "therapeutic cystometry" for intractable overactive bladders. That is, the process of filling the bladder with fluid to measure volume-pressure relationships (cystometrogram) may serve as a therapeutic exercise to increase control of the voiding reflex and improve bladder capacity. An early study with cystometry and the chronically ill elderly yielded much improved or entirely cleared urine symptoms in 43 percent of patients with urine control difficulty and some improvement in an additional 21 percent (Wilson, 1948). A recent study using prolonged bladder distention via cystometry as a treatment for urinary urgency and urge incontinence included four women and one man over 60 (Dunn et al., 1974). The technique involved increasing bladder pressure equal to the patient's systolic blood pressure for four 30-minute periods. Four of the five older patients reported excellent results and the fifth felt improved. Objective evidence indicated that bladder capacity after the cystometry sessions increased from 120 to 620 percent (240 to 410 mL, 50 to 310 mL) and that three of the five had achieved a normal cystometrogram. Three-month follow-ups showed that the improvement had been maintained.

This cystometric treatment is worthy of consideration by urological specialists in the management of continence in the elderly. It is also conceptually similar to a program developed for enuretic children, diurnal bladder tolerance training (Kimmel technique). Sloop (1977) explained the technique and reviewed relevant literature. First proposed in 1960 as a regimen to increase functional bladder capacity, diurnal bladder tolerance training involves the child drinking quantities of fluid during the day and practicing "holding" urine after the urge to void is felt. "Holding" progresses from a 5- to a 45-minute delay. Sloop acknowledges that published reports of this treatment reveal impressive results but that more studies with larger sample sizes are needed. There have been no published studies of systematic urine holding exercises as a treatment plan for urine control in the elderly. However, an unpublished study by Falconer (1979) explored the time between urge to void and need to void in a small sample of elderly, self-ambulant, continent women. She found the mean time over 24 hours was 10 minutes and 25 seconds with a range of 2 minutes and 10 seconds to 31 minutes and 59 seconds. Urine-holding exercises combined with increased fluid intake may be a helpful intervention in continence management for the older person. While such a regimen needs development and clinical testing, nurses might work with older clients in planning personalized exercise programs directed toward increasing voiding delay time.

Sensory Stimulation Stimulation of sensory receptors located in the skin produces a reflex motor response and has been used as a technique to either inhibit or induce voiding (Elizabeth, 1966). Fast brushing on the skin above the pubis for 30 seconds followed by rapid icing for 30 seconds may cause a release of the bladder sphincter and stimulate voiding. Conversely, urinary retention was reported by Elizabeth when fast brushing was applied over peripheral endings of the third and fourth sacral nerves located along the medial area of the buttocks (1966). Bergstrom (1969) tried icing and brushing to stimulate voiding and relieve post-operative urinary retention, thus eliminating the need for catheterization. She studied a small sample of women between the ages of 18 and 65 who had not previously been catheterized and had received general anesthesia during surgery. Standard nursing measures were used to induce voiding up to 8 hours postsurgery. Those patients unable to void were then started on icing and brushing techniques rather than catheterization. An ice cube was rubbed on the skin "from the iliac crests to the groin" for 30 seconds in 2- to 3-second intervals, followed by rapid stroking with a soft, battery-powered brush in the same manner (Bergstrom, 1969, p. 285). Two-thirds of the women voided from 180 to 480 mL following the icing-brushing procedure and one-third required catheterization. Clearly, further investigation of this technique specifically focusing on continence management in the elderly is warranted.

Gynecological and Genitourinal Control Devices Edwards (1975, 1976a, 1976b) reviewed specific devices developed to control urination and noted that these were either mechanical or electrical. Mechanical designs act by occluding urine flow, for males as a clamp across the penis and for females by applying either anterior or posterior pressure against the bladder neck. Such devices should probably not be used for patients with sensory damage and require manual dexterity and mental alertness for self-care. Electrical stimulation of the pelvic floor causes muscle contraction and may serve to increase muscle tone and power. Direct stimulation can be applied through either vaginal or rectal devices for females and via the latter in males. Stimulators can be worn for specified periods or continually but must be removed at frequent intervals for cleaning. Stanton (1979) notes that it is still not clear exactly how such devices work and comments that simply the anatomic support provided and a positive psychological state could account for some successful results. Considerable exploration is current for implantable devices, either electrical or hydraulic. Merrill and Teague (1978) predict that during the next decade a clinically applicable implantable urinary prosthesis to replace absent or abnormal voiding reflexes will be developed.

Behavior Modification and Habit Training

Behavior modification and habit training are two interventions suggested in the literature for continence management in the elderly. The two terms have a similar origin in learning theory but are operationally different. While some might use the terms interchangeably, there is a distinction in practice. Most typically, behavior modification is considered an educative process with the client an active participant in the plan (Bellack and Hersen, 1977). Schaefer and Martin (1975) specify that behavior modification is a useful treatment for improper voiding habits only if psychological forces are solely responsible for the cause. Basic to behavior modification is a plan of social or material reinforcement for correct behavior (Maney, 1976). Habit training is a process of discovering a client's voiding pattern and encouraging a program of regular toilet visiting at those times (Clay, 1978b). In addition, such training usually includes some behavioral reinforcers such as dry pants and perhaps staff praise. Behavior modification includes some reliance on establishing voiding habits. Thus, the two techniques are closely related. In practice habit training is a useful intervention basic to any continence management program; behavior modification is a more complex but equally useful treatment plan which requires guidance from someone skilled in the technique. In-depth discussion of behavior modification is beyond the scope of this chapter. The published studies will be briefly noted with implications for further research. Habit training will be discussed more fully.

Only three publications could be found which utilized behavior modification techniques in elderly patients with urine control difficulties (Carpenter and Simon, 1960; Grosicki, 1968; and Pollack and Liberman, 1974). In all studies, subjects were male and had diagnoses of long-term psychoses, neuropsychiatric disorders, or chronic organic brain syndrome. Carpenter and Simon's (1960) study excluded subjects with possible organic causes for urine control loss and included subjects with age ranges from 33 to 84 years (average 62.1); data are not reported by age. Grosicki (1968) included subjects with cerebral or urological pathology and selected those over age 63 who had become incontinent (four or more times in 24 hours) since admission

to the hospital. Pollock and Liberman's (1974) subjects were 61 years or older; possible urologic pathology was not reported. Considering only the latter two studies with findings exclusive to elderly subjects, it was not found that social and material rewards lessen urinary incontinence. Sample size, 21 and 6, respectively, was small, and inherent design limitations clearly affected the results. Perhaps the most important finding was from Grosicki's control group who significantly decreased incontinence during periods of study time-checks; that is, consistent attention alone reduced incontinence.

These few studies on complex subjects are not sufficient to really evaluate behavior modification technique. Maney's (1976) suggestion that elderly clients for urine control behavior alteration be well oriented and only recently incontinent of urine is sensible. With such clients perhaps the method could be fully developed and adequately evaluated. Certainly on the basis of these early data it would be premature to discard behavior modification for anyone, including the most needy and correspondingly complex clients such as those studied. Further clinical research is very much needed.

Habit training for adults is based on techniques used for children developing bladder control and is an attempt to have clients regain their typical voiding patterns. It will not succeed as an intervention unless staff members throughout the 24 hours understand the process and are committed to its usefulness. The technique requires close observation of voiding frequency to discover the client's pattern and align it with toilet use. Urge to void should be based on bladder capacity and fluid intake. Willington (1975e, 1976) believes that the best measure of true bladder capacity, i.e., not influenced by extraneous psychological and physical factors, is the first incontinence episode during sleep at night. For this reason, he and a colleague have developed a recording device to monitor night incontinence without disturbing the patient (Willington and Ball, 1976). From such accurate data a time plan can be established which sets toileting at periods of bladder fullness. Clay (1978a, 1978b, 1978c) has developed a procedure which is based on client checks and a comprehensive documentation of findings by the nurse. In her plan, clients are initially checked every 2 hours and encouraged to use the toilet whether incontinent or not. As a pattern of bladder emptying appears, the time checks are adjusted to the client's own schedule. Willington (1975e, 1976) would be critical of a procedure which included toileting when the bladder was only partially full or empty, i.e., after incontinence, as sitting on a toilet without proper bladder sensations might inhibit voiding. Nonetheless, Clay (1978c) reports the procedure had only a 15 percent failure rate for a 13-week effort with 20 elderly hospitalized males. Although few, Clay (1978c, p. 24) does note that the failures "did not develop a pattern of micturition." Willington's reasoning is helpful in understanding such training failures and strange urination behaviors sometimes observed in clients.

There are positive and negative stimuli associated with promoting or deterring voiding as a response to a full bladder sensation. Willington (1975e, 1976) states that positive or voiding stimuli are sitting on a toilet-shaped seat, correct position, and the absence of clothing over the genitorectal area. Negative or inhibitory stimuli may be numerous and include pain, lack of privacy, an atypical position, and clean clothes. Willington believes that successful training involves starting with a full bladder, using positive voiding stimuli, and avoiding inhibiting stimuli. He suggests that a bladder program which increases toileting in response to soiling, i.e., shortening toilet intervals to "catch" the voiding, or which involves sitting on the toilet for long sessions may act to inhibit urination behavior because the patient is being asked to void without the proper bladder sensation. Willington postulates that such procedures in combination with the stress of disability and institutionalization can lead the client to be unable to distinguish normal voiding stimuli. In time this can lead to reversal in urination behavior where voiding occurs with normally inhibitory stimulation such as dry sheets and does not occur with normally positive stimuli such as sitting on the toilet (ultraparadoxical inhibition). Newman (1962) described this reversal in urination behavior in an 80-year-old stroke patient after a fractured hip (Newman, 1962). He sees parallels between prisoners of war who often experience coercive indoctrination and chronically ill elderly who are institutionalized, and pleads for a more personalized and sensitive approach to the elderly with urine control difficulty.

It would seem that habit training will be most successful after a thorough description and evaluation of the urine difficulty with remediable action taken as necessary. A good fluid intake and careful observation of output should be documented to look for patterns of bladder fullness noted by large voidings. Regulated toileting before adequate observation works against discerning a true pattern. Whether part of a habit-training program or a regular ward routine, requiring all patients at fixed times to go to the toilet or use an alternative when they do not feel the need seems inappropriate and illogical. In such cases, the only habit being fixed is with staff, and any success in urine control achieved occurs only by chance. Staff time might be better used in individual patient assessment and personalized continence management planning. Proper habit training offers hope for even the most "incurable wetter"; the key to success rests in careful observation and planning, neither of which can occur if staff members feel hopeless or apathetic about continence management.

Drug Management Drug therapy can be highly effective in the management of many voiding problems. An understanding of the specific bladder or bladder outlet disorder is essential to the appropriate selection and desired action of the drug. Bissada and Finkbeiner (1978) classify drugs as those affecting the evacuation or the storage phase of urine. Many prescribed, as well as over-the-counter, drugs alter bladder activity. It is, therefore, important to know all the medications taken by the client with urine control problems.

Cholinergic drugs stimulate bladder activity and enhance bladder emptying (Whitfield, 1977). For example, bethanechol chloride, 50 mg orally every 6 hours, has been found to be useful in patients with atonic bladder but is contraindicated for those with bladder neck obstruction. Anticholinergic drugs inhibit bladder contractility, reduce bladder tone, and increase sphincter tone (Edwards, 1976b). Such drugs may be useful in relieving symptoms or urinary urgency, frequency, urge incontinence, or suprapubic discomfort due to uncontrolled bladder contractions (Bissada and Finkbeiner, 1978).

Three examples of common anticholinergic drugs follow. Propantheline bromide (Pro-Banthine) has been shown to increase bladder capacity. Reports indicate that 30 mg given orally 4 times a day for 7 days is effective in reducing irritative bladder symptoms such as urgency, frequency, dysuria, and nocturia. A single dose at night of nortriptyline hydrochloride (Nortylin, Aventyl) was found successful in controlling enuresis in a small study sample. Emepronium bromide (Cetiprin) is known to reduce urinary incontinence and nocturia; Edwards (1976b) notes that it is often prescribed for cystitis and after bladder surgery.

Antispasmodic drugs also promote bladder relaxation (Bissada and Finkbeiner, 1978). Examples are flavoxate hydrochloride (Urispas) 200 mg orally 4 times a day which is helpful in relieving symptoms associated with cystitis, urethritis, or prostatitis, and oxybutynin chloride (Ditropan) which is effective in reducing bladder spasms induced by a catheter.

In addition, there are drugs thought to involve the vesical neck, posterior urethra, and external sphincter, used to either increase or decrease resistance, depending on the urine control problem (Bissada and Finkbeiner, 1978). While the nurse does not prescribe drugs, a basic understanding of the principles of drug management for urinary control problems is essential. Nursing observation of current medications and voiding patterns including frequency and amount is fundamental to an effective drug therapy program for continence.

MANAGEMENT OF URINE LOSS AND SOILING

External Urinary Collecting Devices These devices are really portable urinals designed to catch and hold urine with comfort and without leakage. They usually consist of a formed cone or cup plus a collecting bag and are available for men and women. Currently available external devices for men may include some useful appliances. Female collecting devices are at a more experimental stage; Lowthian (1975) provides a good review of their current status.

Condom drainage for males is also a form of external urine collection with a variety of materials available (Whyte and Thistle, 1976). Lawson and Cook (1978–1979) report a careful appraisal of such drainage in five patients with spinal cord paralysis; age was not noted. They discovered four specific problems: splitting, detachment, twisting, and stasis of urine within the condom. Useful suggestions included attaching the condom when the penis is clean and dry and not putting it on in humid atmospheres such as the bathroom after a bath. They changed the condom every other day and found that application using adhesive and adhesive tape was best. As noted, condom drainage is not always successful. In addition, great care must be taken to guard against circulatory disruption to the penis because of too tight application; close monitoring of the skin of the genitalia is required to discover possible irritations early.

Internal Urine-Collecting Devices These devices are either suprapubic or urethral catheters; for long-term use the latter are most typically chosen. However, the management of urine control by indwelling catheter most typically lacks a balanced perspective. Either all incontinent clients are catheterized as the standard and only intervention, or else clients never have an indwelling catheter since they are considered harmful and nonprogressive. There is a place for sensible, appropriate long-term catheterization for permanent urine control difficulty in the elderly. Brocklehurst et al. (1978) contend that indwelling catheters can improve the quality of life for individuals with limited prognosis and intractable incontinence at only minimal risk of complications. Another case for catheterization is in those individuals with extensive sacral pressure sores, the healing of which is impossible in a urine-soaked environment. Thus, urethral catheters are a viable option in urine control management with individualized evaluation central to proper use.

The common complication with urethral catheters is bladder infection. Brocklehurst and Brocklehurst (1978) studied indwelling catheters in a small group of long-stay geriatric patients who were predominantly female (17 of 18 subjects). Of 393 urine specimens obtained over a period of 5 to 47 weeks, 79 percent were infected with one organism and 16 percent had mixed bacteria. Response to continuous urinary antiseptics did not significantly impact on the infection incidence. Infection might be thought of as a logical consequence to long-term catheterization. Bacteria can enter the bladder through two routes: via the catheter lumen during the course of catheterization or management procedures such as bladder washouts and by migrating to the bladder along the outside of the catheter tubing (Chambers, 1976). Chambers states that if there is continuous free drainage and a brisk urine flow, the irritation should be minor. Thus, avoidance of drainage tube kinking and a high continuous fluid intake are two sensible measures to reduce infection. Standard antibiotic coverage for those on urethral catheterization is not recommended as it is considered ineffective and likely to result in resistant organisms (Chambers, 1976; Brocklehurst et al., 1978).

Inflammation of the urethra and leakage around catheters are also common catheterization difficulties. Of the catheter materials in use, latex rubber, plastic, and silicon and Teflon-coated latex rubber, the latter are thought to create less urethritis and outflow blockage (Wasting, 1974; Chambers, 1976). While leakage can be due to encrustation along the catheter lumen, Edwards (1976b) notes that reflex contraction of the uninhibited bladder forces urine around a urethral catheter which can not collect such forceful expulsion regardless of catheter size. Since Brocklehurst and Brocklehurst (1978) found that two-thirds of catheter changes in their study were due to leakage, this difficulty needs to be more carefully evaluated. If leakage is due to inherent bladder responses rather than catheter blockage, a change in catheter is unlikely to resolve the problem and may, through recatheterization, increase urine bacterial counts. Careful evaluation of catheter drainage, observation of the leakage process, and consultation with medical colleagues should be primary actions before a catheter is changed due to leakage. Increasing catheter size and/or balloon holding capacity should be carefully considered. Chambers (1976) recommends that size should be as small as practicable and balloon inflation kept at about 10 mL because larger catheters increase the likelihood of urethritis and larger balloon inflation can irritate the bladder as well as compress the catheter outflow. Nursing management of urethral catheters for long-term control of urine in the elderly needs further clinical study.

Protective Garments Elphick (1970) classifies British protective garment designs into (1) pull-on, which resemble ordinary underpants; (2) open-flat, which have press fasteners down each side; (3) combined open-flat and drop front, which enable pad change without garment removal; and (4) pilch style, which resemble a diaper and fasten at the waist with buttons or tapes. American products have not been classified or even identified in an organized manner. Individuals in need of a protective garment or staff seeking such a patient aid are left to exploration of local health supply resources and catalogue review. A major factor to success with any garment is that it fit, especially at the legs, where pad overflow or overfill tends to escape. Garment launder may not be a major home difficulty, but it is in institutions where laundry advice is critical to selection of any washable product. Willington (1975b) lists criteria for a good aid to soiling management and developed a new pant product (Kanga Pant) in 1972 (Willington, 1972). A recent British study compared Kanga Pant with a Swedish garment (Maxi-pant) and found that the latter was preferred (Tam et al., 1978); neither product is presently available in the United States. A great deal of work needs to be done to simply discover and evaluate current American products. Discussion with various health product companies suggests that major development is underway in disposable protective garments.

Protective Pads It is essential to realize that protective pads are not so much protecting clients as they are protecting beds and chairs. The danger in their use is that the quality of care to the furniture may be outstanding while the client suffers from neglect. Few things in life are as demeaning as sitting pantless on a paper, unless it is the added impact of a care provider who incorrectly tells you that it is a suitable place to void: "Go ahead and go; you're on a paper!"

Every nurse ought to experience this humiliation and preferably sit on the soiled paper for at least an hour to learn the sensation of cold, wet urine pools. Clarity might then be acquired in appropriate protective pad use; pads assist with laundry, not urine-control management. In fact, sitting pantless on a paper may inspire individuals to pass urine there, even without inappropriate comment from the staff; therefore, pads may increase lack of urine control. Nonetheless, protective pads can be a significant help to a family's dealing with incontinence at home and can provide protective comfort to the institutionalized elderly who fear soiling the bed.

Willington (1969) lists criteria for a basic incontinent pad: (1) has a waterproof duration of several hours, (2) remains intact wet or dry, (3) has a known absorption capacity, and (4) can be disposed of easily. Unfortunately, most purchase of incontinence pads is based on only one criterion: the largest supply for the least money. That this may be a false economy is not taken into account. That is, the least expensive pad is apt to be the smallest sized with the least absorption capacity, requiring several pads for each use rather than one pad of better quality. Norton (1965) tested three British disposable incontinence pads and concluded that the most desirable was "twenty-four by sixteen inches in size with a non-slippery back (polythene), a dry-barrier top cover, and a fleece and fifteen-ply unbleached cellulose wadding middle." Another pad study has suggested that for restless, demented, or overweight clients a pad 24 by 18 inches is more suitable (Henderson and Rogers, 1971). The latter study also noted that a 17-ply cellulose middle as well as nylon filament cover, similar to Norton's finding, was most successful. An appraisal needs to be made of American disposable incontinence pads. An Australian washable, and thus reusable, absorbent bed pad (Kylie Pad) has been evaluated and appears to offer some advantage over disposable products (Silberberg, 1977).

SUMMARY

It might be helpful to consider four basic principles for urinary continence management in the elderly, as follows:

1. Urinary continence is one definition of adulthood; therefore, threats to or loss of urine control are critical and require prompt nursing action.
2. Always look for a psychological and/or psychosocial disturbance causing or aggravating urine control difficulty; nursing interventions can reduce or resolve many of these problems.
3. Maintain an environment for urinary continence. Through open and positive staff and family attitudes, meaningful activity, structural design, and equipment selection, create an atmosphere which promotes urine control.
4. Even the most difficult cases of urine control disability can be helped; believe in the importance of this clinical problem to clients and that nursing excellence can significantly improve care.

REFERENCES

Adams, George: *Essentials of Geriatric Medicine,* Oxford University, Oxford, 1977.

Agate, John: *The Practice of Geriatrics,* 2d ed., Charles C Thomas, Springfield, Ill., 1970.

Bates, Barbara: *A Guide to Physical Examination,* 2d ed., Lippincott, Philadelphia, 1979.

Bellack, Alan S., and Michel Hersen: *Behavior Modification, an Introductory Textbook,* Williams & Wilkins, Baltimore, 1977.

Bergstrom, Nancy: Ice application to induce voiding, *American Journal of Nursing,* 69(2):283–285, February 1969.

Beyers, Marjorie, and Susan Dudas: *The Clinical Practice of Medical-Surgical Nursing,* Little, Brown, Boston, 1977.

Bissada, Nabil K., and Alex E. Finkbeiner: *Lower Urinary Tract Function and Dysfunction, Diagnosis and Management,* Appleton-Century-Crofts, New York, 1978.

Brocklehurst, John C.: How to define and treat constipation, *Geriatrics,* 32(6):85–87, June 1977.

———: *Incontinence in Old People,* Livingstone, Edinburgh, 1951.

——— **and Susan Brocklehurst:** The management of indwelling catheters, *British Journal of Urology,* 50(2):102–105, April 1978.

——— **and J. B. Dillane:** Studies of the female bladder in old age. I. Cystometrograms in non-incontinent women, *Gerontologica Clinica,* 8(4):285–305, 1966.

——— **and T. Hanley:** *Geriatric Medicine for Students,* Churchill-Livingstone, New York, 1976.

_____ et al.: The prevalence and symptomology of urinary infection in an aged population, *Gerontology Clinics,* **10:**242–253, 1968.

Brod, J.: Study of renal function in the differential diagnosis of kidney disease, *British Medical Journal,* **3**(5767):135–143, July 17, 1971.

Burkitt, Denis P., and Peter Meisner: How to manage constipation with high-fiber diet, *Geriatrics,* **34**(2):33–40, February 1979.

Carpenter, Hazel A., and Ralph Simon: The effect of several methods of training on long-term, incontinent, behaviorally regressed hospitalized psychiatric patients, *Nursing Research,* **9**(1):17–22, Winter 1960.

Chambers, R. M.: Catheters and their management, in F. L. Willington (ed.), *Incontinence in the Elderly,* Academic, New York, 1976.

Clay, Elizabeth C.: Incontinence of urine, *Nursing Mirror,* **146**(9):14–16, March 2, 1978a.

_____: Incontinence of urine, *Nursing Mirror,* **146**(10):36–38, March 9, 1978b.

_____: Incontinence of urine, a regime for training, *Nursing Mirror,* **146**(11):23–24, March 16, 1978c.

Cohen, Stephen: Patient assessment: Examination of the female pelvis, pt. I, *American Journal of Nursing,* **78:**1717–1742, October 1978a.

_____: Patient assessment: Examination of the female pelvis, pt. II, *American Journal of Nursing,* **78:**1913–1941, November 1978b.

_____: Patient assessment: Examination of the male genitalia, *American Journal of Nursing,* **79:**689–712, April 1979.

Coni, Nicholas, William Davison, and Stephen Webster: *Lecture Notes on Geriatrics,* Blackwell Scientific Publications, Ltd., Oxford, 1977.

Cook, William A., et al.: Incontinence in children, *Urologic Clinics of North America,* **5**(2):353–374, June 1978.

Crane, Joyce: Physical appraisal: An aspect of nursing assessment, in J. B. Sana and R. D. Judge (eds.), *Physical Approval Methods in Nursing Practice,* Little, Brown, Boston, 1975.

Dunn, M., J. C. Smith, and G. M. Ardran: Prolonged bladder distension as a treatment of urgency and urge incontinence of urine, *British Journal of Urology,* **46**(6):645–652, December 1974.

Edwards, Lynn: Electronic control, in F. L. Willington (ed.), *Incontinence in the Elderly,* Academic, New York, 1976a.

_____: Incontinence of urine, in J. Blandy (ed.), *Urology,* vol. II, Blackwell Scientific Publications, Ltd., Oxford, 1976b.

_____: Mechanical and other devices, in K. P. S. Caldwell (ed.), *Urinary Incontinence,* Grune & Stratton, New York, 1975.

Elizabeth, Sister Regina: Sensory stimulation techniques, *American Journal of Nursing,* **66**(2):281–286, February 1966.

Elphick, Leonora: *Incontinence, Some Problems, Suggestions, and Conclusions,* Disabled Living Foundation, London, 1970.

Falconer, Paulette Annette: The effects of aging on the time between urge to void and need to void in elderly, self-ambulant, continent, institutionalized women, unpublished master's thesis, University of Rochester, New York, 1979.

Ganong, William F.: *Review of Medical Physiology,* 7th ed., Lange, Los Altos, Calif., 1975.

Glen, Eric S.: Stress incontinence—The turning tide, in E. B. Cantor (ed.), *Female Urinary Stress Incontinence,* Charles C Thomas, Springfield, Ill., 1979.

Glowacki, Gerald: Geriatric gynecology, in W. Reichel (ed.), *Clinical Aspects of Aging,* Williams & Wilkins, Baltimore, 1978.

Goldman, Ralph: Aging of the excretory system, in C. E. Finch and L. Hayflick (eds.), *Handbook of the Biology of Aging,* Van Nostrand Reinhold, New York, 1977.

Greenhill, J. P.: The non-surgical therapy of stress incontinence associated with vaginal relaxation, in E. B. Cantor (ed.), *Female Urinary Stress Incontinence,* Charles C Thomas, Springfield, Ill., 1979.

Grosicki, Jeanette P.: Effect of operant conditioning on modification in neuropsychiatric geriatric patients, *Nursing Research,* **17**(4):304–311, July/August 1968.

Guyton, Arthur C.: *Basic Human Physiology: Normal Function and Mechanisms of Disease,* 2d ed., Saunders, Philadelphia, 1977.

Harris, Charles S.: *Fact Book on Aging: A Profile of America's Older Population,* The National Council on Aging, Washington, 1978.

Henderson, D. J., and W. F. Rogers: Hospital trials of incontinence underpads, *Nursing Times,* **67**(5):141–143, February 4, 1971.

Isaacs, Bernard: The preservation of continence, in F. L. Willington (ed.), *Incontinence in the Elderly,* Academic, New York, 1976.

_____ **and F. A. Walkey:** A survey of incontinence in elderly hospital patients, *Gerontologica Clinica,* **6:**367–376, 1964.

Jaffe, Jack W.: Common lower urinary tract problems in older persons, in W. Reichel (ed.), *Clinical Aspects of Aging,* Williams & Wilkins, Baltimore, 1978.

Jordan, Joe J.: *Senior Center Design: An Architect's Discussion of Facility Planning,* The National Council on the Aging, Washington, March 1978.

Kegel, Arnold H.: The physiologic treatment of poor tone and function of the genital muscles and of urinary stress incontinence, *Western Journal of Surgery, Obstetrics, and Gynecology,* **57**(11):527–535, November 1949.

Kick, Ella Massaro: Rx for incontinence, *ANA Clinical Sessions,* 1972, Detroit, Appleton-Century-Crofts, New York, 1973.

Krauss, Dennis J., Gary J. Schoenrock, and Otto M. Lilien: 'Reeducation' of urethal sphincter mechanism in postprostatectomy patients, *Urology,* V(4):533–535, April 1975.

Lapides, Jack, et al.: Clean, intermittent self-catheterization in the treatment of urinary tract disease, *Transactions of the American Association of Genito-Urinary Surgeons,* 63:92–95, 1971.

Lawson, S. D., and J. D. Cook: An ergonomic appraisal of the use of functional efficiency of condom urinals in the male patient with spinal cord paralysis, *Paraplegia,* 16(3):317–321, November 1978–1979.

Lowman, Edward W., and Judith Lannefield Klinger: *Aids to Independent Living,* McGraw-Hill, New York, 1969.

Lowthian, Peter T.: Portable urinals for women, *Nursing Times,* 71(44):1739–1741, Oct. 30, 1975.

Lye, Michael: Defining and treating urinary infections, *Geriatrics,* 3:71–77, March 1978.

Mandelstam, Dorothy: Support for the incontinent patient, *Nursing Mirror Supplement,* 144(15):xix–xxiii, April 14, 1977.

Maney, Janet Yost: A behavioral therapy approach to bladder retraining, *Nursing Clinics of North America,* 11(1):179–188, March 1976.

Marriner, Ann: *The Nursing Process,* Mosby, St. Louis, 1975.

May, Elizabeth Eckhardt, Neva R. Waggoner, and Eleanor Boettke Hotte: *Independent Living for the Handicapped and the Elderly,* Houghton Mifflin, Boston, 1974.

McLachlan, M. S. F.: The aging kidney, *Lancet,* 2(8081):143–145, July 15, 1978.

Merrill, Daniel C., and Charles T. Teague: A laboratory evaluation of a new hydraulic incontinence device, *Journal of Urology,* 119(1):108–112, January 1978.

Miller, Benjamin F., and Claire Brackman Keane: *Encyclopedia and Dictionary of Medicine, Nursing and Allied Health,* 2d ed., Saunders, Philadelphia, 1978.

Milne, J. S.: Prevalence of incontinence in the elderly age groups, in F. L. Willington (ed.), *Incontinence in the Elderly,* Academic, New York, 1976.

———— et al.: Urinary symptoms in older people, *Modern Geriatrics,* 2:304–311, 1972.

Newman, J. L.: Old folk in wet beds, *British Medical Journal,* i:1824–1827, June 30, 1962.

Norton, Doreen: *By Accident or Design? A Study of Equipment Development in Relation to Basic Nursing Problems,* E. and S. Livingstone, Edinburgh, 1970.

————: Disposable incontinence pads, *British Hospital Journal and Social Science Review,* 75:1907–1909, Oct. 8, 1965.

————, Rhoda McLaren, and A. N. Exton-Smith: *An Investigation of Geriatric Nursing Problems in Hospital,* National Corporation for Old People, London, 1962. Reprinted by Churchill Livingstone, New York, 1976.

Nursing Update, When the woman is incontinent, 7(6):9–14, June 1976.

Pfeiffer, Eric: Use of drugs which influence behavior in the elderly: Promises, pitfalls, and perspectives, in R. C. Kayne (ed.), *Drugs and the Elderly,* University of Southern California Press, Los Angeles, 1978.

Pollack, Donald D., and Robert P. Liberman: Behavior therapy of incontinence in demented inpatients, *Gerontologist,* 14(6):488–491, December 1974.

Robertson, Jack R.: *Genitourinary Problems in Women,* Charles C Thomas, Springfield, Ill., 1978.

Schaefer, Halmuth H., and Patrick L. Martin: *Behavior Therapy,* McGraw-Hill, New York, 1975.

Scottish Home and Health Department: Working party on geriatric accommodation report, unpublished, Edinburgh, 1970.

Silberberg, F. G.: A hospital study of a new absorbant bed pan for incontinent patients, *Medical Journal of Australia,* 1(16):582–586, April 1977.

Sloop, E. Wayne: Urinary disorders, in R. B. Williams and W. D. Gentry (eds.), *Behavioral Approaches to Medical Treatment,* Ballinger, Cambridge, Mass., 1977.

Stanton, Stuart L.: The electronic pessary, in E. B. Cantor (ed.), *Female Urinary Stress Incontinence,* Charles C Thomas, Springfield, Ill., 1979.

Tam, George, John C. Knox, and Margarey Adamson: A cost effective trial of incontinence pants, *Nursing Times,* 74(29):1198–1200, July 20, 1978.

Tarabuley, Edward: Neurogenic diseases of the bladder in the geriatric population, *Geriatrics,* 29(9):123–137, September 1974.

U.S. Department of Health, Education, and Welfare: *Long-Term Care Facility Improvement Study,* Government Printing Office, Washington, 1975.

Walkey, F. A., et al.: Incidence of urinary infection in the elderly, *Scottish Medical Journal,* 12(11):411–414, November 1967.

Wasting, Geoffry: Long-term catheterization, *Nursing Times,* 70(1):17–18, Jan. 3, 1974.

Wear, John B.: Solving selected problems of the aging urinary tract, *Postgraduate Medicine,* 58(6):179–186, November 1975.

Webster's New Twentieth Century Dictionary, unabridged, 2d ed., Collins World, 1978.

Weg, Ruth B.: Changing physiology of aging: Normal and pathological, in D. S. Woodruff and J. E. Birren (ed.), *Aging, Scientific Perspectives and Social Issues,* Van Nostrand, Princeton, N.J., 1975.

Wells, Thelma: Promoting urinary continence in the elderly in hospital, *Nursing Times,* **71**(48):1908–1909, November 1975.

Whitfield, H. N.: Clinical implications of lower urinary tract pharmacology, *Urological Research,* **5**(2):51–54, 1977.

Whyte, John F., and Nancy A. Thistle: Male incontinence: The inside story on external collection, *Nursing '76,* **6**(9):66–67, September 1976.

Willington, F. L.: Management of Urinary Continence, in K. P. S. Caldwell (ed.), *Urinary Incontinence,* Grune & Stratton, New York, 1975a.

_____: Marsupial pants for urinary incontinence, *Nursing Mirror,* **135**(7):40–41 Aug. 13, 1972.

_____: The physiological basis of retraining for continence, in F. L. Willington (ed.), *Incontinence in the Elderly,* Academic, New York, 1976.

_____: The prevention of soiling, *Nursing Times,* **71**(14):545–548, April 3, 1975b.

_____: Problems in the aetiology of urinary incontinence, *Nursing Times,* **71**(10):378–381, March 6, 1975c.

_____: Problems in urinary incontinence in the aged, *Gerontologica Clinica,* **11**:330–356, 1969.

_____: Significance of incompetence of personal sanitary habits, *Nursing Times,* **71**(9):340–341, Feb. 27, 1975d.

_____: Training and retraining for continence, *Nursing Times,* **71**(13):500–503, March 27, 1975e.

_____ and J. A. C. Ball: Electronic monitoring of urinary incontinence in the elderly, *British Medical Journal,* **2**(6028):152, July 17, 1976.

Wilson, Thomas S.: Incontinence of urine in the aged, *Lancet,* **6523**(2):374–377, Sept. 4, 1948.

_____: A practical approach to the treatment of incontinence of urine in the elderly, in F. L. Willington (ed.), *Incontinence in the Elderly,* Academic, New York, 1976, pp. 85–95.

Zacharin, Robert F.: The supervisory mechanism of the female urethra and its practical significance in the surgical management of recurrent stress incontinence, in E. B. Cantor (ed.), *Female Urinary Stress Incontinence,* Charles C Thomas, Springfield, Ill., 1979.

THIRTY-SEVEN

FALLS: A COMMON PROBLEM IN THE ELDERLY

Irene Mortenson Burnside

Many old people have multiple falls, indeed "falling about" is quite a common reason for referral for hospital admissions.
H. M. Hodkinson

LEARNING OBJECTIVES

- Define premonitory falls.
- Define drop attacks.
- List eight causes of falls.
- List four findings in one research study on falls.
- List 12 factors which make the elderly person prone to fall.
- List six intervention strategies which would help prevent falls.

TABLE 37-1
CAUSES OF ACCIDENTAL DEATH, 1978

Type of Accident	Total	Number of Deaths, 65–74 Years	Over 74 Years	Deaths over 64 Years as % of Total Deaths	% of Total Population Aged Over 64 Years
Motor vehicle	51,500	3,100	2,700	11.3	11.0
Pedestrian	9,300	860	1,140	21.5	11.0
Pedalcycle*	1,000	20	20	4.0	11.0
Other types	41,200	2,220	1,540	9.1	11.0
Falls	13,800	1,800	7,900	70.3	11.0
Drowning	6,900	350	250	8.7	11.0
Fires, burns, and deaths associated with fires	6,300	800	950	27.8	11.0
Poisoning by solids and liquids	3,400	200	160	10.6	11.0
Suffocation—ingested object	2,900	450	700	39.7	11.0
Firearms	1,800	90	50	7.8	11.0
Poisoning by gases and vapors	1,700	140	110	14.7	11.0
All other types	16,200	2,100	2,400	27.8	11.0
Total (rounded)	104,500	9,000	15,200	23.2	11.0

* Excluding mopeds.
SOURCE: National Safety Council, Chicago, *Accident Facts*, 1979.

One of the earliest articles in the literature about falls in the elderly appeared in *Today's Health* (Fales, 1959) and lists ideas from Donald Kent: (1) call attention to everyone about the hazards seniors face, (2) train everyone to walk properly and to arrange the environment to prevent falls, (3) teach younger folks about safety with the elders, and (4) start a program to alert people about falls, especially physicians, health departments, safety councils, etc.

Falls among the elderly receive little attention in current literature, yet they are common problems, especially in older women. Some of the falls result in fractures, especially broken hips which may hasten the demise of the individual. There is much stress on staff members, relatives, and peers (the staff members may fear lawsuits) and much time is spent trying to rehabilitate the person who falls and sustains injuries. Even slight falls which do not seem to be serious can jolt an older person considerably. The fear of falling has often been expressed to me by elderly persons who are afraid to leave their home (especially in inclement weather) or venture out of their room in an institution. Unknown turf is one reason, but poor vision and hearing and a staff that move rapidly through the halls may be other reasons.

An example comes to my mind of the fear registered in the face and behavior of an old lady I met as I walked down the street. She was coming toward me slowly and was dragging a wobbly two-wheel shopping cart while her other hand held a cane. Two young boys on skateboards came zigzagging noisily down the sidewalk toward her. She absolutely froze in place as each lad passed her. The fear of being knocked down must have been great, and her precarious balance was obvious.

REVIEW OF MEDICAL LITERATURE

Rodstein (1964) points out that 72 percent of all fatal falls occur in populations 65 years of age and over.

There is one chapter on the subject of falling (Cape, 1978). This geriatrician discusses the management of falls and makes these salient points:

1. Falls should be noted and added to the problem list; the sequence of events which led up to the fall and the time of the fall should be noted.
2. If the cause is a drop attack, a cervical collar should be tried.
3. Arrhythmias should be carefully monitored.
4. The examiner's curiosity should be piqued to find the cause of the fall.

An article about external peer review of skilled nursing care in Minnesota "demonstrated characteristics and needs of patients and produced documented recommendations for Medical Evaluation Studies to strengthen multiple aspects of treatment programs." The subjects were 8917 Medicaid patients. Several problems were identified: (1) large amounts of medications, (2) indwelling catheters, (3) chronic urinary infections, (4) falling incidents, and (5) psychosocial support programs (Miller, Hurley, and Wharton, 1976).

Rodstein (1971) has described conditions which may cause falls in the elderly in an excellent chapter on accidents. He offers many excellent suggestions to help prevent falls that occur in the home and points out that "once the older person starts to fall, he continues to fall." Giorgi's list of considerations (see Chapter 33) will help the reader to change the environment.

See Table 37-1 for causes of accidental deaths due to falls.

English textbooks by geriatricians include some content about falls in the elderly (Devas, 1977; Exton-Smith and Evans, 1977; Anderson, 1977, 1971; Brocklehurst and Hanley, 1976; Caird and Judge, 1977; Hodkinson, 1975, 1976). None of them go into much detail, however.

As early as 1948 Sheldon drew attention to the rising number of falls which occur with advancing age (Sheldon, 1948, 1960). He emphasized that falls are associated with (1) vertigo, (2) the tendency to trip, (3) the difficulty in recovering balance, and (4) the sudden loss of postural control. See Figure 37-1 for the age incidence of falls in elderly men and women.

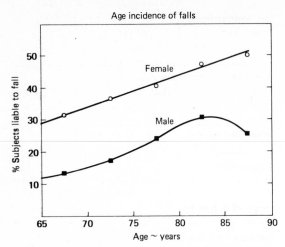

FIGURE 37-1 Age incidence of falls in elderly men and women. ○ = women (*N* = 536); ■ = men (*N* = 427). (*Exton-Smith and Evans, 1977, p. 47.*)

PREMONITORY FALLS

Devas (1977), an orthopedist, states that the commonest fall which causes a fracture is an ordinary trip or a stumble and it usually occurs in the home. The same author writes about "premonitory falls." They are falls which may occur at the onset of any acute illness, especially pneumonia. Falls caused by tripping occur more often in people aged 65 to 74 than those who are aged 75 and over (Exton-Smith and Evans, 1977). Causes for falls in women can be seen in Table 37-2. The falls which resulted in fractures are noted in Table 37-3. Exton-Smith and Evans say that apart from accidental hypothermia,

TABLE 37-2
CAUSES OF FALLS (FEMALES)

Cause	Age 65–74 (*N* = 77), %	Age 75 and Over (*N* = 113), %
Giddiness	6	16
Loss of balance	10	9
Drop attacks	14	12
Tripping	37	22

SOURCE: Exton-Smith and Evans, 1977, p. 48.

TABLE 37-3
FALLS RESULTING IN FRACTURES

	Number with Falls	Number (%) Sustaining Fractures
Men		
65–74	44	10 (18)
75 and over	87	26 (30)
Women		
65–74	77	21 (27)
75 and over	113	46 (40)

SOURCE: Exton-Smith and Evans, 1977, p. 49.

fractures constitute the major consequence of falls in the elderly population. The liability to fall increases with age and so does the age-related increase in the risk of sustaining a fracture during the fall. These findings can be seen in Table 37-2. The same authors remind us that it is worth noting the three common presenting symptoms of disease in elderly clients: (1) falls, (2) mental confusion, and (3) incontinence (1977). These are quite different from the main presenting symptoms in younger persons.

DROP ATTACKS

In the English literature "drop attacks" are given as causes of falls. Drop attacks are falls which occur without warning or loss of consciousness; the aged person is on the floor and often sustains an injury. The reasons for the attacks are not definitely known. Anderson (1971) reminds us that almost any serious illness can cause a fall in the elderly, myocardial infarction, anemia, heart block, latent chest infection, and neoplasm are a few. The fall may be due also to a hypotensive drug. He advises one to find out why the client fell.

Brocklehurst and Hanley (1976) give this list of causes of falls:

1. Environmental causes
2. Inadequate vision

3. Cerebral causes, e.g., epilepsy, drop attacks, and transient ischemic attacks (TIA)
4. Vascular causes, hypotensive drugs, syncope, micturition syncope (rapid emptying of the distended bladder causes a drop in blood pressure and syncope), and the Stokes-Adams attack when consciousness is lost

A fall may be the first indication of a major catastrophe, say these physicians, as in cases of myocardial or cerebral infarction, and it may be the only symptom in the client.

Caird and Judge (1977) warn that it is extremely important to take very seriously a history of falls which come on suddenly and do not have a clear cause in the elderly client.

FALLING ABOUT

Hodkinson (1976) reminds us that painful or deformed feet are a possible cause for immobility and unsteadiness, and he, too, writes about "premonitory falls" which herald an acute illness (Hodkinson, 1975). The same author, in a neat turn of phrase, calls multiple falls "falling about." Women are more vulnerable; they have more falls and are liable to sustain fractures when they do fall—supposedly because they are often osteoporotic. He also reminds us that Parkinson's disease is a cause of falling because of gait abnormalities. The parkinsonian patient may become afraid to walk without help because of being terrified of falling. Fear of falling was also discussed earlier in the chapter.

A perplexing problem in caring for the elderly is the safety factor (Feist, 1978). If activity and independent behavior are to be encouraged in oldsters, then the risk of a fall plays an important role. Many falls which are due to progressive physical and/or mental impairment probably cannot be anticipated or avoided (Feist, 1978).

HIP FRACTURES

The reader is referred to Devas's excellent coverage on hip fractures in the elderly (Devas, 1977). He points out that restoration of function is the most important aim, that the elderly can be jeopardized by staying in the hospital too long, and that bed rest should be as short as possible. Walking is the function most necessary for independence, and it should be achieved at the earliest possible moment.

Devas states that one hears of old people with fractured femurs taking up hospital beds, and he points out that this is a criticism of management and not an excuse. Old people are, by and large, anxious to return home and to be independent.

An old person who presents with a fracture but with no clear history of the fall or injury that caused it has to be examined carefully because some old people do have a drop attack, for no reason apparent to them. This type of injury holds a poor prognosis, "not so much for the part broken but for the integrity of the patient as a whole. Often such a fracture is a symptom of the impending dissolution of the patient."

Other fractures occur in clients who are going about their daily routines, walking, doing household chores; in these one expects a better prognosis because the fracture has been caused by considerable violence.

A misplaced feeling of pity or other emotional reaction must not influence the decision to send the patient home or to cause the patient to be admitted to the hospital. Nothing could be worse. Age alone is no indication for admission to hospital and under no circumstances should admission be merely for rest. The old person has an eternity of rest to follow and to be admitted to hospital to do nothing is the worst possible treatment that could be devised. The whole concept of return to function after a fracture . . . is activity to maintain muscle tone. (Devas, 1977, p. 103)

FRACTURES RESULTING FROM FALLS

An orthopedist states

The old lady who falls on her elbow has a special facility for producing "a bag of bones." This fracture is treated by early movements and a collar and cuff sling.

There is severe pain at first, which is controlled by simple crepe bandaging, but not too tight. A full function of the elbow is unlikely, but the patient does regain a useful arc of movement. (Devas, 1977)

Colles' fracture[1] is one of the most common injuries of the elderly; it should never cause disability and should not necessitate any interruption in the client's home life unless it is a bilateral fracture. An old person will accept a less than perfect looking wrist if it works well and there is no pain (Devas, 1977).

STRESS FRACTURES

Stress fractures are common in the geriatric population, and osteoporosis, if it is accepted as a normal condition of old age, is one of the contributing factors. The most important result of a stress fracture in old age is a complete fracture. If the person has been on steroids, then suspect a stress fracture because of the increase in osteoporosis caused by such drugs. Stress fractures can be bilateral; if one hip has a stress fracture, then the opposite hip must be suspect.

The signs of stress fractures are: (1) local tenderness at the site of the fracture, (2) swelling at the site, and (3) considerable edema. Such fractures occur in the neck of femur and the tibia.

Clients with stress fractures should continue activity as well as possible without experiencing pain from the site of the fracture, and a prophylactic fixation should be done when necessary (Devas, 1977).

REVIEW OF NURSING LITERATURE

The nursing literature on falls is pitifully scant (Feist, 1978; Pinel and Barrowclough, 1973; Shipley, 1975; Brown and Kiss, 1979; Witte, 1979).

---

[1] A fracture of the lower end of the radius, the distal fragment being displaced backward.

An important research article about falls found in the *Journal of Gerontological Nursing,* reports a survey of all the accidental falls which occurred in a small home for the aged (Feist, 1978). The findings of this study were summarized as follows:

1. A few individuals are much more accident prone than others.
2. The first 6 months of residency, and even more the first 6 weeks of residency, are the periods of highest risk.
3. The hours between 6 and 9 P.M. are the period of greatest risk.
4. Less than 3 percent of the falls caused injuries, but of these, 14 fractures resulted in permanent disabilities.
5. The poorly adjusted, confused, or agitated individual is at highest risk.
6. The use of tranquilizers by residents having accidental falls is high; the significance of this is not easy to evaluate.
7. The ambulatory, and the chairbound, are the next to be at high risk.
8. Resident insight into the causes of their falls is usually lacking.
9. Staff evaluation of the causes of falls was only available in one-third of all incident reports.

The experiences and observations of staff members led them to believe that some factors seemed to make the aged more accident prone (Feist, 1978):

1. TIA with vertigo (dizziness), syncope (fainting), or stroke
2. Muscle weakness
3. Interference with the sense of balance
4. Poor eyesight and faulty evaluation of spatial relationships often due to neural deficiencies (see Figure 37-2)
5. Urinary frequency and urgency leading to unsafe maneuvering at toileting
6. Unsteady gait due to pain, fatigue, arthritic changes, or osteoporosis
7. Improper footwear or podiatric difficulties
8. Improper clothing, such as long nightclothes or robes
9. Improper use of wheelchairs and walkers, especially on transfer
10. Mental confusion and faulty judgment

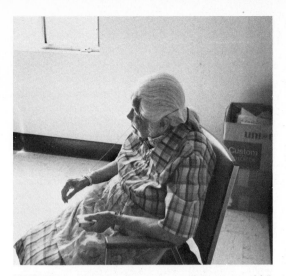

FIGURE 37-2 Visual impairment is one of the causes of falls in the elderly person. Providers of care should not move furniture or objects around in the immediate environment without checking first with the aged individual. (*Courtesy of Anthony J. Skirlick, Jr.*)

11. Mental depression with suicidal tendencies
12. Hostility and anger at confinement with attempts to gain attention

The last factor is a provocative one and reminds me of a woman in a group I once led, as described in the following vignette.

VIGNETTE 1

Mrs. J. was in her seventies and suffering from a depressive state following the suicide of her only child. The staff members had both overtly and covertly suggested that she was to blame for her daughter's death. She took to her bed, and attempts to get her up to walk or to participate in activities were usually futile. She did agree to attend some group meetings. Her behavior was unnerving to me at times, however, as she would stiffen up and begin to slide off her chair. She would also go limp when one was walking with her and appear to go down to the floor in a heap. There was no physical basis for this falling behavior according to the physician. She was never found on the floor alone, and the behavior occurred only when staff personnel attempted to work with her.

Walshe and Rosen (1979) studied the cases of patients who fell from their beds. Legal opinion is that the institution is responsible for patient falls from beds. Their investigation was conducted in a 300-bed community hospital. During the study, 22 percent of all patients admitted were over age 65. The survey source was the mandatory hospital incident report completed by the examining physician and a registered nurse. Of 106 falls during the study, the researchers examined 53 reports. They made specific recommendations for corrective action.

Benedict (1975) reported on a study conducted during a 3-month period in a nursing home. She found that most of the falls occurred in the month of January (the study took place from January through March), usually in the patients' rooms. The 3:00 to 11:00 P.M. shift had the most falls, and they occurred between 4:00 P.M. and 6:30 P.M. (The author noted that the "happy hour" was between 4:00 and 5:00 P.M.) The majority of the patients who fell were ambulatory and alert. No restraints were ordered. All the floors were carpeted. *All the patients were on tranquilizers.*

Gould (1975) stated that poor design of environment was a strong factor in all patient accidents reported in her survey. In the nursing home, she found that most accidents occurred in the residents' rooms during hours when the elderly had trouble distinguishing between light and dark.

In Chapter 20, "Musculoskeletal Problems in Aging," we are reminded that pathological changes in the femur increase the tendency to fall. Hayter (1974) reminds us that the blood vessels in the elderly do not adjust quickly enough to keep an adequate blood supply to all parts of the body as the old person moves from one position to another and that dizziness is common, especially if positions are changed suddenly. Then a fall may occur.

The old person must be taught to sit a bit before standing, then to stand briefly and hold onto something before beginning to walk. Sudden turns or distractions from walking should be avoided so that balance is not lost and a fall result.

CAUTION DURING TESTS

In an article about iron-deficiency anemia, Flynn cautions about the procedures often necessary for diagnosis which involve risk. One of them is the fall which might occur from the sigmoidoscopy table. Another fall could occur from high x-ray tables—especially when there is a small stool to use to get on and off the table. Flynn also points out that dehydration and weakness during periods of fasting for gastrointestinal tests also carry high risk of falling with resultant broken bones (Flynn, 1978).

The same author mentions another type of falls—those which occur when elderly persons are shopping and are mugged and thrown or knocked to the ground. Such falls are not uncommon because of the crimes against old people, many of whom are easy prey because they shop alone (see Figure 37-3a).

During a trip to Malaysia, I asked the nurse in charge of a nursing home if she had problems with broken bones due to falls. She said no because she had taken care of such problems. She then led me to a ward where the first six beds were without bed frames; the mattresses were placed on the floor. She said the ladies had adapted quite well to the mattress on the floor and the low bedside stand. As she explained the solution, two of the nursing home mascots, two large dogs, came bounding in and jumped over the mattresses. The elderly Chinese women smiled at us and were quite unperturbed by the antics of the dogs.

While we do not have a lot of material in the literature regarding implications for nursing intervention, Feist has certainly made a good start. We definitely need more on the care of the people with hip fractures. Wolanin and Holloway (1980) have paved the way in that respect, for they have done intensive work on the confusion, disorientation, and translocation shock which occur in the elderly who have hip fractures. Feist's survey revealed some implications for intervention which are listed here because they are pragmatic, not difficult to implement, do not require new equipment or more money, and focus on prevention of the fall.

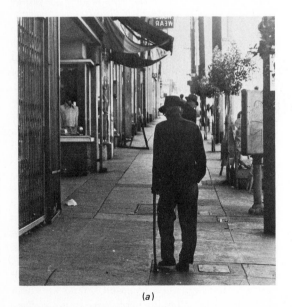

(a)

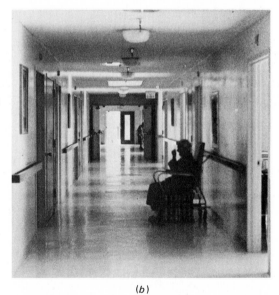

(b)

FIGURE 37-3 Environmental causes of falls may include uneven sidewalks, broken walkways, changes in grade in the sidewalk, or objects lying on the path. (a) Changes in the sidewalk. (b) Highly waxed floors increase the chance of falls, and the glare often hurts the eyes of the visually impaired. [(a) *Courtesy of Richard Davis.* (b) *Courtesy of Will Patton.*]

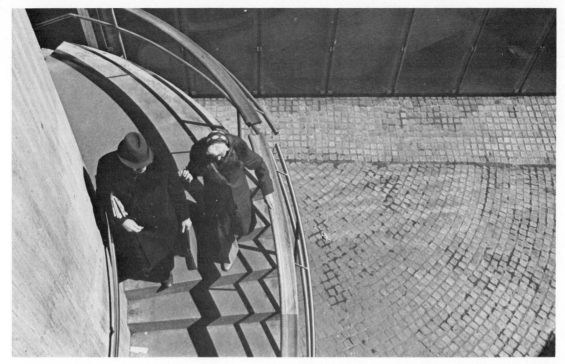

FIGURE 37-4 Falls can be associated with dizziness or the tendency to trip (Sheldon 1948, 1960). Cerebral problems such as transient ischemic attacks (TIAs) or vascular problems from hypotensive drugs, for example, may be reasons for falls. If heights are involved, as in climbing stairs, especially with tricky, hard-to-navigate stairways or stairs that vary in width, there also are increased dangers for the elderly. See the difference in the width of the stairs in the circular staircase pictured here. (*Courtesy of Harvey Finkle.*)

IMPLICATIONS FOR INTERVENTION

The list below is quoted from Feist (1978):[2]

1. Eternal vigilance, close supervision of the confused with individualization of the plan of care for all remains essential.
2. Much reassurance during the initial six months of residency is very important.
3. Early case findings of the accident-prone individual, and concerted efforts by the entire team to minimize unsafe activities and behaviors is essential.
4. Review of medications, especially tranquilizers, as to need, dosage, and side effects must be continuous.
5. Staffing, especially at the most dangerous hours.
6. A safe environment, especially for all ambulatory residents, must be maintained.
7. Attempts to deal with confused and agitated individuals through reality therapy [I am wondering if the author did not mean reality orientation here], behavior modification, and tender loving care.
8. Residents should be taught the safe use of wheelchairs and walkers.
9. The ambulatory resident should be observed for signs of weakness or fatigue and be assisted as necessary.

---

[2] Reprinted with permission of *Journal of Gerontological Nursing,* 4(6):15–17, November–December, 1978. Copyright Charles B. Slack, Inc., Medical Publisher, Thorofare, N.J.

10. Continue to gather further information to initiate a program of accident prevention.

Accident prevention initiated by the nurse may be modified by the client, as happened in the following example.

VIGNETTE 2

A colleague who was working with an elderly woman who lived at home told me this vignette. The nurse had advised the woman to roll up her rugs in the rooms and put them in storage, as there were rolled edges on some of them, and the woman had tripped several times. The nurse went back several times to check on her and the safety suggestion. The lady said, "My dear, I know you mean well, but I have lived with those rugs for most of my life and I cannot bear to roll them up and put them away. But I have listened to you, and now I do not walk across them, I just walk on the bare floor around the rug rather than roll them up."

See Figure 37-4 regarding stairs treacherous for oldsters to nagivate.

SUMMARY

In this chapter, the literature was reviewed on an important problematic area in the care of the elderly: falls. The paucity of the material, and the lack of interest in writing about the problem, make it a prime area for research studies. Some of the serious consequences of this problem when it occurs were briefly discussed. A good portion of the chapter was devoted to interventions which might be implemented by caretakers. The interventions were teased out of the available literature. *Prevention* is still the watchword to avert the consequences of wandering behavior and falls in the elderly.

REFERENCES

Anderson, W. Ferguson: *Practical Management of the Elderly,* 2d ed., Blackwell Scientific Publications Ltd., Oxford, 1971.

———: The role of the physician, in A. N. Exton-Smith and J. Grimley Evans (eds.), *Care of the Elderly,* Grune & Stratton, New York, 1977.

Benedict, Sharon: *Medical Care Evaluation Studies for Utilization Review in Skilled Nursing Facilities,* Hospital Utilization Project, Pittsburgh, Pa., June 1975.

Brocklehurst, J. G., and T. Hanley: *Geriatric Medicine for Students,* Churchill Livingstone, London, 1976.

Brown, Mary H., and Margaraet E. Kiss: A problem-focused approach to nursing audit: patient falls, *Cancer Nursing,* (10):389–391, October 1979.

Caird, F. I., and T. G. Judge: *Assessment of the Elderly Patient,* Pitman Medical Publishing Company, London, 1977.

Cape, Ronald: *Aging: Its Complex Management,* Harper & Row, Hagerstown, Md., 1978.

Devas, Michael (ed.): *Geriatric Orthopaedics,* Academic, New York, 1977.

Exton-Smith, A. N., and J. Grimley Evans: *Care of the Elderly,* Grune & Stratton, New York, 1977.

Fales, Edward D., Jr.: Falls: Threats to oldsters, *Today's Health,* **37**(2):14, February 1959.

Feist, Ruth R.: A survey of accidental falls in a small home for the aged, *Journal of Gerontological Nursing,* **4**(6):15–17, November–December 1978.

Flynn, Kathleen T.: Iron deficiency anemia among the elderly, *Nurse Practitioner,* **3**(6):20–24, November–December 1978.

Gould, G.: A survey of incident reports, *Journal of Gerontological Nursing,* **1**(4):23–26, July–August 1975.

Hayter, Jean: Biologic changes of aging, *Nursing Forum* **13**(3):290–308, 1974.

Hodkinson, H. M.: *Common Symptoms of Disease in the Elderly,* Blackwell Scientific Publications, Ltd., London, 1976.

———: *An Outline of Geriatrics,* Academic, New York, 1975.

Miller, Winston, Sandra J. Hurley, and Elaine Wharton: External peer review of skilled nursing care in Minnesota, *American Journal Public Health,* **66**(3):278–285, March 1976.

Pinel, C., and F. Barrowclough: Accidents in geriatric wards, *Nursing Mirror,* **137**(13):10–11, Sept. 28, 1973.

Rodstein, M.: Accidents among the aged: Incidence, causes, and prevention, *Journal of Chronic Disease,* **17**:515–526, June 1964.

———: Heart disease in the aged, in Isadore Rossman (ed.), *Clinical Geriatrics,* Lippincott, Philadelphia, 1971.

Sheldon, J. H.: On the natural history of falls in old age, *British Medical Journal,* **2**:1685–1689, December 10, 1960.

———: *The Social Medicine of Old Age,* Oxford Univsity Press, London, 1948.

Shipley, S. B.: Let's not let them fall, *RN,* **38**(11):57–61, 1975.

Walshe, Anne, and Harry Rosen: A study of patient falls from bed, *Journal of Nursing Administration,* **9**(5):31–35, May 1979.

Witte, Natalie Slocumb: Why the elderly fall, *American Journal of Nursing,* **79**(11):1950–1952, November 1979.

Wolanin, Mary Opal, and Janet Holloway: Relocation confusion: Intervention for prevention, in Irene Mortenson Burnside (ed.), *Psychosocial Nursing Care of the Aged,* 2d ed., McGraw-Hill, New York, 1980.

THIRTY-EIGHT

THE NEEDS OF OLDER WOMEN

Irene Mortenson Burnside

The older woman is the forgotten woman in our culture—she's considered sexless, powerless and useless.
Adele Rice Nudel

LEARNING OBJECTIVES

- Discuss demographic data regarding women over 65 in the United States.
- List five problems common in the care of elderly women.
- List five diseases more common in older women than men.
- Discuss present problems with Medicare insurance coverage.
- Describe five therapeutic interventions for assisting women who are very recently widowed.
- Describe one aspect of crime prevention for elderly women living in their own homes.

De Castillejo (1973) wrote, "It would seem easy enough for me to write on 'The Older Woman' since I am one, but perhaps it is for that very reason I find it difficult. One can really only see situations clearly when one is outside them, not when one is in the middle of living them. However, there is no help for it. When I have passed the stage of being an older woman I shall also be beyond writing at all." (And now that students also speak of me as an older woman, I am concerned about our plight.) (See Figure 38-1.)

The preponderance of older women in our society is most apparent in public, in the market, in the bank, on the bus, and in a variety of treatment settings. Who knows how many live silently in old hotels or deteriorating neighborhoods? Nurses will have to be increasingly cognizant of the special needs and problems of old women. The very numbers of aged females, and the sad plight of so many of them, are but two of the reasons nurses need to concern themselves with improving psychosocial caring of aged women. Their problems have roots in the psychosocial elements of poverty, living arrangements, vicious crimes against them, plus multiple health problems.

The reader is referred to recent publications about older women (Williams, 1975; Matthews, 1978). I especially recommend an excellent article by Seltzer (1979).

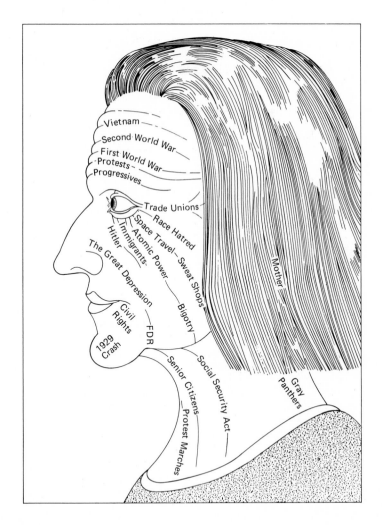

FIGURE 38-1 *Courtesy of Stuart Leeds.*

TABLE 38-1

THE OLDER POPULATION IN THE TWENTIETH CENTURY

Year	Total	Men	Women	Ratio Women/Men
1900	3,080,000	1,555,000	1,525,000	98/100
1930	6,634,000	3,325,000	3,309,000	100/100
1970	19,972,000	8,367,000	11,605,000	139/100
1975	22,400,000	9,172,000	13,228,000	144/100
2000	30,600,000	12,041,000	18,558,000	154/100

SOURCE: U.S. Department of Health, Education, and Welfare, 1976.

DEMOGRAPHIC DATA

Most older persons are women; in fact, in 1977 there were 13.9 million women as compared with 9.5 million men in the 65-and-older age group (Ball, 1977). Between the ages of 65 and 74, there are 130 women per 100 men; after age 74, there are 173 women per 100 men. The average for the total population is 145 women per 100 men. In the year 2000, there will be 154 older women for each 100 men (see Table 38-1).

The data in Table 38-1 tell us something about the need to study the plight of older women *now*. (See Figure 38-2.)

MARITAL STATUS

In 1976 most older men were married (77 percent), but most of the older women were widows (53 percent). There were more than five times as many widows as widowers. Nearly 70

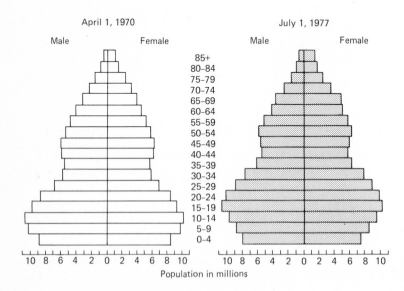

FIGURE 38-2 Age-sex distribution of the United States population, including Armed Forces overseas. (*Metropolitan Life Statistical Bulletin, 1979.*)

percent are widows with little chance of remarriage (Dowling, 1977). Women who are married can expect to live 11 years of their lives in widowhood. It is common knowledge that men tend to marry younger women. In the past, older women have been condemned for marrying men much younger than they, while older men are applauded for marrying young women.

LIVING ARRANGEMENTS

In 1976, 8 in every 10 older men, but only 6 of every 10 older women, lived in a family setting. Approximately three-fifths of older men lived in families that included the wife, but only one-third of older women lived in families that included the husband. More than three times as many older women lived alone or with nonrelatives than did older men (Dowling, 1977).

PERSONAL INCOME

Women and the minority aged are overrepresented among the aged poor; in fact, women 65 years and over are the poorest single group in America. The poorest old women are single women and widows who represent 50 percent of women over 65. It is estimated that widows receive only 50 percent of the pension rights they are entitled to. Retirement benefits for women average only 75 percent of those men receive (National Action Forum for Older Women, Statistical Profile, n.d.) The reader is referred to Baldwin's article (1978) on poverty and older women.

EMPLOYMENT

In 1976, about 20 percent of aged men or 1.8 million and 8 percent of women 65 and over (1.1 million) were in the labor force (U.S. Department of Health, Education, and Welfare, 1976). In the age group of 55 to 64, women's median income is about one-third of their male counterparts (National Action Forum, n.d.).

NATIONAL ACTION FORUM FOR OLDER WOMEN

The National Action Forum for Older Women begins a handout with these lines: "We older women will no longer tolerate our invisibility. We will no longer permit ourselves to be shunted into a corner. We will acquire the power to no longer let ourselves be considered nonpersons."

The Declaration of Older Women from the Houston, Texas, 1977, meeting lists services that "will enable elderly women to live with dignity and security":

- Suitable housing for women living alone, with special concern for their safety.
- Home health and social services, including visiting nurse services, homemaker services, Meals-on-Wheels, and other protective services that will enable older women to function comfortably in their own homes if they so wish instead of moving to institutions.
- Public transportation in both urban and rural areas for otherwise housebound women.
- Efforts to stimulate the elderly woman's interest in life with particular attention to needs of the frail elderly, age 75 and older.
- Bilingual, bicultural programs, including health services, recreation, and other programs to support elderly women of limited English-speaking ability.

Medicare provisions in the Social Security Act should be liberalized by:

- Combining Part B benefits for optional medical services with Part A benefits for hospitalization so that all the elderly receive mandatory coverage for physicians' services as well as for hospital insurance.
- Expanding the Medicare system to include prescription drugs, hearing aids, eyeglasses and eye care, and dental care.

For purposes of organization of psychosocial care in this chapter, each of the services listed above will be discussed.

SUITABLE HOUSING

One of the prime considerations in suitable housing should be safety. Many old women live in deteriorating parts of towns or cities, or on the edges where surveillance by police officers may be low. Break-ins, robberies, and rapes are common news items. I once interviewed a 78-year-old woman who had been raped in her own home and felt lucky that she had not been cut across the face as a woman neighbor of hers had been. Because of her high trust in people, she had difficulty in accepting the public health nurse's suggestions of ways to make her home more secure. In her childhood she never had had to lock doors, and it was difficult for her to grasp how unsafe her neighborhood was even after the rape experience. (See Table 38-2.)

HEALTH AND SERVICES

Stress   Stress is beginning to take its toll in women who have pressure jobs and great responsibilities. In the past year, two acquaintances who are 55 years of age have had cardiovascular accidents. The tension and over-commitment of many working women may be an area for the nurse to intervene. Elevated blood pressures, beginning ulcers, skin rashes, and any other new symptoms that might indicate stress are areas for prevention. The use of the Holmes-Rahe (1967) scale might be one way to quickly note stress-producing events in the older woman's life.

Chronic Illness   About 42 percent of women over 65 have chronic physical conditions limiting normal activities, reports the National Institute on Aging. Women, who are on the average older than men, have higher rates of arthritis, diabetes, hypertension, back impairments, and vision impairments than men who have higher rates of asthma, chronic bronchitis, hernias, ulcers, and hearing impairments (DHEW, 1976). Assessing the situation to keep older women in their own homes is often complicated because families are uneasy and do not wish them to live alone in their own homes, which may be unsafe both internally and externally. Or relatives may be anxious to sell the house for whatever reason.

Sometimes the older woman may handle the sale of her home herself. For example, here is a personal letter regarding a friend who had to help with the house situation:

My friend, who is in the acute hospital, signed a Power of Attorney for me to pay her bills, to sell her house and furniture. I spent ten days going through everything in the house. There were boxes of materials which I gave to her church for quilts, and also what silverware her niece did not take. I gave her flowers to her friends and also other little mementos. I have the house sold, I think. At least, I have a contract for the deed until the abstract, etc., are brought to date. Hopefully in a couple of weeks I will have it off my hands.

LIVING ALONE

Women who live alone in their own homes are subject to lack of feedback, lack of interaction with others, a deteriorating house and/or yard, crime, inability to shop for themselves, and lack of transportation. Falls, broken hips, lying on the floor injured without help, inability to care for personal needs, and slovenly habits may be some specific problems.

Women who are married to men older than they may be caring for a husband who has had a stroke, is blind, or wanders at night. Such women may need tremendous psychological support. A home health aide, a public health nurse, or a visiting nurse may provide such a support.

It is important to encourage the aged woman to renew interests. She may have spent all her life working so hard either raising a family or employed by others that she has denied much of her own creativity and/or enjoyment of leisure. Latent interests and desires need to be discussed. If she lived close to the earth, encourage her in growing flowers and plants. If she enjoyed animals and can still care for them, suggest a pet. Pets do seem to help in the need to nurture—to feel a sense of neededness (see Figures 38-3 and 38-4).

TRANSPORTATION PROBLEMS

It is important for health professionals to be aware that depression occurs in older women who can no longer drive, just as it often does in

TABLE 38-2
INTERVIEW WITH A 78-YEAR-OLD WOMAN

Opening: Interviewer checked vision and hearing with opening of several amenities. Sat close to and vis-à-vis the woman, at a right angle to the class (to decrease anxiety of interviewee).

Interview	Analysis
Interviewer: How long have you been alone? *Mrs. A:* Four years—since 1966. *Interviewer:* And what happened in 1966? *Mrs. A.:* My husband died. (She is crying.)	The elderly will more often cry while talking about deceased spouse or child than at any other point in an interview. Let them cry, as they usually regain composure readily.
Interviewer: It must be pretty painful to think about. It has been 11 years since you lost your husband? (Asked a question.)	Checking the distance from death. (Noting the drop of the voice and the lessening of tears helps interviewer determine the emotion behind content.)
Mrs. A.: Yes. (Said softly, her voice dropped, control of crying.)	
Interviewer: It helps us if you can tell us what is really hard for you. Tell us the hardest part about being alone.	Mrs. A. knew she was participating in a "teaching" interview; she had been asked to help teach about aging.
Mrs. A.: I didn't mind that part—being alone—not right off the bat—but I lost my boy in 1973. (Is crying again.)	Interviewer needs to check dates when they are mentioned for clues of confusion or disorientation.
Interviewer: Can you tell us a little about that? (It took a few moments for Mrs. A. to compose herself at this point. The interviewer waited and held her hand.)	Important to observe how clients regain composure and how long it takes. Watch for nonverbal cues that preceded crying to anticipate future crying episodes in interview. Some old people will blink, others will have trembling lips, still others grimace.
Mrs. A.: Well, he had leukemia and he laid for 3 years in a hospital bed and suffered hell. *Interviewer:* How old was he?	
Mrs. A.: He was 32 when it started and he died when he was 38. When they buried him, it rained on his coffin. And a year later, almost to the day, my daughter died, and I've never gotten over it. (Mrs. A. was quite broken up as she said this.)	Symbolism here strikes a deep note of sadness and pathos as she speaks. ("I've never gotten over it" is a common phrase used by the elderly to describe the throes of grief.) The symbolism of the words, I felt, meant "tears on the coffin, too."
Interviewer: So you think a lot about your son and your daughter and how much you miss them?	Interviewer is acknowledging her sadness, responding to both verbal and nonverbal statements.
Mrs. A.: See, I was here and they were in another state. My husband really got bad. . . . We had to come here because he had bronchial asthma and then it got his heart. He died here. (Mrs. A. mentioned the place where he died, and then went on to discuss all the places she knew in the area and how she got around when she used to drive.)	Interviewer nodded, held her hand.

TABLE 38-2 INTERVIEW WITH A 78-YEAR-OLD WOMAN (*Continued*)

Interview	Analysis
Interviewer: You don't drive anymore?	
Mrs. A.: I gave up driving 'cause I figured I might hurt somebody. Yes, it was hard to give up driving.	
Interviewer: Tell me about the car you learned to drive on.	Pride is involved here. She proudly relates having driven 51 years. Interviewer intentionally moves away from sad theme.
Mrs. A.: You won't believe me when I tell you— a 1925 Reverse Buick. Made in 1925, and I got rid of it in 1926 because nobody could drive it—it was terrible.	
Interviewer: You gave up driving. Because of your eyesight or hearing?	The usual reasons for ceasing driving are hearing and vision loss.
Mrs. A.: Not that . . . I just don't eat and got dizzy. So . . . (broke up crying again).	
Interviewer: You have had a lot of losses in 10 years—husband, son, and daughter. Has anything else serious happened to you in the last few years that has been hard to accept?	Interviewer knew prior to this interview that Mrs. A. had been raped 2 months previously, but was not sure she would be willing to share the information in the classroom.
Mrs. A.: Well, not exactly to me; a close girl-friend's son got killed, and I wasn't able to be with her when she lost him (crying again). She was always with me when I lost my children and husband.	Loyalty to her friends. Importance of confidantes (especially in widowhood).
Interviewer: Are you afraid of living alone?	Crime against elderly women who live alone is often brutal.
Mrs. A.: I was raped and robbed once and he took everything I had—about 2 months ago I had to go to court. The robber is now in jail. He did me and two others. I was beat up—black and blue— terrible. I didn't see him come in. He hit me with his fist and when I came to, he hit me again. I had no way to turn the light on. I couldn't tell who he was. (She then described in detail the other women who were raped and robbed. One had 40 stitches across her face from a knife wound; Mrs. A. felt she had been lucky.) Later officers called and asked me to come and identify him. He got $7 and left my purse on the table with all my papers and I'm glad of that. It cost me $300 to put new bars on my windows. I had to put a new door on with a dead bolt lock.	The importance of money and the extra expenses incurred when one owns a home.
Mrs. A.: I have to wait until my son comes so he can get his stuff out.	(She lived in a bad section of town, and the inter-viewer gently suggested that she is, indeed, in a very unsafe neighborhood.)
Interviewer: (She then discussed her arthritis. She takes 3 tablespoons of mix in a glass with 1 table-spoon of mint-flavored cod-liver oil. She also takes aspirin.)	Interview ended with the focus on Mrs. A. telling the class how she had also "licked the pains of her arthritis." She was paid for helping teach. The goal of the interview was to end with a sense of achievement for her; it had been an interview replete with loss, sadness, and brutality. The objective for the class had been to learn about multiple losses and the crimes against elderly women.

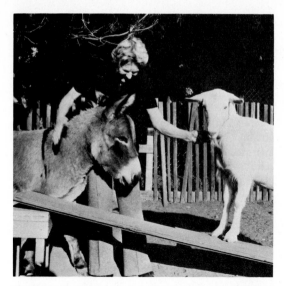

FIGURE 38-3 This woman's fondness for her pets is obvious in the photograph. She is especially fond of Jeremiah, a miniature donkey. Although it is difficult to see Peepers, there is a duck sitting on Jeremiah's back. Peepers, two cats, and a dog are the official welcoming committee for visitors. (*Courtesy of Dadi Noeggerath.*)

men who cannot renew their driver's license. I have observed this especially in women who have driven for many years, who declare with pride that they learned to drive on a Model T or a Model A car! Knowledge of public transportation and resources may be unavailable to them, and so they may become more housebound than is really necessary, because of the lack of knowledge of what is available in their own community. Helping with bus schedules, teaching about services on airlines is helpful. Many older women have never flown and are unaware of services offered by the airlines, such as special diets, escort service, phoning ahead to make connections on another plane, stewardess services.

THE FRAIL ELDERLY

The importance of working with the frail elderly woman was underscored in the declaration of older women quoted earlier (see Chapter 30, "Assessment of the Frail Elderly"). Some frail elderly women are tougher than we give them credit for; often the frailty is overemphasized. Their underlying strengths are not as-

sessed or observed. Even those confined to wheelchairs display amazing qualities of stoicism. Studying octogenarians, nonagenarians, and centenarians could be a fruitful area of research for nurses.

LANGUAGE AND CULTURAL ASPECTS

Hall (1969) states that "people cannot act or interact at all in any meaningful way except through the medium of culture." While future generations may not have the language problems the present aged often do, there continue to be language barriers for some aged who have not learned English fluently enough to negotiate in the medical world or the bureaucratic world. I recall sitting in an income tax office with many little old women about me. Some understood and spoke English poorly and were absolutely addled about why they were there and why they should be paying income tax. With the language problems and the complicated income tax forms, they seemed dazed. They were also somewhat frightened since an authority, the Internal Revenue Service, had called them to appear.

It is difficult to find bilingual persons to assist in psychosocial care; junior colleges, high schools, and universities could be of great help here if they were just tapped or knew about the needs in the community, particularly in nursing homes where many of these persons seem to be.

I am reminded of the story told by a colleague who was in a clinic with a Turkish mother and a sick child. They had waited a long time, and the nurse who was acting as their advocate requested that the instructions be written in Turkish as the mother could not read English. A nurse returned a bit later and handed the advocate instructions in Italian, saying, "Here, you will have to take these; it is all we have now" (Potter, 1978).

MEDICARE

Medicare does not provide payment for prescription drugs, hearing aids, eyeglasses, eye care, or dental care. Lack of prostheses creates many difficulties, and this is one area all old people could benefit from, but especially elderly women, many of whom live alone and at poverty level.

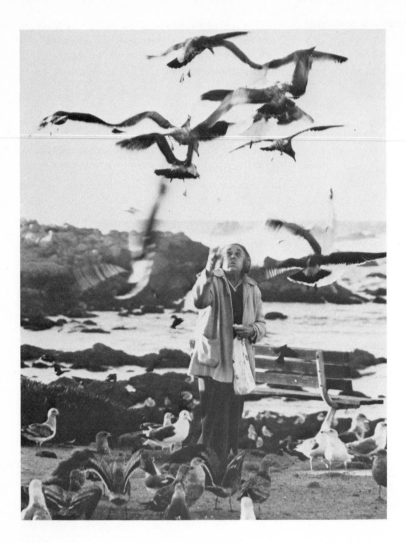

FIGURE 38-4 Feeding wild birds is one pastime some older women truly enjoy; I have observed this habit worldwide. Often they become very possessive and resent others feeding or frightening the birds. This lady was photographed along the Pacific Coast in California. (*Copyright 1979, James Dowgialo.*)

They, indeed, are deprived of the basic aspects of medical care. One has only to observe the caries in teeth and the problems in vision and hearing which ultimately affect communication, friendship, mobility, orientation, and social aspects. One needs to assess the impact the lack of such prostheses has for the older woman. Self-esteem goes skidding when these losses cannot be taken care of or substituted for, even though Otten (1977) says, "Wrinkles will twinkle, fat's where it's at and the sag's in the bag."

A dentist writes, "My observation has been that when the edentulous [toothless] person is provided with a well-fitting denture, especially an upper, there is an immediate improvement in self-concept and behavior. The patient stands erect, smiles more readily, speaks more easily and becomes more willing to socialize. Well-fitting dentures can immeasurably enhance feelings of self-esteem, there aiding a strengthened ego structure" (Epstein, 1976).

SAFETY FACTORS

The Declaration of Older Women of 1977 does not include the problems of the vicious crimes committed against elderly women; however, they must be discussed and prevention considered.

In Columbus, Georgia, during a 4-month period, five elderly women had been strangled in their homes by an intruder who sexually assaulted them. Table 38-2 describes a 78-year-old woman who had been robbed and raped in her home. Another time I interviewed a woman over 80 who had been pistol-whipped when she was in her early seventies and was employed as a restaurant manager. She lost the sight of one eye plus her job as a result.

The time and ability to listen to the brutality described and experienced by these elderly victims are certainly important requirements for nurses—wherever they are working. Rape is an area of concern for older women, especially for the one who lives alone. She may be trusting and open the door without checking first who is there; she may be forgetful and not close windows and doors, or lock them. Old women who live alone in deteriorating neighborhoods have described their fears to me when I was doing home nursing. They also may have illusions and mistake objects for prowlers (Burnside, 1979c).

Whatever nurses can do to encourage the safety of the home environment by checking locks, windows, alarm systems, etc., may ultimately aid the person to continue living at home. The nurse must also listen to the fears expressed by clients. Many elderly women will not leave their apartment or home after dark.

THE INSTITUTIONALIZED AGED

Some years ago, I interviewed elderly women on wards in a large rehabilitation hospital. I asked the women how happy they were these days. These are a few of the replies:

Mrs. L., 93 years old: "Sometimes I get *homesick;* I buried them all—nine brothers and sisters."

Mrs. H., 84 years old: "I am fairly happy; my sister comes to visit, but I feel sad that *I did not pursue my music further.*"

Miss K., 68 years old: "How could you be happy in the hospital?"

Mrs. F., 76 years old: "I am *sad* about losing my husband."

Mrs. D., 70 years old: "I am not too happy because of my *loss of eyesight* and my legs are numb and circulation is poor."

Miss M., 77 years old: "Not very happy; it is due to the *lack of being able to do anything.*"

Note the italicized words and phrases which give some clues to the possible tentative nursing diagnoses which were stated subjectively by the women.

JEALOUS SPOUSES

It has been my experience that elderly women who are admitted to units with their husbands may become quite jealous of their husbands. Nurses will need to use great tact and discretion in caring for the husband, for example, when doing interviews, assessments, dressings, or just leaning in close to explain medication changes. If the wife is suffering from poor vision and/or hearing, she seems to feel even more left out. It is cruel to tease the jealous spouse, but that unfortunately often happens to institutionalized aged persons, regardless of sex. And if the aged woman in the institution is aware of the ratio of women to men in institutions (about 4 to 1), she has good cause to worry! (See Chapter 13 for more about management of jealous spouses.)

EXPRESSION OF GRIEF

Chapter 10 discusses grief reactions, but they are important enough to elaborate on in this chapter, too. A nurse should encourage expression of grief about children, husbands, and siblings. Even though the death may not have been recent, anniversary dates will trigger reactions of depression. "There is something intensely moving in the sight of older women who begin the process of resuming their personal odyssey through the courage of simply holding on" (McLeish, 1976). I have written elsewhere about how often elderly women will mention children they have lost (Burnside, 1979b). One woman told of three daughters dying in infancy (Coles, 1973).

In a lovely, lovely poem about the role of widowhood, Wyse (1978) has expressed the transition.

THE WIDOW
In the beginning
I would look at my watch and say,
"Yesterday he was here."

It has been a long time now since
I looked at my watch,
It has been so long
I do not even look at the calendar.

But in the beginning
People listened to each detail
As if listening confirmed their own mortality.
They were still here at the end of the story.
I guess fresh grief is like fresh milk:
We consume it quickly before it sours.

But grief cannot be worn
Season after season
Like a string of pearls.

Mourning becomes an embarrassment
To those who watch
The seasons of our sorrow.

A well-behaved widow
Does not cry.
(Me? Cry? Just because
I am lonesome for
The only man I ever loved?)

A good widow
Gets on with life.
(I brush my teeth and do not beat
My hands against the wall. I never look up
From my needlepoint and ask, "Why?")

A proper widow
Knows her place.
(Of course, I understand that
You will invite me to the next *party—*
The one with women only.)

A thoughtful widow
Makes no demands on children.
(I smile and tell them yes, go ahead.
I know you have your own life. I do not say,
"Once I had a life.")

I think now as I lie here in the dark
Of all the things we meant to do.
Alone they are nothing. But who wants
To listen to the solo song of widowhood?

No one but another widow, for she
Is the only one who knows the bitter truth.
It never gets better;
It only gets ordinary.

From Lois Wyse, On being a woman, *Woman's Day,* February 3, 1978, p. 87.

Assisting in grief work is commonplace in gerontological nursing. See Chapters 10 and 11 for nursing interventions during grief.

Baldridge (1978) gives practical suggestions for assisting a woman recently widowed:

- The first person you should call is her family lawyer, then the funeral home director. Begin immediate preparations for the funeral and the subsequent services. If there will be church services, the clergyman must be notified, and a time of the service decided.
- If you are in charge, work quietly, efficiently, and rapidly. Have someone else answer telephone calls in her home, give out information about funeral home, services, etc.
- Have friends prepare food for her and her family for the next few days.
- Make a list of everyone close to the family who must be notified by telephone or mailgram, and have someone make the necessary calls (if the widow is agreeable).
- Keep a list of people arriving from out of town. Make sure someone meets them at the airport or stations, have a room reservation if there is not room for them with friends. Transportation will also have to be provided for them.
- If donations to a charity are to be sent instead of flowers, details should be worked out at once.
- Call the newspaper, arrange to have paid notices in the next edition. Give all known funeral details. (In some Protestant services a eulogy may be given by a friend.)
- If there are to be pallbearers, notify them and give instructions. If there are many out-of-town family members and friends, someone could serve lunch after the services.

- It is well to remember that the widow may have hidden strengths. She may wish to attend to many of these details herself. If so, step back and be ready to lend a hand as she proceeds.

CENTENARIAN WOMEN: "THE SMALL CIRCLE OF THE OLD"

It can be noted from the 1970 Census Report in Table 38-3 that centenarian women are outnumbered by males, except in the Negro and other races where the female lives longer. These women have outlived nearly all others. It is important for nurses to become significant persons in the lives of these women and to serve as a catalyst in friendship formation to prevent the loss of confidantes and friendships (Burnside, 1979a).

SEXUAL SELF-IMAGE

Calderone (1975) wrote, "I would hope that older women would begin to command respect and admiration not in *spite* of being older but *because* of it. Their self-images, including their sexual self-image, is at stake here . . . but in the end all older women need to achieve recognition that their bodies, minds, spirits, and sexuality are truly beautiful." Sexuality is covered in Chapter 25 and assessment of sexuality in Chapter 26.

LONGEVITY OF PROMINENT WOMEN

Prominent women, defined as "those who have achieved distinction in a particular field of endeavor," definitely live longer on the average than women of the general population. The conclusion of a study by the Metropolitan Life Insurance Company echoes the findings of a study done 10 years ago about the longevity of prominent men in the United States (*Metropolitan Life Statistical Bulletin,* 1979). Of the 2352 eminent women who were subjects, 539 were educators,

or about 23 percent of the total. Women of letters were the next largest professional group, about 17 percent. This is the first longevity study of prominent women.

A FASCINATING THOUGHT

A writer of science fiction wrote a fascinating article. Le Guin (1976) writes of selecting a friendly native for an arriving spaceship with room for one passenger. The spaceship captain requests a person who would be an exemplary person to typify the race. Le Guin says she would

. . . go down to the local Woolworth's, or the local village marketplace, and pick an old woman, over sixty, from behind the costume jewelry counter or the betel-nut booth. Her hair would not be red or blonde or lustrous dark, her skin would not be dewy fresh, she would not have the secret of eternal youth. She might, however, show you a small snapshot of her grandson, who is working in Nairobi. She is a bit vague about where Nairobi is, but extremely proud of the grandson. She has worked hard at small, unimportant jobs all her life, jobs like cooking, cleaning, bringing up kids, selling little objects of adornment or pleasure to other people. She was a virgin once a long time ago, and then a sexually potent fertile female, and then went through menopause. She has given birth several times and faced death several times—the same times. She is facing the final birth/death a little more nearly and clearly every day now. Sometimes her feet hurt something terrible. She never was educated to anything like her capacity, and that is a shameful waste and a crime against humanity, but so common a crime should not and cannot be hidden from Altair. Anyhow, she's not dumb. She has a stock of sense, wit, patience, and experiential shrewdness, which the Altaireans might, or might not, perceive as wisdom. If they are wiser than we, then, of course, we don't know how they'd perceive it. But if they are wiser than we, they may know how to perceive that inmost mind and heart

TABLE 38-3

ALTERNATIVE ESTIMATES OF THE POPULATION 100 YEARS OLD AND OVER, BY SEX AND RACE: APRIL 1, 1970

Estimation Method	All Classes	White		Black and Other Races	
		Male	Female	Male	Female
Number					
Census count*	106,441	46,015	42,965	8,323	9,138
Medicare records†	7,341	1,508	4,209	513	1,111
Forward-survival:					
From 1960 with 1959–1961 life table rates	3,395	1,109	1,985	121	180
From 1950 with 1949–1951 and 1959–1961 life table rates	3,222	1,090	1,795	136	201
From 1960 with Medicare rates	7,713	1,606	4,263	651	1,193
Population reconstruction:‡					
Stationary assumption	8,211	1,387	3,957	958	1,909
Least squares§	7,854	1,441	4,173	661	1,579
Preferred estimate	4,800	1,250	2,650	300	600
Percent					
Census count*	100.0	43.2	40.4	7.8	8.6
Medicare records†	100.0	20.5	57.4	7.0	15.1
Forward-survival					
From 1960 with 1959–1961 life table rates	100.0	32.7	58.5	3.6	5.3
From 1950 with 1949–1951 and 1959–1961 life table rates	100.0	33.8	55.7	4.2	6.2
From 1960 with Medicare rates	100.0	20.8	55.3	8.4	15.5
Population reconstruction:‡					
Stationary assumption	100.0	16.9	48.2	11.7	23.2
Least squares§	100.0	18.3	53.1	8.4	20.1
Preferred estimate	100.0	26.0	55.2	6.2	12.5

* U.S. Bureau of the Census, 1970 Census of Population, *General Population Characteristics,* Final Report PC(1)-B1, U.S. Summary, Table 50 and Appendix B.

† Persons whose race or sex were not reported have been distributed pro rata; figures include 165 persons whose sex was not reported, 864 whose race was not reported, and 5 persons whose race and sex were not reported.

‡ For Jan. 1, 1970.

§ Fitted equations use four data points except for black and other races females (two points).

SOURCE: *Metropolitan Life Statistical Bulletin,* **60**(1):3–9, January–March 1979.

which we, working on mere guess and hope, proclaim to be humane. In any case, since they are curious and kindly, let's give them the best we have to give.

And as we give them our best, some of us realize, "I see you, old woman. But even as I look, your face turns into my own. We stand at opposite ends of the same long corridor, reflecting the image of one another" (Smith, 1973).

NURSES' DEBT TO OLDER WOMEN

The work that I want to do in my maturity could not be done without the existence of the growing women's culture, or without the support of a women's movement. . . .

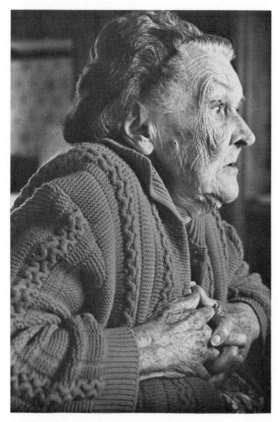

FIGURE 38-5 "I see you, old woman. But even as I look, your face turns into my own. We stand at opposite ends of the same long corridor, reflecting the image of one another" (Smith, 1973). (*Courtesy of Harvey Finkle.*)

We need courage, and we draw on each other for courage, but we have to remember that there have been women who did not have the kind of networks, the kind of culture, the kind of politics surrounding them, that we have. And this in itself is an immense step forward, and it is something we have to protect, we have to further, we have to defend, in order for all of us to do the kind of work we want to do, and that the work needs us to do. (Rich, 1978)

REFERENCES

Baldridge, Tish: What to do if friend has death in family, *San Jose Mercury News,* San Jose, Calif., Contemporary Living Section, Feb. 13, 1978, p. 2.

Baldwin, Doris: Poverty and the older woman: reflections of a social worker, *The Family Coordinator,* **27**(4):448–450, October 1978.

Ball, Robert M.: United States policy toward the elderly, in A. N. Exton-Smith and J. Grimley Evans (eds.), *Care of the Elderly,* Grune & Stratton, New York, 1977.

Burnside, Irene Mortenson: Centenarians: The elitists, in Irene Mortenson Burnside, Priscilla Ebersole, and Helen Elena Monea (eds.), *Psychosocial Caring Throughout the Life Span,* McGraw-Hill, New York, 1979a.

——: Loneliness and grief in senescence, in Irene Mortenson Burnside, Priscilla Ebersole, and Helen Elena Monea (eds.), *Psychosocial Caring Throughout the Life Span,* McGraw-Hill, New York, 1979b, p. 533.

——: Psychosocial caring: Reality testing, relocation, and reminiscing, in Irene Mortenson Burnside, Priscilla Ebersole, and Helen Elena Monea (eds.), *Psychosocial Caring Throughout the Life Span,* McGraw-Hill, New York, 1979c, p. 565.

Calderone, Mary S.: The status of women 1993–1998: Sexual, emotional aspects, in *No Longer Young: The Older Woman in America,* Institute of Gerontology, University of Michigan, Wayne State University, Detroit 1975.

Coles, Robert C.: Una anciana, *The New Yorker,* Profiles, Nov. 5, 1973.

de Castillejo, Irene Claremont: The older woman, in Irene Claremont de Castillejo (ed.), *Knowing Woman,* Putnam, New York, 1973, p. 149.

Dowling, Michael: Developments in aging: 1976, Report of the Special Committee on Aging, United States Senate, no. 95–88, Government Printing Office, Washington, 1977.

Epstein, Sidney: Dental care and the aging, *Perspectives,* **5**(6):14–17, November/December 1976.

Hall, Edward T.: *Hidden Dimension,* Anchor Books, Garden City, N.Y., 1969, p. 188,

Holmes, T. H., and R. H. Rahe: The social readjustment rating scale, *Journal Psychosomatic Research,* **11**:213–218, 1967.

Le Guin, Ursula: The space crone, *The CoEvolution Quarterly,* **10**:108–110, Summer 1976.

McLeish, John A. B.: Naked on the shore, in John A. B. McLeish (ed.), *The Ulyssean Adult,* McGraw-Hill Ryerson Limited, Toronto, 1976, p. 223.

Matthews, Sarah H.: *The Social World of Old Women: Management of Self Identity,* Sage Publications, Beverly Hills, Calif., 1978.

Metropolitan Life Statistical Bulletin: 60(1):3–9, January/March 1979.

National Action Forum for Older Women: A manifesto for older women, a handout (n.d.).

———: Statistical profile of women age 65 and over in the United States (n.d.).

Otten, Jane: Gray chic, *Newsweek,* **90**(23):13, Dec. 5, 1977.

Potter, Barbara: Personal communication, August 1978.

Rich, Adrienne: Quoted in *Forum,* **1**(2):1, National Action Forum for Older Women, fall, 1978.

Seltzer, Mildred M.: The older woman: Fact, fantasies and fiction, *Research on Aging,* **1**(2):140–153, June 1979.

Smith, Bert Kruger: An old woman speaks, in Bert Kruger Smith (ed.), *Aging in America,* Beacon Press, Boston, 1973, p. 198.

U.S. Department of Health, Education, and Welfare: Facts about older Americans 1976, DHEW Publication no. (OHD) 77-20006, Washington (pamphlet).

———: *Health, United States, 1975,* 1976.

Williams, B.: A profile of the elderly woman, *Aging,* Government Printing Office, Washington, D.C., 1975.

Wyse, Lois: On being a woman, *Woman's Day,* Feb. 3, 1978, p. 87.

OTHER RESOURCES

Love It like a Fool: A Film about Malvina Reynolds, film, 28 min/color. Distributor: Red Hen Films, 1305 Oxford St., Berkeley, CA 94709.

Nana, Mom and Me, film by Amalie R. Rothschild, 16 mm, color, 47 min. New Day Films, P.O. Box 315, Franklin Lakes, NJ 07417.

Outsmarting Crime: An Older Person's Guide to Safer Living (booklet), Washington State Office of the Attorney General.

Prime Time: By and for Older Women, a feminist journal which explores problems and solutions for older women. Prime Time, 420 W. 46th St., New York, NY 10036.

Problems of Older Women, audio cassette, 28 min., 1973, Dorothy Tennor and Peggy Nevin, University of Michigan, Ann Arbor.

Social Science Aspects of Clothing for Older Women (booklet), annotated bibliography (2d ed.) by Adeline M. Hoffman and Iva M. Bader, Department of Home Economics and Division of Continuing Education, University of Iowa, Iowa City, March 1977.

Union Maids, documentary film about women organizing in the 1930s, 16 mm, black/white, 48 min., by Julia Reichert, James Klein, and Miles Mogulescu, New Day Films, P.O. Box 315, Franklin Lakes, NJ 07417.

A Woman's Guide to Social Security, booklet, free from Consumer Information Center, Dept. 618F, Pueblo, CO 81009.

THIRTY-NINE

THE DYING AGED PERSON

Irene Mortenson Burnside

I'm lucky to have my own death.
Susan Sontag

LEARNING OBJECTIVES

- List five environments in which nurses may be caring for the dying aged person.
- Define hospice.
- Describe the hospice movement.
- Describe three environments and the problems inherent in each setting if a nurse cares for the moribund aged person in that environment.
- List five criteria which characterize death (as delineated by E. Mansell Pattison).
- List five fears which may occur during the dying process.
- Describe in detail 10 nursing interventions to improve the quality of dying for the aged person.
- Analyze problems with a dying aged patient that could impinge on a similar problem in the student's personal life.

This chapter will examine the whole situation of the dying elderly person—the care of the dying patient, the environment in which the patient dies and its implications for nursing care, the problems of dealing with relatives and survivors, and the support required by health care personnel treating the moribund elderly.

The literature is replete with information on dying, and it has become one of the most popular topics for classes of all disciplines, for workshops, and seminars. While there are many articles on dying and death, the number of articles which focus on the dying aged person are few, and most books on the subject give the aged short shrift. The general concepts for care of dying persons may apply to the aged, but, as in other psychosocial care of the aged, there are differences between care of the aged and of the younger dying person. An effort will be made to explore the differences in this chapter.

Two excellent books of readings are highly recommended: *New Meanings of Death,* edited by Herman Feifel (1977), and *Psychosocial Care of the Dying Patient,* edited by Charles A. Garfield (1978).

The literature on dying is so extensive that I reviewed only articles relevant to care of the dying aged; nothing was reviewed on other age groups. I will discuss only the most relevant articles in this chapter, along with Pattison's theoretical framework, because of its applicability for the nursing profession.

Elizabeth Kübler-Ross's (1969) work on the stages of dying is so well known that it will not be covered in this book. Kastenbaum (1979, p. 583) thoroughly discounts the prevalent idea that old people die in stages. He states that other clinicians have failed to find supportive evidence of the factual status of the stages and further states that "a review of the clinical literature and a recent controlled study again do not support the existence of the pattern sequence that has been claimed." The same author (Kastenbaum, 1978) acknowledges that while Kübler-Ross did not intend misuse of her material, "it is more difficult to recall a defective theory for repairs than a misbegotten offspring from the assembly lines in Detroit" (p. 6). A survey done by *Nursing '75* provided the result that most nurses find it easier to care for middle-aged and elderly terminally ill patients than for dying children or adolescents (Popoff, 1975).

This chapter is divided into seven parts: (1) the character of death—selected principles from Pattison (1967); (2) dying at home; (3) dying during travel; (4) dying in nursing homes; (5) dying in the acute hospital; (6) dying in a hospice; and (7) nursing interventions. While I was struggling to organize the material for this chapter, I was reminded of a little old lady in a nursing home who, as she sat reading the obituary column, nonchalantly asked no one in particular, "How do all of these people die in alphabetical order?"

WHERE DO OLD PEOPLE DIE?

According to Kastenbaum (1978) most older persons live in the community, but most of them die in some type of institution. It is not merely the last few days prior to death, but rather weeks or months, that are spent in an institution. The first such study by Kastenbaum and Candy (1973) indicated that 25 percent of the deaths of people 65 or over occurred in institutional "homes." About five times as many people died in such places as usually are assumed to be living in such places. When all types of institutions are included, the chance that an elderly person will die in the community is less than one in five.

Kastenbaum (1978) suggested that there are four important implications for psychosocial care during the terminal phase of life:

1. The "stigma" of institutionalization.
2. The loss of individual identity, that is, becoming one old person among many in a communal setting.
3. The reduction of self-esteem supports due to the loss of environmental features that helped to maintain continuity, and also reduction in the social contacts with the community.
4. An intensification of all the above once the person is viewed as a dying person.

THE CHARACTER OF DEATH

Pattison's articles (1967, 1978) are useful to better understand the dying process. He has analyzed the types of ego-coping mechanisms which are used in each stage of life and tried to determine the most typical coping mechanisms

TABLE 39-1
QUOTATIONS ABOUT DYING

When a new disability arrives I look around to see if death has come, and I call quietly, "Death is that you? Are you there?" So far the disability has answered, "Don't be silly, it's me."

Florida Scott Maxwell, *Measure of My Days,* 1968, p. 36

Dying is hard work.

Dr. T. S. West, St. Christopher's, in *The Hospice Movement,* Sandol Stoddard, p. 8

You matter because you are you. You matter in the last moment of your life, and we will do all we can not only to help you die peacefully but also to live until you die.

Cicely Saunders, in *The Hospice Movement,* Sandol Stoddard, p. 120

I'm lucky to have my own death.

Susan Sontag, quoted in "Alone against Illness" by Carol Kahn, *Family Health,* November 1978, vol. 10, no. 11, p. 52

A man can't go out just the way he came in. He's got to amount to something.

Arthur Miller, *Death of a Salesman*

For is not philosophy the study of death?

Socrates

> Yes, death is hard, and dark with delay
> before one faces a trace of eternity.
> But the living err in their stark definitions.

Rainer Maria Rilke

I told you I was sick

An epitaph in Medford, Oregon

Rafi: I am a man in the presence of death.
Caliph: There are a thousand paths to the delectable tavern of death, and some run straight and some run crooked.

Flecker

A man's dying is more the survivor's affair than his own.

Thomas Mann, *The Magic Mountain*

I will have many emotions, and I'll say goodbye properly.

Susan Sontag, quoted in "Alone against Illness" by Carol Kahn, *Family Health,* November 1978, vol. 10, no. 11, p. 52

It's not that I'm afraid of dying. I just don't want to be there when it happens.

Woody Allen

> *Ah, I have now learned*
> *what I first feared*
> *that the final pain*
> *is also the greatest.*
>
> *Can no longer work,*
> *have no longer strength,*
> *can no longer direct*
> *the flood of my thoughts.*
>
> *They are over a mountain*
> *to be gathered never more,*
> *and I myself move nearer*
> *to the edge of my grave.*

Bjornstjerne Bjornson, 1906, translated by Marian Rusted, R.N.

Death asks us for identity.

Robert Fulton, *Death and Identity,* Wiley, New York, 1965

---

a dying person uses (Table 39-2). (And incidentally, nurses are often unprepared for the humor that many dying elderly people use in their unique ways to cope with dying.) Pattison (1967) has listed these characteristics of death:

• This stressful event poses a problem which by definition is insoluble in the immediate future.

Dying in this sense is most stressful because it is ultimately insoluble and a problem to which we have to bow rather than solve.
• The problem taxes one's psychologic resources since it is beyond one's traditional problem-solving methods. One is faced with a new experience with no prior experience to fall back on; for although one lives amidst death,

TABLE 39-2

TYPICAL EGO-COPING MECHANISMS OF THE DYING THROUGHOUT THE LIFE CYCLE

Ego-coping Mechanisms	Early Child-hood	School-age Child	Adoles-cence	Young Adult	Middle Age	Aged
Level 1: primitive						
Delusions	+	+				
Perceptual hallucination	+	+				
Depersonalization	+	+				
Reality-distorting denial	+	+				
Level 2: immature						
Projection	++	+++	+		+	
Denial through fantasy	++	+	+			
Hypochondriasis		++	++	++	++	+++
Passive-aggressiveness		+++	++	+++	++	++
Acting-out behavior		+++	++	+++	++	
Level 3: neurotic						
Intellectualization			+++	+	+++	+
Displacement			++	++	+	
Reaction formation			++	+++	+	
Emotional dissociation			+++	+	+	+
Level 4: mature						
Altruism			+		+	++
Humor			+	+	+	+
Suppression			++	+++	+++	+
Anticipatory thought			+++	+++	+++	+++
Sublimation			+	+	++	+++

NOTES: + = occasional use; ++ = moderate use; +++ = considerable use.
SOURCE: Pattison, 1978.

that is far different from confronting one's own death.

- The situation is perceived as a threat or danger to the life goals of the person. Dying interrupts a person in the midst of life, and even in old age it abruptly confronts one with the goals set for one's own life.
- The crisis period is characterized by a tension which mounts to a peak, then falls. As one faces the crisis of death, anxiety begins to mount, rises to a peak during which the person either mobilizes his or her coping mechanisms to deal with this anxiety or experiences disorganization and capitulation to anxiety. In either event, the person then passes to a state of diminishing anxiety as death approaches. Hence, the peak of acute anxiety usually occurs considerably before death.

- The crisis situation awakens unresolved key problems from both the near and the distant past. Problems of dependency, passivity, narcissism, inadequacy, identity, and more are all reactivated by the process of dying. Hence, one is faced not only with the problem of death per se but also of a host of unresolved feelings from one's own lifetime and its past conflicts.

Nurses should also be aware of these other aspects of dying:

- *Fear of the unknown.* The fundamental anxiety might be basic death anxiety. One patient described death as strange and unknown because she had never done it before.
- *Fear of loneliness.* Sickness in and of itself isolates one from the rest of humanity; even more

isolating is the immensity of death. It has been observed that the closer to death the patient came, the slower were the nurses to answer the call light.

- *Fear of loss of family and friends.* This is a loss which must be mourned and worked through.
- *Fear of loss of body.* Bodies are very much a part of our self-image. When illness distorts one's body image, there is not only a loss of function but loss of self, fear of no longer being loved by one's family, fear of rejection, and fear of being left alone.
- *Fear of loss of self-control.* Debilitating disease makes one less able to control one's self, particularly when mental capacity is also affected. It is important to allow and encourage the dying person to retain whatever decisions and authority are possible and to sustain the person in retaining control of small daily tasks and decisions.
- *Fear of loss of identity.* The loss of human contact, the loss of family and friends, the loss of one's body and control are all tied in with the loss of one's sense of identity. There is a threat to one's own ego by losing the feelings for one's own body. In the dying process, one is faced with the crisis of maintaining an integrity of ego in the face of forces moving one toward dissolution and annihilation.

THE ELDERLY WHO DIE AT HOME

Orthothanasia means the appropriate death and involves two important factors: *understanding the meaning of death to a particular individual* and *willingness to provide him or her with whatever gratifications are possible. Euthanasia,* the act of inducing death, will not be covered here; there is simply not space for adequate discussion of such a complex and touchy topic.

Some professionals have found that home is the most appropriate environment for the death of some patients, but Wall (1960) reminds us that it is rare for an individual who is outside of the medical or nursing profession to see an untreated dead person; the dead are usually carefully made up before being viewed by the family.

Terminal care at home in two cultures was studied by French and Schwartz (1973). These authors point out that when long-term illnesses are coped with at home, critical incidents will occur. The authors describe moving a dying Navajo woman from her hogan so that it could be burned. The burning is a part of tribal ritual. The nurse wanted to use two new woolen blankets, as the dying woman seemed very cold. However, the family told the nurse that the blankets could be used only after death.

Such incidents have their roots in the cultures of the person involved. The underlying beliefs can often be identified—either by the nurse or the receiver of the care. If a precise explanation cannot be found, the nurse must respect the personhood of the patient—for that is the right of the one being cared for and the family.

Nursing the dying person at home is a challenging and sometimes frustrating endeavor. The lack of equipment and supplies forces the nurse to improvise constantly. During my employment on a pilot project to ascertain the cost and quality of care involved in maintaining clients in the home, I cared for a dying elderly woman. This vignette describes that experience.

VIGNETTE 1

Mrs. A. was a 70-year-old widow in an acute hospital for terminal cancer. She requested to die in her own home. The public health department contacted the Cancer Society and they provided a bed, a bedpan, and bedpan covers. Mrs. A. was placed in her favorite room, and relatives came—a sister from the Midwest to cook and wash and a daughter to provide moral support, although it turned out she needed more moral support than her dying mother. These were some of the improvisations made for the dying woman's care:

1. Gowns or "johnny coats" were made from men's white shirts with cuffs and collars removed and ties added (and worn backwards).
2. Ice cubes were made smaller (so she could suck on them) by placing them on a paper bag and hitting them with a hammer.
3. Lemon juice and glycerine were made up by her sister (who wanted to help) for her dry lips.

4. During convulsions the physician was called. He arrived without a tourniquet to give an intravenous injection; he was a bit startled when I handed him a yellow douche tube. (The daughter had left the item hanging in the bathroom.)
5. A peanut butter jar was carefully labeled "holy water" for the startled priest when he arrived the first time. (Even the dying woman was amused by her special "Skippy holy water.")

It should be noted here that whatever was lacking in equipment and supplies was more than compensated for by the client's comfort in being in familiar surroundings and with the same persons around, in contrast to the changing shifts, rooms, and beds in acute care facilities.

Mrs. A. was the least of the problems; the distraught relatives were at times more difficult. They were often caustic with one another. Their hostility became rampant. Past grievances arose. Her son would visit and be distressed about his sister's actions (or lack thereof). The sister was often saddened by the deteriorating process and felt everyone was doing "so little for mother." One role I filled was to relieve family members and to listen to each of them separately over a cup of coffee away from the mother's room. The outpouring of feelings was especially noticeable at one point when the physician sent the patient to the hospital for a blood transfusion; the family and Mrs. A. were upset—the disruption and added expense were almost too much for all of them at that point in the dying process. In the follow-up visits to arrange for the return of equipment and to check on the family, even more listening was necessary.

THE ELDERLY WHO DIE WHILE TRAVELING

Because many older people use their leisure time and retirement to travel, it is inevitable for some that their demise will occur in a foreign country. (This is not a common problem with youths who travel.) The complications which arise then were described in a local paper about the death of a traveler abroad in Italy. "The man, usually the humorist in the tour group, had said the day before he died, 'I don't like the smell of this place.' He had undergone heart surgery earlier in the same year. His wife awakened, as she had done frequently since his surgery, to reach over and squeeze his hand, but she got no response. His hand was cold."

The cost to get the deceased person back home was $6420, which included $1200 for a casket, $1000 for embalming, and the rest for "expense" and air freight. One should consider the possibility of death happening abroad; a helpful leaflet is available (Johnson, n.d.). It is also wise for older persons to check with their travel agents and/or an insurance agent to get whatever other helpful information is available.

VIGNETTE 2
A 65-year-old man who had had several coronaries, one of them rather severe, could not give up traveling. He was an excellent photographer and on many of his trips had produced lovely photographs which he had framed and hung in his office. He got up one night in a hotel in a foreign city, walked to the foot of his bed, and collapsed. Again the problems arose of coping with the foreign police and the red tape involved in moving the body out of the hotel and to the man's home country.

The U.S. Consulate in Peking, China, reported in a 5-month period the handling of five medical evacuations and four deaths. All were Americans. Three of the deaths involved persons over 70. The evacuation cases included two broken hips and two cases of pneumonia (Brown, 1980).

THE ELDERLY WHO DIE IN NURSING HOMES

Roberts et al. (1970, p. 119) studied the ways the aged in nursing homes viewed death and dying. For the most part, the aged people spoke matter-of-factly of death, and a few expressed some positive feelings toward the process. The authors ended the article with, "We may not yet know precisely how to ask the questions or what the right questions are to ask, but we do know that the respondents are willing and wanting to answer."

Elizabeth Gustafson (1972, p. 234) studied the career of the nursing home patient. She felt that knowledge of the effects of the different environments and the duration on the career of the dying patient would make for a helpful study. In her summary she wrote, "Medical staff, friends, and relatives, and often patients themselves think of the patient career as an unbroken decline towards death. Instinct and will-to-live cause the patient to fight against the premature social death forced upon him in this situation. The increasing tension makes this a hellish existence for the patient."

Helping the staff in a nursing home face conflicts about death is an important component of in-service education in nursing homes. Academic discussions are usually futile since they do not involve the learner, but role-playing or discussions about recent deaths and depressive states experienced by the staff are usually more helpful. I recall doing research in a 55-bed nursing home. The melancholy air was obvious and was explained to me by the director of nurses who said they had had nine patients die within 1 month; several were long-term residents of whom the staff was very fond. Staff members were obviously feeling the losses. ("I hate to go into Mr. T.'s room now that he is gone," or "I sure miss Mrs. K.'s teasing.") Although they could not help each other, no consultation was sought; in those early years of extended care facilities there was little in-service. There simply were no listeners and no outlet for the grief the staff members were experiencing.

One must also help students to deal with their clients. On one occasion a student came into a conference baffled by the question posed by her aging client. The woman was in a nursing home, and there was not much chance of her ever being discharged. *Both* her first husband and second husband were dead. Since they were both good men (in her eyes), she was quite sure both were in heaven, and she was also certain that heaven would be her destination after death. Her question to the student was, "What

will happen when I die and meet them both in heaven?" Working with the dying person constantly exposes one to some views more or less like one's own and some which are the antithesis. In this case, the student was baffled. One cannot always maintain objectivity when the dying is poignant or painful, and often one does what one has been taught to do in the face of death, even when it might not be what the dying person wants or needs. Singing "Ave Maria" (if you can sing) is fine if the dying person wants it, but others might detest and resent such an intervention.

The sensitive designers of nursing home facilities are to be commended, but often chapels have seemed impractical, uncomfortable, and little used. However, at Mount Royal Hospital in Melbourne, Australia, the unique chapel is used by all denominations. What makes it so unique is that the pews can be turned to face either end of the building; one end is arranged as a Catholic church and the other end as a Protestant chapel. This design allows patients to worship in surroundings that feel familiar.

THE ELDERLY WHO DIE IN ACUTE HOSPITALS

Robert Kastenbaum (1967) studied the mental life of dying geriatric patients and reported on 61 cases of a psychological autopsy series. His study took place with hospitalized geriatric patients over age 65. The study failed to support the assumption that most aged persons are in poor mental contact as they are dying. Positive feelings toward death were heard much more frequently than negative ones of fear and depression. One of the direct implications of the study was that more attention should be given in the psychosocial care of the dying aged patient; that is as true now as when it was written.

A sensitive article by Krant (1972) on the organized care of the dying points out that the terminally ill patient greatly needs psychological support to "die well." The article is recommended for those who work in either nursing homes or acute care hospitals because it contains pragmatic suggestions for intervention.

In a fascinating paper presented at a meeting of the International Congress of Gerontology, Linder (1978), of Uppsala, Sweden, described a study of the last week of life of dying individuals. During a 3-month period each death was studied, and 40 interviews were made. More than 50 percent of the subjects had been in the hospital less than 3 months. Linder found that the main complaints in the last stages of life were: (1) feebleness, (2) pain, (3) difficulty in breathing, (4) anxiety, (5) depression, and (6) agitation.

Conversations in the last week were categorized as shown in Table 39-3.

Kates (1973) has written a poignant account of her mother's demise in a hospital and has described trying to celebrate her mother's one-hundredth birthday while she was in the critical care unit. The article is recommended for nurses who work in acute care hospital settings.

THE ELDERLY WHO DIE IN HOSPICES

The word *hospice* technically means a lodging for traveling (Webster's, 1973); in current usage it is a way station for the dying. Hospices are now springing up across the United States patterned after St. Christopher's in London, which was begun in 1967 by former nurse/social worker Cicely Saunders (1976). However, at this writing the literature yields little about the aged who die in hospices.

TABLE 39-3
CONVERSATIONS WITH THE DYING

	Subject of the Conversation	
	The Disease/ Death	Common Things
Conversations with physicians	11	14
Conversations with nurses	12	22
Conversations with others	9	20

SOURCE: L. Linder, 1978.

Kron (1976) discussed the design of the building for a hospice in the United States. Studies show that patients recover faster in natural light; perhaps they die more comfortably in natural light, too. The architect wrote, "Skylights accentuate the passage of time. The movement of the sun, shadows, rain, snow—it's all palpable. It gives a patient a point of reference to the outside world. . . . Rocking chairs and wing chairs will be standard equipment." He states that the building will be designed with an escape hatch for the staff members to use when they feel the need to slip away; it will be a tiny room, glass-domed and soundproof with no furniture in it.

An inpatient hospice facility provides 24-hour nursing and palliative care. Goals delineated by the Hospice of the Monterey Peninsula (1978) are:

1. To support each patient and patient's family as a unit of care
2. To support each patient with a program of pain and symptom control
3. To encourage family involvement in patient care when appropriate
4. To reduce medical costs for the patient and the health care system
5. To help the patient live as fully as possible

"Not only is the hospice idea novel to the high-technology big-business system of medical care we have, but it embodies a rather rare combination of spirituality and hard medicine, a combination whose uniqueness may not be appreciated until one encounters it in such a person as Cicely Saunders" (Holden, 1978, p. 91).

West (1977, p. B1), deputy director at St. Christopher's, says that the visits of pets are encouraged and described a patient whose son was a circus owner. When a new baby elephant was born, the son drove the elephant to the hospice and the patient was wheeled in his bed to the parking lot to have a look at the elephant. West further stated, "We are willing to go out of the way to please our patients, and this was quite successful." Many elderly people have had pets or animals around them much of their life—we tend to forget that.

The Department of Health, Education, and Welfare has funded 26 hospices in a demonstration project beginning March 1, 1980. It is a 2-year project "to explore the possibilities of making changes in Medicare and Medicaid regulations to provide coverage for hospital services" (*American Nurse,* 1980).

ASSESSMENT

Wolanin (1976, pp. 417–419) reminds us that we should consider the needs of the terminally ill individual in the nursing assessment. The following are her suggestions for assessment:

1. Does this person see his or her health status as life threatening?
2. Is the person concerned with preparation for death at this time or with dying?
3. High-risk elderly persons include:
   a. The elderly person who is alone and who has lost family and friends through death
   b. The elderly person with changes in body function marked either by pain or weakness or by change in body structure
   c. The elderly person who has evidence of terminal illness
   d. The person working toward his or her own self-determined death either by intentional or subconscious means
4. Observations
   a. Does the patient give cues that he or she is thinking of dying and death and wishing to discuss them? Which of the four questions is the patient asking:
      (1) Is this my approaching death?
      (2) Will I be cared for during my dying?
      (3) What is it like to die?
      (4) Will you be honest with me?
   b. Is this person talking of dying?
5. Base-line information
   a. Look to discover:
      (1) The patient's covert or overt references to death. The patient's relationship with at least one other trusted person: family, friend, or a staff member.
      (2) Preparations, if any, which a person has made for death.
      (3) The patient's self-assessment of his or her health.
      (4) Is there evidence that this person is

taking means to determine the time and place of death, either by intentional or subconscious acts?

PROXIMITY OF PATIENT'S PROBLEM

What happens when the dying patient's problems begin to intrude on the nurse's own problems or personal troubles? Let me illustrate: Some years ago in a large hospital, one of the nurses on a medical ward was called cross-country to care for her father who had had a massive coronary. Her father died in her arms. The nurse returned to work earlier than she had planned, because of pressure from administration and shortage of staff. When she returned she requested not to care for coronary patients for awhile. The diabetics, the old men with emphysema, the cancer patients, yes—but not coronaries. On a 4 P.M. to midnight shift a patient had a severe coronary, very much like the one her father had experienced. The patient's problem intruded sharply and painfully on the nurse's own personal space. The sad result in this instance was that the nurse gave a wrong medication later in the shift, a medication with potentially serious consequences.

The point of this, of course, is that caring for dying patients can painfully remind caretakers of their own sufferings and losses, as both nurses and nursing supervisors should constantly be aware (see Figure 39-1).

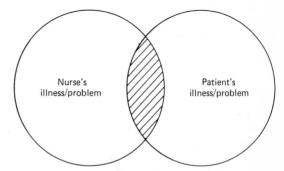

FIGURE 39-1 When the problems of the dying person impinge on memory, emotions, or previous experience of the nurse, it may be a very painful situation for the nurse assigned to the care of the moribund individual.

COMMUNICATION PROBLEMS

Communication with the dying person can be difficult and wrought with problems—whatever the age of the person. The problem of communication with the fatally ill is described in an article by Verwoerdt and Jeffers (1977) about communication between the physician and the family of the dying individual. The article has relevance for nurses. The authors analyze the situation on the basis of ego psychology and psychophysiology and discuss the mechanisms old people might use in facing death. They point out that caretakers need to listen for covert messages, especially when an individual is not discussing dying.

STRUGGLE FOR CONTROL

It has been my observation (both professional and personal) that when dying people begin to lose much control of body and/or life surroundings, they begin to be much more controlling of those individuals around them. Some of my observations based on nursing care are as follows:

Control of Environment

1. Specific criticism is directed at the nurse (or at the aide) concerning the way the bed is made (one patient hated the toe pleats I made in sheets, another hated a pillow at his feet, another hated pillows under the knees), the care given, the bathing schedules. Often bedside stands become battlegrounds as well, as do windows and draperies (how far to open them), the room temperature—anything that is within close range of the person.
2. The closer the item to be controlled is to the person, the more control is exerted. For example, a woman in a nursing home had lovely feminine lingerie given to her by her husband, relatives, and friends during her illness. They were on the closet shelf, while she insisted on wearing her husband's old shirts. At the time I could not understand this behavior at all. It has since occurred to me that, if she was never to have her husband in

bed again (the disease and its effects were too distasteful for him to handle physical closeness with her), perhaps the best she could do to maintain closeness to him was to sleep in his shirt.

Control by the Nurse or Caretaker
One of the ways dying persons can leave legacies and feel needed is by giving advice—becoming sages if their energy level permits. It allows them to be needed, to share something of their own lives, and to give instead of always being on the receiving end during the final phase of life. Nurses need not always resist patients' efforts to control them. They can, for example, take the opportunity to become the patient's ally and advocate when a client says, "Go ask my doctor; find out what that medicine is," or "What did he mean when he made rounds this morning?"

Control by Family
We often control very tightly who visits the dying person, when, and for how long. The aged may need some help here, but often they do not and will state their preferences very clearly. We need to find out their preferences.

Control by the Physician
Though patients may try, frankly most of them do not do very well here since the physician may have difficulty handling death and dying, or may simply have become callous. A physician once related at a conference how difficult the loss of a close colleague had been for him. Finally he went to the hospital to visit his friend carrying a bottle of cold champagne and drank champagne with the patient, who loved it. A similar incident is described by Kean (1974) in his interview with Ernest Becker, who was dying.

Assess *who is in control of the situation* and what can be done to help the patient maintain more control (unless the patient is no longer lucid enough to be in control). Be wary of people who come sashaying in to visit and advise, when the patient is groggy from medication. On occasion I have known dying patients to sign papers who later were not quite sure what they had signed, or did not remember signing. I have also been on private duty in cases where items were removed from the closet shelf by helpful friends or relatives who thought the patient "might not need them anymore so we took them home." On one occasion an executrix called me aside to remind me that the suction machine had not been used and to ask whether we needed it in the room because it was so expensive. (The dying woman knew why it was there and had okayed it.) She pointed out that I was certainly using a lot of Kleenex on the patient, and asked whether I really thought a night nurse was necessary since "she seemed so good." (The patient was terrified of dying at night, and a night nurse was one of the top priorities in my planning care with the moribund woman.)

STATEMENTS FROM THE LITERATURE: GUIDELINES FOR INTERVENTIONS

In an effort to synthesize from the literature, I have listed aspects of the situation of dying elderly people which have significant implications for interventions by nurses.

1. What goals are confronted by the aged persons' impending death (Pattison, 1967)?

2. Are recent (or long past) problems of dependency, passivity, narcissism, inadequacy, self-identity reactivated by the dying person (Pattison, 1967)?

3. Assist the moribund to handle fears: the unknown (explain *all* procedures and interventions thoroughly, honestly, and accurately), loneliness (watch for isolation), the loss of family and friends (encourage the dying person to do grief work), the fear of loss of body (consider the impact of illness and death on the body image), the fear of loss of control. Watch for excessive or unnecessary controlling behaviors in yourself, in the staff, the physician, the relatives (Pattison, 1967).

4. Prepare the family for the sight of a dead person (Wall, 1970).

5. Endeavor to understand the dying persons' culture (French and Schwartz, 1973).

6. Educate would-be travelers about the possibility of a death in a foreign country (Johnson, n.d.).

7. Do not treat "undying" patients in a nursing home as though they are dying residents (Gustafson, 1972).

8. Support nursing-home staff members when

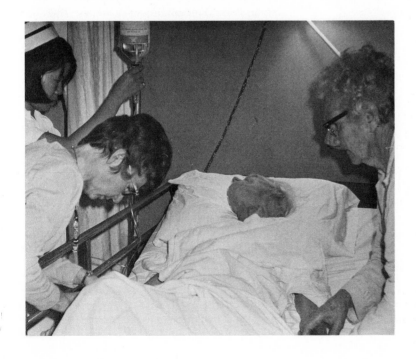

FIGURE 39-2 A dying patient receives an intravenous injection from the nurse-administrator. A resident of the facility is holding the patient's arm and is overheard saying, "Remember that I care." (*Courtesy of Will Patton.*)

they experience bereavement overload due to patient deaths.

9. Most aged patients may be in good mental contact as they are dying; do not assume they are all afraid or depressed (Kastenbaum, 1967).

10. Patients will talk with nurses about disease or death more frequently than with physicians. However, they are more prone to discuss the common things of life and sur-roundings (Linder, 1978). Therefore, nurses must learn to listen for covert messages.

11. The main complaints of dying patients during the last 3 months can be: feebleness, pain, dyspnea, anxiety, depression, agitation (Linder, 1978). Assess constantly for these, intervene appropriately. See Sky and Smith's chart for more definitive interventions in the area of discomforts (Table 39-4).

12. Place dying patients in natural light and also where they can make points of reference to the outdoors (Kron, 1976).

13. Encourage visitation of pets (West, 1977).

14. Nursing instructors assess students for personal problems impinging on professional role (Burnside, this chapter).

15. Provide the dying person with an "ego prosthesis"—that is, psychological support suggested in item 10 (Verwoerdt, 1964; Krant, 1972).

16. "The real issue is not to tell or not to tell, but rather how much to tell and in what manner" (Verwoerdt, 1964, p. 795).

17. Offer the chance to say good-bye properly (Sontag, 1978).

TABLE 39-4
SUGGESTIONS FOR CONTROL OF SPECIFIC SYMPTOMS FREQUENTLY OBSERVED (OTHER THAN PAIN)

Dry Mouth
Review medications (diuretics?)
Decrease or discontinue phenothiazines
Mouth washes, glycerine swabs, 'sour' candies, grapefruit
Ice chips
Topical anesthetic washes for stomatitis

Dysphagia
Pureed food and medication
Small, frequent amounts of food and liquids
Xylocaine jelly for esophagitis

Nausea
Regular antiemetics, antihistamines—oral, rectal, intramuscular

Constipation
Prevent and control by all and any methods and medications

Diarrhea
May be caused by fecal impaction
Kaopectate, Lomotil or related medications

Dyspnea
Calm, quiet surroundings, with constant attention
Proper positioning in bed or chair to achieve maximum comfort
Oxygen
Thoracentesis if pleural effusion
Anxiolytics with analgesics

Bronchospasm
Oxtriphylline (Choledyl)
Salbutamol (Ventolin)
Theophylline by mouth, IV or suppositories

SOURCE: Ruth Sky and David Smith, Continuing care of the terminally ill, *Canadian Family Physician,* vol. 24, May 1978, pp. 461–462. Reprinted by permission of the publisher.

VIGNETTE 3

The best example of sensitive intervention is from a book about hospices. The author describes her dying friend in a hospital. A phone call came for the woman from the man she loved. "The central switchboard had been told no more calls . . . it was too late. Technically, of course it was. Anne was by now far too weak to lift a telephone, even to speak. . . . It was one of the noticing, questioning nurses who intervened. Understanding what must be done for Anne, she fought the switchboard and re-routed the call. Then, holding Anne in her arms and the telephone close to her ear, she stood by until the last words were spoken, so that Anne was able to hear at the very moment of her death, in the beloved voice, 'Anne, I love you'" (Stoddard, 1978, p. 284).

A nurse thanatologist is one who specializes in the care of the dying. Joy Ufema and Judy Urrea-Robertson are both well known for their work. See Table 39-5 for the description of that role.

TABLE 39-5
THE NURSE SPECIALIST FOR THE DYING

- *Formulates* a patient group through personal observation or rounds, or referrals from nursing staff, medical staff, or social service.
- *Assists* nursing staff to plan and implement, with the patient's participation, a care regimen suitable to the patient's needs.
- *Gives* total patient nursing care on a selected basis to formulate a basis for future interaction.
- *Assesses* terminally ill patients to determine their perception of illness.
- *Intercedes* for patient with staff, family, or friends as the patient sees this need.
- *Functions* as a team member with social service and pastoral care on behalf of these patients.
- *Teaches* hospital personnel the dynamics of thanatology.
- *Learns* the dying process, not only from literature seminars and conferences, but especially from dying patients.

SOURCE: Joy K. Ufema, Dare to care for the dying, *American Journal of Nursing*, 76(1):88–90, January 1976.

REFERENCES

The American Nurse, **12**(1):2, January 1980.

Brown, Phil: U.S. tourists' health concerns consulate, *San Jose Mercury,* Feb. 3, 1980.

Feifel, Herman: *New Meanings of Death,* McGraw-Hill, New York, 1977.

Ferguson, Stella: Personal communication, 1976.

French, Jean, and Doris Schwartz: Terminal care at home in two cultures, *American Journal of Nursing,* **73**(3):502–505, March 1973.

Garfield, Charles A.: *Psychosocial Care of the Dying Patient,* McGraw-Hill, New York, 1978.

Gustafson, Elizabeth: Dying: The career of the nursing home patient, *Journal of Health and Social Behavior,* **13**(3):226–235, September 1972.

Holden, Constance: A rare combination, in Sandol Stoddard (ed.), *The Hospice Movement: A Better Way To Care for the Dying,* Vintage Books, Random House, Inc., New York, 1978, p. 91.

Hospice of the Monterey Peninsula: Program description, Carmel, Calif., July 1978.

Johnson, Edward C.: *Death of American Citizens Abroad,* National Funeral Directors Association, 2681 North Orchard St., Chicago, IL 60614, n.d.

Kastenbaum, Robert: Death, dying, and bereavement in old age, *Aged Care and Services Review,* **1**(3):1–10, May/June 1978.

————: The mental life of dying geriatric patients, *Gerontologist,* **7**(2):97–100, July 1967.

————: The physician and the terminally ill old person, in Isadore Rossman (ed.), *Clinical Geriatrics,* Lippincott, Philadelphia, 1979, pp. 576–589.

————, **and S. E. Candy:** The 4% fallacy: A methodological and empirical critique of extended care facility population statistics, *International Journal of Aging and Human Development,* **4**:15, 1973.

Kates, Dorothy D.: The facts of death, *Ms.,* **1**(8):36–38, February 1973.

Kean, Samuel: A day of loving combat, *Psychology Today,* **7**(4):73, April 1974.

Krant, Melvin, J.: The organized care of the dying patient, *Hospital Practice,* **7**(1):101–108, January 1972.

Kron, Joan: Designing a better place to die, *New York,* March 1, 1976, pp. 43–49.

Kübler-Ross, Elizabeth: *On Death and Dying,* Macmillan, New York, 1969.

Linder, L.: Terminal care in a long-term hospital, paper presented at *Eleventh Meeting of the International Congress of Gerontology,* Tokyo, August 1978.

Pattison, E. Mansell: The experience of dying, *American Journal of Psychotherapy,* **21**(1):32–43, January 1967.

————: The living-dying process, in Charles A. Garfield (ed.), *Psychosocial Care of the Dying Patient,* McGraw-Hill, New York, 1978.

Popoff, David: What are your feelings about death and dying? *Nursing,* **5**(8):15–24, August 1975.

Roberts, Jean L., et al.: How aged in nursing homes view dying and death, *Geriatrics,* **25**(4):115–119, April 1970.

Saunders, Cicely: Care of the dying, seven-part series in *Nursing Times,* July 1–Aug. 12, 1976.

Sontag, Susan: Quoted by Carol Kahn, in Alone against illness, *Family Health,* **10**(11):52, November 1978.

Stoddard, Sandol: *The Hospice Movement: A Better Way of Caring for the Dying,* Vintage Books, Random House, Inc., New York, 1978.

Ufema, Joy K.: Dare to care for the dying, *American Journal of Nursing,* **76**(1):88–90, January 1976.

Verwoerdt, Adrian, and Frances C. Jeffers: How the old face death, in Ewald W. Busse and Eric Preiffer (eds.), *Behavior and Adaptation in Late Life,* Little, Brown, Boston, 1977.

Wall, Charles W.: *Helping the Dying Patient and His Family,* Association of Social Workers, New York, 1960.

Webster's New Collegiate Dictionary: G. & C. Merriam Company, Springfield, Mass., 1973.

West, Thomas S.: For whatever life remains . . . *Star Bulletin,* Honolulu, Hawaii, July 8, 1977, p. B1.

Wolanin, Mary Opal: Nursing assessment, in Irene Mortenson Burnside (ed.), *Nursing and the Aged,* McGraw-Hill, New York, 1976.

OTHER RESOURCES

FILMS

The Old Woman, 2 min/color/1973. Central Arizona Film, Arizona State University, Tempe, 85281.

Passing Quietly Through, 26/min/b&w/1970. Distributor: Films, Inc., 1144 Wilmette Ave., Wilmette, IL 66091.

Perspectives on Dying, Concept Media, Costa Mesa, Calif., 1972.

The Parting, 16 min/color/1973. Distributor: Wombat Publications, Inc., Little Lake, Glendale Road, P. O. Box 70, Ossining, NY 10562.

Gramp: A Man Ages and Dies, full-color filmstrip, 86 frames, 16 min, tape cassette or one 12" LP record, Sunburst Communications, Pleasantville, NY 10570. (Teacher's guide included.)

REPORT

"I Want to Die at Home," Katherine Kingsbury. Report of a Churchill Fellowship. Developments in the care of the dying, hospices, the care of the frail aged and the handicapped are discussed. Copies available from Fitzroy Social Planning Office, 239 Brunswick St., Fitzroy, Victoria, 3065, Australia.

RECORDINGS

"Morningside" by Neil Diamond
"Watermelon Wine" by Tom T. Hall
"Old Man River" by Walter Brennan

EIGHT

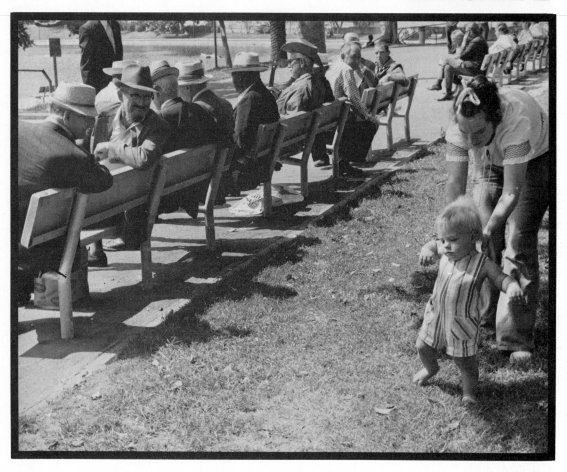

Diane E. Miller

SOCIAL FORCES AND AGING

It's very odd,
But I am beginning to feel, just beginning to feel
That there is something I could understand, if I were
told it.
But I'm not sure that I want to know. I suppose
I'm getting old:
Old age came softly up to now. I felt safe enough;
And now I don't feel safe.

T. S. Eliot
"The Family Reunion"

FORTY

SOCIAL FORCES AND AGING INDIVIDUALS: AN OVERVIEW

Vern L. Bengtson
David A. Haber

Older persons in this society constitute a great national resource, which has largely gone unrecognized, undervalued and unused. The experience, wisdom and competence of older persons are greatly needed in every sector. Creative and innovative ways must be found to enable older people to make their contribution to a new age of liberation. Many older persons have freedom—freedom to think, reflect, and act.

The Gray Panthers
"Age and Youth in Action"

LEARNING OBJECTIVES

- Recite the size and composition of the aged and how these statistics have changed over time.
- List the implications of these changing demographic patterns and speculate on future implications.
- Identify the major changes that one can expect over the course of the life cycle and differentiate changes among different types of reference groups.
- Stimulate discussion on whether a generation gap exists in our society.

The human group, in its many manifestations, is the central focus of all sociology. What human beings do because they are members of groups; how groups are differentiated according to status or function; what characterizes the subgroups that make up the total society—these are the basic questions of sociological analysis.

When sociologists turn their attention to aging and the concerns of gerontology, they are likely to be asking three central questions concerning groups defined by age. The first concerns the *size of the group and the characteristics of its members*. How many aged people are there in a nation such as the United States or in a smaller political unit such as Los Angeles County? What are the characteristics of individuals in this age group, compared with those of other groups? How do such statistics today compare with those of a decade ago? A second basic question concerns the *interactional patterns* within the group. What are the dynamics of interpersonal relations as one grows older—the roles (social positions) and norms (expectations) which define appropriate behavior and which differentiate individuals within the group (high status vs. low status, for example)? The third issue concerns *relations between that group and other groups in the society*. How might one characterize intergroup relations between the young and the old in our society, for example?

These three sociological questions, relevant to the analysis of any group, attempt to describe the regularities of group characteristics and behavior. Gerontologists are faced with an additional complication, however. They must deal with *change over time* in these social characteristics. There are two ways in which this issue is manifest. The first concerns how *individuals* themselves change with the passage of time, how they become different at 40 from what they were at 20, and yet maintain basic elements of identity and continuity. The second involves

how *groups* change, how larger aggregates of human beings such as fraternities, occupations such as nursing, political parties, nations, and civilizations, each exhibit differences and yet have similarities when compared in 1960 and 1970.

The sociologist interested in aging, while describing the characteristics of social behavior that are relevant to aging, must constantly keep in mind the complex perspective of change-vs.-continuity.

This is a complicated set of issues, but as the other chapters in this part attest, they reflect a number of increasingly important social problems. If one is interested in pursuing further the complexity involved with the measurement of social characteristics with the passage of time, the following writings should be consulted: Riley and associates (1971, 1972, 1973), Neugarten and Moore (1968), Maddox (1970), Bengtson and Black (1973), or, for a more introductory discussion, Bengtson (1973), or Atchley (1972).

SIZE AND CHARACTERISTICS OF THE AGED AS A GROUP

The first question a sociologist often asks appears to be simply a manner of counting. "How many are in this particular group? What are they like?" These inquiries constitute the demographic or population perspective of social analysis, an extremely important component of any examination of aging. The answers are more complex than one might suppose.

SIZE

Considering the population of individuals above the age of 65, we are faced with some rather startling figures. According to the 1970 census, there are almost 21 million Americans over the age of 65, which means 1 person out of 10 in our population. These figures are particularly impressive when we compare them with those in 1900, just seven decades ago, when there were only 3.1 million over the age of 65, representing 4 percent of the population. And, when we con-

Preparation of this chapter was assisted by a grant from the RANN program of the National Science Foundation (#GI-ERP-03496), "Sociocultural Contexts of Aging: Implications for Social Policy." We wish to express appreciation to Ann Newman in the preparation of this manuscript.

sider projections into the future, the data are even more dramatic. By the year 2020, when most readers of this chapter will have passed retirement age, there may be about 33 million Americans over the age of 65. Or, if there are major breakthroughs in medical technology and lower fertility rates continue as reflected in some demographic projections, there may be as many as 40 million senior citizens, comprising over 15 percent of the population.

Second, consider life expectancy—the average number of years a person can be expected to live. This has increased from 49 years in 1900 to 70 years today. The increase, however, affects men and women differently. In 1900 women were outliving men by an average of 3 years; in 1970 the difference was widened to 7 years. If this trend continues, some demographers predict that 2 out of 3 aged persons in the year 2020 will be female (Atchley, 1972).

Third, consider the very old, those above the age of 85. According to one recent estimate (Kramer et al., 1973) between the years 1970 and 1980 the percentage of those 85 or older will increase by almost 50 percent.

These statistics are of considerable interest; they suggest we are in the middle of a population revolution regarding the aged. But more urgent are the implications of such statistics in terms of human needs and institutional requirements. As we look ahead, we can foresee an inevitable and dramatic increase in the demands for medical, housing, economic, and other services.

But there is a rather dismal footnote to these facts and projections. Are our current service systems adequate to meet these increases, and are we training enough professionals to deal with the special problems of the elderly? The answer, clearly, is negative. Persons trained in gerontology, persons in the service or medical profession who have some awareness of the needs and characteristics of this group compared with others, are not being produced at a rate commensurate with the population growth of the aged. Nor are there sufficient funds for research of aging. Thus, we face, in 1980 and 1990, a serious crisis in service delivery and knowledge concerning the fastest growing segment of our society.

CHARACTERISTICS

There is, however, another side to the population picture regarding the elderly. Demographers are not only concerned with the size of a given group as discussed above, they are also concerned with the characteristics that describe individual members of the group. Such things as how much education they have achieved, where they were born, what their health and economic status is, what is the proportion of male to female—these data are important in describing a group and in drawing implications for needs and preferences of individual members.

Consideration of these factors suggests there is a "new type of older person" emerging in American society. As described by Cain (1967), there is strong evidence that each successive age-cohort turning 65 is more advantaged than the preceding cohort in a number of characteristics.

For example, if one compares the educational attainment of those who turned 65 between 1938 and 1947, with those who will become 65 between 1978 and 1987, there is a considerable increase. The average 65-year-old in the 1980s will have completed 4 more years of school, including a high-school education. This will have many implications: because of better education they will have had better jobs throughout their lifetimes, they will have enjoyed higher income and command more economic assets, they will have been able to purchase better medical treatment—compared with the average older person of a few decades previous. They will also live longer, and finally, they will have higher expectations regarding what retirement should bring.

To give another example, consider the proportion of immigrants to the native-born in successive age-cohorts. Of those 60 and older in 1960, 18 percent were born in other countries; of the 50 to 59 age group, 10 percent were immigrants; and of those between 40 and 49, less than 5 percent were foreign born (Cain, 1967). When one compares immigrants with native-born, one usually finds the latter to have higher education, better jobs, more stable careers, and higher health status. This again suggests advantages for tomorrow's elderly compared with those of previous decades. Perhaps more important, the cultural adjustments required in moving from one tradition to another are demanding, particularly when making the role transitions of later life as described in the next section. Clark (1967) describes an elderly Polish woman in San Francisco who had adopted what her cultural heritage suggested was the appropriate role for her position—the matriarchal widow, head of her family, consulted by all family members in the making of life decisions. This role, while expected and approved in present rural society, was totally inappropriate in the cultural setting of the New World. Her family resented her intrusiveness; she could not understand their reaction; she developed psychiatric symptoms and was institutionalized. These considerations suggest that being an immigrant and growing old have considerable costs. Given that increasing proportions of tomorrow's elderly will be native-born and raised, it is true that they will have some advantages compared with the average older person in previous decades.

In short, a demographic analysis of the elderly as a group suggests two things; first, that the size of this group has increased dramatically and will continue to grow; second, that they are in many respects more advantaged compared with previous generations of older people. These data suggest important implications in terms of service delivery systems: more and more older people, living longer, who in addition to their numbers and longevity have greater resources and higher expectations and, therefore, will make greater demands on service institutions.

INTERACTION PATTERNS AND INTERPERSONAL RELATIONS

The second question a sociologist often asks in examining a particular group is, "What are the interaction patterns of a person and the group?" Throughout their lives human beings are members of, and act within, an endless succession of groups. Much sociological analysis focuses on the fact that behavior is influenced by the individual's *position* in a group and perceptions of

the *expectations* that go along with such positions. In analyzing social behavior through the course of life, it is important to focus on the changes and continuities in social positions and expectations with the passage of time. We will first consider *losses* in the aging individual's social world; and then examine potential *compensations*.

LOSS

In the sociological analysis of individual behavior over the course of life, three kinds of loss seem evident. The first is *role* loss. Roles are, quite simply, social positions played by individuals. We live our lives in a complex succession of roles: right now you, the reader, might be simultaneously a student, a daughter or a son, a lover, a friend, an employee, a church member, a mother or a father—an intricate package of interpersonal or group positions. A considerable body of sociological research concerns the ways in which various roles mesh or conflict in everyday life and the ways in which these change with the passage of time.

The role losses that occur with age are most dramatically evident in widowhood, when one loses not only a loved confidant but also a social partner. There is also obvious role loss in retirement, when not only income but also a socially valued position is lost. A less visible exit from social position occurs in the middle years for parents when children are "launched" and an effective past function no longer exists. Although this particular loss has not been studied extensively, research by Bart (1968) suggests it may be related to psychiatric disturbance among some women who have been preoccupied with the rearing and socializing of children to the exclusion of other social positions in the middle years of life.

The second aspect of loss from a sociological perspective on growing old concerns *norms* or expectations: social laws, primarily informal, which guide much of what we do in an average day. Norms are obviously related to roles; there are specific expectations concerning work, parental, kin, and husband-wife roles. The lives of adults represent a most complex network of roles, each of which has specific expectations, and problems may arise because of conflicting norms among the various social roles one simultaneously plays. Norms defining optimal performance in the student role may conflict with norms concerning behavior as a spouse or lover or parent (particularly before examinations). In our daily lives we find ourselves constantly juggling the expectations associated with one social position against those attendant to another. To complicate things still further, a single social position involves (simultaneously) many different expectations. For example, it is my observation that the single role of housewife involves the expected performance of the following array of behaviors: cook, therapist, hostess, mistress, chauffeur, lover, manager, and housemaid—to name but a few.

What happens in the middle and later years when roles begin to change? Expectations (norms) also change; there is a greater vagueness and lack of specificity regarding what one is expected to do (Neugarten, Moore, and Lowe, 1965). Put differently, there is a loss of norms with aging, just as there is a loss of roles.

For the middle-aged individual who is working and the parent of dependent children, there are many expectations that govern behavior in day-to-day living. But when the children move away, when a person retires or loses a spouse, normative guidelines become much less specific. What *should* you do when you are retired? What *should* you do when your spouse dies?

In these cases expectations primarily center on what one ought *not* to do. For example, after widowhood the elderly individual should not be too obvious concerning dating; a widow, it would seem, should quietly try to forget about a sexual life. Most important, a woman must not become involved with a man much younger than she is. A movie called *Harold and Maude* depicted in a humorous, yet tragic, way the relationship between an elderly woman and a teen-age boy. It was interesting that some published reviews suggested the movie to be obscene; while American moviegoers may not object to violence or nakedness, they react with indignation to the subject of an old woman and a young man in a sexual and love relationship.

In our humor we see indications of norms that govern everyday life. A current bumper sticker proclaims, "I'm not a dirty old man; I'm a sexy senior citizen." It is of interest to note that, although the carnal old man may be humorous, the sexual older woman is not. Here again is evidence of a norm prescribing loss of sexual activity, a norm that may be inappropriate for many healthy older widows.

A third sociological perspective toward loss in one's interpersonal world concerns changes in *reference group* with aging. We determine much of our behavior from the expectations of the groups to which we refer in judging that behavior. Work organizations or professional groups are important sources of norms specifying appropriate behavior. The religious or ethical tradition with which we identify is another significant source for such expectations. Family and close friends constitute a third, and perhaps most important, reference group.

Longevity can mean that one will outlive one's most relevant reference groups. What happens when people reach their seventies or eighties and most of their friends have passed away?

A while ago we interviewed a man who had just turned 104. In talking about the problems of growing old, he said, "You know, I haven't had a friend since I was 77. That's when my last friend died." To us, living for 27 years without someone who could be termed a confidant represents a significant loss, not only in terms of face-to-face contact and sharing but also in terms of a reference group. To what group can this man refer in judging the adequacy of his behavior? It is inappropriate for him to judge himself by the standards of late middle age, but that is exactly what he does; he exhibits shame and depression in not being able to mow the lawn and care for his garden.

Thus the lives of older people can be characterized by the theme of social loss, as of roles (social positions), of norms (expectations regarding appropriate behavior), and of reference groups. What, then, are the characteristic reactions to such losses?

COMPENSATION

Most investigators who have written about the consequences of the loss of roles and norms in old age have emphasized their *negative* implications. Emile Durkheim, almost a century ago, suggested that one cause of suicide is the feeling of loneliness and estrangement coupled with a condition of being anomic (literally, "without norms") resulting from a marginal social position. We know from more recent research that suicide is often the consequence of loss of roles, norms, or reference groups. The application to problems of aging as discussed above is obvious. It is perhaps no accident that in older age groups, particularly among men, the incidence of suicide surges sharply upward.

How might we compensate for the deleterious results of social losses? This question has intrigued many sociologists writing in the field of social gerontology. Rosow (1967, 1974), articulating one point of view, suggests that encouraging age-homogeneous groupings, from senior citizens centers to "golden-age" apartment or "leisure world" developments, may ameliorate these losses by promoting socialization into old age. He argues that when aged individuals are brought together, norms for appropriate or inappropriate behavior should become more salient, resulting in the creation of an age-appropriate reference group. Anomie, or a feeling of "normlessness," might then decrease.

This would suggest that places such as "Sun City" and retirement hotels have valuable and unanticipated social consequences for the increasing number of aged individuals. Although the issue of age-segregated housing is hotly debated, some data provide evidence that this is one alternative to the negative consequences of social loss in old age.

Positive consequences of the losses that occur with normal aging have received less attention in the gerontological literature. It seems to me, however, that one consequence of the decrease in social expectations may be the *increase* in personal freedom. An average 55-year-old American blue-collar worker devotes 8 hours a day to a job which he may or may not find rewarding, to doing what others may tell him to do, to produce something he may never see as a finished product. He may spend another several hours worrying about his adolescent son who is dropping out and his daughter who is turning on. A continual worry is the financial responsibility for a houseful of consumers. Many roles and expectations govern the behavior of

this middle-aged man, and as a consequence he may find he has relatively little freedom.

Consider the same man at age 65, retired. No longer does anyone tell him how he must spend 40 hours of his week. His children are grown and he no longer has the responsibility for educating and launching them. Although he has less income, he also has fewer financial responsibilities. From a sociological perspective, the aging man has lost roles and has less clear-cut expectations governing behavior. But he also has considerably more freedom and greater opportunity to do what he himself wants to do with his time. In short, his formal social loss represents potential personal gain—if he has the resources to take advantage of the opportunity.

Consider a second kind of loss, one that is even more personally painful: widowhood. The grief and bereavement associated with loss of a lifelong mate is one of the most tragic aspects of growing older. However, it is of some interest to us that often, after a period of mourning, persons who have lost a spouse appear to be establishing a satisfying new life-style.

In this regard many studies have suggested that some marriages of long duration are sufficiently unhappy that the partners find little pleasure together. The relationship may have been so demanding that each individual's creativity was hampered. In such cases, the death of a spouse after a long and unsatisfying marriage may present an opportunity for many new kinds of freedom. For instance many men and women enrolled in continuing education programs are widowers and widows. Close questioning sometimes reveals that they felt uncomfortable about taking such courses during their marriage and are now in a position to do so.

We are not, of course, suggesting that bereavement is ever easy, and much less that any significant proportion of middle-aged individuals welcome the loss of a mate. Rather we are noting that the role losses associated with aging—even widowhood—may not necessarily have negative consequences; the decrease in normative expectations can be viewed as an opportunity for gains in freedom and individual development. This potential has too infrequently been acknowledged or communicated by those in service-delivery positions with respect to the elderly.

Thus the pattern of interpersonal and interactional changes associated with aging is characterized by *loss;* but with the proper resources—economic, health, and most important psychological, the consequence of such loss may be increased *freedom* to choose more for oneself in the later stages of the life cycle than ever before in adulthood.

INTERGROUP RELATIONS: THE YOUNG AND THE OLD

The third question a sociologist is likely to ask in examining a particular group is, "What about relations with other groups? What kinds of similarities and contrasts are evident between this collectivity and others in the society?" This question has received a great deal of attention in American sociology where comparisons of social class, of ethnic groups, of males and females have led to a vast literature on social stratification. It is only quite recently, however, that systematic attempts have been made to characterize relations among *age* strata (Riley, 1971, and 1973; Riley et al., 1972).

In fact, this issue was raised in the mass media long before it became of interest to many sociologists, as the debate concerning the "generation gap" became a highly visible issue by the early 1960s. At that time there appeared to be an unprecedented and widening cleavage in American society between groups defined by age (Bengtson, 1970). First there was the civil rights movement which attracted national attention. Then the free-speech movement at Berkeley in 1964 was followed by a wave of campus protests concerning student rights (curricula, grades, administration, living arrangements). But these developments were quickly overshadowed by the mounting protest against the Vietnam war. By 1968 more than three-fourths of American universities had been the scene of significant protest activity. And finally, during the 1960s there emerged among the young a constellation of values and life-style so distinctive it was dubbed the "counterculture." Although its more exotic manifestations involved setting up rural communes and the

rising incidence of hallucinogenic drugs, the clothes, music, sexual behaviors, and antiestablishment orientations of this style of life quickly spread to larger groups of youth across the world (Bengtson and Starr, 1974).

These developments have led many sociologists to consider more seriously relations and contrasts between groups defined by age. And, although much of the generation gap literature was sensationalistic or founded on questionable data, the result has been some useful and current information about contrasts and continuities between the young and the old. Much of the new data question widely held assumptions regarding the nature of age-strata differences.

VALUES

One's general orientations concerning desirable goals serve as standards for making choices among specific courses of action. These general orientations, or *values,* appeared to vary considerably among age groups in the 1960s, according to some observers. At least one large-scale study, however, questions this assumption (Bengtson, 1975).

In this research, 2044 individuals who were members of three-generation families were asked to rank-order in importance 16 values ("things people find important in life"). The results were analyzed in terms of three generational groups: youth (average age 19), middle-aged (average age 44), and elderly (average age 67). There were two value dimensions that emerged from the 16 items. One, which reflected materialism vs. humanism, was composed of such items as possessions, financial comfort, and respect, as opposed to a world at peace, equality of mankind, and service. On this dimension significant age-group differences did *not* appear. The middle-aged were slightly more humanistic than were the youth. These findings are certainly not consistent with the stereotype of the older generation being less concerned with matters of peace and equality than the younger.

On a second value dimension however, there *were* significant age-group differences. This orientation, collectivism vs. individualism, consisted of items such as patriotism, loyalty, and religious participation, as opposed to freedom, an exciting life, and skill. The youth were the most individualistic, the elderly most collectivistic, and the middle-aged intermediate. One can say that there are significant contrasts between age strata on this dimension.

What causes such intergroup differences? There are two interpretations. The first can be called the *maturation,* or aging, explanation: the young people are more open to freedom, doing their own thing, establishing their own identity, while older people more highly value established institutions. If one follows this interpretation, one would predict that the youth will change their orientation with age and become more collectivistic when they are in their middle and late years. But a second explanation can be given: a *cohort-historical* or generational interpretation. Because of events in the 1960s, the young people came to value individualistic orientation more highly than the two other age groups; to a lesser extent the same phenomena occurred during the 1940s (explaining the current orientation of the middle-aged). One might say this evidences a trend toward the romanticism of individualism, as opposed to the institutionalism of collectivism in our culture, but it shows up in age groups differently. Unfortunately there is no way of telling which is more influential, the maturation or the cohort-historical explanation, until many more years have gone by, but to simply assume that youth will be "just like their elders" when they grow up would be inappropriate and would ignore one of the major forces of social change (Bengtson, 1973).

A final point is indicated in this study. Not only were the age group differences the largest on the individualism/collectivism value, but also there was the greatest indication of parent-child transmission on this value dimension. This is rather surprising, but it can be explained quite simply. The most salient issues between generations today are not along lines of materialism/humanism, but rather collectivism/individualism; not only are there significant age-group differences in perspectives, but also parents and children talk about such issues more. Thus the generations are more similar in many families; and in other families there may be more direct rebellion. In any case, the generation gap is not always what it seems to be.

FAMILY RELATIONS

A second area in which "inter-age" relations have been trenchantly debated recently involves the quality of parent-child relationships. Here again we have many stereotypes: youth feeling estranged from their parents more than ever before in our fast-changing society; elderly parents isolated from and neglected by their adult children; the "isolated nuclear family." And here again careful research suggests some alternative perspectives.

In the three-generation study described above, respondents were asked how much of a generation gap they felt within their families. They were also asked, in various ways, to describe the quality of relationships within the family. None of the three generations indicated that they experienced much "gap" within their families. The middle-aged parents as a group reported they felt slightly closer to the youth than the youth, in turn, reported. The elderly parents, likewise, reported slightly higher feelings of closeness to their middle-aged children than the middle-aged felt towards them. But on all scales, for almost all individuals, the message was clear: warm and supportive family relations, no gap in *our* family.

We also asked about interactions and exchanges among the three generations. Here it may be surprising for some to note how much interchange there was among the three age groups. Over two-thirds of the elderly said they saw their children more often than once a week. The elderly slightly overestimated the amount of assistance they received from their children, but both generations reported substantial exchange. And what stands out in the data is how many activities are shared with family members of other generations.

Certainly the elderly, in this study at least, did not feel isolated and abandoned from their families, nor did the youth feel estranged from their parents. Other studies have suggested similar patterns. This is not to ignore the reality of family quarrels and the fact that many families do not get along, but it is to suggest that some of our stereotypes about the generation gap and feelings of estrangement may be unfounded, at least as regards family relations.

CONFLICT BETWEEN AGE GROUPS

Perhaps it is not surprising that youth feel close to their parents or that the elderly are in close contact with their own children. How about at a more general level: the feelings different age groups have about each other when they are not related? How deeply do youth feel that "you can't trust anyone over 30"? What potential is there for the development of an old-age political movement based on sentiments that the elderly are fighting the middle-aged and the young for scarce economic resources?

There are unfortunately little data on these issues, and some issues are in the process of emerging at this time—as is the problem of old age political action. What does seem evident, however, is that the prospect of conflict between age groups seems minimal. There is less rivalry between age groups than was the case a decade ago; and although this may change due to such organizations as the Gray Panthers, age-group membership does not appear as a salient cleavage issue in politics or opinion.

The preceding discussion has, in summary, concerned three important issues of relevance from a sociological perspective of aging. First, in recent decades there has been a dramatic increase in the *size* of the population of the aged, and some significant changes in the *characteristics* of the average older person. Such changes will continue, according to population projections, well into the year 2000. Second, an analysis of the *interaction patterns* associated with the course of aging suggests loss of roles, norms, and reference groups in old age. But these losses can be countered in various ways, and there is an intriguing prospect of increased *freedom* in old age, which, in an increasingly active and vigorous population of seniors, reflects potential opportunity frequently ignored.

Third, an analysis of *relations between age groups* suggests that many stereotypes in regard to the generation gap and the neglected aging family member are inaccurate. Intergroup relations, defined by age, are generally close and rewarding within the family and nonconflictual at the broader cultural level.

There are many implications for practitioners in the medical and social service professions from data such as these, many of which are spelled out adequately in other chapters of this book. But there are two conclusions which we think must be emphasized. The first is the necessity for more realistic assessment of the sociological characteristics of the aged: the size of the group they represent, the characteristic changes with the life cycle, their relations with other groups. Few policymakers, to say nothing of the public at large, are aware of the population revolution in aging. Not only is old age a relatively unexamined frontier in terms of research, it also is an immense and growing social problem. In the absence of adequate data, program planning cannot be effective. In the absence of wide dissemination of such data, inaccurate stereotypes will continue.

To go a step further, we professionals in the field of aging have to advocate, disseminate information, and even agitate for programs and research needed by the elderly. Such programs in the past have been among the first to suffer from budgetary cuts, especially at the local and county level. In the light of the astonishing population revolution among the elderly in our society, such economies may be disastrous. We should recognize the potential political strength represented by the elderly and draw on this resource. Certainly the fact that 15 million voters in our nation are over age 65 offers a promise of political muscle which might be flexed in their and our behalf, for all of us, whatever our age, are inevitably growing older.

REFERENCES

Atchley, R.C.: *The Social Forces in Later Life: An Introduction to Social Gerontology,* Wadsworth, Belmont, Calif., 1972.

Bart, P.: Social structure and vocabulary of discomfort: What happened to female hysteria? *Journal of Health and Social Behavior,* **9:**188–193, 1968.

Bengtson, V. L.: The generation gap: A review and

typology of social-psychological perspectives, *Youth and Society,* **2:**7–32, 1970.

_____: On the socialization of values: Report to the National Institutes of Mental Health Contract no. 18158, December 1975.

_____: *The Social Psychology of Aging,* Bobbs-Merrill, Indianapolis, 1973.

_____, **and K. D. Black:** Intergenerational relations and continuities in socialization, in P. Baltes and W. Schaie (eds.), *Personality and Socialization,* Academic, New York, 1973.

_____, **and J. M. Starr:** Continuity and contrast: A generational analysis of youth in the 1970s, in R. J. Havighurst and P. Dryer (eds.), *N.S.S.E. Yearbook, 1975: Youth in the Seventies,* University of Chicago, 1975.

Cain, Leonard: Age status and generational phenomena: The new old people in contemporary America, *Gerontologist,* **7:**83–92, June 1967.

Clark, M.: The anthropology of aging: A new area for studies of culture and personality, *Gerontologist,* **7**(1):55–64, 1967.

Kramer, M., C. Taube, and R. Redick: Patterns of use of psychiatric facilities by the aged: Past, present and future, in C. Eisdorfer and M. Lawton (eds.), *The Psychology of Adult Development and Aging,* American Psychological Association, Washington, 1973.

Maddox, G.: Themes and issues in sociological theories of human aging, *Human Development,* **13:**17–27, 1970.

Neugarten, B., and J. Moore: The changing age status system, in B. L. Neugarten (ed.), *Middle Age and Aging,* University of Chicago, 1968.

_____, _____, **and J. Lowe:** Age norms, age constraints, and adult socialization, *American Journal of Sociology,* **70:**232–235, 1965.

Riley, M. W.: Aging and cohort succession: Interpretations and misinterpretations, *Public Opinion Quarterly,* **37**(1):35–49, Spring 1973.

_____: Social gerontology and the age stratification of society, *Gerontologist,* **11**(1):79–87, 1971.

_____, **A. Johnson, A. Foner, and Associates:** *Aging and Society: A Sociology of Age Stratification,* Russell Sage Foundation, New York, 1972.

Rosow, I.: *Social Integration of the Aged,* Free Press, New York, 1967.

_____: *Socialization to Old Age,* University of California, Berkeley, 1974.

FORTY-ONE

RETIREMENT

Robert C. Atchley

And this our life, exempt from public haunt, finds tongues in trees, books in the running brooks, sermons in stones, and good in everything.
William Shakespeare
As You Like It

LEARNING OBJECTIVES

- Define role.
- Describe the social role of retirement.
- Describe three general expectations of the retired person.
- Discuss phases of retirement.
- List four ways retirement can affect other roles for the retired individual.
- Discuss difficulties that could occur in retirement.
- Discuss one phase of retirement and how a nurse might intervene.

Retirement is many things. It is a phase of the occupational career cycle, following a socially defined minimum period of employment, in which occupational responsibilities and often opportunities are at a minimum and in which the individual is entitled to an income independent of a job. Retirement is also a social role which systematically helps to place people in the structure of society by specifying their rights, duties, and relationships with other people in their environment. Retirement is also a process through which the individual prepares for, takes up, adjusts to, plays, and eventually relinquishes the retirement role.

Thus, retirement is not an all-or-nothing state. It is a phase of life which is approached, lived through, and given up. *It is important for those who serve retired people to recognize the complex nature of the retirement process and how the various phases of retirement interact with other aspects of an individual's life.* This chapter seeks to provide an overview of the retirement role, the phases of retirement, and some personal consequences of retirement. It ends with a discussion of the implications of retirement for nursing.

THE RETIREMENT ROLE

Just as retirement is a complex concept, *role,* too, has several aspects. First, role can refer to the culturally transmitted, general expectations governing the rights and duties associated with a position in society (judge, woman, retired person, father, etc.). The rights of a retired person include the right to income without holding a job (but at the same time without the stigma of being regarded as dependent on society, as in the case of the unemployed), the right to freedom to manage one's own life, and sometimes more specific rights such as the right to use company or union facilities, to hold union office, and to retain various privileges.

Retirement duties represent a particularly neglected aspect of the retirement role. Job roles are most often discussed in a context of detailed, interrelated tasks, each of which is necessary to the operation of a system. Yet job roles are always more than that. To a greater or lesser degree, job roles also include man-

nerisms, ways of thinking, and generalized skills which people make part of themselves. They are expected to continue to be the *same type of persons* after retirement as they were before. People are also expected to retain their job skills, and sometimes they are expected to provide free service now that they are retired. A retired accountant recently told me that within a month after he retired he was approached by several voluntary associations and churches that wanted him to do their books. This expected continuity of behavior constitutes a major set of expectations facing the retired person. The *ability* of the retired person to live up to these expectations often depends on being able to remain able-bodied with a level of income reasonably consistent with preretirement levels. The *necessity* for living up to these expectations is strongest for the 96 percent of retired people who remain in the same community following retirement.

In addition, the retired person is confronted with other general expectations. The most general and important of these is that the retired person will assume responsibility for managing his or her own life. For a great many jobholders, the employer or the work schedule decides how much insurance is adequate, when to get up in the morning, when to go on a trip, what kind of clothes to wear, and even what to do for recreation. For a great many people, jobholding means playing the game by the rules, not only on the job but in other areas of life as well. For these people, retirement brings a great deal of new decision-making responsibility. Also, part of the time formerly devoted to the job must be set aside for these new decision-making duties. That is, in retirement there is little mandatory structure to the individual's relationships with time, space, and people. The individual must decide these matters; thus, not all the time made available by leaving the job is available for leisure. And for even the most responsible and autonomous jobholders, retirement represents an increase in decision making about their *personal* lives and the affairs of their households.

Also, retired people are expected to manage to live within their income, regardless of its level. Many people cannot, usually through no fault of their own, but the expectation is there nevertheless.

Retired people are expected to avoid becoming dependent either on their families or on the community. And just as income without jobholding is a reward for retirement, being looked down upon is punishment for those retired people who become dependent. Consider the difference in reaction to the dependency of a 55-year-old retired person as opposed to the reaction to the same dependency of an 80-year-old retired person. We expect the retired persons to fend for themselves, but we allow the elderly persons more dependency.

Finally, retired people are expected to stay out of the job market. This expectation is even built into social security regulations. A little part-time employment is okay, but if the individual earns more than is allowed, then social security retirement pension is cut back 1 dollar for every 2 dollars earned over the allowable amount.

To the extent that individuals want to take up *new* roles to adjust to retirement, they are expected to select from among leisure roles or volunteer roles. For most retired people, selecting leisure roles is both feasible and desirable, but volunteer roles often represent problems. Not only are volunteer roles for retired people not plentiful, but many of them are menial, depreciating positions which occupy time but provide little sense of accomplishment or self-worth. Also, there often is little choice among the tasks volunteers are allowed to do. For volunteer roles to provide satisfaction they must be *responsible* positions which both the volunteers *and* paid staff respect. Society is only just beginning to recognize this. The success of the Retired Senior Volunteer Program has shown that volunteer roles can be a viable option for both retired people and agencies in the community.

Role can also be defined as a relationship between individuals in a concrete situation. In this framework the retirement role is the relationship between the retired person and those who are still employed, either in a particular profession or in a particular organization. The crux of the relationship is the fact that both the retired person and the person still on the job tend to identify themselves in terms of the same job or work organization. Thus, the position of retired person is similar to that of alumnus. As with alumni of a given school, people recently retired from a job may be envied by those they left still on the job, and interaction centers around shared past experiences. The alumnus-type retirement relationship is tougher for the retired person if those still on the job are very negative about retirement. However, the longer the elapsed time in the retirement role, the fewer the number of friends still on the job, and the relationship becomes characterized less in terms of shared past experience and more in terms of general identity and loyalty. Contacts between retired people and those still on the job are seldom courted on a regular basis, but they are frequent enough that most retired people experience this particular aspect of the retirement role. And this is particularly true for those who remain in the same community.

Retirement is thus a complex social role which is composed of both general and specific privileges, expectations, and relationships. As compared with most job roles, the retirement role is more flexible and qualitative. In the past there has been a pronounced tendency to lament the absence of very programmatic and specific norms for the retirement role. More recently, however, the vagueness of the retirement role has come to be seen as a possible advantage. Given the fact that retired people differ considerably from one another in terms of physical, mental, and financial capability, it is perhaps useful to have a retirement role that is vague enough to allow each retired person to interpret it within a unique set of physical and social limitations. This leaves the retired person free to *negotiate* a detailed role definition with the significant persons in his social environment.

PHASES OF RETIREMENT

When retirement is viewed as a social role, it is useful also to consider the various phases through which the role is approached, taken, and relinquished. What follows is an attempt to sketch out the phases, with the understanding that our knowledge is quite tentative in this area (see Figure 41-1).

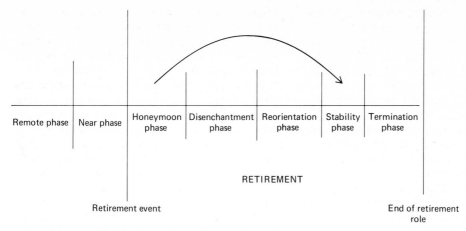

| Remote phase | Near phase | Honeymoon phase | Disenchantment phase | Reorientation phase | Stability phase | Termination phase |

RETIREMENT

Retirement event

End of retirement role

FIGURE 41-1 Phases of retirement.

PRERETIREMENT

The preretirement period may be divided into two phases: remote and near. In the *remote phase,* retirement is defined by the individual as a vaguely positive phase of the occupational career which is still a good distance in the future. This phase can begin even before the individual takes on his or her first job, and it ends when the individual realizes that retirement is near. Even in the remote phase, most people expect to retire. Very few expect to die before they reach retirement age and very few expect to work until they die. Few dread retirement, but few see retirement as requiring rational planning. Information-gathering tends to be unsystematic and only rarely intentional. Employers seldom expose their employees to any sort of formal retirement planning program during the remote phase. Thus, preparation for retirement in this phase may include positive attitudes and beliefs gained through experience. It may also include negative stereotypes. Because socialization in this phase is informal and unsystematic, the outcome is understandably unpredictable. It also leaves to chance several issues, such as financial resources and leisure skills, which must be dealt with if the individual is to satisfy the prerequisites for successfully taking up the retirement role.

Socialization is intended not only to teach people how to play a role but also to alert them to the prerequisites. Thus, high school not only prepares students for college by attempting to teach them how to learn, but it also provides students quite systematically with detailed knowledge concerning what it takes to get into college. Most high schools attempt to provide this information early enough so that students will know the prerequisites in time to satisfy them.

The retirement role also has prerequisites. *Retirement income adequate for the style of life one wants is an important prerequisite which requires long-term preparation.* People who want an expensive life-style in retirement must do a great deal of prior financial planning. Financing retirement is expensive and is accomplished best through long-range planning. Most people require a supplement to whatever retirement pensions they receive in order to sustain their desired life-style. But in order to provide for this supplement, the individual must be aware of the need very early in the occupational career.

Developing leisure skills is another prerequisite of the retirement role. These skills can sometimes be learned in later phases of retirement, but developing a wide variety of leisure skills is easier to accomplish during the early years of adulthood for two reasons. First, settings for learning are generally more available to younger people, and, second, younger people are somewhat more likely to seek new leisure skills. Ties to the community through participation in various types of organizations are also easier to develop earlier rather than later in adulthood.

A third important prerequisite of the retirement role is good health. While this variable is to some extent outside the individual's control, a good preventive health-care regimen in young and middle adulthood can definitely increase the odds favoring a vigorous and healthy retirement. A healthy status or being able-bodied is particularly important because retired people are expected to be independent, and because physical dependency cuts into the individual's field of choices.

Smooth adjustment to retirement is associated with financial security, personal adaptability, and good health. Yet at present, very little systematic effort is devoted toward making people aware of the need for developing these characteristics during the remote phase of preretirement. A good case can be made for the need of such efforts, especially among working-class people. Information about the prerequisites of retirement should be part of every student's experience in secondary and higher education. Otherwise, millions of people will continue to remain unaware of the prerequisites until it is too late.

The *near phase* of preretirement begins when the individual becomes aware that he or she will soon take up the retirement role. This phase is often initiated by an employer's preretirement program. It may also be initiated by the retirement of slightly older friends. For women, it is often initiated by their husband's retirement. Women often marry men a few years older than they are, and as a result, their husbands may retire a few years before. This brings home to these women the fact that retirement is near for them.

Attitudes toward retirement generally become more negative during the near retirement phase because the realities of retirement become clearer and because so many individuals currently are faced with not having met the financial prerequisites. Yet there are many who remain quite positively oriented toward retirement during this phase. Preretirement planning programs help to offset the negative stereotypes concerning retirement, and there are many whose financial outlook is quite good. The leisure-skill issue is particularly of concern to working-class people during this phase because they often realize at this point that they have no skills for dealing with big blocks of leisure.

Preretirement programs most often are offered to people in the near phase of preretirement. The range of topics varies, but financial planning and the use of leisure time are the two most common topics. *Preventive health care is often neglected in these programs.* Preretirement programs are successful in reassuring people and reducing their anxieties about retirement. But at this late stage it is usually impossible to remedy large deficiencies in preretirement socialization. It is especially difficult to do much about inadequate financial planning at this stage.

During the near phase, people begin to gear themselves for separation from jobs and the social situation within which they carried out those jobs. They may adopt a "short-timer's" attitude. They may begin to notice subtle differences in how they are viewed by others around them. Participation in retirement planning programs, retirement ceremonies, presence of an on-the-job trainee for replacement, and sometimes "promotion" into a less essential job are all mechanisms which serve to publicly define a person as being in the near phase of preretirement. In job situations where retirement is viewed negatively, people can be expected to avoid these symbolic indicators of status decline. In job situations where retirement is viewed positively, then people can be expected to welcome these symbolic indicators of a gain in status.

One way that people prepare for upcoming events is by projecting themselves into the setting and "living out" that situation in their imaginations. Thus, during the near phase of preretirement, many people develop a detailed fantasy, an imaginary living out, of their projected life in the retirement role. These fantasies may be quite accurate pictures of the future or they may be totally unrealistic. There is always an element of idealization in fantasy, but there is also a great deal of difference between pragmatic idealism based on knowledge and romantic idealism based on wishful thinking. To the extent that fantasy is realistic, it can serve as a "dry run" which may smooth the transition into retirement by identifying issues that require advanced decision making. To the extent that fantasy is unrealistic, it may thwart a smooth transition into retirement by setting up a detailed but unrealistic set of expectations. A prime goal of preretirement education is to provide essential facts which can be used to construct a realistic fantasy. Nurses may be able to listen to persons who are doing a "dry run" regarding their future retirement, and they should be able to recognize the process.

THE HONEYMOON PHASE

The retirement event is often followed by a rather euphoric period in which the individual wallows in newfound freedom of time and space. It is in this phase that people try to "do all of the things I never had time for before." The honeymoon period tends to be a busy time, filled with a wide variety of activities, all done at the same time. A typical person in this phase might say, "What do I do with my time? Why, I've never been so busy!" The person in the honeymoon period of retirement is often like a child in a room full of new toys, flitting from this to that, trying to experience everything at once. Not everyone has a honeymoon. Some people cannot afford it. Others find that their field of choices is pretty limited—by finances, by life-style, by health, or by family situation.

The honeymoon period may be quite short or it may extend for years, depending on the individual's resources and imaginativeness in using them. However, most people find that they cannot indefinitely keep up the pace of the honeymoon period, and they then settle into some sort of routine.

The nature of the routine which follows the honeymoon period is important. If the individual is able to settle into a routine that provides a satisfying life, then that routine tends to stabilize. Many people whose off-the-job lives were full prior to retirement are able to settle into a retirement routine fairly easily. For these people, choices among activities and groups and plans to live were made earlier. All that remains is to realign one's time in relation to those choices.

THE DISENCHANTMENT PHASE

However, for many people it is not so easy to adjust to retirement. After the honeymoon is over and the pace of life begins to slow down, many people experience a period of let-down, disenchantment, or even depression. The depth of this emotional letdown is related to a number of factors. People with few alternatives, people who have little money or poor health, people who were overinvolved in their jobs, those who are unaccustomed to running their own lives, people who experience other role losses in addition to retirement, people who leave communities where they have lived for many years—these are the types of people who are apt to experience deep and lengthy periods of depression following the honeymoon period. *The typical symptom during this phase is overwhelming self-pity.*

The honeymoon period represents a reality test of the preretirement fantasy. The more unrealistic the preretirement fantasy turns out to have been, the more likely the individual is to experience a feeling of emptiness and disenchantment. The failure of the fantasy represents the collapse of a structure of choices, and what is depressing for the individual is that he or she must start over again to restructure life in retirement. "So traveling turned out to be a drag when done constantly, now what?" The disenchantment phase also results from the failure of anticipatory socialization for retirement. Somehow the individual developed a concept of the retirement role that was either too unrealistic or too vague to be workable. Such failures are common. Quite often the individual's fantasies of slots he or she is about to occupy are inadequate. This problem is usually solved by on-the-job training. Likewise, most people eventually work their way through the disenchantment phase, but some do not. Those who remain in this phase need help in moving into the reorientation phase.

THE REORIENTATION PHASE

A reorientation phase is necessary for those who are unable to develop a satisfying routine in retirement. During the reorientation phase, those who are depressed "take stock" and "pull themselves together." Otherwise they must remain in the disenchantment phase. This process involves using direct experience as a newly retired person to develop a more realistic view of the alternatives, given a particular set of resources. It also involves exploring new avenues of involvement. Groups in the community sometimes help during the reorientation phase. For example, many people become involved in senior center activities for the first time during this phase. Outreach programs of community agencies and churches also sometimes help.

But for the most part people are on their own during the reorientation phase, and if they seek help it is most often from family and close friends. The goal of the reorientation process is to find a set of realistic choices which can be used to establish a structure and a routine for life in retirement which will provide a life that is satisfying at least some of the time.

THE STABILITY PHASE

Stability here refers to the development of routine criteria for dealing with change, not to the absence of change. In the stability phase of retirement, the individual has a well-developed set of criteria for making choices, and these allow the person to deal with life in a reasonably comfortable, routine fashion. Life may be busy, and it may have exciting moments, but for the most part it is predictable and satisfying. Many people pass into this phase directly from the honeymoon phase; others reach it only after a painful reassessment of personal goals; others never reach it.

People in the stability phase have mastered the retirement role; they know what is expected of them; they know what they have to work with, what their capabilities and limitations are. They are self-sufficient adults, going their own way, managing their own affairs, unduly dependent upon no one. Being retired is for them a serious responsibility, seriously carried out.

During this phase the individual inevitably encounters physical declines which change the level of functioning. But these changes, too, can usually be incorporated into the routine without changing the criteria for making choices. Sometimes, however, physical disabilities or losses of

other roles are serious enough to cause a need for a new routine. At this point, the individual may again encounter a reorientation phase.

TERMINATION PHASE

Many older people die rather abruptly with no lengthy period of disabling illness. But people lose the retirement role in other ways. Often it is canceled out by illness and disability. An individual who is no longer capable of engaging in major activities, such as housework, self-care, and the like, moves from the retirement role to the sick and disabled role. This transfer is based on the loss of able-bodied status and the loss of independence, both of which are required for adequately playing the retirement role. It is not so much that the individual stops being a retired person, but rather that being a sick or disabled person begins to take priority in how the individual is treated by others. Another way that an individual may lose the status as a retired person is to lose financial support. At that point, the person ceases to be retired and becomes dependent. Of course, still another way to lose the retirement role is to take a full-time job.

The increasing dependence forced by old age usually comes gradually enough that the retirement role is given up in stages. But if the person becomes institutionalized, independent choices threaten to become so trivial as to remove totally the dignity that adheres to the retirement role. In health-care institutions it is especially important to be alert to areas where the dignity and decision making of the disabled can be maintained.

RETIREMENT AND OTHER ROLES

There is no universal point of retirement, just as there is no universal point at which one becomes old or loses responsibility for adult children. There is thus no way to tie the retirement role specifically to a particular chronological age or to other phases of the life cycle. Yet retirement can affect other roles in at least four ways: (1) by increasing the time available for playing other roles, (2) by affecting eligibility for playing other roles, (3) usually by changing the economic wherewithal available for playing other roles, and (4) sometimes by changing the manner in which the person plays other roles.

The increase in time results from the fact that the decision-making and management functions which make up the retirement role do not require all the time freed by loss of the job. This is particularly true once the stability phase of retirement is reached.

Retirement sometimes affects eligibility for playing other roles. For example, many jobs allow and require involvement in community affairs. And the community often courts such involvement because the individual has an advantageous occupation such as banker, lawyer, or plant manager. Upon retirement, the influential position in community affairs often goes to one's successor on the job. A similar process also sometimes operates in unions, professional associations, and voluntary associations.

Retirement income often necessitates curtailment of expensive leisure pursuits such as golf, boating, or travel. It may also limit continued participation in voluntary associations. It may force the family to relocate.

Probably most important is the change which occurs in the *quality* of other role playing, especially in the family. Retired men inevitably seem to play a bigger part in taking care of the household. This increased involvement may be wanted or it may not. For example, some wives welcome their husband's increased time spent around the house; others do not. As one woman put it, "I married my husband for better or worse, but not for lunch." Middle-class wives usually welcome this trend, but working-class wives often do not. Retirement usually involves negotiating a new routine in the household, a routine that encompasses more contact and cooperation between spouses.

SOME DETAILED CONSEQUENCES OF RETIREMENT

A great many people see retirement as a social problem. This view is usually based on the idea that giving up one's job precipitates a major identity crisis for the individual. According to those who subscribe to this view, the job is *the* major source of identity in American society, and retirement signifies the individual's inability to perform in his or her most highly prized role. Retirement is thought to trigger an identity breakdown which hamstrings the older person in efforts to cope with life without a job. As plausible as this argument may seem, research from a wide variety of sources indicates that it does not fit the experience of the vast majority of retired people. About 20 percent have difficulty adjusting to the loss of job or decline in income. Another 10 percent have problems in retirement, such as poor health or loss of spouse, but these do not result from retirement per se.

The fact of the matter is that Americans are increasingly looking at retirement as a period of life when individuals can enjoy a high degree of well-earned autonomy over their lives. By far the majority of retirements occur *before* the mandatory age. Also, many workers see the mandatory retirement age as welcome social permission to retire.

Yet retirement is not trouble-free. There are people who encounter difficulties in retirement. The crucial problem is to separate those difficulties which arise from the operation of the system from those which arise out of unique, individual factors.

It may be useful to begin by dispelling some myths concerning the effect of retirement. Retirement seldom triggers an identity breakdown. Most people have many identities. In addition, people retain their job identities in retirement. Retirement has no significant effect on self-esteem. *Retirement has little effect on physical health. If anything, removal of job demands tends to improve health. Retirement may also make life easier for the mentally ill by allowing them to stay away from demanding, highly structured situations* (Atchley, 1976, 1980).

Retirement tends to produce no change or to increase social participation. Only in a small minority of cases does retirement contribute to loneliness or social isolation. Social participation outside the family in retirement is to a great extent a function of occupation as opposed to being a purely individual matter. A key determinant of social participation in retirement is having had an orderly work career which allows the development of ties with the community.

Retirement results in an increased participation in leisure pursuits, and increasingly this move toward leisure is being defined by retirees and the general public as a positive move.

Retirement also has situation consequences. To the extent that retirement produces poverty, it restricts the individual's options, particularly in terms of reduced food energy. Poverty also drastically reduces allotments for recreation and travel.

Retirement itself seldom produces changes in the community of residence. However, it may precipitate a search for more suitable housing within that community. Only about 2 percent of those who retire will ever move across state lines. However, as the general educational level of the retired population increases, this proportion can be expected to increase.

Somewhere around 40 percent of the women who retire are widows, and most couples have encountered the "empty nest" by the time of retirement. To the extent that increased involvement with the job is used as a mechanism for adjusting to widowhood or the empty nest, retirement may produce a delayed crisis of adjustment to those situational factors as well as to retirement itself. Retirement has a positive impact on couples in general, but among working-class couples, retirement often produces conflict.

There are three types of problems associated with the institution of retirement that arise as a result of the system. All these problems arise out of the nature of jobs. Jobs which demand the total energies of people leave them ill prepared for retirement. The professions, high-level management positions, and some types of self-employment are most likely to demand too much of workers in a sense that they leave them no time to develop alternatives to the job for giving meaningfulness and structure to their lives. Two prime prerequisites for successful retirement are prior involvements in a wide range of activities and leisure skills. Jobs which literally absorb the individual's energy prevent him from satisfying these prerequisites.

Some jobs produce poverty in retirement. Many of these are the same jobs that do not pay a living wage for the worker. Others have no pensions attached to them or pension systems with so many loopholes that many workers lose

their pensions. On the *average,* income drops 50 percent following retirement; for many retired households, it drops a lot further than that. The realities of retirement income show that 80 percent of retired American couples are trying to exist solely on social security, which averages just above the poverty line.

Finally, some jobs have mandatory retirement provisions attached to them. While mandatory retirement provisions are not nearly as universal as many people think, such provisions do create a problem for the capable older worker who wants to, or needs to, stay on the job.

IMPLICATIONS FOR NURSING

As individuals, of course, nurses need to satisfy the prerequisites for successful retirement for themselves just as anyone else does. *In fact, since they often deal primarily with those retired people who are physically or mentally ill, nurses tend to have very negative views of retirement.* Such negative views can and should be modified through in-service educational programs which present a more balanced view of the promise of retirement.

Retirement is apt to inject itself into the situation the nurse faces on the job in a couple of predictable contexts (and, of course, some unpredictable ones, too). There are people who fearfully regard retirement as a great unknown. Some of these people deal with this fear by hiding behind the sick role. Psychosomatic illness can be an effective ploy for ducking the responsibilities of retirement and for intruding on adult children and becoming dependent on them. This pattern is particularly likely to occur among working-class retirees.

Another common situation which nurses can expect to encounter is that in which the disenchantment phase of retirement compounds the treatment problem for retired clients. It is often literally true that until people are helped to reorient themselves positively toward retirement, they have little motivation for recovery.

In both of these situations *someone* has to help clients develop a viable concept of a meaningful retirement. It may not be the nurse, but nurses are in a good position to identify people in need of this kind of help, and to refer them to various community resources.

Nurses also encounter people who are in the process of relinquishing the retirement role for a more dependent role. Americans are taught to prize independence and to guard it. As a result, most adults rebel at the idea of becoming physically dependent on others. This rebellion is understandable and inevitable. It is not directed only toward nurses, but nurses, because they have the jobs they have, are often the most convenient target. The most understanding and helpful thing a nurse can do for people in such situations is to avoid treating physically dependent people like children, not to be patronizing, and to make as few *choices* for the person as possible.

Nurses are employed in retirement villages, and often care for the elderly frail living there who manage to stay in the retirement complex because of home visits by the nurse and the 24-hour nursing care available.

RETIREMENT: A COMPLEX SOCIAL ROLE

Retirement is not a vacuum. It is a complex social role which involves rights, duties, and relationships. It involves processes whereby the individual prepares for, takes up, adjusts to, and relinquishes the retirement role.

Retired people are expected to remain consistent with their past, to assume decision-making responsibility over their own lives, to avoid dependency, and to live within their limited incomes. If they add new roles in retirement, they are expected to select them from among available leisure and volunteer opportunities. Retired people receive pensions and various privileges in return for accepting these responsibilities. The relationship of retired people to their former jobs is similar to that of alumni. *People in American society generally respect retirement and retirees, and this is becoming increasingly true.*

Socialization for retirement involves satisfying prerequisites at least as much as it does developing specific knowledge or skills. It ideally should take place in the remote preretirement phase, but it seldom does. Instead, the remote phase tends to be typified by a haphazard collection of both information and misinformation. In the near phase of preretirement, the individual develops a detailed fantasy of what life in retirement will be like and uses this fantasy to make decisions about retirement. In the honeymoon phase just following retirement, retirees try to live out this fantasy. If they are successful in living out retirement plans, they develop a stabile routine built around a detailed set of criteria for making everyday decisions. To the extent that the retirement fantasy is unworkable, retirees become disenchanted. Most people move from disenchantment into a reorientation phase in which a new and stabile set of decision-making criteria is sought. The retirement role enters the termination phase when retirees encounter severe illness or disability or are forced to become financially dependent.

Retirement generally does not have negative consequences for health, self-esteem, social participation, social isolation, or residential mobility. However, retirement often produces drastic reductions in income, and at the same time income is the most difficult thing to do anything about on an ad hoc basis. Retirement can also be a problem for those already in poor health, those who were overinvolved in their jobs, and those who experience role losses in addition to retirement.

Yet, overall, retirement is becoming a more positive and promising experience for Americans, and as we begin to learn more about retirement, we hope we can help make it an even more positive and challenging experience.

REFERENCES

Atchley, Robert C.: *The Social Forces in Later Life,* Wadsworth, Belmont, Calif., 1980, chap. 8.
————: *The Sociology of Retirement,* Schenkman Publishing Co., Inc., Cambridge, Mass., 1976.

FORTY-TWO

ETHNICITY AND AGING

Sharon Y. Moriwaki

We have met the enemy and he is us.
Walt Kelly

LEARNING OBJECTIVES

• Describe a sociocultural model for understanding ethnic elderly attitudes and behaviors.
• Describe some of the pitfalls of statistical and cultural stereotypes of ethnic minority elderly.
• Identify similarities and differences among ethnic elderly in requesting or utilizing services.
• Discuss modification of standardized intake forms which would facilitate identification of problems and solutions to more effectively help ethnic elderly patients and their families.

All of us will grow old, but the response to our aging, whether successful or not, depends on many factors other than the stresses of the current situation. Ethnicity is one of these factors. Mr. W. was a 71-year-old Japanese man. He had spent the last 10 years watching his wife's physical decline, caring for her until her death less than a year ago. Now he was alone, although he still lived with his eldest son's family. His other children visited him every couple of weeks, but they were all married with their own families to care for. He began losing interest in all his usual activities. He stopped reading the Japanese newspaper and watching television (which he could not understand anyway). He could no longer get excited about the occasional fishing trip. He became more distressed with his physical difficulties—his neck hurt, his skin itched, his prostate bothered him. He doubted whether he would ever get well. He had watched his wife's extended illness; he did not want to be a burden in the same way. Shortly after his hospitalization for an operation—within a year of his wife's death—Mr. W. was found hanging in the garage of his son's home (Reynolds, 1971).

Suicide was Mr. W.'s response to old age, his strategy for coping with the biological, social, and psychological losses of aging. A sad end to a life story which began with so much hope for the future. Many of our ethnic minority elderly came to this country as young adults, hoping to carve out a successful life for themselves and their families. But for some, perhaps for too many, aging has not been as they had expected. Could knowing Mr. W.'s ethnic culture further our understanding of his adjustment to aging?

WHAT IS ETHNICITY?

To determine whether knowing one's ethnic background is important in understanding behavior and attitudes toward aging, we must first define ethnicity. Using the more categorical definition of the Bureau of the Census and other information systems, we should examine the statistics on suicide to determine whether Mr. W., a Japanese elderly man, would be expected to take his own life. Surprisingly, these statistics indicate that there are very few suicides among our Japanese Americans. Reynolds (1974) tabulated the number of reported suicides in Los Angeles County in 1970 from data obtained from the coroner's office (see Table 42-1). The data indicate that Caucasians had the highest rate of

TABLE 42-1
REPORTED SUICIDES BY ETHNICITY AND AGE, LOS ANGELES COUNTY, 1970

Age	Ethnic Group			
	Black	Japanese	Mexican	Caucasian
10–19	10	1	4	74
20–29	33	7	20	223
30–39	22	1	10	141
40–49	13	2	6	183
50–59	5	2	7	214
60–69	4	0	0	138
70–79	0	0	2	75
80 and over	0	0	0	39
Age unknown	1	0	0	1
Total	88	13	49	1088
Rate per 100,000 (approximate):				
Total	12	12	4	23
60 years and older	6.7	0.0	2.5	31.5

SOURCE: Adapted from Reynolds, 1974, and U.S. Bureau of the Census, 1972.

suicide, nearly twice that of Japanese and blacks, and over four times that of Mexican Americans. Looking at the data for those 60 years and older, again the Caucasian rates were highest (31.5 per 100,000), approximately 5 times higher than blacks and more than 10 times higher than Mexican Americans. There were no reported suicides among the Japanese elderly. From these data, we would not have expected Mr W.'s suicide.

However, it must be recognized that these data are official statistics and many suicides may go unrecorded. Kalish and Reynolds (1972) cite data on death and bereavement among four ethnic groups in Los Angeles which indicate that Japanese Americans most frequently tended to conceal suicides; one in five respondents knew of a suicide that was "covered up." These findings suggest that suicides do occur among Japanese Americans, and we cannot rely solely upon statistical and categorical definitions of ethnicity.

To understand the importance of ethnicity in influencing behavior, we must go beyond the purely categorical definitions. We could not predict Mr. W.'s suicide merely by knowing that he was Japanese. We need to know more of the meaning of his present life conditions—that he was socialized in a culture that revered the elderly and that sought advice from them on all important matters; that he had not achieved status in the larger dominant society, which was still unfamiliar and foreign to him; that he had watched his only social support linger on for 10 years, dying a gradual death; that he felt he could no longer contribute to his son's family in any way now that he, too, was physically declining. Lacking the status he had hoped to achieve

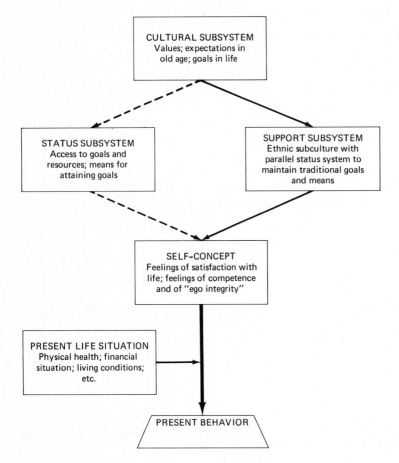

FIGURE 42-1 Components of ethnicity as related to individual behavior.

in his younger years and the social supports to buffer his failure, Mr. W. was left in an unbearable situation that seemed to worsen with age. He took the acceptable Japanese strategy of coping.

Ethnicity is a complex social variable which can be viewed as involving three components: the cultural, the social status, and the support subsystems. Together they influence the individual's self-concept, and, in turn, interact with the individual's present life circumstances to produce a unique pattern of adjustment to aging (see Figure 42-1). *We cannot understand the elderly ethnics' behavior without first understanding something of their values and expectations, their past experiences and achievements in the larger societal network, and their relations to ethnic peers and progeny.*

THE CULTURAL SUBSYSTEM

Ethnicity provides some understanding of the behavior and attitudes of ethnic elderly through identifying the culturally conditioned beliefs, values, and attitudes of their heritage. For first-generation immigrants, their world view and language derive from a country different from the one in which they are now old. They learned early, by observation, how their parents and other community members treated others, how they related to each other, how they treated their elderly. Simone de Beauvoir (1972) depicts the differences between the Hopi and Navajo cultures in their treatment of the elderly. Because Hopi culture was derived from a struggle against an unpredictable world, the present was all-important. Nonfunctional members, such as the elderly, were excluded from the tribe. In contrast, nature was less overwhelming for the Navajo who developed a culture based on past knowledge and experience. They attended to and cared for their elders, for they thought them to be endowed with supernatural powers which could affect their lives. Similarly for the Japanese immigrants who came primarily from small farming villages in southwestern Japan, ancestor worship was important in tying the land to genealogy. The aged directed ceremonies and were highly respected, since they would soon become ancestors who would watch over the

family. They were a symbol of order and predictability.

Cultural Changes It is important to understand the culture in which our ethnic elders were socialized, for their initial world view seems to be what is best remembered in old age. The problem for many of our immigrant elderly, however, stems from their growing old in an environment much different from that of their beginnings.

Kalish and Moriwaki (1973), in an article examining the elderly Asian American, suggest that for the Japanese and Chinese elderly, who

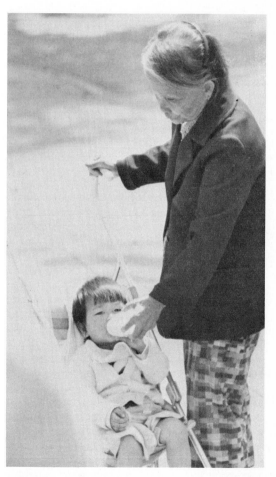

FIGURE 42-2 The problems of many of our immigrant elderly stem from their growing old in an environment much different from that of their beginnings. (*Courtesy of Anthony J. Skirlick, Jr.*)

initially anticipated returning to their homelands, the maintenance of values and customs of the old country was very important. They transplanted their values, language, and rules of behavior and transmitted them to their children so as to facilitate their adjustment on their return home. But streets in the new country were not lined with gold and the Asian immigrant was to grow old in a foreign land, with children socialized in a different country and a different time.

Two ethnic groups, however, did not follow the pattern of immigration, arrival, prejudice, and acceptance: the American Indian, who was already here, and the black, who was captured and brought unwillingly to toil on the Southern plantations. The histories of these two groups differ from the other ethnic minorities, and consequently, the elderly of these groups have had different cultural experiences. Pinckney (1969) discussed the situation of black Americans. When they were uprooted from their native lands and tribes and randomly sold to Southern plantation owners, they were unable to keep intact their tribal customs and organizations. Few aspects of Negro life today stem from their past native culture with the possible exception of religious life.

The similarity between these ethnic groups lies in the differences in value orientations between the elders and the younger generations, be it the grandchildren of immigrants, the Indians who have moved off the reservations into the cities, or the blacks who have migrated to the North or out of the ghettos.

A study of the mental health characteristics of the Mexican-American community in Los Angeles demonstrates this generational difference even in perceptions of mental illness. Edgerton and Karno (1971) found no significant differences in the definitions and perceptions of mental illness between Anglos and Mexican Americans. However, when they examined the responses of the Mexican-American group only, they found greater variations between those who were English-speaking as compared with those who were Spanish-speaking. These findings point to the necessity of looking at generational differences, particularly between younger members more assimilated into the dominant society and their elders who are not.

THE SOCIAL STATUS SUBSYSTEM

This perspective is the one with which we are most familiar; we treat people according to visible physical characteristics; and in the past, more so than today, it was the basis for ascribing status and life chances. Those who were dark-skinned were inferior and denied opportunities for education and higher status occupations; those who were yellow-skinned were thought to be unassimilable and inscrutable aliens to be carefully controlled and definitely not allowed to own property nor to become citizens (Kalish and Moriwaki, 1973). These features of minority group experiences—of discrimination and prejudice, of the maintenance of separate subcultures in ethnic enclaves (the ghettos, barrios, Chinatowns, etc.), and of the development of various institutionalized coping mechanisms (the black church, the Mexican family, the Chinese benevolent societies, etc.)—are the underlying similarities among all ethnic minority groups (Moore, 1971; Kent, 1971). Their minority status in the American social system, ascribed primarily by physical traits, has consequences for aging and responses to old age.

The National Urban League's approach that "today's aged Negro is different from today's aged white because he is Negro . . . and this alone should be enough basis for differential treatment . . ." focuses on the minority situation and ethnic stratification as the means for acquiring resources in the larger social network. The white majority is seen as controlling the resources which are valued by all; the nonwhite minority is seen as having fewer resources and fewer opportunities to obtain them. They have had fewer educational opportunities and lower-level occupations and incomes; consequently, they have had lower life chances.

One product of the status subsystem is the development of stereotypes or prejudgments about individuals who have similar physical characteristics. Perhaps because of our need to order our complex world and to find some efficient way of interacting with others, we categorize people who look alike as similar and treat them alike, with such labels as "all blacks are lazy" or "all Asians are inscrutable." Such categorizations, however, can be misleading and deleterious to the individual, for one can only think of the very startling illustration of the self-fulfilling prophecy in the cases of mistaken diagnoses. Normal children diagnosed as mental retardates and placed in institutions can quickly learn and exhibit all the symptomatic characteristics. *Diagnosis is helpful to some extent in providing effective treatment; however, misdiagnosis can have devastating effects on the individual so misclassified.* So it is with stereotyping; its disadvantage is that it prevents looking beyond the physical appearance of the individual toward more precise and accurate explanations for his behaviors.

Status Changes In examining the effects of minority status on the elderly, we must not over-look the effects of time. With succeeding generations assimilation occurs which affects the group's status or position in society. Societal attitudes may also affect the minority situation. Moore (1971) notes that discriminatory practices and stereotypes are now being attacked and displaced. Not only do changes in status occur with succeeding generations, they may also occur as a result of international events.

The racial distance studies by Bogardus (1959) reflect the changing attitudes toward ethnic groups over a 30-year period. He reported data on the status of 30 ethnic groups in 1926, 1946, and 1956. His data indicated that social changes occur which raise or lower the status of the entire ethnic group. For example, the Japanese were highest on the social distance scale during World War II (1946), but after their defeat and their shift toward democracy (1956), relations toward them improved, with social distance decreasing.

These differences in the social milieu between the now elderly and their progeny create intergenerational conflicts and have consequences for the elderly's adjustment. The difference between young and old is reflected in the ethnic elders not being able to communicate with the younger generation nor to understand their "violence" and unruliness, and the old claim that their life is better now than it has ever been.

THE SUPPORT SUBSYSTEM

For the ethnic elderly, the last component is, for want of a better term, the "support" subsystem—the buffer against discrimination, prejudice, and the unfamiliar customs, language, and institutions of the dominant society. The ethnic group acts as a reference and membership group with which people identify and through which they find self-worth. Our identity or self-image depends on how we define ourselves in terms of the values and attitudes that have been learned and accepted; but it is also modified by how we are treated by others, particularly by those who are significant in our lives. The Mexican immigrant might not be upset with the degradation and ill treatment by Anglo society because he sees his basic self-worth through identifying with his home village

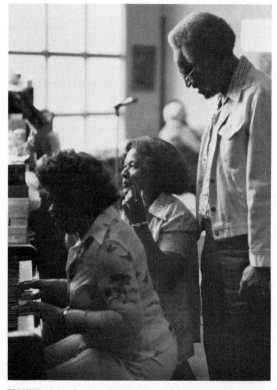

FIGURE 42-3 One product of the social status subsystem is the development of stereotypes for those individuals with similar physical characteristics. The disadvantage of stereotyping is that it prevents looking beyond the physical appearance of the individual toward more precise and accurate explanations for behaviors. For one of elderly minority status, it has a double impact: being old and of different ethnic origin. (*Courtesy of Anthony J. Skirlick, Jr.*)

in Mexico, disregarding the actions of the "loco gringo."

But ethnicity may have little influence on the behaviors and attitudes of people who identify with the dominant Anglo society rather than with their ethnic group. If they are trying to assimilate into the dominant society but are not accepted, such an affront to their egos may be extremely damaging. The negative effects of marginal status, of belonging to a minority status group but identifying with the dominant one, was found among Chippewa Indian children. Those who were most likely to develop neurotic traits and inconsistent self-concepts identified most with American standards, but were most likely to be rejected because of their physical appearance (Kerckhoff and McCormick, 1955). For the marginal person who aspires to membership in the higher status group but meets impermeable barriers, the losses of aging are even more stressful.

For the elderly who live in close-knit communities which have maintained their transplanted values and traditions, and who have been able to transmit these values to their children, their aging is a successful one. *But for those elderly who have no family or children or are estranged from them, and who are isolated from their ethnic communities, aging is a lonely and defeating battle.*

These three subsystems of ethnicity give us different lenses through which to view and understand the behavior and attitudes of ethnic minority elderly. In the medical care system the social status perspective is most often used, i.e., hospital statistics are tabulated by race categorically; however, to provide quality care that is accepted by the elderly ethnic client, all three perspectives must be considered, particularly as they influence the client's self-identity.

UTILIZATION OF SERVICES: WHO GETS HEALTH CARE?

There is little comprehensive and detailed information about the relative health and health care needs of ethnic elderly nationwide

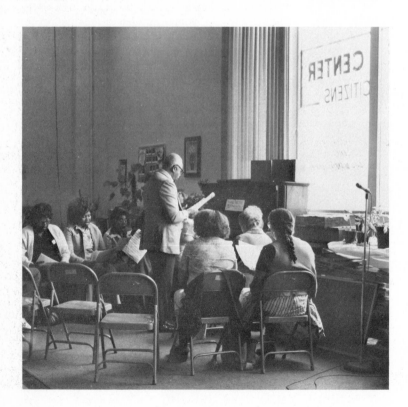

FIGURE 42-4 The ethnic group acts as a reference and membership group with which people identify and through which they find self-worth. This is especially meaningful for the ethnic elderly. (*Courtesy of Anthony J. Skirlick, Jr.*)

(Weaver, 1977; Jackson, 1978). What do exist are national health statistics (National Center for Health Statistics, 1973a; USDHEW, 1976) and a few studies in selected geographic areas (Hirsch et al., 1972; Weeks and Darsky, 1968; Valle, 1978). Statistics gathered by the National Center for Health Statistics can be used as suggestive evidence of who gets into the medical care system. They do not tell us the actual health condition of a particular ethnic group, nor do they adequately portray the age and ethnicity of the patient and the patient's health condition and needs. However, these data do reflect, to an extent, the discrepancy between the white and nonwhite rates of utilization.

Weaver (1976) provides the most comprehensive work on health care services to ethnic minorities, particularly in terms of health problems and strategies for using the social structures within ethnic communities to alleviate these problems. However, his presentation at the Fourth Institute on Minority Aging (Weaver, 1977) focuses more specifically on ethnic minority elderly. Here he discusses the differential morbidity patterns of various ethnic groups, based on the data which are available. For some groups such as the Native American elders, very little is known. Weaver states, "In fact, and bluntly speaking, there's damn little *anyone* knows about the numbers, conditions, or needs of Native Americans" (Weaver, 1977, p. 52). Of major importance is Weaver's emphasis on the heterogeneity of the populations "lumped together as non-Anglos," underscoring the need for service providers and planners to be aware of the peculiarities and similarities of constituent groups of minority aged, if useful and effective assistance is to be provided.

Weaver (1977) cites national health statistics which indicate that although more than twice the proportion of nonwhites are in poor health, suffering 40 percent more days of restricted activity, they have fewer contacts with physicians. In contrast, Hirsch et al. (1972) reported that, among their sample of low-income black and white aged in Pennsylvania, black elderly were not significantly different in health status, and, in fact, 60 percent of both white and black elders were not limited by health conditions. However, their data corroborate Weaver's findings that a greater proportion of whites (50

percent) had visited a physician in the past year, as compared with blacks (20 percent).

Reasons for the underutilization of health care services may be due to adherence to folk medical beliefs and practices (Weaver, 1976; Nicodemus, 1977; Wilson and Heinert, 1977) as well as to cost factors (Weeks and Darsky, 1968; Special Committee on Aging, 1971; Weaver, 1977). A study by Weeks and Darsky (1968) of low-income white and black elderly in Detroit reported that over 40 percent of the black elderly, as compared with about 14 percent of the white elderly, reported that they had an unmet health need. Asked their reasons for failing to obtain attention, 70 percent of the black and 59 percent of the white sample cited financial problems. Jackson (1978) reports changes in this trend, perhaps due to factors such as desegregated medical facilities, neighborhood clinics, increase in the number of black physicians, and Medicare and Medicaid, which have diminished the previously negative effects of race and income on physician visits.

Other reasons stated by minority elderly community residents involved the service providers. Hirsch et al. (1972) indicated the lack of communication to be one of the less favorable aspects, with health personnel, at times, assuming a greater medical sophistication among the elderly than really existed and at other times totally disregarding the social needs of the elderly patient. Thus, although the patient's medical needs were well-diagnosed and treatment appropriately prescribed, the "hoped-for medical therapy" was negated.

Similar findings regarding the insensitivity of the service system were reported by the San Diego Center on Aging studies of ethnic elderly, in particular that on the black elderly (Stanford, 1978) and on the Latino elderly (Valle and Mendoza, 1978). Among the Latino sample 30.7 percent and among the black 17.8 percent indicated they were in poor health. However, reasons for not seeking medical help were not only financial. Both blacks and Latinos shared their mistrust of doctors and medical personnel as well as their fear of illness and its consequences. One Latino elder was quoted as saying, "Why go to the doctor? One will only find more things wrong. These will only be more trouble and it will all cost more money" (Valle and Mendoza,

1978, p. 51). The health services system is thus seen as foreign to many of the ethnic elderly, who have not had ongoing contact with health care professionals, and is ever more problematic for those who are non-English-speaking.

ACUTE GENERAL HOSPITAL CARE

The data available for the number of patients 65 years and older discharged from nonfederal short-stay hospitals reveal that of the approximately 6 million discharges in 1972, 80.7 percent were white, with 6.5 percent being nonwhite. Further examination indicates that not only were the nonwhites less represented, but when they did seek medical care they tended to be more severely ill, having a longer stay in the hospital (see Table 42-2).

LONG-TERM CARE

The rising cost of health care affects the entire population but hits more severely the elderly, and in particular the ethnic minority elderly. In the face of limited and fixed incomes during inflationary periods, the elderly with chronic health conditions in need of medical assistance are most severely burdened. Thus, on the national level, the Administration on Aging (1978) is beginning to focus on the continuum of need and care of the elderly, especially those 75 years and older who are most vulnerable. The propor-

tion in this age group is increasing rapidly, and the increases are greatest for the nonwhite population. Comparison of data from the 1960 and 1970 censuses indicates that in all age groups over 60, the increases in the nonwhite elderly population were greater than those in their white counterparts. Looking at the vulnerable age categories, the nonwhite population growth has been significant: in the 75 to 79 age category, there was an increase of 32.5 percent among nonwhites, reflecting a 2.7 percent higher rate of increase than that which occurred among the white elderly for the same decade. Again for the same decade, in the 80 to 84 age group, the increase of nonwhites was great, 32.5 percent, with a 19.3 percent higher rate of increase than for the white elderly in the same age group. Finally for those 85 years and older, the increase was almost double the 1960 figure, 99.2 percent, and 25.8 percent greater than the increase among the white elderly in this age group. These increases in the proportion of the "old old" among the ethnic elderly emphasize the need for developing culturally relevant long-term care programs.

Although 89 percent of nursing and personal care home residents are elderly, the proportion of the total elderly population in such institutions is only 3.8 percent (see Table 42-3). Examination by race indicates underrepresentation by the nonwhite elderly; with residents representing 3.9 percent of the white elderly but only 1.6 percent of the nonwhite elderly of the

TABLE 42-2
PATIENTS 65 YEARS AND OLDER DISCHARGED FROM NONFEDERAL SHORT-STAY HOSPITALS BY ETHNICITY, 1972

| | Patients Discharged | | | |
Ethnic Group	Number	Percentage	Rate per 1,000 (Approximation Based on 1970 Population)	Average Length of Stay, Days
White	5,356,000	80.7	291.7	12.2
All other	432,000	6.5	249.0	14.0
Color not stated	847,000	12.8		11.7
Total	6,635,000	100.0	326.4	12.2

SOURCE: Adapted from the National Center for Health Statistics, 1973b, and U.S. Bureau of the Census, 1973.

TABLE 42-3

RESIDENTS IN NURSING AND PERSONAL CARE HOMES BY AGE AND
ETHNICITY, JUNE–AUGUST 1969

Age	White		All Other		Total	
	Ethnic Group					
	Number	Percent	Number	Percent	Number	Percent
Under 65	83,500	90.0	9,300	10.0	92,800	100.0
65 years and older	694,900	96.2	27,300	3.8	722,200	100.0
Total	778,400	95.5	36,600	4.5	815,000	100.0
Percentage of ethnic population (approximation based on 1970 population)		3.9		1.6		3.8

SOURCE: Adapted from National Center for Health Statistics, 1973b, and U.S. Bureau of the Census, 1973.

total 815,000 residents in 1972, 95.5 percent were white as compared with only 4.5 percent in the "all other" category. This includes blacks, Asians, American Indians, and any other race, with blacks making up the largest single component, i.e., 92.9 percent of this category. Clearly, this reflects underutilization by the ethnic elderly.

Although the utilization rates for other ethnic groups are not known, Yamaguchi (1973) has estimated the utilization of nursing homes by the Japanese elderly in Los Angeles to be very small, approximately 0.2 percent of the Japanese elderly. We do not know whether utilization is low because of the cultural tradition of "filial piety" (i.e., reverence and care for one's elders), the lack of adequate institutions for the ethnic minorities, or the lack of accessibility to them. The disproportionately low numbers of ethnic minority elderly in long-term care facilities may also be indicative of the greater support networks via extended families and neighbors (Maldonado, 1975; Kitano and Kikumura, 1976; Solomon, 1976). What is not known, however, is the extent to which the family is able to care for its elderly when they have become chronically ill and frail. At what point does the family decide that the stresses are too great and that institutionalization is the only alternative? An exploratory study of the frail elderly in Hawaii, where 76 percent of the state's population is nonwhite, indicated that 79 percent of the elderly 60 years and older living in

the community had one or more chronic conditions. Although data were not available on the number of chronically ill elderly living with their families, interviews with service providers suggest the need for greater community supportive services such as home health care, day-care services, homemaker chores and home-delivered meals, as well as respite services for caregivers (Moriwaki, 1979). These recommendations reflect the growing need for various long-term care alternatives.

The need for institutional care as well seems to be growing. Yoshida and Endo (1969), in a study of the adult children of parents placed in a Japanese nursing home, found that although children felt the guilt of placing parents in a nursing home, they felt their present lifestyle prohibited keeping elderly parents in their own homes. Thus even among a group that heretofore has been seen as a closely knit unit that "cares for its own," the need for long-term care is great. In fact, at Keiro, the only nursing home in Los Angeles available for the Japanese elderly, there are seldom any vacancies and always a long waiting list. It seems, then, that if facilities are available which provide needed services, they will be used by ethnic groups, regardless of past cultural mores.

The growing numbers of "old old" ethnic elderly may also contribute toward the increase in the use of long-term care facilities. Table 42-4 reflects the rise in the proportion of nonwhite elderly residing in long-term facilities. During a

TABLE 42-4
COMPARISON OF WHITE AND NONWHITE NURSING HOME RESIDENTS, 1969 AND 1973–1974

| Ethnicity | Number of Residents | | Percent Increase |
	1969*	1973–1974†	
White:			
Under 65	83,500	99,200	18.8
65 and older	694,900	911,300	31.1
Nonwhite:‡			
Under 65	9,300	15,100	62.4
65 and older	27,300	50,200	83.9

* Data from National Center for Health Statistics, 1973a.

† Estimates of nonwhite elderly based on U.S. Department of Health, Education, and Welfare, 1977.

‡ Includes black and Spanish-speaking as well as all other nonwhite groups.

4- to 5-year period (1969 and 1973–1974), the nonwhite elderly nursing home resident population increased by almost 84 percent, as compared with 31 percent among the white elderly group. If these data are any indication of future trends, we can expect to see an increase in the need for institutional care by the ethnic elderly who have become too frail to maintain themselves in the community.

Although long-term care facilities are less utilized by the ethnic elderly than are short-term care facilities, they are the focus of this chapter, since the discomforts of the medical regimen can be tolerated if the stay is short. However, the problem is greatly intensified for the person suffering from debilitating chronic conditions. A return to normal life outside the institution is questionable; thus the client's institutional care and treatment become more salient concerns.

TREATMENT

But why are ethnic elderly so underrepresented in long-term nursing care facilities and other institutions? Is it that they are much healthier and do not need such care? Is it that they cannot afford these services? Or is it that their needs are not being met by the institutions available?

Thornton (1973), chairperson of the board, Los Angeles Indian Free Clinic, succinctly stated the reasons for the low utilization of services by Indian elderly: "cost, language, insult." Ito (1974) further emphasizes the importance of language as well as culture in the care and treatment of elderly patients:

In Los Angeles there is one Japanese hospital and one nursing home that can treat elderly Japanese patients. Or more correctly, every hospital and nursing home in Los Angeles claims they can treat these Japanese but only two facilities of over 800 in Los Angeles County can meet their particular cultural, language, and dietary needs.

LANGUAGE AND CULTURAL EXPECTATIONS

Language is important in terms of acquiring information as well as in understanding the values and expectations of the elderly. Getting them to the facility requires that they know of the service, that they want the service, and that they can easily obtain it. A study of outreach approaches in dealing with Chinese immigrants in Los Angeles (Chao and Chan, 1974) found that neither direct personal contacts nor indirect mail contacts were effective. These immigrants were unfamiliar with the bureaucratic red tape and filling out of forms necessary to obtain services. They wanted immediate help, particularly during the first few months after their arrival. They were disenchanted with the forms to be filled out which consumed their time but brought little or no results.

The experiences related by Brown et al. (1973) in a mental-health facility in the Los Angeles Chinatown area again emphasize the ethnic differences in expectations for services. They found that their Chinese clients were not familiar with the once-weekly scheduled appointments. Clients came unannounced or very late for scheduled interviews. Instead of the

50-minute interview, they sometimes took 2 hours of the social worker's time. They terminated treatment after they felt they were satisfied with their situation, regardless of the clinician's judgments.

Such differences between the expectations of ethnic group members and the present system of medical care are even more problematic for the elderly ethnics who are ill and must enter a long-term institution. They have fewer resources and less freedom to leave if dissatisfied.

INSTITUTIONALIZATION

Most studies on institutionalization speak of its negative effects on the elderly, their psychological losses, alienation, and withdrawal. However, we do not know whether this is the result of institutionalization per se, or of admission policies; i.e., they get to the institution only when they cannot manage alone in the community or their families are no longer able to care for them.

The problem for all elderly entering long-term institutions is the foreign and impersonal environment where life is totally regulated and routinized (Goffman, 1961; Reynolds and Kalish, 1974) for an indefinite time period. For the ethnic elderly who do not know the language and have expected to remain in their children's care until their last days, the institution can be a totally devastating experience, with the individual withdrawing completely to the extreme of taking his or her own life. For those elderly with no family or other social resources, the institution is a prison rather than their "home." But when physical care is paramount and the facility understaffed, little time remains for personal responsiveness.

Yamaguchi (1973) emphasizes the trauma of institutionalization for the elderly Japanese, stemming primarily from cultural values of filial piety, where children were expected to care for their parents, and the family disgrace of having an elder become a ward of the government. They were socialized during a period where the elderly, regardless of physical disability, were kept in the family's home until death. Institutionalization for them is not only unfamiliar, it is a personal disgrace.

FILLING OF FORMS

The bureaucracy adds to the impersonalization of the institution, particularly in its form-filling procedure upon admission. The ethnic elderly have problems enough with the language without having to undergo the barrage of questions on age, social security number, name, etc. Most information sought is used for summary statistics in reports to the boards, etc., or not used at all. Along these lines I would recommend that admissions procedures be more informal and mutually satisfying for both client and staff. A bilingual and bicultural staff member should conduct this initial interview, or if not available, a volunteer or aide with a background similar to the client. The importance of ethnic and cultural similarities between client and practitioner in effective treatment has been emphasized by several investigators (Brown et al., 1973; Edgerton and Karno, 1971; Wolkon et al., 1973).

In addition to the necessary medical and demographic information which is not already available in past records, the admissions interviewer would obtain information more helpful to the staff in relating to clients and understanding them, and in providing more adequate care and a more satisfying institutional life. For example, the following types of information could be taken on admission to determine whether the client's needs could be adequately met by the resources available at the facility.

CLIENT DATA FORMAT

1. Client's present condition
   a. Physical disabilities in terms of patient's perceived symptoms and functioning
   b. Degree of concern over illness and surgery
   c. Present emotional status
   d. Client's assessments of personal assets and liabilities
   e. Client's goals, values, satisfactions, and dislikes
   f. Client's resources—degree of social supports available
   g. Attitudes regarding institutional living and expectations from the facility

2. Cultural background of the client
   a. Place of birth—if not in United States, year of arrival in United States
   b. Important values stressed in homeland concerning old age, illness, care
   c. English-language facility and language of preference
   d. Likes and dislikes in diet; the meaning of mealtime rituals as well as other daily routines or religious ceremonies
   e. Degree of ethnic identification—particularly being the only ethnic in the institution.
3. Social background of the client
   a. If an immigrant, past immigration experiences and responses to them; if not, past life experiences
   b. Past crises and how handled
   c. Former living arrangements, particularly degree of privacy and control desired
   d. Past experiences with agencies and institutions—attitudes and responses toward them
4. Client treatment plan (based on above information and medical diagnosis)

Such a client-facility contact gives clients a sense of having more control over their lives and a better rapport with staff once accepted. Gathering the above kinds of information may take more than one session, but if the interviewer could then be assigned as the contact in the institution throughout the client's stay, this could provide some continuity and personal contact in the life of the elderly client.

ETHNIC INFLUENCES IN INSTITUTIONS

One study by Dominick and Stotsky (1969) examined more than a hundred nursing homes to determine whether there were ethnic differences in these homes. They highlighted some of the differences in an anecdotal manner, relating their impressions and observations of staff and clients. They were particularly concerned with the ethnic influences on the social environment of nursing homes, specifically those relationships between the culture-bearing client and caregivers. Observations of behavior of various ethnic groups in 10 nursing home settings were detailed. Although their findings are based on subjective evaluations, these investigators did provide some evidence that ethnic groups do demonstrate different behavioral patterns, depending on size and organization of the home as well as ethnicity of the clients and staff. What is implied is the need for the supportive presence of other members from one's own ethnic group. For example, the Armenians, Italians, and Jews in a predominantly ethnic setting all retained their traditions through group solidarity. Even in a heterogeneous home, a group of Chinese men adjusted well through group support and interaction. *It seems that one's support system does not necessarily have to be one's own family; if these are not available, clients can accommodate if persons with similar backgrounds are present.*

The positive effect of social supports on the ethnic client in an alien environment is further exemplified by Brown et al. (1973). They relate a case of a Chinese patient who was diagnosed as psychotic, i.e., "isolated, seclusive, and withdrawing from contact." These symptoms were noted as continuing, with the client remaining in his room for all but scheduled activities, until another Chinese patient was admitted. Thereafter, there was no further mention of the client's seclusiveness. Thus, the behavior of the client may have been the result of imposed isolation, being in an unfamiliar environment, not knowing the rules of proper social behavior, and deprived of his ethnic support system.

The effect of lifetime minority status also influences the adjustment of ethnic elderly to institutional settings. Dominick and Stotsky (1969) found black patients to be impersonal, docile, and apathetic in a home where fewer than half of the patients were white and the entire staff was black. They conclude:

The Negro patients had grown up at a time when racial prejudice was strong. Subservience, submissiveness, and inconspicuousness keynoted their adjustment to a white society and carried over to relationships with their Negro nurses. . . . The white patients, less accustomed to this mode of adjustment but now dependent upon a Negro staff, were less well adjusted.

Weinstock and Bennett (1968), however, report different results from interviews with 19 elderly residents (11 white and 8 black) in a 200-bed racially heterogeneous nursing home, with the entire staff being black except for the chief administrator and his secretary. They found the black clients to be enthusiastic and highly positive toward the nursing staff. White clients, however, deviated from the normative mode of communicating their needs by bypassing the nurses to complain to the white administrator. Whether the negative responses of the white clients and the positive responses by the black were due to the ethnicity of the staff or to other factors unique to this particular facility, only a more rigorously designed study would be able to determine. However, these findings do suggest the importance of the staff-patient interaction in the treatment of elderly clients.

STAFF-PATIENT COMMUNICATION

Regimentation and the impersonal custodial care of total institutions fail to provide the personal contact and concern that is so necessary for positive self-image and morale. The problem becomes more acute for ethnic elderly who can understand neither the system nor the language. We have yet to learn whether the "life review" is a process in which all elderly must engage prior to their death (Butler, 1963; Culbert, 1968; Moriwaki, 1973); but, if so, many ethnic elderly in institutions must live their last days with no one to share their thoughts and feelings of their past achievements and life experiences. Bilingual and bicultural paraprofessionals and volunteers—perhaps ethnic community elderly—could visit with clients, giving them the emotional support which can facilitate their adjustment to an alien environment.

Feedback, or explaining treatment and medical status to patients, is also important in appeasing some of their fears. In a study by Koenig et al. (1971) of black and white elderly patients in an acute general hospital in Detroit, patients were asked what kind of physician they preferred. Seventy-eight percent said their physician's race was not important, with no significant differences between blacks and whites. Only 13 percent of the black patients indicated a preference for a doctor of their own race. However, descriptions by patients of the ideal physician were a person "who tries to treat everyone the same, who talks encouragingly to them. . . . One who explains their illness and lets a man know what shape he is in."

What this study suggests is the importance for all elderly, regardless of ethnicity, to have feedback and personal encouragement from the physician. It helps patients to understand their condition and feel some security and control over their environment. It is even more important in terms of the patient's activities and daily routine. When clients are not told in advance that their conditions require dietary changes, activity changes, or relocation, they suffer from a feeling of helplessness; they feel totally dependent in an environment that is not only unfamiliar but unpredictable and hostile.

In another study by Kalish and Reynolds (1972) of four ethnic groups on attitudes toward death, most ethnics wanted to be told of their own deaths, again stressing the client's desire for honesty and concern by staff. Their data also suggest the importance of the family. Of the Mexican Americans, 56 percent as compared with 44 percent of the Anglo-Americans, 36 percent of the Japanese Americans, and 32 percent of the blacks stated they wanted their family to be near at the time of their death, regardless of inconvenience. Perhaps in these instances, family members, together with physician, nurse, and other staff supports, should discuss with clients their medical status. In addition, staff should deal with some of the feelings of adult children and spouse as well as of the client.

KEIRO NURSING HOME: A MODEL OF AN ETHNIC-ORIENTED INSTITUTION[1]

Opened in 1969 through funds donated by individuals in the Japanese-American community, Keiro Nursing Home is a unique 87-bed facility

---

[1] The author wishes to acknowledge the assistance of Art Ito, assistant administrator at Keiro Nursing Home, in providing data on Keiro for this chapter.

located in Los Angeles. It is the only nursing home in the United States specifically geared to meet the language, dietary, and cultural needs of the Japanese (Ito, 1974). It provides care for the elderly Japanese who are physically handicapped and need extended nursing care.

Yamaguchi (1973) relates how the institutional life at Keiro is adapted to the needs of the elderly Japanese client by providing a Japanese cultural environment. For example, the physical environment has been landscaped so as to provide a familiar setting. Further, Japanese food and utensils as well as baths (*ofuro*) are adapted features of the traditional nursing routine. Recreational and educational activities such as Japanese movies, flower arranging, *go* (the traditional Japanese game), and Japanese reading materials, that have meaning for the Japanese patients, are also provided to meet the cultural needs of the client.

Keiro provides for both language needs and quality nursing care by using Japanese speaking aides (many of whom were nurses in Japan) who communicate the patient's needs to nurses, and by using community resources, such as regular visits by ministers representing the various Japanese congregations in the community and visits during traditional holidays by civic organizations and youth clubs (Ito, 1974).

What Keiro offers to the Japanese community is a cultural environment that is familiar to the elderly and which makes the trauma of institutional living less severe. Adaptations to the nursing routine and concern for the past lifestyle of the elderly are integral parts of program planning (Figure 42-5).

It must not be overlooked that Keiro is exclusively geared to the Japanese elderly. Individuals who are not familiar with the cultural life-style may feel as alienated and incompetent in this environment as ethnics in an Anglo institution. The model presented by Keiro, however, suggests that long-term facilities must provide care beyond the medical and custodial needs of clients; they must provide care adapted to their cultural and individual needs.

Ethnicity is one crucial variable in uncovering clients' self-concept and their satisfaction with their life situation in old age. It is only *one* of many variables, however well it may predict the probability of certain attitudes and behav-

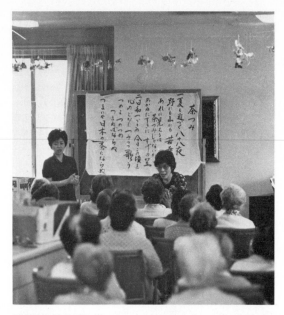

FIGURE 42-5 The importance of using the native language of the elderly cannot be overemphasized. At Keiro Nursing Home, the language needs are met by using Japanese-speaking aides who communicate the client's needs to nurses and by utilizing Japanese-speaking individuals from community resources. This photo depicts a group singing a song about harvesting tea leaves. (*Courtesy of Anthony J. Skirlick, Jr.*)

iors. Three dimensions—the cultural, social status, and support subsystems—of ethnicity have been discussed. To understand ethnic elderly individuals, we must view them as a composite of these various forces rather than according to a purely categorical definition.

The medical care system is often impersonal and degrading to the elderly who do not know what is going on and already have a low evaluation of themselves and of their ability to control the environment. Thus, bilingual staff should work with ethnic clients and their families and other social supports to obtain client input for more appropriate care, to familiarize them to the institution and its regimen, and to provide feedback to clients regarding their medical status or daily schedule changes. Working together with clients, allowing them to make decisions, even if we start with simple matters such as meal planning and scheduling of activities, would offer them a more meaningful environment.

The negative effects of the total institution could be somewhat alleviated by opening the doors to input from the surrounding community. Volunteers who have similar backgrounds and language might spend more time with the patient to provide personal and informal contact beyond the necessary custodial care.

The concept of institutional care must be extended to include an atmosphere that demonstrates concern for the elderly client as a meaningful human being with abilities as well as needs. Helping is a two-way process, best achieved when there is a sharing between client and staff. We can provide for the ethnic elderly's needs only by understanding the client and his or her cultural background, past experiences, and present situation.

REFERENCES

Administration on Aging: *Meeting the Long-Term Care Needs of the Elderly—A Background and Issues Paper,* November 1978.

Bogardus, Emory E.: *Social Distance,* Antioch Press, Yellow Springs, Ohio, 1959.

Brown, Timothy R., et al.: Mental illness and the role of mental health facilities in Chinatown, in Stanley Sue and Nathaniel Wagner (eds.), *Asian-Americans: Psychological Perspectives,* Science and Behavior Books, Inc., Ben Lomond, Calif., 1973, pp. 212–231.

Butler, Robert N.: The life review: An interpretation of reminiscence in the aged, *Psychiatry,* **26**:65–76, February 1963.

Chao, Clara, and Diana Chan: A study of the familiarization process of recent Chinese immigrants, unpublished master's thesis, University of Southern California, Los Angeles, 1974.

Culbert, S. A.: *The Interpersonal Process of Self-Disclosure: It Takes Two to See One,* Renaissance Editions, New York, 1968.

de Beauvoir, Simone: *The Coming of Age,* Putnam, New York, 1972.

Dominick, Joan R., and Bernard A. Stotsky: Mental patients in nursing homes, *Journal of the American Geriatrics Society,* **17**(1):63–85, January 1969.

Edgerton, Robert B., and Marvin Karno: Mexican-American bilingualism and the perception of mental illness, *Archives of General Psychiatry,* **24**:286–290, March 1971.

Goffman, Erving: *Asylums,* Anchor Books, Doubleday, Garden City, N.Y., 1961.

Hirsch, Carl, Donald P. Kent, and Suzanne L. Silverman: Homogeneity and heterogeneity among low-income Negro and white aged, in D. Kent, R. Kastenbaum, and S. Sherwood (eds.), *Research Planning and Action for the Elderly,* Behavioral Publications, New York, 1972, pp. 484–500.

Ito, Arthur K.: Institutionalization: Ethnic elderly need more than medical care, paper presented at the Institute of Minority Aging, San Diego, Calif., June 7, 1974.

Jackson, Jacquelyne J.: Special health problems of aged blacks, *Aging,* (287–288):15–20, September-October 1978.

Kalish, Richard A., and Sharon Y. Moriwaki: The world of the elderly Asian American, *Journal of Social Issues,* **29**:187–209, 1973.

——, and David K. Reynolds: The meaning of death and dying in the Los Angeles Mexican-American Community, in *Proceedings, Sixth International Association for Suicide Prevention,* Mexico City, December 1972, pp. 291–295.

Kent, Donald P.: The elderly in minority groups: Variant patterns of aging, *Gerontologist,* **11**:26–29, 1971.

Kerckhoff, Alan C., and Thomas C. McCormick: Marginal status and marginal personality, *Social Forces,* **34**:48–55, 1955.

Kitano, Harry, and A. Kikumura: The Japanese American family, in C. H. Mindel and R. W. Habenstein (eds.), *Ethnic Families in America: Patterns and Variations,* Elsevier Scientific Publishing Co., New York, 1976.

Koenig, Ronald, et al.: Ideas about illness of elderly black and white in an urban hospital, *Aging and Human Development,* **2**:217–225, 1971.

Maldonado, David: The Chicano aged, *Social Work,* **20**(8):213–216, 1975.

Moore, Joan: Situational factors affecting minority aging, *Gerontologist,* **11**:88–93, 1971.

Moriwaki, Sharon Y.: Self-disclosure, significant others and psychological well-being in old age, *Journal of Health and Social Behavior,* **14**:226–332, September 1973.

—— (ed.): *Hawaii's Vulnerable Elderly: Needs and Needed Resources,* Hawaii Gerontology Center, Honolulu, 1979.

National Center for Health Statistics: *Characteristics of Residents in Nursing and Personal Care Homes, U.S., June-August 1969,* HSM 73-1704, series 12, no. 19, February 1973a.

——: *Utilization of Short-Stay Hospitals: Summary of Non-Medical Statistics, U.S., 1970,* Department of Health, Education, and Welfare Publication (HRA) 74-1765, August 1973b.

Nicodemus, Mildred: Indian culture, *Proceedings of Workshop on Cultural Health Traditions: Implications for Nursing Care,* William A. Lang (ed.), Sept. 29, 1977, pp. 32–34.

Pinckney, Alphonso: *Black Americans,* Prentice-Hall, Englewood Cliffs, N.J., 1969.

Reynolds, David K.: Japanese American aging: A game perspective, paper presented at the Society for Applied Anthropology, Miami, 1971.

———: Suicide among ethnic groups in Los Angeles with focus on Japanese Americans, testimony presented at the hearings on suicide prevention before the California Legislature, Senate Committee on Health and Welfare, Subcommittee on Medical Education and Health Needs, Los Angeles, April 6, 1974.

———, **and Richard A. Kalish:** The social ecology of dying: Observations of wards for the terminally ill, *Hospital and Community Psychiatry,* 25(3):147–152, March 1974.

Solomon, Barbara B.: *Black Empowerment: Social Work in Oppressed Communities,* Columbia, New York, 1976.

Special Committee on Aging, U.S. Senate: *The Multiple Hazards of Age and Race: The Situation of Aged Blacks in the United States—A Working Paper,* Washington, September 1971.

Stanford, E. Percil: *The Elder Black,* Center on Aging, San Diego State University, San Diego, 1978.

Thornton, Louella: Unpublished presentation at Ethnicity and Aging Seminar, Andrus Gerontology Center, University of Southern California, Los Angeles, July 1973.

U.S. Bureau of the Census: *1970 Census of Population: Characteristics of the Population,* vol. I, U.S. Summary, pt. 1, sec. 2, June 1973.

———: *1970 Census of Population and Housing, Los Angeles-Long Beach,* pt. 1, PHC(1)-117, May 1972.

———: *1960 Census of Population: Characteristics of the Population,* vol. I, *U.S. Summary,* pt. 1, 1964.

U.S. Department of Health, Education, and Welfare: *Characteristics, Social Contacts, and Activities of Nursing Home Residents—United States: 1973–74 National Nursing Home Survey,* Rockville, Md., May 1977.

———: *Health—United States: 1975,* Health Resources Administration Publication, Rockville, Md., 1976.

Valle, Ramon: *A Cross-Cultural Study of Minority Elders in San Diego,* nos. 1–8, Companile Press, San Diego University, San Diego, Calif., 1978.

——— **and Lydia Mendoza:** *The Elder Latino,* Center on Aging, San Diego State University, San Diego, Calif., 1978.

Weaver, Jerry L.: *National Health Policy and the Underserved: Ethnic Minorities, Women and the Elderly,* Mosby, St. Louis, 1976.

———: Personal health care: A major concern for minority aged, *Comprehensive Service Delivery Systems for the Minority Aged, Proceedings of the Fourth Institute on Minority Aging,* Center on Aging, San Diego State University, San Diego, Calif., 1977, pp. 41–62.

Weeks, Herbert, and Benjamin J. Darsky: *The Urban Aged: Race and Medical Care,* University of Michigan, School of Public Health, Ann Arbor, 1968.

Weinstock, Comilda, and Ruth Bennett: Problems in communication to nurses among residents of a racially heterogeneous nursing home, *Gerontologist,* 8(2):72–75, Summer 1968.

Wilson, Holly S., and Jose Heinert: Los viejitos: The old ones, *Journal of Gerontological Nursing,* 3(5):19–25, September-October 1977.

Wolkon, George H., Sharon Y. Moriwaki, and Karen J. Williams: Race and social class as factors in the orientation toward psychotherapy, *Journal of Counseling Psychology,* 20(4):312–316, 1973.

Yamaguchi, Yoshiko: The elderly Japanese and his institutionalization, paper presented at *Ethnicity and Aging Seminar,* Andrus Gerontology Center, University of Southern California, Los Angeles, July 1973.

Yoshida, Jane, and Paula Endo: An exploratory study of the impact of aging on the Japanese-American family, unpublished master's thesis, University of Southern California, Los Angeles, 1969.

OTHER RESOURCES

FILMS

Asian American

On Lok—Where the Old Keep on Growing, sponsored by Social Rehabilitation Services, DHEW, available via National Audio Visual Center, Sales Branch, Washington, 20036.

Sam, produced by Indiana University. Available via University of California, Extension Media Center, Berkeley, CA 94720.

Wataridori: Birds of Passage, produced by Visual Communications. Asian-American Studies Central, Inc. Available via Amerasia Bookstore, 338 East 2d St., Los Angeles, CA 90012.

Black American

A Man Named Charlie Smith, produced by N. H. Comines. Available via (Macmillan) Audio Brandon, 1619 North Cherokee St., Los Angeles, CA 90028.

A Well Spent Life, produced by Les Blank and Skip Gerson. Available via Flower Films, 11305 Q-Ranch Road, Austin, TX 78757.

Fannie Bell Chapman: Gospel Singer, produced and distributed by Center for Southern Folklore, 1216 Peabody Ave., Memphis, TN 38104.

I'm the Prettiest Piece in Greece, produced by Richard Wedler. Available via North Texas State University, Gerontological Film Collection, Main Library, Denton, TX 76203.

Me and Stella, produced by Geri Ashur. Available via Phoenix Films, 470 Park Ave. South, New York, NY 10016.

New Wings for Icarus, produced by Lutheran Television, Box 14572, St. Louis, MO 63178.

Old, Black, and Alive!! Released by The New Film Co., Inc., 331 Newberry St., Boston, MA 02115.

Taking Care of Mother Baldwin, 20 min/b & w/16 mm. Produced by Victor Nunez. Distributor: Perspective Films. Available via Viewfinders, P.O. Box 1665, Evanston, IL 60204.

Uncommon Images, 22 min/color/16 mm. Produced by Evelyn Barron. Available via Filmmaker Library, Inc., 290 West End Ave., New York, NY 10023.

With Just a Little Trust, produced by Teleketics Films (Tony Frangakis). Available via Teleketics, Franciscan Communications Center, 1229 South Santee, Los Angeles, CA 90015.

Hispanic

Agueda Martinez, 16 min/color/16 mm, Moctesuma Esparaza Production Film distributed by Educational Media Corp., 2036 Lemoyne Ave., Los Angeles, CA 90026.

Artesanos Mexicanos, 22 min each/color/16 mm, available in Spanish or a bilingual English version. A group of three films produced by Judith Bronowski and Robert Grant available from The Works, 1659 - 18th St., Santa Monica, CA 90404.

Manuel Jimenez—Wood Carver, produced by Judith Bronowski, Available via The Works, 1659 - 18th Street, Santa Monica, CA 90404.

Mario Sanchez: Painter of Memories, produced by Jack Ofield. Available via Bowling Green Films, Inc., Box 384-D, Hudson, NY 12434.

Pedro Linares—Folk Artist (Artesano Cartonero), produced by Judith Bronowski. Available via The Works, 1659 - 18th St., Santa Monica, CA 90404.

Sabina Sanchez and the Art of Embroidery (Artesana Bordabora), available via The Works, 1659 - 18th St., Santa Monica, CA 90404.

Native American

Alice Elliott, 11 min/color/16 mm. Produced by Extension Media Center, University of California, Berkeley, CA 94720. Rental $14.

Annie and the Old One, a Greenhouse Films production from a book by Miska Miles (Little, Brown). Available via BFA Educational Media, 2211 Michigan Ave., Santa Monica, CA 90404.

Legend Days Are Over, produced by Robert Primes. Paulist Productions, P.O. Box 1057, Pacific Palisades, CA 90272.

PAMPHLET

A Language Guide for Patient and Nurse, compiled by Edith M. Pritchard, Eli Lilly and Company, Indianapolis, Ind., n.d.

FORTY-THREE

ENVIRONMENT AND THE AGED PERSON

Robert J. Newcomer
Michael A. Caggiano

Life is like music; it must be composed by ear, feeling, and instinct, not by rule.
Samuel Butler

LEARNING OBJECTIVES

- Identify stress-reducing results of changing lighting levels in client bedrooms and client recreation rooms, and compare differing behavior in each setting.
- Describe the effects on the client of color stimuli added to the environment.
- Contrast the behavior of the client in a solitary setting with that in a social setting when stimulating an awareness of time, e.g., daytime with covered vs. unshaded windows, introduction of holiday objects.
- Identify how client percepts are modified by means of manipulating environment as above with the end results of reducing stress in an institutional setting.

Over the past decade or so, a new discipline has begun to emerge. The discipline is variably called *environmental psychology, transactional psychology, ecological psychology,* and *man-environment relations.* Simply stated, the purpose of these endeavors is to understand better how environment influences human behavior and well-being. Such understanding will enable designers, administrators, and others to match individuals with environments suited to their abilities. In the field of nursing and nursing-home administration, these notions readily translate into such things as patient screening criteria, ward rules and regulations, furniture selection, and therapy programs. In effect, environments are formed by physical surroundings, rules, and other people.

For hospital-confined persons, especially those of diminished physical or mental capacity, the type and quality of environment created by these elements can be extremely important. The intent of this chapter is to increase sensitivity to environmental conditions affecting the daily lives of institutionalized patients, and encourage imaginative nursing staff intervention into those inadvertent environmental situations which may have untapped therapeutic potential or even may be causing difficulty for patients.

Discussion is focused on two basic human needs: variety and privacy. Within this framework we will examine the effects of furniture and room design, noise, color, smell, temperature, and certain administrative policies. Illustrations of successful environmental intervention are included.

PEOPLE-ENVIRONMENT CONGRUENCE

The human adaptability to a variety of situations has frequently been observed. *The ability to adapt diminishes as competence diminishes.* If a new situation requires an individual to respond beyond his or her capabilities, stress and anxiety result. New admissions often find themselves in such circumstances. It has been reported by Lieberman (1969) and others that it may take as long as 6 months for adjustment to occur. Sickness, depression, even increased mortality have been found to be associated with institutionali-

zation. Once the relocation effects and the newness wear off, another malaise may develop—understress or understimulation. In this circumstance, ability exceeds the demands made by the environment. When understressed, patients experience daydreaming and sleepiness. Hallucinations even may occur as psychological attempts to combat this situation. Care must be taken to avoid confusing these symptoms with those of withdrawal caused by overstimulation. More capable patients may resort to overt displays of emotion in an attempt to produce variety in their lives. Cantankerousness and aggressive acts may be symptoms of these needs. If we anticipate this, we can minimize the need for drugs or special counseling by manipulating the environmental variables. Something as simple as temperature change of a room can affect the patient's mood.

If we would graph the daily activity of an individual together with a fixed level of environmental stimulus, it would look something like Figure 43-1. If we could match stimuli to the individual's capabilities, it would be possible to avert psychological crises.

Control can be effected with relative ease by the nurse. The time it takes for the trained professional to anticipate an environmental confrontation and modify it would be a fraction of the time it takes to deal with an emotional problem through conventional therapy. In addition, it presents a creatively stimulating, problem-solving situation for the nurse.

When people are in a mismatched or incongruent situation, there are at least three possible ways of restoring congruence between their abilities and environmental resources, according to Lawton and Nahemow (1973).

1. Individual ability can be prosthetically supplemented without changing the environment. The use of eyeglasses and false teeth illustrate this approach. Medication, though often overused, is another alternative.
2. Individual rehabilitation in the form of physical therapy or education can be used to enhance capability.
3. The often-ignored approach, basic to this chapter, is alternation of environmental circumstances so that they are compatible with the individual.

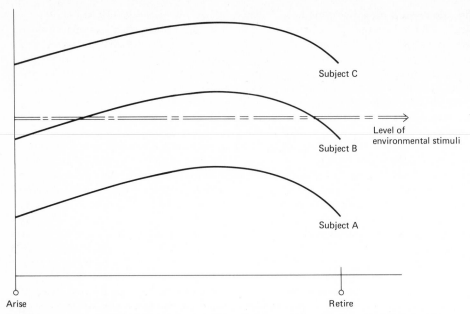

FIGURE 43-1   The hypothetical relation between each of three variables and a constant level of environmental stimuli.

A simple example may further highlight the difference between these approaches. Consider a bed patient who is too weak to lean from the bed to the bedside table to get a drink of water. Getting a drink is the behavioral outcome that is important. An extreme medical model may be to provide intravenous feeding. Staff or other patients can provide help, additional examples of augmenting individual ability. A patient's inability to reach the water pitcher often generates negative staff reaction that the patient is simply seeking attention. Such an attitude only increases the patient's stress. Moving the water to an overbed table so that the individual can get it without assistance though not always practical, is a slight environmental modification that permits the patient to function better independent of external prosthetic supports.

If environmental planners and designers have successfully anticipated patient and staff needs, the staff should easily be able to unobtrusively augment the patient's abilities for self-help. If enough flexibility and variety are planned into the facilities, a broad range of "custom-designed" spaces will result (Figure 43-2). Within some logical economic constraints, the planners would provide a variety of environmental conditions to eliminate the stereo-

type "hospital green" and ceramic tile surfaces of years ago. For instance, vinyl-covered wallboard is available in many colors, textures, and designs to enhance the patient's room.

The more conventional prosthetic supports a space contains, the more institutional (hence, less human) the environment will appear to patients, staff, and visitors. Fear of institutionalization is recognized universally as a retardant to successful psychophysical therapy.

There are no clear-cut measures for knowing precisely which intervention technique is best for every individual in every situation. Sensitivity to needs and experimentation with alternatives are essential if the optimum technique is to be used.

IMPORTANCE OF PLANTS AND LANDSCAPING

A universally accepted common denominator for a pleasing environment is landscaping, and patients' rooms are often adorned with cut flowers. Many institutions are even allowing potted plants in patient spaces. Wherever possible, the facilities should be heavily landscaped with a

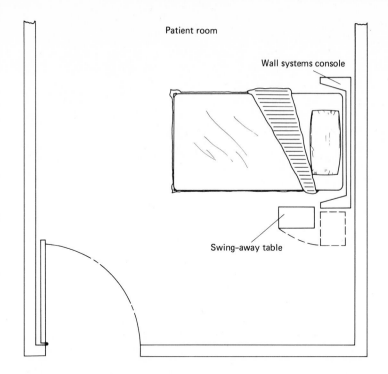

Patient room

Wall systems console

Swing-away table

FIGURE 43-2 **A swing-away bed-side table attached to a wall systems console allows the patient to position the table at his or her own convenience.**

variety of shapes, sizes, textures, and colors, easily visible from patient areas. Interaction with landscape and outdoor spaces should be encouraged. Sun decks should be converted to sun-and-shade decks. The most obvious advantages are oxygen, temperate climate, and variety. Other, more subtle, advantages are gained through association: emotionally soothing, spiritual, interesting (see Figure 43-3).

Having developed a rudimentary conceptual framework of human-environment interaction, subsequent sections will relate spatial behavior

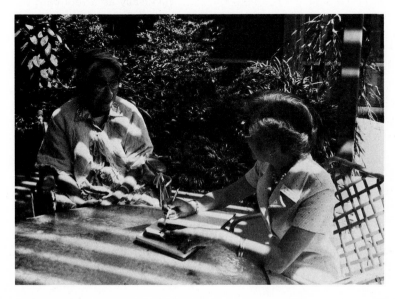

FIGURE 43-3 **Sun-and-shade decks. Patient areas should provide interesting patterns, textures, colors, and aromas.** (*Courtesy of Anthony J. Skirlick, Jr.*)

in institutional settings with environmental stimuli, and discuss strategy for dealing with these factors.

TERRITORIALITY AND WARD BEHAVIOR

Have you ever paid much attention to the way people use space, the way they sit around tables or on couches, or their relation to other people when conversing? The relative position in which people arrange themselves in space communicates information to other people. Where one sits is a signal to others as to whether they are invited to join or not. The proximity of one to another also communicates the degree of intimacy desired. These behavior patterns are learned and are culturally specific demonstrations of territoriality. An awareness of territorial needs can be helpful in understanding behavioral manifestations. One such manifestation occurs in the use of patient space and ward common spaces (Sommer, 1969).

Frequently, relatively competent long-term patients appear eccentric with regard to items under their direct control. Bedside tables are meticulously arranged, everything with its exact place. Pity the uninformed individual who should disturb this balance. Patients also acquire "favorite" chairs or tables in the day room and in the dining room. Their claim to this territory is established through frequent use. The "owner" of this space often will not hesitate to tell any intruder to leave. Other people will not only recognize this personal territory, but will also act to protect it from intruders, "Please don't sit there. That is so-and-so's chair." We have all come in contact with this phenomenon and the daily activity in accordance with its dictates. Yet, we remain insensitive to the manifestation of this activity among institutional patients, perhaps because it requires "special handling" in each case if we are taught that efficient nursing service precludes such individual consideration. This problem has a simple solution. If we can encourage social interaction on a higher social level by manipulating the environmental setting, we can raise the level of efficiency while achieving a higher level of therapeutic patient activity.

Possessiveness traits are most in evidence when the individual has few controls of options over environmental circumstances. Hence, patients with private rooms become less concerned about bedside tables and "favorite" furniture than those in shared rooms (Ittleson et al., 1970). Persons in shared rooms are less possessive of personal effects if they have furniture or other objects which clearly identify a space as theirs. Stress occurs only when there are no

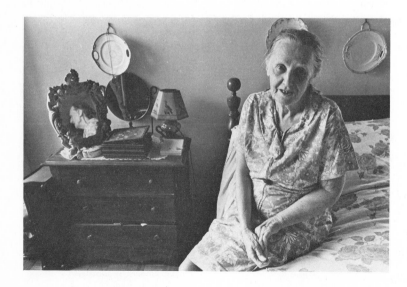

FIGURE 43-4 If environmental planners and designers have successfully anticipated patient and staff needs, the staff should easily be able to unobtrusively augment patients' abilities to help themselves. Note the personal items in the room of this elderly woman. (*Courtesy of Harvey Finkle.*)

clear-cut territorial boundaries or when territory is invaded.

If a well-located common space is poorly used, it would be appropriate to examine the extent to which furniture design, arrangement, or patient needs has established this area as either a place to visit with others or where entry would constitute invasion of the private domain of a few users. One person can dominate a setting by his position in the middle rather than at the side. The use of such a space by others can be increased by the selection of more "democratic" furniture or manipulating the furniture so there is no "middle," just as King Arthur achieved democracy at the round table.

PERSONAL SPACE AND PRIVACY

Related to the notion of territoriality is a concept called "personal space" (Hall, 1966; Sommer, 1969). This refers to a "space bubble" around the individual. Being within less than an arm's distance or even touching signifies intimate contact. About an arm's length produces a normal conversational distance. This can vary depending on the setting. Normal distance can be greater in a large room or an outdoor space. Under most circumstances the distance outside the conversational distance is neutral. People use this distance to recognize and invite entry into more personal contact. While uninvited intrusion into this public-aggressive space is not overly threatening, it has been observed, among mental patients especially, that the frequency of entry into personal space is important. Potential intruders must be recognized while they are at a public-aggressive distance, usually 5 to 10 feet. Entry into more proximate contact is by invitation only. Violation of this code causes agitation and anger. These characteristics are based on an average for middle-class, American culture. *Ethnicity, mental competence, and educational level may vary these patterns.*

Personal space is not limited to physical contact or proximity. Eye contact and sound can also represent invasions. When the individual cannot control invasions into personal space, invasions of privacy occur.

Privacy, as the ability to control the quantity and quality of social interaction, is vital to the individual (Pastalan, 1970). If one is under the constant surveillance of others, if the physical setting does not permit respite from such surveillance, if roles or moods cannot be changed by varied circumstances, then there is a necessity to always be "on." People need to get off stage in order to attain emotional variation and release. Continuous performances can be psychologically exhausting.

Four techniques for accomplishing emotional variation have been identified by Pastalan (1970):

1. Visual separation to achieve solitude
2. Small-group involvement in which it is at least an acoustically protected setting
3. Development of a sense of anonymity by becoming "lost" in a crowd
4. Psychological withdrawal into oneself, a condition described as reserve

In the interpretation of patient behavior, staff and other patients easily recognize acting out behavior, e.g., demands for personal attention, crabbiness, and general talkativeness. Most staff members would attribute these behaviors to loneliness , as often they are. Are sullen, inactive patients depressed or psychologically incompetent? Perhaps this is true, but we should consider the possibility that some of this behavior is in response to constant invasion of the need for privacy and is, therefore, correctable by "environmental therapy." *Attempts at forced social interaction, which is often considered to have a positive value, may be counterproductive.* The provision and utilization of optional choice for the patient would likely produce optimum results.

A description of social design problems in each of the major ward spaces follows:[1]

- Entrance lobbies are often densely occupied if seating is provided. Many patients, particularly the less ambulatory, like to cluster for long periods to watch the behavior of others. More mobile individuals will make their "rounds" at shorter intervals.

---

[1] Much of this material has been more elaborately described by M. Powell Lawton of the Philadelphia Geriatric Center (1973).

Nurse stations and heavy-traffic corridors often serve similar functions because of all the activity centered there. These areas may also attract people who are more competent, because any aggregation of people is a precondition for social interaction. Because the "sitting and watching" syndrome occurs when there is heavy staff or public traffic, many administrators frequently discourage such assemblies. Some even remove chairs or forbid "loitering." These actions may give the institution a more orderly image, but it is detrimental to the social life of the patient unless alternative activity foci can be produced. The result is a rigid, institutional feeling that perpetuates fear of incarceration.

PRIVACY OF TERMINAL PATIENTS

In the case of terminal patients' privacy, we are often guilty of overreaction. Terminal sections become "tiptoe-and-whisper" wards. Segregation of terminal patients falls under the heading of "ecology of competence." Even though the environment may not exhibit hopelessness, the "atmosphere" too often does.

There have been many documented cases of spontaneous remission in terminal patients where the principals all testified afterward that they could not bring themselves to believe there was no hope and acted accordingly.

If "terminal sections" are necessary, gloomy surroundings are inappropriate. Most experienced nurses recognize that there is no valid reason why bedside manner of nursing service should be any different from other areas of nursing care.

PHYSICAL ENVIRONMENT

Within the ward setting there exist many physical features which can be used to enhance or reduce the patient's functional or emotional ability. To this point, discussion has concentrated on the relatively well-researched phenomena of territoriality and personal space. Many environmental factors exist that are tangential to these dimensions, influencing positive or negative patient response. Following are descriptions of the major environmental factors.

LIGHT

Light, for the sighted, is an integral part of the physical environment. *Few architects and fewer building owners have any real understanding of how illumination can affect human experience.*

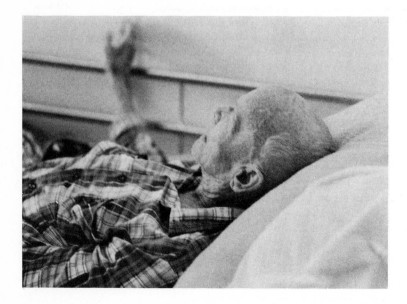

FIGURE 43-5 In providing privacy for terminal patients, we are often guilty of overreaction. Terminal sections become "tiptoe-and-whisper" wards. Segregation of terminal patients falls under the heading of "ecology of competence." Even though the environment may not exhibit hopelessness, the atmosphere too often does. (*Courtesy of Anthony J. Skirlick, Jr.*)

Light can affect mood, orientation, and functional ability. Existing lighting criteria are based on technical specifications such as footcandles and lumens. These criteria continually increase after "new discoveries" by lighting-industry research of our human needs. It makes one wonder how we ever managed without the fluorescent light. These notions fail to appreciate the human value of variation in intensity, shape, or color. As a consequence, many institutions rely upon fluorescent lighting because of its seemingly low operating cost and efficiency, although most maintenance engineers will testify to the high maintenance cost. The glare and eyestrain produced by such lighting have been given scant attention. Reliance upon so narrow a set of design criteria ignores the importance of lighting for different human activities. In restaurants, for example, it has been observed that high illumination levels increase customer turnover. Softer, low-keyed lighting slows turnover and reduces the loudness of conversations. This indicates a definite relation of behavior to environment.

A decrease in illumination and a well-designed combination of lighting systems can decrease operational costs and enhance the patient environment. As evidenced by our current energy conservation programs, we can certainly get along with a fraction of the light that the industry has told us we need.

In institutional settings, other lighting problems arise due to the overlapping goals and activities of many spaces. Dining rooms can be for meals, meetings, or crafts; day rooms for meals, reading, or sleeping. Variations in lighting could enhance each of these varied activities, but often the fixed lighting system precludes such options. A woman who normally worked on her oil painting during the day was shocked at the off-color results of one night's painting by electric light. Yet, the light was appropriate and pleasant for evening mealtime just a few hours before.

Further complicating the design process is that the brightness of daylight, differing weather conditions, different temperatures, and different times of the day all can affect the amount and quality of artificial light needed. Some sort of average level is adopted which may, under varied conditions, be totally inappropriate for patient needs. More likely, a situation is created in which there is virtually no change of pace from bright lighting. Designing around the average does not readily complement needed variation in mood or "atmosphere" for patients.

Variation is healthy, and it makes good sense to allow people some opportunity for control and choices. These may take form either through direct individual control or conscious attempts by staff to vary the perceptual stimuli. Dimmers can often be inexpensively added to light fixtures. Curtains or room dividers can help break up a room and permit more individual control over large lighting systems. Individual fixtures with separate controls can be strategically placed in rooms to supplement a general light system.

Combinations of materials and colors can also be used to good advantage. *Care should be taken to guard against the possibilities of excessive heat and reflected glare when selecting or locating these materials.* A frequent error is the use of unpainted, smooth concrete surrounding shuffleboard courts. If overhead shade is not provided, the courts will remain unused because of glare.

Glare can be a major factor in patient disorientation. One does not have to be old to experience visual disorientation. One can have this experience while driving in a rainstorm looking for street signs or a house number, and the glare from lights through the rain causes distortion and disorientation. When confronted with a sudden case of "sensory deprivation," we become disoriented and confused, possibly frustrated and frightened. But most very old people do not really experience these feelings suddenly, mainly because sensory acuity decreases very gradually. They learn to avoid situations that require higher levels of sensory performance than they are capable of. Building surfaces and windows that might produce glare will probably be sources of discomfort and will ultimately be areas that are avoided.

For the older person especially, it is important to be sensitive to potential problems. Studies by Pastalan, at the University of Michigan (1973), illustrate how changes in the eye associated with aging make the older person more vulnerable to glare. Color contrast ability is diminished so that white-on-white surfaces, in particular, such as those of a white dining table with white dishes, lack sufficient contrast for patients to clearly distinguish table from dish. The adverse effect this might have on apparent patient competence or on self-confidence should be obvious.

COLOR

Color investigations of the psychological correlates of different types and degrees of color are more numerous than studies of light. These two dimensions are not, of course, independent. Differential responses including anxiety, arousal, subjective temperature perception, and degree of comfort have been noted with red, white, and blue light. A list of such responses to red and blue follows (Hayward, 1974):

Red: Exciting, stimulating, defiant, contrary, hostile, hot, passionate, active, fierce, intense, happy, sometimes irritating

Blue: Calm, peaceful, soothing, tender, secure, comfortable, melancholy, contemplative, subduing, sad, dignified, restful

Again, as with lighting, the multiple demands made upon institutions are such that they typically are designed to satisfy some median response. Studies of possible color effects on specific individuals provide some means for anticipating or diagnosing the likely consequence of specific schemes.

Variation of colors enhances moods and orientation. A recent example in hospital design illustrates one innovative approach to the use of color (Chaney, 1973). Recognizing that warm colors such as reds, oranges, and yellows can act as stimulants which raise blood pressure and pulse rates, and that cool-tone blues and greens may be too relaxing, this group sought to find exciting neutral colors for patient areas. Grays and browns were used in bold patterns. Walls, draperies, and bedspreads were all incorporated in this schema. As an added touch, these patterns were varied for each patient's room, alternating from floor to floor. These efforts had the effect of making rooms more personal, while enhancing visitor and patient orientation as they moved along the corridors. In public spaces, bold colors, graphics, and prints were used to increase orientation and to provide greater visual stimuli.

Color research data are made available through the American Inter-Society Color Council, NASA, the Navy, and universities.

Cheskin et al. (1974) indicate that a color psychologist's recommendations for a hospital might include halls and entrances painted a warm, gentle apricot or peach for a calming effect; father-to-be waiting rooms painted cool greens and blues; physical therapy areas painted stimulating orange-reds; convalescent rooms painted yellow to create cheer and optimism. Pink and peach in operation recovery rooms reflect a healthy-looking color to the patient's skin and have a beneficial psychological effect.

When comprehensive color variation is impractical, there are simple means for achieving some effects. Many facilities are reportedly introducing art displays in the form of mosaics, woodcuts, paintings, sculpture, and other forms of art expression. Local talent is actively boosted. In addition, permanent collections are assembled for display throughout the facility. Large displays and single pictures are changed or rotated periodically. Many art museums rent or lend consigned artwork. Significant psychological benefits to patients and staff, as well as visitors to the facility, have been reported as a consequence of these changes.

NOISE

Noise is often a neglected feature of the ambient environment. For years, human factors engineers, and others concerned with instrument design, confined their concern to physiologically harmful decibel levels. As a result, today, very few major appliances or other properly tuned machines exceed established noise limits. But, alas, high-intensity sound is not the only requisite component of noise, not if one defines noise as any unwanted sound. *There is increasing evidence that unwanted sound can be harmful emotionally and physically* (Farr, 1967).

The annoyance value of sound can be categorized in the following five self-explanatory qualities: (1) unexpected, (2) interfering, (3) inappropriate, (4) intermittent, and (5) reverberating. Self-generated sound, regardless of which category has a much higher tolerance than sounds generated from other sources.

The multiplicity of sounds which surround us every day—radio, television, and many simultaneous conversations—produces few problems for those with high discriminatory ability. The older person who has suffered diminished hearing acuity (presbycusis) can be especially susceptible to noises resulting from interference and inappropriateness. For these individuals, the complexity of heterogeneous background noises may make it impossible to select desired sounds. Sound entering a ward from movement of equipment, street traffic, or staff conversations can further compound noise intensity.

Little attempt has been made to improve designs and select construction materials that provide acoustical control. Selection of sound-absorbing furniture and getting rid of noise-making "music" may help rectify some of the design mistakes.

ODORS

Odors can have an emotional effect. The sense of smell has been found to be intimately linked with memory, emotion, and judgment. Many people have expressed association of pleasant memories with the smell of perfume, suntan lotion, burning leaves, and a variety of other aromas. Although the sense of smell becomes less acute with age, it has been shown that there can be broad variation of sensitivity to smells at all ages, depending upon the individual.

It has been demonstrated that the olfactory function can produce a broad range of behavior in human beings (Gibson, 1974). The problem with smell stimulus is that it is difficult to control the drift range of smells. An aroma that is pleasant to one person may be offensive to another, so that caution should be exercised in experimentation.

FURNITURE AND SURFACES

Furniture and surfaces, which have been frequently alluded to as a means of rectifying mistakes in environmental design, have received little research interest. Other than to recommend selection of sound-absorbing seating, and non-glare, moderate contrast surfaces on table-tops and other furnishings, few specific recommendations can be made. As interest in the subject of specialized furnishings for the elderly increases, product designers and manufacturers will undoubtedly advance their efforts to develop new products. To date, however, few significant advances have been made.

The case of carpeting vs. resilient floor coverings is an exception to product research neglect. It offers some insight into the multiplicity of planning considerations and the trade-offs which have to be made in any design decision.

The main issues in the floor-covering debate have concerned slip hazard, noise, soil and bacteria transportation, fire hazard, wheeled-vehicle resistance, wear, and maintenance. The National Bureau of Standards (1969) has compiled data from field evaluations of these floor coverings.

In general, it has been found that carpets reduce noise and the incidence of slips and falls. Even when falls do occur on a carpeted floor, there is less risk of injury. Further, there has been no evidence of increased bacteria transportation when carpeting is used. Following are some difficulties that have been experienced:

1. Carpets are much less functional for rolling heavy-wheeled equipment, such as beds, wheelchairs, and stretchers, and in "dirty" or abnormal spillage areas.
2. Static electricity becomes a problem when the relative humidity is low.
3. Vacuum-cleaner noise can be irritating to both staff and patients. Because the cleaning routine requires daily vacuuming of each room and corridor, there may be noise on the nursing unit for up to 5 hours per day.
4. Vacuum-cleaner cords and hoses can create safety hazards.
5. Food spills, vomit, and urine require prompt cleaning and repeated deodorizing; unpleasant odors may be retained for several days.

Noise and safety inconveniences are partially offset by a reduction of other harsh noise. Voices, footsteps, wheeled vehicles, and telephones are all reportedly less irritating in carpeted units. Noise-baffling containers for vacuum cleaners or central vacuum systems also help offset noise and problems. Floor surface glare reduction is another direct benefit. *An important guideline is that patients generally respond positively to carpeting.*

In spite of all the difficulties and subjectively measurable benefits, the basic issue seems to be reduced to this: Positive patient and staff response to carpeting is due to the elegant appearance and pleasant atmosphere it creates. The presence of odors and spots concerns administrators, staff, and patients. Not enough is yet known to quantify the positive psychological advantages and to contrast them against the real economic costs of a "dirty" appearance in attracting new patients. Thus, in this example, as in all the others discussed in this chapter, a willingness to experiment and innovate seems to be the most reasonable recommendation to make. Taking no action on these matters is not a viable solution or approach to problem solving.

When we are concerned about environmental influences on the older person, we must consider two basic questions: What do we mean by environment? What do we need to understand about the older person in order to evaluate possible environmental effects? If it is recognized that behavior is influenced every time capabilities are matched against environmental situations, an important first step has been made in gaining sensitivity to the positive and negative consequences that might be expected.

While some suggestions can be made for methods to maximize an individual's life quality within any given setting, the relative newness of human-environment research does give cause for caution. It is essential that great care be given to evaluation of suspected individual needs, and that equal care be given to the environmental modification made. With any modification, behavioral responses should be carefully, and unobtrusively, monitored. Nurses are in key positions to do such monitoring.

The complexity of environmental effects, especially within group settings, is a creative challenge—one that demands constant experimentation and variation. A demonstrated willingness to act may, in itself, produce positive effects.

THE HAWTHORNE EFFECT

One prominent example of this axiom is the classic study of lighting variation at the Hawthorne, California, plant of Western Electric (Roethlisberger and Dickson, 1939). In this study, employee work performance was evaluated. Performance was first monitored under normal lighting levels. The level of illumination was increased and work performance increased. This pattern was repeated, each time with the same results. These experiments had apparently confirmed a direct relationship between the level of illumination and performance, until someone decided to reverse the process. When the highest level of illumination in the first test was decreased, work performance again increased. With each subsequent decrease in illumination, there was an incremental increase in work performance. The researchers ultimately concluded that, within the limits of lighting tested, it was not light per se that influenced performance, rather, employees' awareness of some special attention paid to them by management that seemed to be the real stimulus. This phenomenon, now widely known as the "Hawthorne effect," implies that environmental manipulation is the medium for expressing concern.

Thus, to the extent that experimentation, variation, and options are perceived as "messages" of concern, everyone benefits. To the extent that these changes also satisfy basic individual psychophysical needs, additional benefits are gained. With such prospects for positive effects, it seems reasonable to encourage nurses to consider environmental alteration as a major technique in the day-to-day functions of any institutional setting.

REFERENCES

Chaney, P.: Decor reflects environmental psychology, *Hospitals,* June 1, 1973.

Cheskin, Louis, et al.: Color psychology: Rainbow in your mind, in *The Family Creative Workshop,* Plenary Publications International, Inc., New York, 1974.

Farr, L.: Medical consequences of environmental home noise, *Journal of the American Medical Association,* pp. 171–174, October 1967.

Gibson, John E.: Do you know about your sense of smell? *Family Weekly,* July 28, 1974, p. 10.

Hall, E. T.: *The Hidden Dimension,* Doubleday, Garden City, N.Y., 1966.

Hayward, D. G.: Psychological factors in the use of light and lighting in buildings, in J. Lang et al. (eds.), *Designing for Human Behavior,* Dowden, Hutchinson and Ross, Stroudsburg, Pa., 1974.

Ittleson, W., H. Proshansky, and L. Rivlin: Bedroom size and social interaction in the psychic ward, *Environment and Behavior,* pp. 255–270, December 1970.

Lawton, P., and L. Nahemow: Ecology and the aging process, in C. Eisdorfer and P. Lawton (eds.), *The Psychology of Adult Development,* American Psychological Association, Washington, 1973.

Lieberman, M.: Institutionalization of the aged: Effects on behavior, *Journal of Gerontology,* pp. 330–340, July 1969.

National Bureau of Standards evaluated performance of hospital floor coverings, *Hospitals,* pp. 72–73, May 1969.

Pastalan, L.: How the elderly negotiate their environment, in T. Byerts (ed.), *Housing and Environment for the Elderly,* Gerontological Society, Washington, 1973.

————: Privacy as an expression of human territoriality, in L. Pastalan and D. Carson (eds.), *Spatial Behavior of Older People,* University of Michigan Press, Ann Arbor, 1970.

Roethlisberger, F., and W. Dickson: *Management and the Worker,* Harvard University Press, Cambridge, Mass., 1939.

Sommer, R.: *Personal Space: The Behavioral Basis of Design,* Prentice-Hall, Englewood Cliffs, N.J., 1969.

FORTY-FOUR

RELIGION AND THE AGED

Gerald A. Larue

Do not go gentle into that good night,
Old age should burn and rave at close of day;
Rage, rage against the dying of the light.
Dylan Thomas

LEARNING OBJECTIVES

- Distinguish between toxic and nourishing religious influences.
- Identify relevant nourishing biblical passages.
- Describe ways in which ancient and new ethical materials may be utilized by the healing professions.

We have inherited from the ancient past through Judaism and Christianity ways of thinking about aging and the aged that are both an affirmation of life and a denial of life. Attitudinal responses are programmed into our thinking and behaving from infancy by home, synagogue, church, and society. Sometimes the influence is open and direct; often it is subtle and inferential. Because we are shaped to some degree by what we believe about ourselves, it is important for those who work with the aged to be aware of positive and negative influences that may operate subconsciously in the thinking of the aged person. In this chapter it is not our intention to discuss how religious organizations attempt to meet the needs of retired or older communicants through counseling or special programs; it is enough to note that these institutions tend to segregate individuals by age and work with groups according to age rather than individuals according to need. Our intention is to discern, insofar as possible, how religious beliefs may affect and determine attitudes of personal identity and worth and thereby influence the way an individual thinks about aging.

Life-affirming factors enhance life, give meaning and purpose to existence, strengthen one's feelings of self-worth, encourage self-actualization, and are health-giving and life-sustaining. Life-denying influences restrict or enclose life patterns, limit experiences and associations, place burdens of guilt on individuals, encourage feelings of unworthiness, and are generally health-denying and life-inhibiting. Often the two are intermingled. Our concern is with recognizing ways to emphasize and encourage nourishing and life-affirming concepts and to diminish the effects of toxic or life-denying influences.

The principal source for authoritative religious teachings in Judaism and Christianity is the Bible which includes Hebrew Scriptures (Tanach or the Old Testament), Christian Scriptures (the New Testament), and for Roman Catholics and Eastern Orthodox churches certain deuterocanonical books called the Apocrypha by Jews and Protestants. Individual groups may have additional interpretive materials. For example, Muslims accept the Koran in addition to the Bible, Mormons utilize the *Book of Mormon,* Christian Scientists have *Science and Health with Key to the Scriptures,* and so on. The religious cult is the central conveyor and interpreter of biblical concepts through ritual, preaching, teaching, and interaction with the home and society. Biblical literature is believed to be divinely revealed, and hence supernatural authority is given to precepts, principles, values, attitudes, and life-styles implicit in the sacred writings or affirmed by cult expositors. So powerful is the effect of biblical teaching that some persons become burdened with feelings of "ought" and with guilt should they fail to reach idealized objectives; for others the regulations provide guides for meaningful living.

Of course, how the Bible is interpreted is important. For example, certain "science of health" groups such as the Church of Christ, Scientist, stress the illusory nature of pain, disease, and death. The real human is not the "mortal" being but is a divine reflection of God; the world of senses is unreal, a matter of belief. Healing is explained metaphysically, religiously, and biblically, and although teachings are health-oriented, there is a tenacious denial of medical and pharmaceutical practices, of many public-health measures, and of scientific research into health knowledge. The Bible, used as a source book and explained metaphysically, is interpreted to support cultist attitudes. Little is gained in debate about the merits of different interpretations or versions of the Bible; individuals believe what they believe. However, many enlightened followers of metaphysical cults operate in the spirit of the Hebrew sage Ben Sira, whose wisdom is included in Roman Catholic Bibles but not in the King James Version accepted as authoritative by Christian Scientists. Ben Sira acknowledged that all healing came from God but was administered by physicians. The wise man went on to say:

The Lord created medicines from the earth and a sensible man will not despise them. (Ecclus. 38:4)

We will concentrate on the ways religious concepts affect patterns of life and living and mind-sets and attitudes.

THE GOOD DIE YOUNG

Some religious systems include the concept of "fate" and teach that certain things happen (including illness and death) because of patterns set in motion in a previous life (karma) or in this life by powers beyond human control. Muslims use the phrase *inshallah,* signifying "if Allah wills"; Christians speak of resignation to the "will of God." Quietistic acceptance of fate may develop a nonresistant attitude toward the frailties of old age to the extent that simple wheelchair exercises prescribed by therapists to discourage atrophy of joints and muscles are ignored or treated with indifferent tolerance. Religious beliefs may encourage a *que será será* (what will be, will be) attitude toward infirmity and become harmful influences interfering with healing processes. After all, if the infirmity is an expression of divine judgment, what is the point in fighting it? If one's time has come, why not accept it?

There are those who are convinced that the human life-span is limited by divine decree, and they find support for their belief in the Bible. A Psalmist wrote "Our lifespan is seventy years, or, if heaven decrees, eighty" (Ps. 90:10). Of course some biblical personages lived longer. Preflood heroes lived for centuries, time periods that most biblical scholars believe are a literary device designed to fill long historical periods concerning which nothing was known.

In Hebrew thought, longevity was a reward for obedience to religious teachings. The modern adage "the good die young" was not part of ancient world thought where the good died old as a recompense for fidelity. Abraham, the model of faith, was 75 and Sarah 66 when they left their homeland to journey in faith to Canaan (Gen. 12:4). Sarah is described as a woman so beautiful and so sexually desirable that she became a member of the Egyptian ruler's harem (Gen. 12:11). Age was no detriment to beauty. Abraham was 85 when his first son, Ishmael, was born to Hagar, the maidservant (Gen. 16); his second son, Isaac, was born to Sarah when she was in her nineties and Abraham was 100 (Gen. 17:17). Sarah died at 127 (Gen. 23:1); Abraham remarried at about 135, and his new wife Keturah bore him six sons (Gen. 25:1). He died at 175 (Gen. 25:7). Beauty, sexual vigor, leadership, response to challenge were not limited by age in the Abraham story. Other heroes also lived long lives (Gen. 35:28; 47:28; 50:22). When Moses died at 120 years, he possessed good eyesight and was still sexually vigorous (Deut. 34:7).

But heroes are exceptions and represent those singularly blessed because of obedience to divine instruction. Their stories teach that adherence to revealed commands as interpreted by the cult yield long, full lives. This belief encountered difficulty when the good died young, when suffering came to obedient believers, and when wicked scoffers enjoyed longevity and good fortune. The Bible provides a number of responses to this dilemma. For example, emphasis on corporate identity moved Hebrew thought away from a stress on individuality. A person was a member of a group and so entwined with the group that it was impossible to affirm any real identity apart from membership in the whole. Personal misfortune might be caused by another. For example, if a parent violated a divine law and escaped punishment, retribution could be exacted of the children, grandchildren, great-grandchildren, and so on (Deut. 5:9). Of course, the concept of corporate personality was challenged, and it was taught that individuals suffered for their own sins (Ezek. 18). If neither theory fitted a situation, when someone suffered as Job did for no apparent reason, the sufferer could only protest against injustice, keep the faith, and hope that somehow the deity would set matters right. Nor does the New Testament offer an answer to the problem of suffering by the innocent. A young man born blind was presented to Jesus with the query: "Who sinned, this man or his parents?" Jesus replied, "Neither this man nor his parents have sinned," and He healed the man. He did not respond to the implied question about the reason for suffering.

The good did not always die old, nor did the wicked always die young. Ben Sira commented that an individual's life-span should be considered great if it reached 100 (Ecclus. 18:9), and a prophet dreamed of an ideal Jerusalem where it could never be said that "an infant lives only a few days or an old man failed to complete his life span. The child will die at one hundred years, and whoever fails to reach one hundred is cursed" (Isa. 65:20). The reality never matched the vision, and Judaism developed beliefs in life after death with rewards and punishments to be meted out in an afterlife. Righteous individuals who failed to receive blessings in this life were assured that they would be rewarded in the next; the wicked who enjoyed prosperity and health in this life were warned of judgment and punishment in the next (Dan. 12). This belief was inherited and developed by Christianity.

Today a believer enjoying good health and longevity might feel rewarded for adherence to the faith. On the other hand, disablement, pain, misfortune, financial loss might induce guilt and a search through past experiences to determine "what have I done to deserve this?" *Guilt, grieving over past misdeeds, and anger about present misery generally tend to be life-denying, harmful and a waste of energy, making it difficult to help individuals change and focus on potentials in the present or on life-affirming alternatives.*

For some, promises of blessing in a future life may make infirmities bearable and the thought of death tolerable. But beliefs about suffering and afterlife vary. In some forms of Buddhism, death marks a transition from the world of human beings to the world of spirits, where social structures and values prevail similar to those of the world of the living. Spirits mete out rewards and punishments to both living and dead, and public disaster or personal illness, brevity of life or sudden death may be interpreted as punishment. In Hinduism, judgments are reflected in reincarnation and karma whereby a believer receives in this life recompense for thoughts and actions in a previous life. Some Jews do not believe in an afterlife and consider death terminal and illness as a mark of physical frailty to be met with proper medical and health care; other Jews (Orthodox) believe in an afterlife with rewards and punishments. For Christians there is judgment in the next life, with heaven and hell as alternatives and punitive cleansing in purgatory included for Roman Catholics.

For some, belief in future punishments and rewards provokes feelings of guilt and fear. It is not surprising to find that older persons often become deeply concerned about religion and the afterlife. If these persons are Bible-oriented, as most Jews, Roman Catholics, and Protestants are, emphasis on biblical passages stressing forgiveness (such as Isa. 1:18; Matt. 6:14; 26:28) may give reassurance and provide chaplains and nurses with opportunity to redirect thoughts toward life-enhancing objectives. On the other hand, those who "long to be with their Lord in heaven" may be reacting against intolerable situations so that heaven is an escape from misery. If the unhappiness stems from family or social conditions, then love, attention, and reassurance are of paramount importance; if the death wish is due to pain and physical suffering, then medical expertise, love, attention, and reassurance are all that can be given.

YOU MATTER

Surveys have shown that, for many, retirement from gainful employment is a traumatic experience. The gold watch, the plasticized testimonial, the farewell party, the induction of a successor form part of a rite of passage, marking the termination of a relationship and the inauguration of a new phase of living. Nor can there be any return. The result is, often, loss of a sense of significance.

At present, society has given only limited attention to preparation for retirement (see Chapter 41 on retirement). Some programs assist the retired to adjust to new roles, but little has been done in preretirement training, in developing nourishing, life-affirming attitudes to the "gold watch" syndrome and postemployment days. Not everyone can enjoy the healthful attitude of a retired 70-year-old schoolteacher who exclaimed:

No classes to prepare for. No alarm clock to tell me I must get up and be on time. No code to conform to. I have never been so free. I get up when I feel like it. I go to meetings if I feel like it, and if I am late, it doesn't really matter. I am more myself than I have ever been. I am not afraid to say what I think. It is simply wonderful to be old.

Family ties do not always meet the psychic crisis of the feeling of uselessness. Some families integrate members so that everyone feels wanted, needed, and loved; others do not. Indian and Oriental families have traditionally esteemed the aged, but in recent times the respect is becoming more token than real. Where old cultural habits endure, the aged are made to feel important and are treated as persons of honor; in other situations older persons are very much on their own. Biblical law demanded that parents be honored and communal standards placed pressure on all to conform (Exod. 20:12; Lev. 19:3; Deut. 5:16). Present-day attitudes are different; the aged are not considered wise or even knowledgeable about rapid societal changes; they are, simply, "not with it." In the past, social changes came slowly and life patterns tended to be carried on from generation to generation by families living in the same community. Today, change is rapid and young families differ markedly in attitudes, interests, and mores. Older people are "a drag." Fragmented families, separated by distance, live in nuclear modules. Generation clashes encourage fewer visits. The aged are "better off" on their own; young families prefer to develop their own lifestyles without advice and argument. Without involvement in work patterns where the individual is important to society, without involvement in familial decisions, older adults feel they no longer matter. The result can only be psychologic disintegration. Enfeebled elderly are placed in nursing homes. Those who can pay the high costs enter retirement communities where varied programs are designed to keep members busy and, one hopes, interested in living actively. *Because we have discovered that it is easier to deal with individuals if they are incorporated in an amorphous group, we tend to forget that each of us needs to feel loved and important to survive as a human.*

Illness and hospitalization may increase feelings of helplessness and dependency for some; for others the special nursing care provided may be the first expression of concern for their well-being experienced in a long time. Illness brings response from family and attention from professionals.

Every situation that moves individuals into new roles and relationships is alive with possibilities for growth, including illness and confinement. To be inert, not to change and grow, is to stagnate. If the patient has religious orientations, the chaplain may encourage feelings of self-worth and help to develop nourishing attitudes for the posthospital period. Obviously a heavily sedated person or one in extreme pain is in no condition to reflect on opportunities for personal growth. Preparation for the problems and infirmities of aging must begin in childhood, for what individuals express or discover in invalidism depends upon what they brought with them to that situation. Chaplains and nurses can only encourage development of nourishing, life-sustaining attitudes.

Biblical teachings place value on all persons and a special emphasis on honoring the elderly. The New Testament teaches that the very hairs of one's head are numbered (Luke 12:7), that if the deity is concerned about the welfare of birds and natural things, it can be assumed that God has a greater concern for humans (Luke 12:6–7; 22–31). Ben Sira depicted the elderly as sources of wisdom and good judgment and worthy of honor:

> How beautiful judgment is in gray-haired men and knowledge of what to advise in the elderly. How attractive wisdom is in the aged and understanding and counsel in honorable men. The crown of the elderly is rich experience and their boast is the fear of the Lord. (Ecclus. 25:3–6)

Teachers advised their pupils:

> Pay attention to your father who begot you and don't despise your mother when she is old. (Prov. 23:22)

The old were to be heard and in the story of Job, young, impatient Elihu waited until the older wise men had spoken before introducing his ideas (Job 32:6–22). A New Testament writer urged youth to treat older persons like parents and denounced those who would rebuke an older man (1 Tim. 5:1–2).

We live in different times and situations. The aged are no longer repositories of wisdom. Modernization brings much that makes old wisdom obsolete. The past is easily retrievable through videotape recordings or through well-documented and illustrated history books. There is no particular magic in the accumulation of years: A stupid oldster is no more tolerable than a stupid youngster. Nor has an older person automatically earned respect by becoming old, no more than a youth can be denied respect by the fact of being young. Some elderly persons may have something of worth to share as they contemplate life, and some older persons with family ties may have something unique to contribute.

Some older individuals have been elevated to a greater status by the growing interest in family history. Young people, fascinated by backgrounds, by discovering "who they are," and where they came from, collect family memorabilia, tape-record interviews with parents, grandparents, and other relatives and unearth old letters, diplomas, and documents. The experience has brought families together in an adventure of shared discovery. For example, one woman taped interviews with her mother and father talking about their childhood, courtship, marriage, and the problems, failures, and successes associated with each. The father was under treatment for throat cancer which was at that time in a state of remission. A generation gap had existed between parents and daughter for some time. As the interviews progressed, as the young woman read her parents love letters, diaries, and other source materials, as she listened to their reminiscences, her appreciation of them as people deepened; their understanding of her as a person grew; the gap closed. As she interviewed her grandparents new bonds were formed. In her mother and grandmother she discovered feelings of rebellion similar to her own. She understood them better. "Suddenly," she said "they became human." The older persons became figures of significance, bearers of unique memories. As they opened themselves to her, she knew and loved them as never before. The situation became a growing and continuing nourishing of personalities catering to emotional and psychologic health. Old controversial issues became part of family history and were treated with calmness that served to heal wounds long hidden but still open. Unfortunately, in the rush of life, few have time to listen and discover the identity and humanity of the elderly.

Up to this moment, religious organizations have not found truly adequate ways to give support and meaning to lives of older persons. People are segregated by age. It is assumed that each group has unique interests, character, mind-set, and potency.

There are strengths and weaknesses in grouping systems. The strengths are obvious: sharing of similar interests, attitudes and concerns, and the reinforcing of group mind-sets. The weaknesses are often overlooked. The multiple dimensions of being human are confined or channeled into predetermined limits that provide the basis for criticism for nonconformity. For example, an older woman joined a youth group in folk dancing. She became the subject of covert condemnation by her age peers who thought she "should act her age," the assumption being that there are fixed behavioral patterns for differing age groups. Interests of older groups are not always health-giving or life-enhancing. A retired college administrator refused to attend monthly meetings of the "over 65" group of colleagues because each meeting opened with a register of the ill, incapacitated, or recently deceased. "The meetings were demoralizing and downright poisonous. I would come away feeling I was next on the list. I would go in feeling great and come out feeling terrible. No more for me."

Older individuals, with so much life experience to share often feel frustration, as expressed by Mardelle Dressler Dobbins (1974) in her poem:

> Not rich enough
> to buy an organ
> reroof a church
> pay a preacher
> build a mission far or near
> replace ghetto homes
> endow a school
> provide perpetual scholarships
>
> Not poor enough
> to beg for food
> for clothing worn or new
> to voice a need
> to bask in sympathy
> real or condescending
>
> Not good enough
> to radiate brilliance
> attract notice and reward
> and working hard
> gain the limelight

Not bad enough
to excite a wish to save
punish and scold
lock up and fine
and completely scorn

Brimming with wealth
of thoughts and wisdom
stored high I hope through years
I cannot share these riches
when no one listens

THE CLERGY, THE CHURCH, AND THE ELDERLY

Pastoral psychology is currently included in the academic curriculum of most seminaries. Some clergy take special courses in counseling and working with the aged. Some have, in turn, provided education for lay persons enabling them to assist in the ministry to the aged. Such trained individuals may provide nourishing support for the work of members of the medical profession.

On the other hand, untrained persons may become toxic influences. For example, one well-intentioned pastor, while visiting an ailing elderly man, asked the patient for his favorite scripture passage. The man replied "John 14." Without bothering to ask why this passage was selected, and without pausing to reflect that this passage was used regularly in funeral services, the pastor began to read. The man became emotionally upset, began to sob violently and vomited his medicine. The pastor was a bit put out with the nurse's impatience with him as she responded to his urgent call which required cleaning up, comforting, and remedicating the patient.

If the pastor had been sensitive to the patient's situation, he might have asked why this passage was a favorite. He would have learned that it had meaning for the man because it was associated with the funerals of his mother, father, wife, and eldest daughter. It had provided comfort in moments of dire distress. In the present situation it assumed foreboding qualities. It reminded the patient of his own mortality and seemed to imply that his present infirmity might be fatal (which it was not). The pastor, in his eagerness to give scriptural comfort,

ignored the patient and developed a toxic environment.

Trained clergy are sensitive to clients' needs and to the responsibilities of those in charge of clients' health and well-being. They direct conversation to humanistic concerns such as the client's feelings, needs, attitudes, and relationships. Consequently, such trained clergy assume adjunctive roles in the healing process.

Some churches have trained older adults for visitation with the elderly who are confined to nursing homes or who are invalid. At times considerable stress is laid upon evangelizing the ill, and some converters become so eager to bring clients to their particular interpretation of religion or to their brand of faith that the emotional, physical, and psychic needs of clients become secondary. For the well-being of clients, hospitals and homes for the elderly cannot be permitted to become hunting grounds for evangelical recruitment and conversion. The most effective church workers among the elderly are those who have had their consciousness raised concerning the physical, emotional, intellectual, and psychic needs of the elderly and who are aware of the nature of the work of medical professionals. Such persons move quietly and confidently among the elderly to develop a nourishing, life-enhancing environment. Some are excellent conversationalists. Some read stories or novels. One visitor discovered that an elderly woman had grown up happily in a town where the visitor had relatives. It was a simple matter to arrange to have the local town paper delivered. Correspondence with relatives brought up-to-date news about persons and old familiar places.

Unfortunately only small steps have been taken in spanning age differences. In some churches teen-agers have been given special training to enable them to visit elderly indigents with something other than "entertaining them" in mind. These young people have been taught to engender conversations that reflect genuine personal interest in and concern for the individual. They have been trained to listen with patience, to ask relevant questions, and to help the older person experience some sense of self-worth in the opportunity to convey to a new generation wisdom gained through years of living. In one such visit, a college student sat with a lonely, isolated man whose communication with the nurses and hospital personnel had been limited to gestures and a few words in broken English. The student recognized the patient's accent—he spoke Italian. Because she had spent two semesters studying abroad in Italy, they were able to converse. "What that man knew about Italian art and culture blew my mind," she reported. A genuine friendship developed, and hospital staff and patient regularly welcomed this young person who brought nourishing strength to a man who had been physically, emotionally, and linguistically isolated.

Outside the established communities for the aged, some churches have initiated programs designed to develop communication across age barriers. A film is shown to a mixed-age group—often a somewhat controversial film. The larger group is broken into units of five, each composed of a teen-ager, a young married person, a middle-aged person, a late-middle-aged person, and one elderly (70 years or older) individual. They talk about what they have seen. Often interesting interpretive bonds are formed. For example, an older person discovers that some one who has lived a fifth of a century in our technologically geared society may have links with those who have lived three-quarters of a century and have witnessed some of the most rapid and dramatic changes in society that the world has ever known. Demolition of barriers among individuals and groups, and establishment of respect and understanding for persons regardless of age, give promise of nourishing results for the future.

POTENTIALS FOR A NEW ETHIC

Through the centuries religious organizations have varied emphases and found within sacred Scriptures support for their actions. For example, in the Bible there have been found bases for asceticism and social action, for pacificism and war, for slavery and antislavery, and so on. In each instance certain passages were interpreted as attitudes approved by the deity and as guides for action. The Western world has accepted a work ethic supported by religion that teaches that only as one is productive, only as one continues to labor and contribute to human survival and advancement, only as one earns one's way is one entitled to the benefits of society. Little or no emphasis has been placed on enjoying life for what it is, on draining the cup of pleasure rather than filling a measure of social responsibility; on using leisure time and retirement years to explore human potentials for enjoyment of love, beauty, and happiness. It is not surprising to find some persons almost apologetic for retirement, for not being involved in wage-earning, for accepting social security or other benefits which are their right. Nor has the social environment made them feel otherwise. Retired persons are "old fogies" with meager incomes, out-of-style clothes and ideas—the withered, tired, bored and boring, inactive, dependent, the helpless. Is it any wonder that older retired persons regard their situation with such low esteem? Old age is an indignity. How can religion and religious organizations and nursing become involved in changing the image? Perhaps by developing alternatives to the work ethic, that will be taught at all age levels. Potential emphases might include:

1. Acceptance of individuals as "wholes." Age divisions have some validity, but they tend to become fixed and develop stereotypes. Only by accepting persons as persons, rather than as members of an age group, can the fixed images be broken.
2. Encouraging exploration of innate qualities of being human including response to curiosity through open inquiry so that life may become a continuing adventure in learning and experiencing; stressing potentials of human awareness as we move from space to space rather than emphasizing differences as we move from age to age.
3. Placing new emphasis on human potentials and less on human limitations; more on new ways of experiencing life and less on sin for violating some concept that was useful several thousand years ago; giving less heed to rules that inhibit and produce guilt and placing more importance on possibilities for self-awareness and self-realization.
4. Placing more emphasis on humor inherent in much that occupies and absorbs the human

situation and less on obscure ultimate meanings.

5. Discussing aging as a process that begins at birth and placing less emphasis on age groupings, age behavior patterns, age limitations.

6. Talking openly of death as termination of life that can occur at any age, and, whether or not the particular religious group believes in an afterlife, stressing potentials and alternatives to experiencing life now.

Aging is part of the natural process of living. Retirement is earned time. Social security is earned money. Medicare is earned medical protection. Such benefits belong to every elderly person as partial recognition to contributions made (no matter how small) to the continuing health, wisdom, and existence of the community, the nation, the world.

Should proof texts be needed to support the emphasis upon living in a nourishing, fulfilling manner, the Bible supplies many, including advice to people to eat, drink, and find pleasure in the work they do under the sun during the few days God has granted them, for that is their destiny (Eccles. 5:18), and Jesus' invitation to the young man, who having kept all the religious commandments was still unhappy, to forsake his present life-style and enter into a new adventure in living with Jesus and his followers.

REFERENCES

Dobbins, Mardelle Dressler: Notes from an old church member, *A.D.,* United Church of Christ edition, May 1974, p. 74.

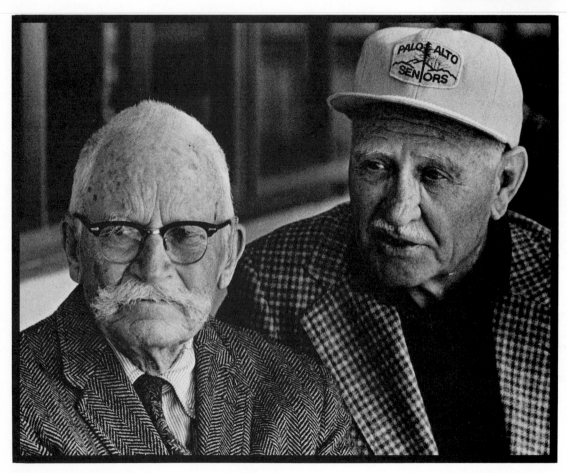

NINE

Richard Wisdom,
for San Jose Mercury News

RESEARCH

DEFINITION OF AN ELDER
An elder is a person who is still growing, still a
learner, still with potential and whose life continues
to have within it promise for, and connection to the
future. An elder is still in pursuit of happiness, joy
and pleasure, and her or his birthright to these
remains intact. Moreover, an elder is a person who
deserves respect and honor and whose work it is to
synthesize wisdom from long life experience and
formulate this into a legacy for future generations.

The Live Oak Project

The old man wraps his years
Around him as a cloak
Against a world grown cold
And warms himself within
By memories and dreams,
As he sits
To await
His completion.

Ross Allen McClelland

FORTY-FIVE

GERONTOLOGICAL NURSING RESEARCH

Linda Dold Robinson

Research is to teaching what sin is to confession; without one, you have nothing to tell in the other.
William R. Allen

LEARNING OBJECTIVES

- List three sources for retrieval of gerontological nursing research.
- Discuss two problems in locating nurse-authored research.
- Discuss theoretical frameworks which provide conceptual bases for gerontological nursing research.
- Discuss common methodologies in gerontological research.
- Describe three landmark research studies in gerontological nursing.
- Compare trends in gerontological nursing research from 1966 to 1975 and 1975 to 1979.

Nursing research on aging is a relatively new endeavor, and few definitive studies have been produced. However, the quantity and quality of geriatric nursing research have shown steady growth over the past decade. A search of the geriatric nursing literature was conducted in order to identify the body of gerontological research. Select aspects of trends in research in the field of gerontology and geriatrics were discussed, but considerably more research is needed in order to provide a body of scientific knowledge upon which to base the practice of geriatric nursing and the teaching of nursing students.

The purpose of this chapter is to present a review of published research on aging and aged persons. The literature search will be described and the studies composing the body of nursing research on aging will be discussed. Select aspects of the substantive problem areas, underlying frameworks, methodologies, and findings will be presented to identify trends and suggest areas needing further investigation.

THE LITERATURE REVIEW

A systematic review of gerontology and geriatric nursing literature published in English was undertaken to identify research conducted by nurses alone or in conjunction with members of other disciplines. No attempt was made to evaluate the quality of the studies. Because the ultimate goal was to acquaint nursing students and practitioners with studies completed, in progress, and readily available, the search was confined to published materials. Hence, no attempt was made to review unpublished master or doctoral dissertations. (The reader is referred to *Dissertation Abstracts International* for these materials.) The search began with the literature published in 1966 and continued through February 1975. The main bibliographic sources utilized for the search were the *International Nursing Index* (published as a quarterly cumulation) and the Abstracts which are published in each issue of *Nursing Research* and indexed annually.

The search for nurse-authored research on aging and the aged was complicated by two problems. In nonnursing publications the professional affiliation of an author could not al-

ways be ascertained, even by inspection of any accompanying biographic footnotes. The presentation of some studies was found to be extremely brief or confined solely to narrative based on findings without mention of methodology or other information to identify it as a piece of proper research. Hence, it is possible that some of the nursing research on aging has not been identified.

GERONTOLOGICAL NURSING LITERATURE

The body of gerontological nursing literature has grown rapidly in quantity and quality. A preponderance of the articles consist of "how-to-do-it" advice and moralistic declarations of "shoulds" and "oughts" based on anything ranging from limited clinical experience to documented research. More recently, a number of excellent detailed case studies of theory-based deliberative nursing interventions with elderly persons have been published. These experiential writings provide a valuable source of problem areas needing research.

Another important segment of the gerontological nursing literature has been concerned with the delivery of various health-care services to the aged. The number of innovative demonstration projects described in narrative form has increased sharply.

TRENDS IN GERONTOLOGICAL NURSING RESEARCH

The volume of nursing research on aging and the aged has steadily increased. The search of the literature published between 1966 and February 1975 yielded 36 reports of research conducted by nurses utilizing study populations composed entirely of aged persons. Five studies were found in which attempts were made to discover differences in manifestations of phenomena by comparing persons over the age of 55 with younger persons. The attitudes of nursing students and staffs toward aging and the aged continue to provide a research arena. Five studies were found which dealt exclusively with the attitude problem. An additional pair of research reports was found in which investigation of the attitudes of nursing staff toward aging patients, toward certain kinds of unacceptable patient behavior, and toward dying patients and their care was a portion of a larger study.

THE SUBSTANTIVE AREAS

Inspection of the substantive areas from which the research problems have been derived revealed that direct patient care has been the major area of concern, followed closely by patient variables influencing care. Half the studies were in these two areas. The other half was divided among four areas: care delivery systems, attitudes toward aging and the aged, the nursing process, and setting variables influencing care. The substantive areas will be referred to again in a later section.

THE THEORETICAL FRAMEWORKS

The frameworks underlying the gerontological research have been drawn from a broad range of theoretical and conceptual bases. A few studies were found to be based on theories derived from the physical sciences. The behavioral and social sciences have provided the framework for the majority of the studies. However, the vast majority of the research has been reported without reference to an underlying theoretical framework. Although not all types of research require a theoretical or conceptual framework, such a framework is necessary in order to relate and integrate the findings within a larger body of scientific knowledge.

Concepts from physiology and physics provided the framework for a study designed to identify patients at risk of developing pressure sores (Hicks, 1971). Cybernetics and energy exchange theories have been used in the development and testing of a model of nurse-patient interaction (Putnam, 1971). Two studies have been grounded in the research on aging changes in nerve impulse transmission (Panicucci et al., 1968; Greenberg, 1973). Sensory deprivation has been used as the theoretical base for one intervention study (Carlson, 1968) and for a large-scale exploratory study of deprivation phenomena and effective nursing interventions (Ellis et al., 1968). Investigations based on the phenomenon of social disengagement and its associated theory have been reported by two nurses (Levine, 1969; Reed, 1970). Communication theory has been used as a basis for a survey of the perceptions of retired persons about a specific disease entity (Zornow, 1973).

Two experiments in patient teaching reported conceptual frameworks derived from learning theory. In one study a role-delineated approach was developed (Ankenbrandt and Tanner, 1971), while the other involved a decision-making approach (Hallburg, 1970). Learning theory has also been used in the development of various forms of behavior therapy, one of which is operant conditioning. This framework underlies an experimental study of nursing intervention in incontinence (Grosicki, 1968).

Several theories were merged to form the framework of a piece of basic research on cognitive development and person perception in the aged (Muhlenkamp, 1972). The modal form of theoretical framework underlying those gerontological research studies which have frameworks has been composed of theories and concepts borrowed from other disciplines. An alternative to this mode is to develop conceptual frameworks grounded in the phenomena encountered in nursing practice. One example of this type of framework was found (Weiss, 1968).

What is most striking about the framework underlying the gerontological research is the lack of duplication. It is rare to find two studies, even when concerned with the same problem areas, which utilize the same theoretical framework. Although it would be possible to ground the investigations of various phenomena in the same theoretical framework and thereby build a more coherent body of knowledge, nurses appear to prefer to conduct completely original research.

THE METHODOLOGIES

A number of methodological trends have also emerged during the review of research in these fields. An increase in collaboration between nursing and other disciplines has been reflected in the selection of problem areas for study and in joint authorship of publications. More experimental studies have been reported, although the predominant research design has continued to be exploratory. There have been few replication or follow-up studies. In addition, there have been few instances in which data collection tools have been modified, refined, or even utilized in subsequent studies. Only one study (Schwartz, Henley, and Zeitz, 1964) has been cited by a number of nurse researchers as the basis for later studies—Gimble, 1968; Hallburg, 1970; Neely and Patrick, 1968—the last being a replication. One additional replication study was found (McKnight, 1970).

The captive populations of mentally or physically ill elderly patients in institutional settings (psychiatric or general hospitals or nursing homes) have been the source of data for the vast majority of studies. However, in 10 of the more recent studies, non-ill aged or aging individuals in the community have been the subjects. On the whole, sample sizes have tended to be small and the duration of the studies brief.

LANDMARK STUDIES

The body of gerontological nursing research contains three landmark studies. The first of these to be published was *The Elderly Ambulatory Patient* (Schwartz, Henley, and Zeitz, 1964). This was an extensive study of the nursing and psychosocial needs of elderly ambulatory clinic patients and an exploration of how best to meet those needs. The impact of this project continues to be manifested as a basis for subsequent studies by other nurses and also as the foundation for significant changes in health-care delivery in the original study setting (Wang and Brayton, 1970; Wang, 1970; Schwartz, 1973).

The second basic study was *Nurses, Patients, and Social Systems* (Weiss, 1968). This represents the first published rigorous, quantitative investigation of the effects of the introduction of skilled nursing care upon chronically ill older patients in a variety of institutional settings (nursing homes). It has been of great interest to this reviewer that the search of the literature yielded only one later study (Brown, 1970) based upon this one.

The most recent of the three landmark studies to be published was *The Aged Ill* (Jaeger and Simmons, 1970). This research identified some critical problems in geriatric nursing care related to coping with illness, infirmity, and dying; de-termined how these problems were being dealt with by staff in select institutional settings; and compared the current practices with recommendations obtained from certain nursing leaders as to how the problems should be handled.

The ultimate purpose of research is to provide new knowledge—valid answers to questions or valid solutions to problems, verification of facts, and development of theories. In order that this be accomplished, the final step in the research process must be the making public of the findings and the means by which the findings were obtained. Small studies of brief duration have limited generality and not much ability to add greatly to the body of scientific knowledge. However, clusters of replication studies or studies arising from closely related problem areas and utilizing rigorous and systematic designs and methodologies have the potential for expanding the body of knowledge and assisting in the development of theory. The published reports of each of the three landmark studies cited above are very detailed and comprehensive. Sufficient information has been presented to enable another researcher to replicate either one section or the entire study. Data collection tools and analysis schedules have been included, as well as suggestions for revisions and recommendations for additional research.

THE SUBSTANTIVE AREAS REVISITED

This section has been designed to highlight the gerontological nursing research studies in each substantive area and to challenge the reader to peruse the studies at their primary sources. Time and space limitations do not permit presentation of full discussion of each of the studies.

DIRECT-PATIENT CARE

Therapeutic Nurse-Patient Interactions (One-to-One)

"Personalization of the institutionalized older patient" (Brown, 1970)

"Nurse-patient interchange in the arrest of psychosocial atrophy of aged, institutionalized patients" (Brown and Brown, 1971)

"Therapeutic interaction: A means of crisis intervention with newly institutionalized elderly persons" (Robinson, 1974)

"Effects of individualized nursing intervention on senile status and self-care achievement of institutionalized patients" (Thomas, 1968)

Nurses, Patients, and Social Systems (Weiss, 1968)

Broad Approach Interventions

The Aged Ill (Jaeger and Simmons, 1970)

The Nursing Home and the Aged Psychiatric Patient (Stotsky, 1970)

"Older patients and their care: Interaction with families and public health nurses" (Adams, 1969)

Health-Care Teaching

"Role-delineated and informal nurse-teaching and food selection behavior of geriatric patients" (Ankenbrandt and Tanner, 1971)

"Oral medications and the older patient" (Gimble, 1968)

"Teaching patients self-care" (Hallburg, 1970)

"Expanded speech and self-pacing in communicating with the aged" (Panicucci et al., 1968)

Interventions for Specific Patient Problems

"Collagenase debridement" (Barrett and Klibanski, 1973)

"Selected sensory input and life satisfactions of immobilized geriatric female patients" (Carlson, 1968)

"Suggestions for the care of eye surgery patients who experience reduced sensory input" (Ellis et al., 1968)

"Effect of operant conditioning on modification of incontinence in neuropsychiatric geriatric patients" (Grosicki, 1968)

PATIENT VARIABLES INFLUENCING CARE

Patient Characteristics as Predictors of Phenomena

"Urinary incontinence in the acute phase of cerebral vascular accident" (Adams, Baron, and Caston, 1966)

"An assessment tool to identify pressure sores" (Gosnell, 1973)

"An incidence study of pressure sores following surgery" (Hicks, 1971)

"Predictors of longevity: A follow-up of the aged in Chapel Hill" (Palmore and Stone, 1973)

Manifestations of Social Involvement and Disengagement

"Disengagement in the elderly: Its causes and effects" (Levine, 1969)

"Social disengagement in chronically ill patients" (Reed, 1970)

"Social involvement of elderly studied in relation to mental health status" (Thomas, 1970)

Determinants of Health-Care Needs

"Reaction time in the elderly" (Greenberg, 1973)

"Older adults: A community survey of health needs" (Managan et al., 1974)

"Relationship of patients' responses to nursing history questions and selected factors: A preliminary study" (McPhetridge, 1973)

The Elderly Ambulatory Patient (Schwartz, Henley, and Zeitz, 1964)

Patient Knowledge about Self-Care

"The hospital patient and his knowledge of the drugs he is receiving" (Marks and Clarke, 1972)

"Problems of aged persons taking medications at home" (Neely and Patrick, 1968)

"Perceptions of residents of retirement communities about osteoarthritis" (Zornow, 1973)

Theory Development

"Getting around with emphysema" (Fagerhaugh, 1973)

"Cognitive developmental aspects of person perception in the aged" (Muhlenkamp, 1972)

SETTING VARIABLES INFLUENCING CARE

"Effects of institutionalization: A comparison of community, waiting list, and institutionalized aged persons" (Prock, 1969)

"Wine in the treatment of long-term geriatric patients in mental institutions" (Mishara and Kastenbaum, 1974)

"Beer and TLC" (Volpe and Kastenbaum, 1967)

"The effects of introducing a heterosexual living space" (Silverstone and Wynter, 1975)

"Suggestions for the care of eye surgery patients who experience reduced sensory input" (Ellis et al., 1968)

THE NURSING PROCESS

"Nursing observation and care planning for the hospitalized aged" (Hefferin and Hunter, 1975)

"Nurse awareness and psychosocial function in the aged" (Putnam, 1973)

"Supplementary regulation of environmental interchange: An operational approach to the study of nursing" (Putnam, 1971)

HEALTH-CARE DELIVERY SYSTEMS

Providing In-Home Care

"Older patients and their care: Interaction with families and public health nurses" (Adams, 1969)

Public Health Nursing for the Sick at Home (Holliday, 1967)

"Services to the aged by the Canadian public health nurse in the official health agency" (Schwenger and Sayers, 1971a)

"A survey by Canadian public health nurses of the health and living conditions of the aged" (Schwenger and Sayers, 1971b)

Providing Care in Institutional Settings

"Rehabilitative psychiatric nursing for chronically ill, elderly patients" (Gelper, 1973)

Nursing Home Research Study: Quantitative Measurement of Nursing Services (McKnight, 1970)

The Nursing Home and the Aged Psychiatric Patient (Stotsky, 1970)

ATTITUDES TOWARD AGING AND THE AGED

Held by Nursing Students

"Specialty preferences and characteristics of nursing students in baccalaureate programs" (DeLora and Moses, 1969)

"Students' attitudes towards geriatric nursing" (Gunter, 1971)

Held by Nursing Staffs

"Patient variables associated with nurses' preferences among elderly patients" (Brown, 1971)

"Factors affecting nurse-patient interaction in a geriatric setting" (Burchett, 1968)

"Study of the attitudes of nursing personnel toward the geriatric patient" (Campbell, 1971)

"Attitudes of nursing personnel toward the aged" (Gillis, 1973)

The Aged Ill (Jaeger and Simmons, 1970)

The Nursing Home and the Aged Psychiatric Patient (Stotsky, 1970)

And toward the Dying Patient

The Aged Ill (Jaeger and Simmons, 1970)

The Nursing Home and the Aged Psychiatric Patient (Stotsky, 1970)

HEURISTICS

Nursing research on aging conducted over the past 10 years has provided a small body of scientific knowledge upon which to build. Much remains to be done, especially in the area of patient care research or clinical research. Past reviews of nursing research and the gerontological nursing literature have resulted in ample recommendations relative to substantive areas needing investigation and how to proceed to get the research done (Basson, 1967; Schwartz, 1969; Abdellah, 1970).

Of considerable importance to any organized research venture is the availability of persons prepared to conduct the research project. Only a few programs exist to prepare nurses in geriatric nursing at the master's level. Perusal of the *International Directory of Nurses with Doctoral Degrees* (American Nurses' Foundation, 1973) reveals a total of 13 nurses whose dissertations dealt with the subjects of aging, the aged, or geriatric nursing. Clearly, the need is great for nurses prepared at the doctoral level.

The geriatric nursing literature is replete with descriptions of experiences of nurses dealing with a wide range of patient needs, behavior problems, and patient responses to aspects of medical treatment and nursing care. Here is a valuable source of problems that need solutions.

Useful methodologies, as well as additional problem areas worthy of investigation, can be found in the larger body of nursing research conducted with middle-aged subjects. Some of the completed studies might provide a basis for comparison of phenomena and determination of age-related differences.

At present there is still a great need to delineate the specific body of knowledge underlying clinical geriatric nursing practice. Systematic descriptions of the responses of elderly persons to their health problems and to specific nursing interventions are needed. There has been little written about the way patients manage their health problems. Additional descriptions are needed of the variable effects of treatment settings and of deliberative alterations in the environment upon aged clients. Specific nursing interventions need to be tested and evaluated in terms of patient outcomes. Guidelines for patient assessment and nursing intervention need to be developed and rigorously tested.

A number of descriptions of demonstration projects of innovations in the delivery of health care to elderly clients have been published recently. Now there is need for evaluative studies to determine the impact upon the patient of the innovations. Included among the innovations are the expanded role and functions of the gerontological nurse practitioner.

GERONTOLOGICAL NURSING RESEARCH: 1975 to 1980

This portion of the chapter is an overview of nurse-authored research on aging and the aged published from 1975 to 1980 in the United States. The author has been deliberately brief in order to stimulate the reader to seek out the original studies either in the library or from the researchers themselves.

The literature search began with material published in March 1975 and continued through November 1979. The review has followed the same criteria as previously stated in the chapter with one exception. The main bibliographic source was the abstracts published in *Nursing Research.*

The search for nurse-authored research on aging and the aged was again complicated by the same two problems: (1) difficulty identifying nurse-authors and (2) brevity of presentation. It is highly likely that some of the nursing research in aging has not been identified. In addition, some excellent literature reviews which constitute theoretical and conceptual frameworks for generating researchable questions have been omitted from this presentation. The tendency to publish studies piecemeal militates against the more rapid development of a body of gerontological nursing research.

TRENDS IN GERONTOLOGICAL NURSING RESEARCH

The volume of nursing research on aging and the aged has continued to increase. The search of literature published between March 1975 and November 1979 yielded 71 studies, plus a critical British study (Norton, McLaren, and Exton-Smith, 1975) which was too important to omit. Collaborative efforts have increased. Of the studies 21 were authored by two or more nurses while 22 studies represented interdisciplinary authorship. Many more studies were conducted with funding beyond the researcher's own purse. This trend follows a tendency toward more experimental designs, more attention to tighter controls, more sophisticated statistical data analyses, and computerized data treatments. Better funding makes possible more complex research designs. So also do better research designs attract greater financial support. Funding sources have included local institutions, private foundations, Sigma Theta Tau, Western Interstate Commission for Higher Education, and a variety of federal agencies—National Institute of Mental Health, Nursing Division of National Institutes of Health, Health Services Research and Development, and the Department of Health, Education, and Welfare.

Six replication studies have been found in this search. Two (Franck, 1979; Hain and Chen, 1976) were derived from Managan et al. (1974). The other four replications dealt with four separate questions (Foote, 1979; Kayser and Minnigerode, 1975; McGlone and Kick, 1978; and Muhlencamp, Gress, and Flood, 1975). The appearance of ongoing research efforts and clusters of studies has been particularly noteworthy. These studies have addressed specific nursing interventions (Baltes and Zerbe, 1976; DeWalt, 1975; DeWever, 1977); properties of the elderly (Muhlencamp, Gress, and Flood, 1975; Lester and Baltes, 1978; Spasoff et al., 1978); and the testing of an assessment tool (Fitzpatrick and Donovan, 1979).

Informed consent Probably the most critical issue in research on the elderly is that of competent informed consent. Berkowitz (1978) has dealt definitively with the problem in terms of resources within the law and a variety of alternative solutions. To advance a research-based body of knowledge in gerontological nursing mandates increasing use of aged persons as subjects. Of the studies presented in this paper, 56 involved the elderly—20 studies of community residents and 36 studies of institutionalized patients. The majority of these studies dealt briefly with special precautions taken to ensure competent informed consent.

Another trend worthy of mention is the increase of studies designed specifically to develop and test assessment tools and guidelines. Three such studies were found (Fitzpatrick and Donovan, 1979; Brink et al., 1978; Kupfer et al., 1978). A concomitant trend is the reporting of high levels of validity and reliability of original tools. Replication studies should increase in the future with persistent attention to this and other methodological issues.

Inspection of the substantive areas from which the research problems have been derived revealed two main areas of concern: patient variables influencing care (30 studies) and direct patient care (21 studies). The focus has shifted to patient and family outcomes as opposed to prior years' focus on nurse and system inputs. (See Table 45-1.)

Patient Characteristics: Predictors of Phenomena Closer inspection of the substantive areas for study revealed categories that differed from those appropriate to the prior decade of studies. Patient variables influencing care contained four subcategories. The first, patient characteristics as predictors of phenomena, dealt with community residents (Bullough, Bullough, and Mauro, 1978; Muhlencamp, Gress, and Flood, 1975; Edsall and Miller, 1978; Lally

TABLE 45-1
AREAS OF STUDY IN GERONTOLOGICAL NURSING RESEARCH

Topic	No. of Studies
Patient variables influencing care	30
Direct patient care	21
Attitudes toward aging and the aged	8
Evaluation of health care programs	5
Education for gerontological nursing	4
Miscellaneous	3
Total	71

et al., 1979; Grier, 1977) and included a new focus on sexuality (Brower and Tanner, 1979; Friedeman, 1979; Kaas, 1978). Patient characteristics as determinants of health care needs continued the investigations of community residents (Franck, 1979; Hain and Chen, 1976; McGlone and Kick, 1978; Schank, 1977). Responses of the elderly to hospitalization (Munoz and Mesick, 1979; Mezey, 1979) and to institutionalization (Chang, 1978; Gioiella, 1978; Hughes, 1979; DeWever, 1977; Spasoff et al., 1978; Miller and Beer, 1977; Francis and Odell, 1979; Snyder et al., 1978; Feist, 1978) involved studies particularly well grounded in theory. Responses to deliberate environmental change were the fourth subcategory of studies and dealt with relocation (Wolanin, 1978; Dimond, King, and Burt, 1979; Thomas, 1979) and a host of critical issues for planning (O'Donnell, Collins, and Schuler, 1978; Lester and Baltes, 1978; Johnson, 1979; Alverman, 1979).

The second major substantive area was direct patient care. Investigations of interventions for specific problems focused on recovery from hip fracture (Lamb, 1979; Mikhail, Sonn, and Lawton, 1978; Williams et al., 1979); confusion (Walsh, Walsh, and Melaney, 1978; Voelkel, 1978; Hogstel, 1979); preventive health care teaching (Conrad, 1977; Foote, 1979); and a set of unrelated studies all well grounded in theory (Norton, McLaren, and Exton-Smith, 1975; Baltes and Zerbe, 1976; DeWalt, 1975; Gerber and Van Ort, 1979; Wichita, 1977; Dufault, 1978). There has been increasing concern with drug use (Dittmar and Dulski, 1977; Garetz et al., 1979;

Raskind, Alvarez, and Herlin, 1979), problems in self-medication (Raskind, Kitchell, and Alvarez, 1978), and appropriate prescribing (Sorensen, Sorensen, and Zimmer, 1979; Requarth, 1979; Brown et al., 1977).

Evaluation of Health Care Programs The third substantive area of investigation was the evaluation of health care programs. The major innovation here has been the focus on patient outcomes (Chekryn and Roos, 1979; Kahn et al., 1977; Sherr and Goffi, 1977; Sullivan and Armignacco, 1979; Uman, 1979).

Attitudes The fourth major substantive area was attitudes toward aging and the aged, with minimal concern for RN attitudes (Taylor and Harned, 1978; Dye, 1979) and concentration on nursing students. Here the focus has moved from attitude assessment only to testing deliberative ways to change students' attitudes toward the positive (Heller and Walsh, 1976; Kayser and Minnigerode, 1975; Robb, 1979; Tobiason and Knudsen, 1979; Wilhite and Johnson, 1976; Chamberland et al., 1978; Hart et al., 1976).

The specific studies bearing on education for gerontological nursing were closely related to those bearing on attitudes. Brower (1977, 1979) has done extensive work on content needs plus program analysis and evaluation at the graduate level. *No studies were found that addressed undergraduate issues in education for gerontological nursing.* However, one study did deal with the impact of nursing staff attitudes on geriatric nurse practitioner students (Tharp, Baker, and Brower, 1979). Dye and Sassenrath (1979) tested a variety of health care professionals and made recommendations concerning educational needs based on errors made in their assessments of specific physiological and functional conditions.

SUMMARY

Several years ago Gortner and Nahm (1977) analyzed the state of the art of nursing research in the United States in terms of historical perspectives, contributions of nursing research to practice, and resources which had fostered the growth. There was a notable lack of geriatric and/or gerontological nursing impact in their findings. However, in that same year, Gunter and Miller (1977) concluded that the number of studies reported in the nursing journals was still far too limited to support the existence of a nursing gerontology grounded in nursing research. They did, however, conclude that the beginnings of a nursing gerontology were present in the multidisciplinary field of applied gerontology along with nursing research having application to the care of the elderly. Hence the key to gerontological nursing in the future lies in the foci and quality of research. As nursing knowledge of aging and the aged increases, there will be accompanying changes and improvements in clinical practice and education, but only when the new knowledge is disseminated to geriatric nurse practitioners, educators, and researchers in the field.

REFERENCES

Abdellah, Faye G.: Overview of nursing research 1955–1968, pt. I, *Nursing Research,* **19:**6–17, January–February 1970; pt. II, **19:**151–162, March–April 1970; and pt. III, **19:**239–252, May–June 1970.

Adams, Mary: Older patients and their care: Interaction with families and public health nurses, in *Fourth Nursing Research Conference March 1968,* American Nurses' Association, New York, 1969, pp. 128–160.

————, **Martha Baron, and Mary Ann Caston:** Urinary incontinence in the acute phase of cerebral vascular accident, *Nursing Research,* **15:**100–108, Spring 1966.

Alverman, Mary M.: Toward improving geriatric care with environmental intervention emphasizing a homelike atmosphere: An environmental experience, *Journal of Gerontological Nursing,* **5:**13–17, May–June 1979.

American Nurses Foundation: *International Directory of Nurses with Doctoral Degrees,* New York, 1973.

Ankenbrandt, Marguerite D., and Linda K. Tanner: Role-delineated and informal nurse-teaching and food selection behavior of geriatric patients, *Nursing Research,* **20:**61–64, January–February 1971.

Baltes, Margret M., and Melissa B. Zerbe: Independent training in nursing-home residents, *Gerontologist,* **16:**428–432, October 1976.

Barrett, Daniel J., and Aron Klibanski: Collagenase

debridement, *American Journal of Nursing*, **73**:849–851, May 1973.

Basson, Priscilla H.: The gerontological nursing literature: Search, study, and results, *Nursing Research*, **16**:267–272, Summer 1967.

Berkowitz, Sandra: Informed consent, research, and the elderly, *Gerontologist*, **18**:237–243, June 1978.

Brink, T. L., et al.: Hypochondriasis in an institutional geriatric population: Construction of a scale (HSIG), *Journal of the American Geriatrics Society*, **26**:557–559, December 1978.

Brower, H. Terri: A study of content needs in graduate gerontological nursing curriculum, *Journal of Gerontological Nursing*, **5**:21–28, September–October 1979.

———: A study of graduate programs in gerontological nursing, *Journal of Gerontological Nursing*, **3**:40–46, November–December 1977.

——— **and Libby A. Tanner:** A study of older adults attending a program on human sexuality: A pilot study, *Nursing Research*, **28**:36–39, January–February 1979.

Brown, Martha M.: Personalization of the institutionalized older patient, in *ANA Clinical Conferences 1969 Atlanta/Minneapolis*, Appleton Century Crofts, New York, 1970, pp. 118–124.

———, **and Patricia R. Brown:** Nurse-patient interchange in the arrest of psychosocial atrophy of aged, institutionalized patients, in *Sixth Nursing Research Conference, San Diego, CA, April 1970*, American Nurses' Association, New York, 1971, pp. 1–32.

Brown, Martha M., et al.: Drug-drug interactions among residents in homes for the elderly: A pilot study, *Nursing Research*, **26**:47–52, January–February 1977.

Brown, Myrtle I.: Patient variables associated with nurses' preferences among elderly patients, in *Fifth Nursing Research Conference, New Orleans, March 1969*, American Nurses Association, New York, 1971, pp. 176–195.

Bullough, Vern, Bonnie Bullough, and Maddalena Mauro: Age and achievement: A dissenting view, *Gerontologist*, **18**:584–587, December 1978.

Burchett, Dorothy E.: Factors affecting nurse-patient interaction in a geriatric setting, in *ANA Regional Clinical Conferences 1967 Philadelphia/Kansas City*, Appleton Century Crofts, New York, 1968, pp. 123–130.

Campbell, Margaret Eleanor: Study of the attitudes of nursing personnel towards the geriatric patient, *Nursing Research*, **20**:147–151, March–April 1971.

Carlson, Sylvia: Selected sensory input and life satisfactions of immobilized geriatric female patients, in *ANA Clinical Sessions 1968 Dallas*, Appleton Century Crofts, New York, 1968, pp. 117–123.

Chamberland, Gerry, et al.: Improving students' attitudes toward aging, *Journal of Gerontological Nursing*, **4**:44–45, January–February 1978.

Chang, Betty L.: Generalized expectancy, situational perception, and morale among institutionalized aged, *Nursing Research*, **27**:316–324, September–October 1978.

Chekryn, Joanne, and Leslie L. Roos: Auditing the process of care in a new geriatric unit, *Journal of the American Geriatrics Society*, **27**:107–111, March 1979.

Conrad, Doris: Foot education and screening programs for the elderly, *Journal of Gerontological Nursing*, **3**:11 ff., November–December 1977.

DeLora, Jack R., and Dorothy V. Moses: Specialty preferences and characteristics of nursing students in baccalaureate programs, *Nursing Research*, **18**:137–144, March–April 1969.

DeWalt, Evelyn M.: Effect of timed hygienic measures on oral mucosa in a group of elderly subjects, *Nursing Research*, **24**:104–108, March–April 1975.

DeWever, Margaret K.: Nursing home patients' perception of nurses' affective touching, *Journal of Psychology*, **96**:163–171, July 1977.

Dimond, Margaret, Kathleen King, and Mildred Burt: Forced relocation and the elderly: Identifying facilitators and barriers to adjustment, *Clinical and Scientific Sessions*, American Nurses' Association, Kansas City, Mo., 1979, pp. 134–153.

Dittmar, Sharon S., and Theresa Dulski: Early evening administration of sleep medication to the hospitalized aged: A consideration in rehabilitation, *Nursing Research*, **26**:299–303, July–August 1977.

Dufault, Sister Karin: Urinary incontinence: United States and British nursing perspectives, *Journal of Gerontological Nursing*, **4**:28–33, March–April 1978.

Dye, Carol J., and Dorothy Sassenrath: Identification of normal aging and disease-related processes by health care professionals, *Journal of the American Geriatrics Society*, **27**:472–475, October 1979.

Dye, Celeste A.: Attitude change among health professionals: Implications for gerontological nursing, *Journal of Gerontological Nursing*, **5**:31–35, September–October 1979.

Edsall, Jean Oswald, and Lee A. Miller: Relationship between loss of auditory and visual acuity and social disengagement in an aged population, *Nursing Research*, **27**:296–302, September–October 1978.

Ellis, Rosemary, et al.: Suggestions for the care of eye surgery patients who experience reduced sensory input, in *ANA Regional Clinical Conferences 1967 Philadelphia/Kansas City*, Appleton Century Crofts, New York, 1968, pp. 131–137.

Fagerhaugh, Shizuko Y.: Getting around with emphysema, *American Journal of Nursing*, **73**:94–99, January 1973.

Feist, Ruth R.: A survey of accidental falls in a small

home for the aged, *Journal of Gerontological Nursing,* **4:**15–17, November–December 1978.

Fitzpatrick, Joyce J., and Michael J. Donovan: A follow-up study of the reliability and validity of the motor activity rating scale, *Nursing Research,* **28:**179–181, May–June 1979.

Foote, Dianne F.: A relaxation technique as a preventive health measure for an aging population, *Clinical and Scientific Sessions,* American Nurses' Association, Kansas City, Mo., 1979, pp. 115–122.

Francis, Gloria, and Shirley H. Odell: Long-term residence and loneliness: Myth or reality, *Journal of Gerontological Nursing,* **5:**9–11, January–February 1979.

Franck, Phyllis: A survey of health needs of older adults in northwest Johnson County, Iowa, *Nursing Research,* **28:**360–364, November–December 1979.

Friedeman, Joyce Sutkamp: Development of a sexual knowledge inventory for elderly persons, *Nursing Research,* **28:**372–374, November–December 1979.

Garetz, Floyd K., et al.: Efficacy of nylidrin hydrochloride in the treatment of cognitive impairment in the elderly, *Journal of the American Geriatrics Society,* **27:**235–236, May 1979.

Gelper, Eve Arlin: Rehabilitative psychiatric nursing for chronically ill, elderly patients, *Journal of American Geriatrics Society,* **21:**566–568, December 1973.

Gerber, Rose Marie, and Suzanne Rowe Van Ort: Topical application of insulin in decubitus ulcers, *Nursing Research,* **28:**16–19, January–February 1979.

Gillis, Sister Marion: Attitudes of nursing personnel toward the aged, *Nursing Research,* **22:**517–520, November–December 1973.

Gimble, Josephine G.: Oral medications and the older patient, in *ANA Regional Clinical Conferences 1967 Philadelphia/Kansas City,* Appleton Century Crofts, New York, 1968, pp. 138–151.

Gioiella, Evelynn C.: The relationships between slowness of response, state anxiety, social isolation and self-esteem, and preferred personal space in the elderly, *Journal of Gerontological Nursing,* **4:**40–43, January–February 1978.

Gortner, Susan R., and Helen Nahm: An overview of nursing research in the United States, *Nursing Research,* **26:**10–33, January–February 1977.

Gosnell, Davina J.: An assessment tool to identify pressure sores, *Nursing Research,* **22:**55–59, January–February 1973.

Greenberg, Barbara: Reaction time in the elderly, *American Journal of Nursing,* **73:**2056–2058, December 1973.

Grier, Margaret R.: Living arrangements for the elderly, *Journal of Gerontological Nursing,* **3:**19–22, July–August 1977.

Grosicki, Jeanette P.: Effect of operant conditioning on modification of incontinence in neuropsychiatric geriatric patients, *Nursing Research,* **17:**304–311, July–August 1968.

Gunter, Laurie M.: Students' attitudes towards geriatric nursing, *Nursing Outlook,* **19:**466–469, July 1971.

——— **and Jeanne C. Miller:** Toward a nursing gerontology, *Nursing Research,* **26:**208–221, May–June 1977.

Hain, Sister Mary Jeanne, and Shu-Pi C. Chen: Health needs of the elderly, *Nursing Research,* **25:**433–439, November–December 1976.

Hallburg, Jeanne C.: Teaching patients self-care, *Nursing Clinics of North America,* **5:**223–231, June 1970.

Hart, L. K., et al.: Changing attitudes toward the aged and interest in caring for the aged, *Journal of Gerontological Nursing,* **2:**23–26, July–August 1976.

Hefferin, Elizabeth A., and Ruth E. Hunter: Nursing observation and care planning for the hospitalized aged, *Gerontologist,* **15:**57–60, February 1975.

Heller, B. R., and F. R. Walsh: Changing nursing students' attitudes towards the aged: An experimental study, *Journal of Nursing Education,* **15:**9–17, January 1976.

Hicks, Dorothy J.: An incidence study of pressure sores following surgery, in *ANA Clinical Sessions 1970 Miami,* Appleton Century Crofts, New York, 1971, pp. 49–54.

Hogstel, Mildred O.: Use of reality orientation with aging confused patients, *Nursing Research,* **28:**161–165, May–June 1979.

Holliday, Jane: *Public Health Nursing for the Sick at Home,* Visiting Nurse Service of New York, 1967.

Hughes, Elizabeth: Institutionalized older adults and their future orientation, *Journal of the American Geriatrics Society,* **27:**130–134, March 1979.

Jaeger, Dorothea, and Leo W. Simmons: *The Aged Ill,* Appleton Century Crofts, New York, 1970.

Johnson, Freddie Louise Powell: Response to territorial intrusion by nursing home residents, *Advances in Nursing Science,* **1:**21–34, July 1979.

Kaas, Merrie Jean: Sexual expression of the elderly in nursing homes, *Gerontologist,* **18:**372–378, August 1978.

Kahn, Kenneth A., et al.: A multidisciplinary approach to assessing the quality of life in long-term care facilities, *Gerontologist,* **17:**61–65, February 1977.

Kayser, Jeanie Schmit, and Fred A. Minnigerode: Increasing nursing students' interest in working with aged patients, *Nursing Research,* **24:**23–26, January–February 1975.

Kupfer, David J., et al.: Electroencephalographic sleep recordings and depression in the elderly, *Journal of the American Geriatrics Society,* **26:**53–57, February 1978.

Lally, Maureen, et al.: Older women in single room occupant (SRO) hotels: A Seattle profile, *Gerontologist*, **19**:67–73, February 1979.

Lamb, Karen: Effect of positioning of postoperative fractured-hip patients as related to comfort, *Nursing Research*, **28**:291–294, September–October 1979.

Lester, Pamela B., and Margret M. Baltes: Functional interdependence of the social environment and the behavior of the institutionalized aged, *Journal of Gerontological Nursing*, **4**:23–27, March–April 1978.

Levine, Rhoda L.: Disengagement in the elderly: Its causes and effects, *Nursing Outlook*, **17**:28–30, October 1969.

Managan, Dorothy, et al.: Older adults: A community survey of health needs, *Nursing Research*, **23**:426–432, September–October 1974.

Marks, Janet, and Margaret Clarke: The hospital patient and his knowledge of the drugs he is receiving, *International Nursing Review*, **19**:39–51, 1972.

McGlone, Frank B., and Ella Kick: Health habits in relation to aging, *Journal of the American Geriatrics Society*, **26**:481–488, November 1978.

McKnight, Eleanor M.: *Nursing Home Research Study: Quantitative Measurement of Nursing Services*, Government Printing Office, Washington, 1970.

McPhetridge, L. Mae: Relationship of patients' responses to nursing history questions and selected factors: Preliminary study, *Nursing Research*, **22**:310–320, July–August 1973.

Mezey, Mathy: Stress, hospitalization, and aging, *Clinical and Scientific Sessions*, American Nurses' Association, Kansas City, Mo., 1979, pp. 123–133.

Mikhail, S. F., M. Sonn, and A. H. Lawton: Optimism in the management of hip fracture in elderly patients, *Journal of the American Geriatrics Society*, **26**:39–42, January 1978.

Miller, Dulcy B., and Susan Beer: Patterns of friendship among patients in a nursing home setting, *Gerontologist*, **17**:269–275, June 1977.

Mishara, B. L., and Robert Kastenbaum: Wine in the treatment of long-term geriatric patients in mental institutions, *Journal of the American Geriatrics Society*, **22**:88–94, February 1974.

Muhlenkamp, A. F.: Cognitive developmental aspects of person perception in the aged, in Betty K. Mitsunaga (ed.), *Fifth Annual Nurse Scientist Conference, April 1972*, University of Colorado Medical Center, Denver, pp. 113–141.

———, Lucille D. Gress, and Mary A. Flood: Perception of life change events by the elderly, *Nursing Research*, **24**:109–113, March–April 1975.

Munoz, Rodrigo A., and Betty Mesick: Hospitalization of the elderly patient for acute illness, *Journal of the American Geriatrics Society*, **27**:415–417, September 1979.

Neely, Elizabeth, and Maxine L. Patrick: Problems of aged persons taking medications at home, *Nursing Research*, **17**:52–55, January–February 1968.

Norton, Doreen, R. McLaren, and A. N. Exton-Smith: *An Investigation of Geriatric Nursing Problems in Hospital*, Churchill Livingstone, Edinburgh, 1975.

O'Donnell, John M., Joseph L. Collins, and Susan Schuler: Psychosocial perceptions of the nursing home: A comparative analysis of staff, resident, and cross-generational perspectives, *Gerontologist*, **18**:267–271, June 1978.

Palmore, Erdman B., and Virginia Stone: Predictors of longevity: A follow-up of the aged in Chapel Hill, *Gerontologist*, **13**:88–90, Spring 1973.

Panicucci, Carol L., et al.: Expanded speech and self-pacing in communicating with the aged, in *ANA Clinical Sessions 1968 Dallas*, Appleton Century Crofts, New York, 1968, pp. 95–102.

Prock, Valencia N.: Effects of institutionalization: A comparison of community, waiting list, and institutionalized aged persons, *American Journal of Public Health*, **59**:1837–1844, October 1969.

Putnam, Phyllis A.: Nurse awareness and psychosocial function in the aged, *Gerontologist*, **13**:163–166, Summer 1973.

———: Supplementary regulation of environmental interchange: An operational approach to the study of nursing, *Seventh Nursing Research Conference, Atlanta, Ga., 1971,* American Nurses' Association, New York, 1971, pp. 81–94.

Raskind, Murray A., Carrol Alvarez, and Susan Herlin: Fluphenazine enanthate in the outpatient treatment of late paraphrenia, *Journal of the American Geriatrics Society*, **27**:459–463, October 1979.

———, Margaret Kitchell, and Carrol Alvarez: Bromide intoxication in the elderly, *Journal of the American Geriatrics Society*, **26**:222–224, May 1978.

Reed, Dixie L.: Social disengagement in chronically ill patients, *Nursing Research*, **19**:109–115, March–April 1970.

Requarth, Connie H.: Medication usage and interaction in the long-term care elderly, *Journal of Gerontological Nursing*, **5**:33–37, March–April 1979.

Robb, Susanne S.: Attitudes and intentions of baccalaureate nursing students toward the elderly, *Nursing Research*, **28**:43–50, January–February 1979.

Robinson, K. D.: Therapeutic interaction: A means of crisis intervention with newly institutionalized elderly persons, *Nursing Clinics of North America*, **9**:89–96, March 1974.

Schank, Mary Jane: A survey of the well-elderly: Their foot problems, practices, and needs, *Journal of Gerontological Nursing*, **3**:10 ff., November–December 1977.

Schwartz, Doris R.: Aging and the field of nursing, in M. W. Riley (ed.), Aging and Society, vol. II: Aging and the Professions, Russell Sage Foundation, New York, 1969, pp. 79–113.

————: Steps leading to a Primex program, in *ANA Clinical Sessions 1972 Detroit,* Appleton Century Crofts, New York, 1973, pp. 50–54.

————, **Doris Henley, and Leonard Zeitz:** *The Elderly Ambulatory Patient,* Macmillan, New York, 1964.

Schwenger, C. W., and L. A. Sayers: Services to the aged by the Canadian Public Health nurse in the official health agency, *American Journal of Public Health,* **61:**1846–1852, September 1971a.

———— **and** ————: A survey by Canadian public health nurses of the health and living conditions of the aged, *American Journal of Public Health,* **61:**1189–1195, June 1971b.

Sherr, Virginia T., and Sr. Maria Teresa Goffi: On-site geropsychiatric services to guests of residential homes, *Journal of the American Geriatrics Society,* **25:**269–272, June 1977.

Silverstone, Barbara, and Lolita Wynter: The effects of introducing a heterosexual living space, *Gerontologist,* **15:**83–87, February 1975.

Snyder, Lorraine Hiatt, et al.: Wandering, *Gerontologist,* **18:**272–280, June 1978.

Sorensen, Andrew A., Donna I. Sorensen, and James G. Zimmer: Appropriateness of vitamin and mineral prescription orders for residents of health related facilities, *Journal of the American Geriatrics Society,* **27:**425–430, September 1979.

Spasoff, Robert A., et al.: A longitudinal study of elderly residents of long-stay institutions: I. Early response to institutional care, II. The situation one year after admission, *Gerontologist,* **18:**281–292, June 1978.

Stotsky, Bernard A.: *The Nursing Home and the Aged Psychiatric Patient,* Appleton Century Crofts, New York, 1970.

Sullivan, Judith A., and Felice Armignacco: Effectiveness of a comprehensive health program for the well-elderly by community health nurses, *Nursing Research,* **28:**70–75, March–April 1979.

Taylor, Kathleen Heitzeg, and Thomas Lee Harned: Attitudes toward old people: A study of nurses who care for the elderly, *Journal of Gerontological Nursing,* **4:**43–47, September–October 1978.

Tharp, Terril Stone, Brydie Jo Baker, and Terri Francis Brower: Nursing staff attitudes toward the geriatric nurse practitioner student, *Nursing Research,* **28:**299–301, September–October 1979.

Thomas, Ellen G.: Morbidity patterns among recently relocated elderly, *Clinical and Scientific Sessions,* American Nurses' Association, Kansas City, Mo., 1979, pp. 154–165.

Thomas, Frances J.: Effects of individualized nursing intervention on senile status and self-care achieve-

ment of institutionalized patients, in *ANA Regional Clinical Conferences 1967 Philadelphia/Kansas City,* Appleton Century Crofts, New York, 1968, pp. 152–162.

————: Social involvement of elderly studied in relation to mental health status, *Nursing Research Report,* **5:**1, 3–4, 6, September 1970.

Tobiason, Sara Jane, et al.: Positive attitudes toward aging: The aged teach the young, *Journal of Gerontological Nursing,* **5:**18–23, May–June 1979.

Uman, Gwen C.: Pre-retirement health planning, *Clinical and Scientific Sessions,* American Nurses' Association, Kansas City, Mo., 1979, pp. 105–114.

Voelkel, Donna: A study of reality orientation and resocialization groups with confused elderly, *Journal of Gerontological Nursing,* **4:**13–18, May–June 1978.

Volpe, Anne, and Robert Kastenbaum: Beer and TLC, *American Journal of Nursing,* **67:**100–103, January 1967.

Walsh, Arthur C., Bernice H. Walsh, and Catherine Melaney: Senile–presenile dementia: Follow-up data on an effective psychotherapy-anticoagulant regimen, *Journal of the American Geriatrics Society,* **26:**467–470, October 1978.

Wang, Mamie K.: A health maintenance service for chronically ill patients: An exploratory project for expanding the nurses' role in the ambulatory clinic, *American Journal of Public Health,* **60:**713–721, April 1970.

————, **and Robert G. Brayton:** Health maintenance service for the high-risk chronically ill, *Nursing Clinics of North America,* **5:**199–210, June 1970.

Weiss, J. M. A. (ed.): *Nurses, Patients, and Social Systems,* University of Missouri Press, Columbia, 1968.

Wichita, Carol: Treating and preventing constipation in nursing home residents, *Journal of Gerontological Nursing,* **3:**35–39, November–December 1977.

Wilhite, Mary J., and Dale M. Johnson: Changes in nursing students' stereotypic attitudes toward old people, *Nursing Research,* **25:**430–432, November–December 1976.

Williams, Margaret A., et al.: Nursing activities and acute confusional states in elderly hip-fractured patients, *Nursing Research,* **28:**25–35, January–February 1979.

Wolanin, Mary Opal: Relocation of the elderly, *Journal of Gerontological Nursing,* **4:**47–50, May–June 1978.

Zornow, R. A.: Perceptions of residents of retirement communities about osteoarthritis, in Marjorie V. Batey (ed.), *Communicating Nursing Research: Collaboration and Competition,* vol. 6, Western Interstate Commission for Higher Education, Boulder, Colo., 1973, pp. 177–184.

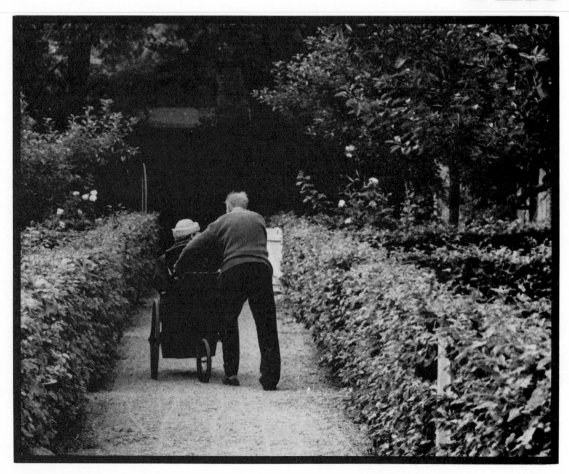

TEN

E. Mandelmann, reprinted with permission
of the World Health Organization

EPILOGUE

We must not ask where science and technology are taking us, but rather how we can manage science and technology so that they can help us get where we want to go.

René Dubois

FORTY-SIX

PAST, PRESENT, AND FUTURE

Irene Mortenson Burnside

Do not resent growing old; many are denied the privilege.
Anonymous

As we are constantly reminded whenever we turn on the television, open a magazine, or walk down the street, we live in a youth-oriented culture. In the future, nurses will have to struggle like everyone else in our society to shake off that idolization of youth. Halleck (1968) has observed that in drifting into a youth-oriented culture we have ignored the teachings of philosophers who since the time of Plato have emphasized the need to revere maturity. We are often told that our youth are our future. Yet, unless we can create a world which offers the possibility of aging with grace, honor, and meaningfulness, no one can look forward to the future.

As I noted at the beginning of this volume, there are signs that we are gaining a new awareness of old age as a special state with its own dignity, capabilities, and value. The decrease in forced retirement based solely on age is one such sign, as is the growing number of gerontological nursing programs. Let me illustrate this awareness with a vignette taken from a student's paper which describes the student helping a tough old lady home from the store.

VIGNETTE

She was carrying a sack of groceries which also held a carrier containing her parakeet, Bobby, which she takes with her every place she goes. She is short and heavy and walks with a cane, is slightly hard-of-hearing, and does not wear glasses. I offered to carry the sack and she accepted reluctantly. During the hour it took to walk the eight blocks uphill to the externally presentable building in which she has a light-housekeeping room, she told of several occasions when relatives, acquaintances, and sometimes strangers had "borrowed" or stolen some of her possessions.

On the way she spied an empty Coke bottle, stopped and considered it soberly for a moment, and then bent and picked it up. She placed it in the sack and said with some satisfaction that "a body could get some good money out of empty bottles," and that once she found 30 cents on the sidewalk, so she's learned to "look sharp." She said she could carry more if she could leave Bobby home, but she does not dare, because there might be a fire in the building when she is

away. There was a small fire several months ago.

We took the tiny, creaky elevator to the fifth floor. We walked down the corridor, and she unlocked a door that revealed a short corridor with a bathroom and three other rooms opening off from it. She said the kitchen was on the main hall. Her room had one window that opened onto a narrow ventilation well. The room was cold and had colorless, faded, torn wallpaper, a bare floor, a rough, unpainted little table in the middle piled high with corroded pans and small bits of staple groceries. But the bed was made and the floor had been swept. She uncaged her beautiful, serene little parakeet, and cried, "Bobby, we're home!" (Aker, 1967)

A pessimist, hearing that story, might well point out all the past and current problems of the aged which can be glimpsed in it—the loneliness of many old people living in the alien or even hostile environment of our cities, the lack of adequate recreation and health care services in the community, the lack of psychosocial support services, etc. The litany of such problems is surely familiar to anyone who has read this far through this book. Yet I am sure that most readers react to the story the same way I did, with admiration for that lady's courage, resourcefulness, and sheer ability to cope. That humane response, a recognition of our common humanity and common future, is the basis of what I see as a new awareness of the special state of being old.

GROWING POPULATION, GROWING PROBLEMS

That new awareness will be crucial if we are to solve the problems presented by a growing population of old people. In recent years, people have been living longer (living to be older) and have been less healthy in old age.

It is as sure as any prediction of the future that the number of old people will continue to increase (see Figure 46-1), both because of improvements in health care and because the largest generation in American history, those

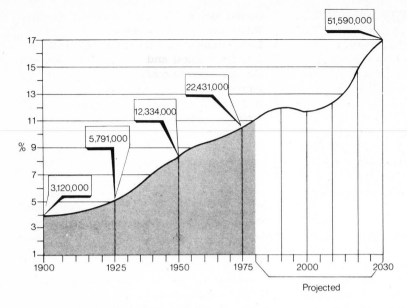

FIGURE 46-1 Age gauge. Chart shows the percentage of the American population 65 and older from 1900 to 1975, with predictions for 1980 to 2030. (*U.S. Census Bureau.*)

born between 1945 and 1955, will turn 65 between the years 2010 and 2020. Makanodin (1978) believes that this trend may cause severe economic problems for the government. There will be increased need for medical, psychiatric, social, and economic assistance in the future.

Spengler (1969) considers some of the reasons that the future of the aged could be bleak:

1. The society of the future will be a "society of so-called secular values."
2. The age composition of the future American population will not be favorable to productivity.
3. Inflation will continue to erode the purchasing power of old people who live on fixed incomes.
4. Unemployment will increase.
5. Employment opportunities will deteriorate.
6. People's health problems are being intensified, especially those caused or exacerbated by the environment.

Brotherston (1969), writing about the National Health Service in the United Kingdom, stated that the major phenomenon of the elderly in the health service is underdemand, not overdemand. Future generations of elderly may experience better health because of having had a better environment in their earlier years, but Brotherston suggests they will not be so stoic in facing disabilities or use medical services so sparingly as the present generation. His words remind one of Curtin's (1972) statement: "If you are going to be stranded on a desert island, you better hope that at least one person in the group is plenty old, because the rest of us have learned very little about survival."

QUALITY OF LIFE

A discussion of the growing problems which may be associated with an increasingly large population of old people may sound bleak. But there are also grounds for optimism in the simple fact that we are increasingly aware of the potential problems. A number of years ago, Heron and Chown (1967) wrote: "It seems that alarm bells must ring variously and continuously before the world awakes fully to the implications of health measures which are leading to a doubling of the world's population within a single short generation!"

This awareness has had the effect of turning many people's efforts away from simply developing techniques for extending life and to-

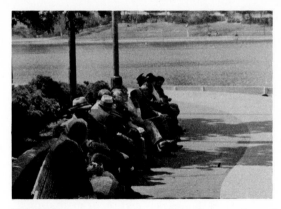

FIGURE 46-2 A new awareness of the sheer numbers of older persons should remind us all of our common future. (*Courtesy of Diane E. Miller.*)

ward the quality of life of the aged. Butler and Lewis (1973) have made this point forcefully: "Simply extending human life for more and more years is folly and even inhumane unless the quality of life can be improved. Yet very little research in this nation concentrates either on fundamental biological processes of aging or on the social and psychological supports for old age."

More research in the areas Butler and Lewis suggest, and greater attention to the quality of life when providing medical and nursing care, can be expected to alleviate many of the potential problems mentioned above. Emphasis, for example, can be shifted to the control of chronic diseases, and Laurie Gunter and Jeanne Miller (1977) have argued that the need for research in the psychosocial area of gerontological nursing is critical.

PREVENTION

Prevention of disease is one of the most obvious, and most important, ways of improving the quality of later life. (For a complete discussion of prevention, see Chapter 32.) Some prevention measures are very basic, but the constant role of teaching them will fall to nurses of the future just as it does present-day nurses, and so they bear repeating.

1. The diet should be low in cholesterol and saturated fats.

2. Do not smoke.
3. Do not become overweight.
4. Regular moderate exercise is important.
5. Regular medical and physical examinations are necessary to control such factors as high blood pressure, diabetes, etc.
6. Regular eye examinations and dental care are also important.

EDUCATION OF NURSES

With such a vision of the future, what should nursing education emphasize? Most nurses would agree with Butler and Lewis (1973) that extending human life for many years can be inhumane, especially since nurses are the likely ones to have to take care of the withering person during that span of life.

Geropsychiatric nurses are a rarity at this writing, but their role may well emerge in the next decade. Many present-day nurses in nursing homes were educated in diploma programs and were taught skilled nursing in acute hospital settings; education in long-term care included such training as a rotation on a rehabilitation ward or a tuberculosis ward. It will take some unlearning and relearning on the part of present older nurses to come to grips with the philosophy of gerontological nursing.

One exploratory study of registered nurses working in nursing homes in California concentrated on the way they perceive themselves and their role (Gorenberg, 1979). The data created a profile of these nurses as middle-aged, married women who hold administrative positions and who graduated from diploma schools of nursing with little or no preparation in gerontology or administration. The data also revealed that the nurses primarily choose the nursing home for personal reasons; they stay in the setting longer than most geriatric nurses. The perceptions of the nurses' self-image and their role expectations of the ideal geriatric nurse differed. They perceived the ideal geriatric nurse as one who possessed more positive attributes than they attributed to themselves.

Sometimes nursing seems to be divided into two camps—those who believe in long-term care and those who believe only in the elderly residing at home. We need excellent nurses caring for the aged in both areas.

OPTIMISM AND PROFESSIONAL SUPPORT

The need for a more optimistic posture toward the aged by the nursing profession becomes increasingly apparent. So long as nurses are apologetic to their peers about working on geriatric settings, the image of geriatric nursing is not likely to be improved.

The work of many geriatric nurses goes unwritten, undocumented, and, unfortunately, often unnoticed. Borlaug (1974) and Acord (1974) described elderly individuals admitted to their facilities in severely regressed states. The intensive work and interest of dedicated staff members brought these old people out of their shells. Such optimism, hopefulness, and nursing care goes by unrewarded for the most part. It is not dramatic; it is not sudden; and often there are no spectators to marvel at the nursing care

benefits accomplished against extraordinary odds. It is the reward of the instructor to be privy to such results and accomplishments of students. Placing student nurses in nursing homes will help improve care of the residents. (The complaints of nursing home residents can be seen in Figure 46-3.)

If there is an increase in the emotional problems of the aged, the curricula of future nursing classes will have to be weighted more heavily in one-to-one relationship therapy (adapted to the aged client), group work (also adapted to the aged), crisis intervention, family therapy, the dynamics of depression and other mental problems, and intervention in these problems.

Education of nurses is costly, especially in the field of aging. Few nurses are interested in the subject, so that elective classes tend to be small. This makes them expensive to teach. Often planned classes are canceled because of lack of enrollment. This is also true of workshops on aging; many lose money because of lack of attendance. Providing interesting and challenging classes and educational methods is not only

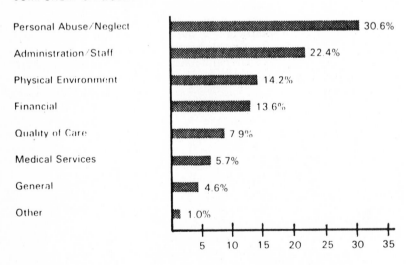

COMPLAINT
COMPONENT CATEGORY

Category	%
Personal Abuse/Neglect	30.6%
Administration/Staff	22.4%
Physical Environment	14.2%
Financial	13.6%
Quality of Care	7.9%
Medical Services	5.7%
General	4.6%
Other	1.0%

Frequency in Terms of %

FIGURE 46-3 Frequency of categories of complaint components during fiscal year 1977–1978. [*State Nursing Home Ombudsman Committee, Annual Report of the Nursing Home Ombudsman Committee 1978, Tallahassee, Fla., 1978, p. 41; reprinted by permission from Nursing Leadership 2(1):11, March 1979.*]

a current problem but may also be a great challenge for nursing educators of the future.

Teaching for change is also difficult. The problems nurses face today in caring for the aged are not the same problems that nurses of the future will have to solve. As Bengtson and Haber pointed out in Chapter 40, the future generations of elderly will be more educated, will have lived in more affluent times (although at this writing those affluent times may be waning), and will have had different life-styles than the aged people of the present. The education of the present nurse in caring for the elderly will most likely be obsolete in a few years.

NURSING AS A PROFESSION

Samuel Kellams (1977, p. 31) argues that "colleagues respect the professional judgment of one another and develop standards for identifying and rectifying incompetent or unethical practice. . . . One profession never takes orders from another profession. If this occurs, the subordinated profession is called a paraprofession." Kellams further believes,

If [nursing] is to continue to emerge in its own right, nursing will have to develop its

own unique "expertise." This expertise will have to be different in kind than that used by other medical professionals. . . . The meaning of this dual focus is that nurses are not controlled by the patient, by physician, by colleagues or by lone organizational authority. To be controlled fully by any one or all of these groups would be tantamount to the loss of professional autonomy.

Gerontology is an area in which nursing should develop a particular professional expertise if only because of the lack of qualified personnel from all professions. I believe that many nurses have the special expertise, compassion, and philosophy needed to care for old people.

NEED FOR FURTHER RESEARCH

The body of research in this field has grown noticeably even since the first edition of this book, and I have tried to incorporate as much of that new research as possible in this edition. I have also tried to point out, in various chapters throughout the book, specific topics for further research. In addition, Laurie Gunter and Jeanne Miller (1977) have called attention to the general

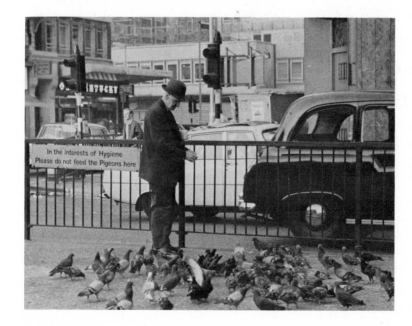

In the interests of Hygiene
Please do not feed the Pigeons here

FIGURE 46-4 When aged persons cannot have pets in their places of residence, they often feed birds or wild animals. Sometimes they defy the local ordinances, as this Londoner has done. (*Courtesy of Diane E. Miller.*)

need for research in the whole psychosocial area of gerontological nursing. The National Institute on Aging has pinpointed the same need. In a flyer entitled *Guide to NIA Programs and Awards* (1976), they write,

> The Institute is concerned with the impact of psychosocial problems on the health of the elderly. This includes a consideration of probable future age-structures of the population and their impact on health problems, studies of cognitive function as a function of aging, studies of the health impact of interpersonal relations and work life and retirement in the aging and aged, and studies of the impact of housing and institutional care on health.

Nurses will also need to do more research on problems that concern and disturb them as they care for the aged person. Such areas include (1) sensory stimulation; (2) sensory deprivation; (3) the dying aged person and hospices; (4) continence; (5) individuals with organic brain syndrome; (6) nutrition; (7) learning abilities in the aged; (8) energy levels of the aged person; (9) drug abuse in aged persons; (10) use of touch and its impact on the aged; (11) improving environments; (12) use of prosthetics in the aged person; (13) sexuality; (14) successful curricula in gerontological nursing; (15) data about the products of present gerontological nurse programs; (16) effectiveness of treatment modalities in dementia cases, e.g., reality orientation, music therapy; (17) pets and the elderly; and (18) the well aged and the life-styles that have promoted wellness, vitality, and longevity.

BEING OLD: "A HOLY TASK"

An observation of Hermann Hesse (1974) can help nurses understand the perspective of older clients, and it is a proper ending for this book because it is an eloquent summary of a humane awareness of the dignity, grace, and value of old age. That awareness will, in the long run, do more than any particular strategy or technique to improve our care of the aged.

> Being old is just as beautiful and holy a task as being young, learning to die and dying are just as valuable functions as any other—assuming that they are carried out with reverence toward the meaning and holiness of all life. A man who hates being very old and gray, who fears the nearness of death, is no more worthy a representative of his stage of life than a strong young person who hates and tries to escape his profession and his daily tasks. . . . I can . . . name some of the gifts that old age bestows on us. To me the dearest of these gifts is the treasury of pictures which after a long life one carries in one's memory and to which one turns, as activity decreases, with a quite different interest than ever before. Human figures and faces that for sixty or seventy years have no longer existed on earth go on living within us, they belong to us, provide us with company, look out at us from living eyes. We see houses, gardens, cities that have since disappeared or are wholly changed as they once were, and distant mountain ranges and seacoasts that we once visited on journeys decades ago we find fresh and colorful in our picture book. Noticing, observing, contemplating become more and more a habit and exercise, and imperceptibly the mood and attitude of the beholder permeate our whole behavior.

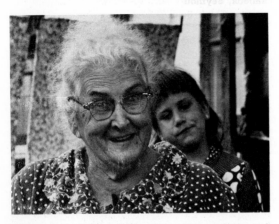

FIGURE 46-5 "Being old is just as beautiful and holy a task as being young" (Hesse, 1974). (*Courtesy of Harvey Finkle.*)

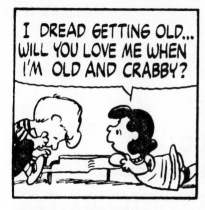
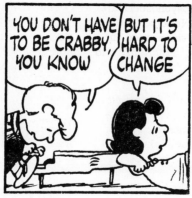
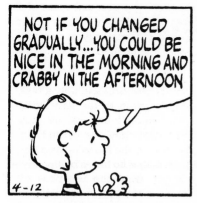
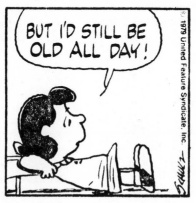

FIGURE 46-6 © United Feature Syndicate, Inc., 1979.

REFERENCES

Acord, Lois: Personal communication, 1974.

Aker, Guila M.: Survey and report on facilities and resources for the aged in San Francisco, unpublished manuscript, 1967.

Borlaug, Jolana: Personal communication, 1974.

Brotherston, J. H. F.: Change and the National Health Service, *Scotland Medical Journal,* **14:**130, 1969.

Butler, Robert N., and Myrna I. Lewis: *Aging and Mental Health: Positive Psychosocial Approaches,* Mosby, St. Louis, 1973.

Curtin, Sharon R.: *Nobody Ever Died of Old Age,* Little, Brown, Boston, 1972, p. 74.

Gorenberg, Bobbye: Study of characteristics, self-image, and role expectations of registered nurses working with the elderly in nursing homes, unpublished master's thesis, San Jose State University, San Jose, Calif., 1979.

Guide to NIA Program and Awards, DHEW, National Institute on Aging, Bethesda, Md., 1976.

Gunter, Laurie M., and Jeanne C. Miller: Toward a nursing gerontology, *Nursing Research,* **26**(3):209–221, May/June 1977.

Halleck, Seymour: Why they'd rather do their own thing, *Think,* **34**(5):7, September–October 1968.

Heron, Alastair, and Sheila Chown: *Age and Function,* Little, Brown, Boston, 1967.

Hesse, Hermann: Old age, in Theodore Ziolkowski (ed.), *My Belief: Essays on Life and Art,* translated by Denver Lindley, Farrar, Straus & Giroux, New York, 1974, pp. 269–271.

Kellams, Samuel E.: Ideals of a profession: The case of nursing, *Image,* **9**(2):30–31, June 1977.

Makanodin, Takahashi: In-service lecture, class at American Lake Veterans' Administrative Hospital, Tacoma, Wash., April 18, 1978.

Sandburg, Carl: *The People Yes,* Harcourt, Brace, New York, 1936, p. 284.

Spengler, Joseph J.: The aged and public policy, in E. W. Busse and E. Pfeiffer (eds.), *Behavior and Adaptation in Late Life,* Little, Brown, Boston, 1969.

APPENDIX A

PROFESSIONAL JOURNALS

American Journal of Nursing, 10 Columbus Circle, New York, NY 10019.

American Journal of Psychiatry, 1700-18th St., N.W., Washington, DC 20009.

Geriatric Nursing, American Nurses' Association, 10 Columbus Circle, New York, NY 10019.

Gerontologist, Gerontological Society, 1 Dupont Circle, Washington, DC 20036.

Journal of Gerontological Nursing, Charles B. Slack, Inc., 6900 Grove Rd., Thorofare, NJ 08086.

Journal of Gerontology, Gerontological Society, 1 Dupont Circle, Washington, DC 20036.

Journal of Long Term Care Administration, American College of Nursing Home Administrators, 4650 East-West Highway, Washington, DC 20014.

Long Term Care and Health Services Administration Quarterly, Panel Publishers, 14 Plaza Rd., Greenvale, NY 11548.

Medical Care, J. B. Lippincott Company, East-Washington Square, Philadelphia, PA 19105.

Nurse Practitioner, Health Sciences Media and Research Services, Inc., 3845 42 Ave., N.E., Seattle, WA 98105.

Nursing Homes, 4000 Albemarle St., N.W., Room 504, Washington, DC 20016.

Nursing Research, American Journal of Nursing Company, 10 Columbus Circle, New York, NY 10019.

Nursing Times, Macmillan Journals, Limited, IV Essex St., London, WC2R 3LF, England.

Patient Care, Miller and Fink Corporation, 16 Thorndal Circle, Darien, CT 06820.

APPENDIX B

RECOMMENDED READING AND FILMS

AUTOBIOGRAPHY AND BIOGRAPHY

Baruch, Bernard M.: *Baruch: My Own Story,* Holt, New York, 1957.

Buck, Pearl S.: *A Bridge for Passing,* John Day, New York, 1962.

Cousins, Norman: *Dr. Schweitzer of Lambarene,* Harper, New York, 1960.

de Beauvoir, Simone: *A Very Easy Death,* Putnam, New York, 1966.

Goudeket, Maurice: *The Delights of Growing Old,* Farrar, Straus & Giroux, Inc., New York, 1966.

Hodgins, Eric: *Episode: Report on the Accident Inside My Skull,* Atheneum, New York, 1964.

Jacobs, Ruth Harriet: *Life after Youth: Female, Forty, What Next?,* Beacon Press, Boston, 1979.

Jones, Ernest: *The Life and Work of Sigmund Freud, 1919–1939,* vol. 3, Basic Books, New York, 1957.

Jury, Mark, and Dan Jury: *Gramp,* Grossman Publishers, New York, 1976.

Laurence, Margaret: *The Stone Angel,* Knopf, New York, 1964.

Moses, Anna Mary Robertson: *Grandma Moses: My Life's History,* Harper, New York, 1952.

Scott-Maxwell, Florida: *The Measure of My Days,* Knopf, New York, 1969.

Vining, Elizabeth Gray: *Being Seventy: The Measure of a Year,* Viking, New York, 1978.

NOVELS

Arkell, Reginald: *Old Herbaceous,* Harcourt, Brace, New York, 1951.

Bagnold, Enid: *The Loved and the Envied,* Doubleday, Country Life Press, New York, 1951.

Balzac, Honoré de: *Père Goriot,* Modern Library, New York, 1950.

Bennett, Arnold: *The Old Wives' Tale,* Harper, New York, 1950.

Bermant, Chaim: *Diary of an Old Man,* Holt, New York, 1967.

Bromfield, Louis: *Mrs. Parkington,* Harper, New York, 1943.

Cary, Joyce: *To Be a Pilgrim,* Harper, New York, 1942.

Cather, Willa: *Death Comes for the Archbishop,* Knopf, New York, 1955.

Chase, Mary Ellen: *The Plum Tree,* Macmillan, New York, 1949.

Colette: *The Last of Cheri,* Farrar, Straus & Cudahy, New York, 1953.

Cooper, James Fenimore: *The Prairie,* Dodd, Mead, New York, 1954.

Corbett, E.: *Our Mrs. Meigs,* Lippincott, Philadelphia, 1954.

Cox, Joseph A.: *The Recluse of Herald Square,* Macmillan, New York, 1964.

Cozzens, James Gould: *By Love Possessed,* Harcourt, Brace, New York, 1957.

Eldridge, Paul: *The Second Life of John Stevens,* Yoseloff, London, 1960.

Gallico, Paul: *Mrs. 'arris Goes to Paris,* Doubleday, Garden City, N.Y., 1958.

Hemingway, Ernest: *The Old Man and the Sea,* Scribner, New York, 1962.

Hilton, James: *Good-bye Mr. Chips,* Little, Brown, Boston, 1934.

Jansson, Tove: *The Summer Book,* Pantheon Books, New York, 1974.

Laurence, Margaret: *The Stone Angel,* Knopf, New York, 1964.

Michener, James: *The Fires of Spring,* Random House, New York, 1949.

Ruark, Robert: *The Old Man and the Boy,* Holt, New York, 1953.

Sarton, Mae: *As We Are Now,* Norton, New York, 1973.

Spark, Muriel: *Memento Mori,* Lippincott, New York, 1959.

Topkins, Katharine: *Kotch,* McGraw-Hill, New York, 1965.

Van Velde, Jacoba: *The Big Ward,* Simon and Schuster, New York, 1960.

Walker, Mildred: *The Southwest Corner,* Harcourt, Brace, New York, 1951.

Wallant, Edward Lewis: *The Human Season,* Harcourt, Brace, New York, 1960.

Wilson, Angus: *Late Call,* Viking, New York, 1965.

Zola, Emile: *Earth,* Dufour Editions, Philadelphia, 1955.

POETRY

Browning, Robert: "Rabbi Ben Ezra," in Jacob Zeitlin and Clarissa Rinaker (eds.), *Types of Poetry,* Macmillan, New York, 1926.

Burnside, Irene M.: "Baroque Pearls," *American Journal of Nursing,* **73**(12):2061, December 1973.

Deutsch, Babette: "Heard in Old Age," in *Coming of Age,* Indiana University Press, Bloomington, 1959.

Eliot, T. S.: "Gerontion," in *Collected Poems 1909–62,* Harcourt, Brace & World, New York, 1963.

———: "Lines for an Old Man," in *Collected Poems 1909–62,* Harcourt, Brace & World, New York, 1963.

Holmes, Oliver Wendell: "The Last Leaf," in Jacob Zeitlin and Clarissa Rinaker (eds.), *Types of Poetry,* Macmillan, New York, 1926.

Jeffers, Robinson: "Age in Prospect," in Louis Untermeyer (ed.), *Modern American and British Poetry,* Harcourt, Brace, New York, 1955.

Kavanaugh, James: "Old Man," in *There Are Men Too Gentle to Live among the Wolves,* Nash Publishing, Los Angeles, 1970.

Maclay, Elise: *Green Winter, Celebrations of Old Age,* Reader's Digest Press, Thomas Y. Crowell, New York, 1977.

Merriam, Eve: "A Conversation against Death," *Ms.,* September 1972.

Thomas, Dylan: "Do Not Go Gently into That Good Night," in James Laughlin (ed.), *Collected Poems of Dylan Thomas,* New York, 1953.

Wood, Nancy: *Many Winters,* Doubleday, Garden City, New York, 1974.

SHORT STORIES

Arkin, Frieda: "The Light of the Sea," in Martha Foley and David Burnett (eds.), *Best American Short Stories,* Houghton-Mifflin, Boston, 1962.

Aumonier, Stacy: "Old Fags," in *Master Stories of the Twentieth Century,* selected by Herbert Van Thal, Parr Books, London, 1963.

Brown, Dr. John: "Rab and His Friends," in Phyllis and Albert Blaustein (eds.), *Doctor's Choice,* Fink, New York, 1957.

Broyard, Anatole: "Sunday Dinner in Brooklyn," in William Phillips and Philip Rahv (eds.), *Avon Book of Modern Writing No. 2,* Avon, New York, 1953.

Calisher, Hortense: "A Wreath for Miss Tatten," in *Best American Short Stories, 1952,* Houghton-Mifflin, Boston, 1952.

Clark, Walter Van Tilburg: "The Wind and the Snow of Winter," in *Best American Short Stories, 1915–1950,* Houghton-Mifflin, Boston, 1952.

Dinesen, Isak: "Sorrow Acre," in Bernardine Kielty (ed.), *A Treasury of Short Stories,* Simon and Schuster, New York, 1947.

Dreiser, Theodore: "The Lost Phoebe," in *Fifty Best American Short Stories, 1915–1965,* Houghton-Mifflin, Boston, 1965.

Granat, Robert: "My Apples," in Paul Engle (ed.), *Prize Stories, 1958: The O. Henry Awards,* Doubleday, Garden City, N.Y., 1958.

Hale, Nancy: "The Great-Grandmother," in *Short Stories from the New Yorker,* Simon and Schuster, New York, 1940.

Hill, Elizabeth Starr: "The Old Dog," in *New World Writings,* Lippincott, Philadelphia, 1961.

Mosher, John: "In Honor of Their Daughter," in *Short*

Stories from the New Yorker, Simon and Schuster, New York, 1940.

O'Connor, Frank: "The Storyteller," in Bernardine Kielty (ed.), *A Treasury of Short Stories,* Simon and Schuster, New York, 1947.

Sansom, William: "Old Man Alone," in *Master Stories of the Twentieth Century,* selected by Herbert Van Thal, Parr Books, London, 1963.

Tyler, Anne: "The Baltimore Birth Certificate," *The Critic,* **21**(4), February–March, 1963, St. Thomas More Association.

Webber, Howard: "Games," *The New Yorker,* March 30, 1963.

Welty, Eudora: "A Worn Path," in *Selected Stories,* Modern Library, New York, 1954.

Yezierska, Anzia: "A Window Full of Sky," *The Reporter,* **31**(1), July 2, 1964.

Zugsmith, Leane: "The Three Veterans," in *Short Stories from the New Yorker,* Simon and Schuster, New York, 1940.

FILMS

The Autobiography of Miss Jane Pittman, TV film, directed by John Korty, 1974.

Harold and Maude, directed by Hal Ashby, 1971.

Harry and Tonto, directed by Paul Mazursy, 1974.

I Never Sang for My Father, directed by Gilbert Cates, 1970.

Kotch, directed by Jack Lemmon, 1971.

Little Big Man, directed by Arthur Penn, 1970.

Love, directed by Karoly Makk.

The Shameless Old Lady, directed by Rene Allio, 1969.

Wild Strawberries, directed by Ingmar Bergman, 1957.

TEACHING FILMS

The Art of Age, produced by Leonard S. Berman Films, 1972; 27 min, 16mm, color. The philosophy of four elderly people is shown in the lives of a mailman, an artist, a former businessman, and a teacher.

Don't Count the Candles: An Essay by Lord Snowden. Problems of aging are seen through the eyes of rich and poor, famous and humble persons. "CBS News Special," Wilbein K. McClure; 60 min, 16mm, black & white, 1968.

Minnie Remembers, 5 min, 16mm, color, 1976. A film based on a poem reflecting the loneliness of an older woman. Distributor: Mass Media Ministries, 2116 North Charles Street, Baltimore, MD 21218.

Nell and Fred, produced by National Film Board of Canada, distributed by McGraw-Hill Films; 29 min, black and white. The film documents the experiences of an aged couple as they made the decision to move into a senior citizen's home.

Peege, produced by David Knapp and Leonard Berman, 28 min, 16mm, color, 1974. The central theme of the film is the breaking of communication barriers to reach those isolated by age and failing mental capacities.

The String Bean, directed by Edmond Sechan, 1964; 17 min, black and white with color. An excellent film about an old woman who cultivates a string-bean plant with tender loving care.

Three Grandmothers, 28 min, 16mm, black and white. Depicts the lives of three grandmothers, one in an African village, one in a hill city in Brazil, and one in a rural community in Canada. Produced by Findley Sleigh; educational supervisor, Isme Benne.

APPENDIX C

CATALOGS OF FILMS ON AGING

About Aging: A Catalog of Films, Millie V. Allyn, Editor, Publications Office, Andrus Gerontology Center, University of Southern California, Los Angeles, CA 90007.

Administration on Aging Catalogue of Films on Aging, Government Printing Office, Washington, DC 20402 (59-page annotated bibliography of films, slides, plays, and television programming on aging—stock number 1762-00070).

Aging. A Filmography, by Judith Trojan, Educational Film Library Association, New York, NY 10023 (annotated films on both psychology and biology of aging).

Basic Bibliography, Gray Panthers, 3700 Chestnut St., Philadelphia, PA 19104.

Film Resources, National Council of Senior Citizens, Washington, DC 20005.

Selected Films on Aging, Johanna Wiese, Editor, Institute of Gerontology, University of Michigan, Ann Arbor, MI 48104.

APPENDIX D

REFERRAL ORGANIZATIONS, GERONTOLOGY CENTERS, AND GOVERNMENT PROGRAMS

NATIONAL ORGANIZATIONS

Action for Independent Maturity (AIM), 1909 K St., N.W., Washington, DC 20049.

Advisory Committee on Aging, Administration on Aging, Social and Rehabilitation Service, Washington, DC 20201.

American Association of Homes for the Aging, 1050 17th St., N.W., Washington, DC 20036.

American Association of Retired Persons, 1909 K St., N.W., Washington, DC 20049.

American Foundation for the Blind, Inc., 15 West 16th St., New York, NY 10011.

American Health Care Association, 2500 15th St., N.W., Washington, DC 20015.

Gerontological Society, 1 Dupont Circle, Washington, DC 20036.

Gray Panthers, 3700 Chestnut St., Philadelphia, PA 19104.

International Federation on Aging, 1909 K St., N.W., Washington, DC 20049.

International Senior Citizens Association, Inc., 11753 Wilshire Blvd., Los Angeles, CA 90025.

Jewish Association for Services for the Aged, 222 Park Ave., S., New York, NY 10003.

National Alliance of Senior Citizens, Box 40031, Washington, DC 20016.

National Association of Jewish Homes for the Aged, 2525 Centerville Rd., Dallas, TX 75228.

National Caucus on the Black Aged, 1730 M St., N.W., Washington, DC 20036.

National Council on the Aging, 1828 L St., N.W., Suite 504, Washington, DC 20036.

National Council for Homemaker—Home Health Aide Services, 67 Irving Pl., New York, NY 10003.

National Council of Senior Citizens, 1511 K St., N.W., Rm. 202, Washington, DC 20005.

National Federation of Grandmother Clubs of America, 203 North Wabash Ave., Chicago, IL 60601.

National Geriatrics Society, Inc., 212 West Wisconsin Ave., Milwaukee, WI 53203.

National Institute on Aging, Bethesda, MD 20014.

National Institutes of Health, Bethesda, MD 20014.

National Retired Teachers Association, 1090 K St., N.W., Washington, DC 20049.

Pennsylvania State University Gerontology Center, University Park, PA 16802.

San Jose State University Gerontology Center, San Jose, CA 95129.

Southern California, University of, Andrus Gerontology Center, Los Angeles, CA 90007.

South Florida, University of, Institute on Aging, Tampa, FL 33620.

Syracuse, University of, All University Gerontology Center, Syracuse, NY 13210.

PROFESSIONAL ORGANIZATIONS

American Geriatrics Society, 10 Columbus Circle, New York, NY 10019.

American Nurses' Association, Inc., Division on Geriatric Nursing Practice, Kansas City, MO 64108.

International Congress of Gerontology, Hamburg, Germany.

United States Gerontology Society, Washington, D.C.

Western Gerontology Society, San Francisco, California.

GERONTOLOGY CENTERS IN EDUCATIONAL INSTITUTIONS

Boston University Gerontology Center, Boston, MA 02215.

Brandeis University, Florence Heller School, Waltham, MA 02154.

Chicago, University of, Adult Development and Aging Program, Chicago, IL 60637.

Duke University, Center for the Study of Aging and Human Development, Durham, NC 27710.

Florida, University of, Center for Gerontological Studies, Gainesville, FL 32611.

Michigan, University of, Institute of Gerontology, Ann Arbor, MI 48109.

North Texas State University, Center for Studies on Aging, Denton, TX 76203.

GOVERNMENT PROGRAMS

Foster Grandparents, ACTION, Washington, DC 20525.

IESC (International Executive Service Corps),[1] 545 Madison Ave., New York, NY 10022.

Operation Mainstream Programs: Green Thumb (men)/Green Light (women), National Farmers Union, 1012 14th St., N.W., Washington, DC 20005 or Manpower Administration, Operation Mainstream, Department of Labor, Washington, DC 20212.

Senior AIDES, National Council of Senior Citizens, 1511 K St., N.W., Washington, DC 20005.

Senior Community Service Programs: National Council on the Aging, 1828 L St., N.W., Washington, DC 20036.

Senior Community Service Aides: National Retired Teachers Association, 1225 Connecticut Ave., N.W., Washington, DC 20036.

Peace Corps, ACTION, Washington, DC 20525.

RSVP (Retired Senior Volunteer Program), ACTION, Washington, DC 20525.

SCORE (Service Corps of Retired Executives), ACTION, Washington, DC 20525.

VISTA (Volunteers in Service to America), ACTION, Washington, DC 20525.

---

[1] Independent organization supported by government and non-government funds.

NAME INDEX

NAME INDEX

Page numbers in **boldface** indicate entries in References sections.

Dodd, Marylin J., 193, 195, **198**
Dohrenwend, Barbara Snell, 86, **97**
Dohrenwend, Bruce P., 86, **97**
Dominian, J., 508, **517**
Dominick, Joan R., 71, **84**, 130, **136**, 624, **627**
Donezky, Raymond M. P., 458
Donovan, Michael J., 661, **664**
Dowling, Michael, 563, **573**
Downs, Florence S., 401, **402**
Drachman, D. A., 23, **28**
Drake, Charles G., 456, 458, **464**
Driscoll, P. W., 285, **293**
Droller, H., 319, **321**
Drummond, Linda, 203–207, **209**
Drye, R. C., 151, **155**
Dudas, Susan, 534, **545**
Dufault, Sister Karin, 661, **663**
Duffy, C., 25, **29**
Duhme, D. W., 357, **359**
Duling, Brian, 456, **464**
Dulski, Theresa, 661, **663**
Dundee, J. W., 355, **359**
Dunn, Halbert L., 451, 452, **464**
Dunn, M., 539, **546**
Durkheim, Emile, 596, **601**
DuVries, Henri L., 296, **305**
Dyck, J., 509, **517**
Dye, Carol J., 662, **663**
Dye, Celeste A., 662, **663**
Dymock, I. W., 312, 317, **322**

Eastwood, H. D. H., 318, **321**
Ebersole, Priscilla, 99, 107, **112**
Edgerton, Robert B., 616, 623, **627**
Edsall, Jean Oswald, 661, **663**
Edwards, Lynn, 540, 542–544, **546**
Edwards, Willie M., 13, **18**
Egan, Gerard, 79, **84**
Ehrlich, George, 286, **293**
Eide, Imogene, 461, **465**
Eisdorfer, Carl, 23, **29**, 44, 50, 56, **68**, 128, **136**, 159, **165**, 172, 187, 195, **198**, 469, **490**
Eisenberg, Howard, 455, **465**
Eissler, K. R., 129, **136**
Elizabeth, Sister Regina, 540, **546**
Ellis, Rosemary, 656, 658, 659, **663**
Elphick, Leonora, 536, 537, 544, **546**
Endo, Paula, 621, **628**
Engen, Trygg, 487, **490**
Epstein, F. H., 358, **361**
Epstein, Leon, 128, **136**, 187, **198**, 354, 355, **359**
Epstein, Sidney, 568, **574**
Erickson, Roberta, 389
Erikson, E. H., 100, 105, **112**, 194, **198**
Ernst, Philip, 178, 195, **198**, 205, **209**, 212, **220**
Esberger, Karen, 398, **402**
Estes, E. Harvey, 10, **18**
Etigson, E., 102, **113**
Evans, J. Grimley, 550, 552, **558**
Everitt, A. V., **321**
Ewy, G. A., 351, 357, **359**
Exton-Smith, A. N., 11, **19**, 159, 165, **167**, 453, **464**, 536, **547**, 550, 552, **558**, 660, 661, **665**

Fagerhaugh, Shizuko Y., 658, **663**
Fairbairn, J. F., 297, **305**
Falconer, Paulette Annette, 540, **546**
Fales, Edward D., Jr., 550, **558**
Falk, J. M., 101, 102, 109, **112**, **113**
Farberow, Norman, 145, **156**
Farr, L., 638, **641**
Farrah, Shirley, 507, **517**
Faye, Eleanor E., 469, **490**
Feifel, Herman, 576, **587**
Feinberg, I., 182, **198**
Feinstein, P. A., 288, **293**
Feist, Ruth R., 553, 554, 557, **558**, 661, **663**
Ferguson, Stella, **587**
Fernsebner, Wilhelmina, 472, **490**
Festinger, L., 104, **112**
Few, A., 25, **28**
Field, N., 441, 443, **449**
Fields, W. S., 458, **465**
Fikry, M. E., 311, **321**
Finch, Caleb, 24, 26, 27, **28**, 147, **155**
Finkbeiner, Alex E., 524, 535, 542, 543, **545**
Finkel, R. M., 319, **322**
Finkle, A., 371, **372**
Finkle, Betty C., 61, **69**
Fischer, Roland, 195, **198**
Fischer, Trudy, 195, **198**
Fitzgerald, Alice M., 399, **402**
Fitzpatrick, Joyce J., 661, **664**
Flekkøy, Kjell, 193, **198**
Flood, Mary A., 660, 661, **665**
Florini, J. R., 24, **28**
Flurkey, K., 25, **28**
Flynn, Frances, 13, **18**
Flynn, Kathleen T., 329, 330, 333, 334, 336, **347**, 556, **558**
Folsom, James C., 204, 208, **209**
Foner, A., 593, 598, **601**
Foote, Dianne F., 660, 661, **664**
Foraker, A. G., 243, **257**
Fordtran, J. S., 312, **322**
Foster, J. R., 24, **28**
Foster, T. A., 358, **359**
Fowler, Marsha D., 299, **305**
Fox, N., 377, **379**
Fozard, James L., 479, **490**
Francis, Gloria, 66, **68**, 661, **664**
Franck, Phyllis, 660, 661, **664**
Frank, L., 365, **372**
Frank, Lawrence K., 508, **517**
Frankl, Viktor, 104, **112**
Fras, I., 317, **322**
Freedman, S. Saul, 500, **501**
French, Jean, 579, **587**
Freud, Sigmund, 12, **18**, 58, **68**
Friedeman, Joyce Sutkamp, 661, **664**
Friedman, Erika, 80, **84**
Friedman, J. S., 377, **379**
Friedman, Sandor A., 298, **305**, 351, **360**
Friedman, T., 440, **449**
Fritz, E., 27, **29**
Froelicher, Victor F., 458, **465**
Frolkis, V. V., 26, **28**
Fromm-Reichmann, Frieda, 62, **68**
Frost, Monica, 181, **198**
Fulton, Robert, 577

Gaitz, C. M., 438, **449**
Ganong, William F., 523, 524, **546**
Garetz, Floyd K., 56, **69**, 330, 335, **347**, 661, **664**
Garfield, Charles A., 576, **587**
Gebhard, P. H., 365, 370, **373**
Gedan, Sharon, 72, **84**
Gee, J. B. L., 235, **257**
Gelper, Eve Arlin, 659, **664**
Gerber, Rose Marie, 661, **664**
Gerhards, Michael, 459, **465**
Germican, A., 309, **321**
Gerson, Samuel, 56, **68**
Getty, R., 25, **28**
Gibson, J. J., 480, **490**
Gibson, John E., 639, **641**
Gillis, Sister Marion, 12, **18**, 659, **664**
Gimble, Josephine G., 657, 658, **664**
Ginsberg, Leon H., 335, **347**
Gioiella, Evelynn C., 661, **664**
Giorgi, Elsie A., 462, **465**
Glass, R., 370, 372, **372**
Glasser, G., 101, 109, **112**
Glen, Eric S., 521, 522, **546**
Glover, B., 419, **421**
Glowacki, Gerald, 416, **421**, 526, 535, **546**
Godber, Colin, 179, 180, 185, **198**
Godbole, Anil, 79, **84**
Goddard, Don, 459
Goffi, Sister Maria Teresa, 662, **666**
Goffman, Erving, 397, **402**, 623, **627**
Goldfarb, Alvin I., 49, **50**, 55, **68**, 177, **198**, 222, **228**, 353, 354, **360**, 397, **402**, 444, **449**
Goldfischer, S., 25, **28**
Goldman, Ralph, 327, **347**, 351, **360**, 412, 419, 420, **421**, 525, **546**
Goldstein, Kurt, 175, 177, 192, **198**
Goldstein, S., 178, **199**
Gollicker, Jacqueline, 71, **84**
Goodchilds, J., 329, **346**
Gooddy, W., 182, **198**
Goodhill, Victor, 483, **490**
Gordon, D., 413, **421**
Gordon, Susan K., 105, **112**
Gordon, Thomas, 90, **97**
Gorenberg, Bobbye, 673, **677**
Gorney, J. E., 105, **112**
Gorney, S., 370, **372**
Gortner, Susan R., 662, **664**
Gosnell, Davina J., 343, **347**, 658, **664**
Gotestam, K. Gunnar, 59, **68**, 182, **198**
Gould, G., 555, **558**
Goulding, M. E., 151, **155**
Goulding, R. L., 151, **155**
Gramlich, Ed, 134, **136**, 138, **142**
Grauer, H., 160, 165, **167**
Green, H. L., 458, **465**
Green, R., 378, **379**
Greenberg, Barbara M., 63, **68**, 223, **228**, 504, **517**, 656, 658, **664**
Greenblatt, D. J., 355, 357, **359**, 360
Greenblatt, R., 365, **372**
Greenhill, J. P., 531, 538, 539, **546**
Gregerman, R. I., 359, **361**
Gress, Lucille D., 660, 661, **665**
Gribbin, Kathy, 42, 43, 48, **50**
Grier, Margaret R., 661, **664**
Griffith, Elizabeth W., 387, **402**

Wylie, C. M., 288, **294**
Wynter, Lolita, 659, **666**
Wyse, Lois, 570, **574**

Yamaguchi, Yoshiko, 621, 623, 626, **628**
Yasargil, M. Gazi, 458

Yiengst, M. J., 24, **29**
York, Jonathan L., 59, **69**
Yoshida, Jane, 621, **628**

Zacharin, Robert F., 526, **548**
Zarit, Steven H., 185, 187, **199**

Zboralski, F. F., 310, **322**
Zeiger, Betty L., 107, **113**
Zeitz, Leonard, 657, 658, **666**
Zerbe, Melissa B., 661, **662**
Zimmer, James G., 662, **666**
Zivin, I., 355, **361**
Zornow, R. A., 656, 658, **666**
Zuidema, George D., 343, **347**

SUBJECT INDEX

SUBJECT INDEX

Page numbers in **boldface** indicate entries in the References sections; page numbers in *italic* indicate illustrations or tables.

Absorption, problems of, 314–315
Accident prevention, 460
   (*See also* Safety of home)
Acidosis, 331
Acute brain syndrome, 172, 203
Acute illness, 412
Administration on Aging, 620, **627**
Advocacy, 82, 336
Aeration, 391–392
Affect in organic brain syndromes, 172
Affective states in group work, 227
Aged, the:
   attitudes toward, 12, 13, 27, 28, 39
   frail (*see* Frail elderly)
   future for, 6–7
   as a group (*see* Groups, aged)
   population: growth and problems,
      671–672
      projections of, 5–6
   as teachers, 17
   very old (*see* Very old, the)
   well (wellness in), 676
Ageism, 12
Aging:
   nutritional status and, 324
   social forces and, 591–601
Aging and Addiction in Arizona, **464**
Aging changes:
   body organs, decreased weight of, *36*
   body potassium, changes in, *37*
   Bouchard's nodes, 39
   breasts, 418
   cervix, 418
   chest, 419
   climacteric, 25–26, 368, 369, 417–418
   dental, 34–35
   differentiating normal and abnormal,
      409–421
   digestive system, 308–318
   height loss as, 32
   kidneys, 260–261
   muscles, 35
   nervous system, 308
   normal, 31–40, 410
      differentiating from abnormal,
         409–421
   ocular, 34
   pigments (lipofuscins), 25, 36
   reproductive system, 362–373, 417–
      419
   research in, 12, 13
      biological theories, 23–28

(*See also* Research gerontological
   nursing)
   beneath the skin, 35–36
   skin and subcutaneous tissue, 32–34
   time-related pathological events and,
      38–39
   tongue papillae, 326–327
Aging pigments (lipofuscins), 25, 36
Alcoholism, 158, 312, 333, 355, 459
   in frail elderly, 430
   paranoid state and, 160
Alkalosis, 331, 415
Alzheimer's disease, 126, 172, 175, 203,
   339
   brain atrophy in, 182
   first case, 182
   life-span, 182
   neurofibril tangles in, 182
   nursing literature on, 181
   nutrition and, 339
   occurrence in men, 182
   occurrence in women, 182
   personal hygiene and, 182
   plaques in, 182
   rate of, 175
   sleep and, 182
   vital statistics on, 182
Ambulation, 410
   in frail elderly, 435
American Nurse, The, 583, **587**
American Nurses' Association (ANA), 5,
   10, 17, **18**, 303, **305**
American Nurses Foundation, 659, **662**
Analgesics, 179
Anemia, 203, 330
   folate deficiency, 330
   in frail elderly, 423, 434
   macrocytic, 330
Anger:
   in frail elderly, 433
   at suicidal clients, 150
*Annals of the New York Academy of
   Sciences*, **40**
Anorexia, 330, 410, 412
Anticholinergic drugs (atropine-like
   drugs), 354–355
Antihypertensive drugs, 272
Antiparkinsonian drugs, 179
Anxiety, 59–64, 90–91
   anxiety-producing situations, 61
   death and, 578
   frail elderly and, 433

in group members, 191
in group therapy, 92
manifestations of, 62–64
   during physical examinations, 62
overt signs of, 62–64
reduction of, 75–84
   regarding coleadership, 90
   retirement home residents and,
      91
AOA Fact Sheet, **346**
Apathy, 174, 212
Aphasia, 74
Applanation tonometry, 473
Arcus senilis, 413
   defined, 34
Arrhythmias, 240–241, 354
Arteriosclerosis, 34–35
   defined, 34
Arteriosclerotic lesions, 411
Arthritis, 411
   of feet, 297
   treatment of, 286–288
   (*See also* Osteoarthritis; Rheumatoid
      arthritis)
Assessment:
   of bowel problems, 396
   of elimination function, 395, 396
   of foot, 299–303
   of frail elderly, 422–436
      agitation during, 430
      approach in, 428
      attention span during, 432
      confusion during, 429
      data base and, 430
      dying elderly, 583
      existing history and, 430
      explanations and, 428
      eye contact during, 428
      fatigue level during, 432
      fear of, 428
      hope restored during, 428
      initial approach, 428–429
      laboratory studies in, 430
      mobilization of resources during,
         428
      priorities in, 432
      self-image improvement during, 428
      trust and, 428
   of homebound (*see* Home assessment)
   mental status, 187, 433
   nutrition, 324, 333, 341–343, 346
   pain (*see* Pain)

Crisis (continued)
  dementia and, 197
  family therapy and, 118
Crystallized intelligence, 43, 185, 417
Culture (see Ethnicity; Social forces and aging)
Cumulative Index to Nursing and Allied Health Literature, 71, **84**
Curricula, gerontological nursing, 13, 16, 17, 674–675

Day-care centers, 461–462
Deafness, admission to group and, 88
Death:
  anxiety and, 578
  assessing reactions to, 583
  death rates, 7, 144
  privacy needed, 636
  of spouse, 87
  talking openly about, 650
  (See also Dying; Suicide)
Decubitus ulcer, 303, 356
Dehydration, 356, 357, 419
  diagnosis of, 357
  edema, in frail elderly, 430
  electrolyte imbalance, 430
  in frail elderly, 433
  renal failure, 430
Delirium, 353, 354, 412
  due to digitalis, 412
Delusions of persecution, 158
Demented client, 512–513
  use of touch with, 512–513
Dementia, 126, 172, 410, 417
  activities and sensory stimulation, 194–195
  case studies of, 180, 186
  cerebrovascular disease and, 179
  cognitive impairment, testing, 187
  communication with clients, 192–194
  communication disorders and, 207
  crises and, 197
  defined, 172
  depression and, 126, 179, 191
  diagnostic issues, 178
  drugs and, 179, 187, 195, 352–354
  fatigue and, 189
  feeding problems and, 341
  grooming and, 187
  group work and, 195
  hearing evaluation and, 179
  hypnotics and, 179
  hypotensives and, 179
  lack of language initiative, 185
  librium and, 179
  magnitude of problem, 172
  manipulation of environment, 195
  meanings of, 172
  medications and, 179, 187, 195
  memory loss and, 191
  nursing care of patients, 168
  nursing homes in, 173
  nursing research areas, 197
  paranoid attitudes in, 190
  plan of management, 179–181
    living alone, 179–180
    living with others, 180
  poverty of words, 185

prevention strategies in: accidents, 196
  acute stress, 196
  agitation, 196
  burnout, staff, 196
  choking, 196
  decubiti, 196
  dehydration, 196
  disease, 196
  falls, 196
  immobility, 196
  infections, 196
  injuries to self and others, 196
  malnutrition, 196
  Sundowner's syndrome, 196
  translocation shock, 196
  prognosis, 182
  qualities of therapist, 192
  retaliatory behavior and, 190
  scope of problem, 202
  self-esteem, increase of, 194
  sensory losses and, 190
  sensory stimulation, 194–195
  sleep disturbances, 182, 187
  social graces and, 187
  suicide and, 178
  therapist's behavior and, 191–192
  tranquilizers and, 179
  treatment modalities and, 191
  in United Kingdom, 172
  use of drugs, 179, 187, 195
  Valium and, 179
  vision evaluation, 179
  visual aids and, 208
  visual problems and, 191
  vitamin deficiencies, 331
  wandering and, 181–182, 192
  (See also Presenile dementia; Senile dementia)
Denial, 124–125, 189
  depression and, 124
  by frail elderly, 428, 432
Dental care, preventive, 458–459
Dental changes, 34–35
Dental status, 333
Dentures, 208, 326–327, 330
Dependency:
  on group leader, 89
  reduction of, 89
Depression, 76, 82, 120, 122–132, 158, 330, 417, 498, 512
  affective disorder, 123
  agitated, 123
  atypical, 123
  bipolar, 123
  cardinal features of, 123–124
  communication and, 129
  contagious quality of, 128
  defined, 123
  dementia and, 126, 179, 191
  depressive equivalent, 123
  endogenous, 126
  exogenous, 123
  faulty nutrition and, 330
  follow-up, 124
  frail elderly and, 434, 435
  guide for diagnosis, 127
  of health professionals, 131
  individual, profile of, 124

involutional melancholia, 123
  manic depressive psychosis, 123
  masked, 123, 125
  neurotic, 123
  of nurse, 131
  nutrition and, 330, 339
  pain and, 489
  psychotic, 123
  reactive, 123, 125, 126
  reasons for relief, 130
  rehabilitation, 127
  relief of, 130
  reserpine and, 358
  retarded, 123
  statistics of, 123
  suicide and, 150, 152, 153
  unipolar, 123
Dermatology (see Skin)
Diabetes mellitus, 276, 331, 415
Diabetic retinopathy, 469, 475
  microaneurysm, 476
  treatment of, 476
Diagnostic and Statistical Manual of Mental Disorders, 196, **198**
Diet:
  refusal of, 339
  (See also Nutrition)
Dietary surveys, 325–326
  calcium, 326
  calories, 326
  niacin, 326
  protein, 326
Digestive system, 308
  duodenum, 313
  esophagus, 309, 311
  small bowel, 313–314
  stomach, 311–313
  teeth and mouth, 309
Digitalis toxicity, 356–357
Digoxin, 179, 357
Disorientation, 189, 202
  defined, 202
  of person, 187, 189
  of place, 189
  of time, 189
Diuretics, 179, 331, 357–358
Diverticulosis, 321
Dizziness, organ of Corti, 413
Drug abuse, 676
Drugs, 349–361, 459
  affecting primarily cardiac system, 246–248
  affecting primarily pulmonary system, 248–249
  antihypertensive, in treatment of uremia, 272
  central nervous system depressant, 356
  dementia and, 179, 187, 195, 352–354
  distribution in body, 351
  drug disposition, 350–351
  drug therapy, 333
  drug toxicity, 435
  elimination of, 351
  inducing delirium, 353–356
  insulin, 359
  intoxication from, 203
  mechanisms in delirium, 354
  medication errors, 351–352

Loneliness, 64–67, 97
  causes of, 66–67
  in dementia, 178
  interventions in, 66–67
  journal articles, 65
  mental health and, 54, 64–67
  privacy and, 178
  related to nutrition, 64
Longevity, 6–7, 6, 7
Long-term memory, 23
Loss:
  compensations for, 596–598
  of memory (see Memory loss)
  of norms, 595–596
  sensory (see Sensory losses)
  of social world, 595–596
  of spouse, 138
  suicide and, 146
  of teeth, 458–459
Lung cancer, 243
Lungs, 419
  (See also Cardiopulmonary system)

Macular degeneration of eye, 469,
    474–475
  implications for care, 474
Male sexuality (see entries beginning
    with terms: Sexual; Sexuality)
Malnutrition, 326, 329, 330, 335
  in frail elderly, 423, 430
    alcohol-related, 430
  in organic brain syndrome, 331
Masked depression, 123, 125
Masturbation, 196
Meals-on-Wheels, 328–329, 335
Medical-surgical nursing standards of
    practice, 408
Medical World News, 465
Medicare insurance, 563, 567–568
Medication:
  errors: adverse drug reactions and,
      351–352
    in nursing homes, 352
  of frail elderly, 423, 430, 431
  self-administered, 351
    frail elderly, 423
  (See also Drugs)
Memories, 102–103
  adaptive, 109
  catalysts for, 104, 109
  of centenarians, 105, 109
  development of, 193–194
  earliest, 102, 109
  exciting, 109
  as genealogy, 109
  high frequency of, 109
  immediate, 203
  memorabilia, 109
  oral history, 109
  pilgrimages, 109
  recent, 203
  reconstruction of, 103
  to regain identity, 109
  remote, 203
  reunions, 109
  salient, 109
  sex differences and, 105, 109
  strokes, effect on, 23

  taped, 109
  (See also Reminiscing)
Memory:
  attention to, in interview, 73
  long-term, 23
Memory chains, 82
Memory development, 193–194
  cues and, 193–194
  learning conditions, 193–194
  meaningful materials, 193–194
  overarousal, 194
  (See also Reminiscence)
Memory impairment:
  group admission and, 88
  lack of progress as self-fulfilling
    prophecy in, 207
Memory loss, 174–175, 417
  compensations for, 174
  dementia and, 191
  of name, 187
  problems in, 86
  as a sign of confusional state, 202
  as a symptom of confusional state,
    202
Menopause, 25–26, 368, 369, 417–418
Mental changes, 412
Mental health, 53, 69, 455–456
  boundaries of, 55
  defined, 55
  facilities, 56–58
    nurses employed in, 57
  loneliness and, 54, 64–67
  positive characteristics of, 55
  problems in conceptualization, 55
Mental health status questionnaire
    (MSQ), 189
Mental illness, 55–58
  iatrogenic, 58
  nursing homes in, 56, 58
  problem, extent of, 55–56
  problems in seeking help, 58
  suicide of mentally ill aged, 55–56
  (See also name of specific condition or
    syndrome)
Mental status, assessment of, 187, 433
  precision essential in, 187
Mental status examination, modified, 89
Mentation, 412
Merck Manual of Diagnosis and Therapy,
    202, 209
Meta-memory, 417
Metabolic conditions, 203
Metaphors in group psychotherapy, 90
Metropolitan Life Statistical Bulletin, 6,
    7, 18, 562, 571, 574
Milieu for reality orientation, 205
Minerals, 328
Minority groups (see Ethnicity)
Mobile Life-Line, 490
Mobility, 303
  (See also Muscles; Musculoskeletal
    disorders)
Modified mental status examination, 89
Mönckeberg sclerosis, 35
Mood, 126
  depressed, 126
  swings in, 214
Morale in elderly, variables in studies,
    55

Mortality (see Death; Dying; Suicide)
Mouth lesions, 414
MSQ (mental status questionnaire), 189
Multidimensional assessment, 75
Multiphasic screening, 456–457
Muscles:
  aging changes, 35
  cramps, 415
  disorders, 283–284
    implications for nursing, 289–293
Musculoskeletal disorders, 282–294,
    303
  (See also name of specific disease)
Music:
  as catalyst, 141
  management of grief reactions and,
    139
  as therapy, 137–142, 676
    defined, 138
    guidelines for, 142
Myocardial infarction, 23, 412, 416
  in frail elderly, 423
  silent, 423
Myocardial ischemia, 411
Myocardium, 36

National Academy of Sciences, 327, 328,
    347
National Action Forum for Older
    Women, 563, 574
National Association of Hearing and
    Speech Agencies, 484, 485, 490
National Bureau of Standards, 639, 641
National Center for Health Statistics,
    619–622, 627
National Dairy Council, 324, 328, 331,
    347
National Institute on Aging Information
    Office, 324, 347
National Society for the Prevention of
    Blindness, Inc. and Affiliates, 470,
    472, 474, 490
Need to be needed, 82
Negativism, 174, 221
Nervous system changes, 308
Nervous system depressants, 355
Neurological findings, 334
  nutrition assessment in, 334
Neuron damage, 411
Neurosyphilis, 172
Newsweek (magazine), 363, 373
Nihilistic attitudes, 178
Nocturia, 411, 420
Nocturnal confusion, 206
  (See also Sundowner's syndrome)
Nocturnal dyspnea, 411
Nonverbal communication, 75–76, 82
Nonverbal cues, 76, 211, 509
Normal aging:
  changes, 31–40, 410
    differentiating normal from abnor-
      mal, 409–421
  historical and cultural perspectives,
    363
Normal intelligence and memory, 23
Nurse(s):
  as advocate, 298, 299
  aides, 196

Parkinsonism, 302–303
  drugs, 187
"Partnership for Older Americans," 64,
  69
Pelvic examination, 418
Penis, 418
Perceptual deprivation, 493
Peritonitis, 416
Perseveration, 177
Pets, 676
  importance of, 80
  paranoid persons and, 163–164
  relation of pet ownership to coronary
    disease, 80–81
Pharynx, 414, 419
Physical assessment of the aged, normal
    vs. abnormal, 409–419
Pick's disease, 172
Pneumonia, 356, 416, 420
  in frail elderly, 430, 434
Podiatry (see Foot)
Point of maximal impulse (PMI), chest,
    411
Population growth and problems, 671–
    672
Post–White House Conference on
    Aging Reports, 8, **19**, 324, **347**
Potassium, body, decline in, 37
Power of attorney, defined, 461
Presbycusis, 413, 484
Presbyopia, 469
Presenile dementia, 172, 181, 182
  (See also Alzheimer's disease)
Prevention:
  assessment of factors in, 451–465
  disease, 673
  epidemiological approach to, 451
  high-level wellness and, 452
  injury, 462–463
  levels of, 451
  multiphasic screening as, 456
  primary, 451
  primary prevention of depression, 131
  protective services, 460–461
  theoretical framework for, 451
Prostate, 418
  cancer of, 418
  nodular hyperplasia, 418
  prostatism, 268–269
Prosthetics, 496, 676
Pseudodementia, 127–128
Psychosocial care in musculoskeletal
    diseases, 292–293
Psychosocial examination, 202
Psychotherapy, 79–80
  telephone, 80
  (See also Family therapy; Group psy-
    chotherapy)
Public Health Service Office on Smoking
    and Health, **465**
Pulmonary system (see Cardiopulmo-
    nary system)
Pulse rate, 411
Pyelonephritis, 264

Quadriceps paralysis, assessment of,
    302
Quality of life, 208, 673

Rales:
  atelectatic, 419
  basilar, 419
Rape, 375
Reactive depression, 123, 125, *126*
Reality orientation, 196, 204
  aids in, 216
  classroom, 205
  clues and, 204
  environment and, 204
  nurse as key person, 205
  personal interactions in, 204–205
    twenty-four-hour, 204
  research and, 676
  structure of time, 205
Reality testing, 82, 196
Relationship:
  defined, 211
  working (see Working relationship)
Relationship therapy, 70–84
  anxiety reduction in, 75–84
    client's, 82
    nurse's, 82
  assessment of therapist's feelings, 75
  charting of progress, 75
  communication with staff and rela-
    tives, 75
  confidante, role of nurse as, 75
  confidentiality in, 75
  contract in, 72
    constituents of, 72
  coordination of services in, 75
  defined, 71
  good-byes, 79
  growth potential of, 79
  guidelines for intervention, 81–84
  as helping relationship, 71
  honesty in, 82
  instructions to client, 77
  low client self-esteem, 82
  modifications necessary, 74–75
  options explained, 82
  pace (timing) in, 79
  pain control, attention to, 82
  pseudofamily role of therapist, 75
  questions for therapist self-
    evaluation, 83
  reminiscing strategies, use of, 82
  role modeling of nurse, for staff, 75
  termination of, 79
  touch during, 75
Religion and the aged, 642–650
  clergy, 648
  death and, 644–645
  developing a sense of self-worth
    through, 645–647
  life-affirming factors and, 642
  life-denying factors and, 642
  potentials for a new ethic in, 649–650
Relocation:
  stages in move to retirement home,
    96
  stress and, 87
Reminiscence:
  characteristics of, 104–105
  chronic brain syndrome and, 111
  cognitive dissonance and, 104
  confusional state and, 207
  conversational, 109

Reminiscent, the:
  age of, 103
  defined, 99
Reminiscing, 90–113, 493
  adaptive function of, 101
  as antidote to boredom, 106, 493
  art therapy and, 107
  as basis for communication, 109
  catastrophic reactions from, 111
  defined, 99
  dissertations on, 100
  encouragement of, 111
  free-flowing, 105–106, 109
  high school students as chroniclers of
    old peoples' lives, 108–109
  inner mental process as, 109
  in-service classes on, 111
  mechanics of, 109
  nurse contributions to, 106, 109
  as oral history, 109
  as a phenomenon, 101
  as providing diagnostic clues, 108
  quotations on, *99*
  with regressed aged, 106
  relation of chronological age to, 105
  as sagas, 109
  sensory stimulation and, 102, 112
  sex differences and, 105, 109
  stress and, 102
  structured, 109
  student experience with, 108–109
  theoretical frameworks for, 99
  use of props, 110–112
  use in therapy, 104, 108
  verbal, 109
  written, 109
Renal abnormalities, 258–281
  fluid output of renal patients, 273–
    274
  fluids and, 269–271
  intrarenal problems, 264–267
  postrenal problems, 267–269
  prerenal problems, 263–264
  (See also Kidneys)
Renal failure, 266
  in frail elderly, 423, 430
Renal insufficiency, 417
Reproductive system:
  dysfunction, 370–371
  female anatomy and physiology,
    367–368
  male anatomy and physiology, 366–
    367
  normal aging changes, 362–373,
    417–419
  (See also entries beginning with terms:
    Sexual; Sexuality)
Research, gerontological nursing, 653–
    666
  areas of study in, *661*
  attitudes: of staff, 659
    of student nurses, 659
    toward aging and aged, 662
  direct patient care, 657–658
  evaluation of health care programs,
    662
  health-care delivery systems, 659
  heuristics, 659–660
  informed consent, 661